Essentials of Pediatric Nutrition

Edited by

Patricia Queen Samour, MMSc, RD

Director, Nutrition Services and Dietetic Internship Program
Beth Israel Deaconess Medical Center
Boston, Massachusetts

Kathy King, RD, LD

Private Practitioner
Publisher
Helm Publishing
Lake Dallas, Texas

JONES & BARTLETT
LEARNING

World Headquarters
Jones & Bartlett Learning
5 Wall Street
Burlington, MA 01803
978-443-5000
info@jblearning.com
www.jblearning.com

Jones & Bartlett Learning books and products are available through most bookstores and online booksellers. To contact Jones & Bartlett Learning directly, call 800-832-0034, fax 978-443-8000, or visit our website, www.jblearning.com.

Substantial discounts on bulk quantities of Jones & Bartlett Learning publications are available to corporations, professional associations, and other qualified organizations. For details and specific discount information, contact the special sales department at Jones & Bartlett Learning via the above contact information or send an email to specialsales@jblearning.com.

Production Credits
Publisher, Higher Education: Cathleen Sether
Senior Acquisitions Editor: Shoshanna Goldberg
Managing Editor: Amy Bloom
Editorial Assistant: Agnes Burt
Production Manager: Julie Champagne Bolduc
Production Editor: Jessica Steele Newfell
Associate Marketing Manager: Jody Sullivan
VP, Manufacturing and Inventory Control: Therese Connell
Composition: Circle Graphics
Cover Design: Scott Moden
Photo Researcher: Sarah Cebulski
Permissions and Photo Research Assistant: Lian Bruno
Cover Image: © Lana K/ShutterStock, Inc.
Printing and Binding: Malloy, Inc.
Cover Printing: Malloy, Inc.

To order this product, use ISBN: 978-1-4496-5291-3

Library of Congress Cataloging-in-Publication Data
Essentials of pediatric nutrition / edited by Patricia Queen Samour, Kathy King.
p. ; cm.
Abridged version of: Pediatric nutrition / edited by Patricia Queen Samour, Kathy King. 4th ed. c2012.
Includes bibliographical references and index.
ISBN 978-0-7637-8449-2 (pbk. : alk. paper)
I. Samour, Patricia Queen. II. King, Kathy, RD. III. Pediatric nutrition.
[DNLM: 1. Child Nutritional Physiological Phenomena. 2. Infant Nutritional Physiological Phenomena. 3. Child Nutrition Disorders. 4. Child. 5. Diet Therapy. 6. Infant Nutrition Disorders. 7. Infant. 8. Needs Assessment. WS 115]
LC–classification not assigned
618.92—dc23

2011033472

6048

Printed in the United States of America
15 14 13 12 11 10 9 8 7 6 5 4 3 2 1

Essentials of Pediatric Nutrition *is dedicated to all pediatric caregivers who strive to improve the nutrition status and health outcomes of our infants and children. Children are our future, and, in order to realize this future, we need practitioners to meet the challenges of the obesity epidemic, health care reform, and other opportunities facing us in creating a healthy population.*

A special thanks to my parents, Lillian and Emmett Queen, who taught me to have "high aims and ideals always."

—Patricia Queen Samour

This book, Essentials of Pediatric Nutrition, *is dedicated to my parents, Iris and Lee King. Mother died in 1996, and I miss her dearly. She talked me into majoring in dietetics and was my business sounding board, manuscript copyeditor, and new product critic. She modeled high energy, jumping on new ideas and sticking with a job until it was at a standard of which I was proud. My dad, Lee, was an instructor pilot in the Army Air Corps in WWII and then became an architect and engineer; he passed away in 2011. He was always methodical and cautious, not an early adopter, but always supportive and proud of my various new ventures. They are the flowers in my garden.*

—Kathy King

Contents

Preface

Essentials of Pediatric Nutrition contains the most practical "key elements" that practitioners need at their fingertips to work in pediatric nutrition with various age groups and diseases/conditions. The purpose of *Essentials of Pediatric Nutrition* is different from that of the fourth edition of *Pediatric Nutrition*, which is a complete textbook that includes evidence-based research, discussion behind the clinical decisions, and best-practice guidelines. *Essentials of Pediatric Nutrition* covers the core best-practice guidelines on the most needed information on the normal child, from preconception through adolescence, as well as infants and children with diseases/conditions affecting nutritional status.

This book is intended to be used by students learning about pediatric nutrition in all disciplines and by practitioners managing the nutrition of pediatric groups and individuals. Normal growth and development is always the goal for all infants and children. As pediatric practitioners, we assess growth, evaluate nutrition status and intake, and strive to achieve maximal health status. The growth charts, screening and assessment parameters, and routes of feeding may vary with age and disease states or other conditions, but the desired outcomes remain the same. Chapters of this text have been written to help the reader apply these key pediatric nutrition practices and principles.

The appendices contain core figures, tables such as the Centers for Disease Control and Prevention growth charts, the Tanner stages of sexual development, the RDA/DRI tables, commonly used lab value norms, and equations for calculating energy needs. These appendices are available online via access code.

Case studies are included in most chapters using the standardized language of the nutrition care process from the third edition of *The International Dietetics and Nutrition Terminology* (IDNT) published in 2009 and available online at http://www.eatright.org.

Highlights of This Text

Chapter 1, "Prenatal Nutrition," includes the recommended weight gain during pregnancy guidelines and key nutrient concerns during pregnancy. Important pregnancy issues such as diabetes, obesity, hypertension, and polycystic ovary syndrome also are addressed, as well as food safety concerns.

Chapter 2, "Physical Growth," provides an overview of growth and maturation and their assessment, as well as practical tips on how to accurately obtain height/length, weight, and head circumference measurements. Practical examples on how to plot on a growth chart and use the BMI charts are included; these are essential tools for all pediatric nutrition providers.

Chapter 3, "Assessment Basics," addresses the key basic concepts of nutrition screening and assessment that are needed for all infants and children. Essential topics include the definitions of obesity, malnutrition, and failure to thrive and the how-to's in determining nutrient and energy needs.

Chapter 4, "Premature Infant Nutrition," addresses the unique nutrient concerns and management considerations of these high-risk neonates. Key issues for this population include the use of intrauterine and premature infant growth charts. The use of human milk, premature infant formulas, and parenteral nutrition are addressed. Other topics include growth assessment and monitoring of parenteral and enteral nutrition.

Chapter 5, "Infant Nutrition," addresses the recommended feeding practices for healthy full-term infants and common feeding problems encountered during the first year of life. The basics of normal infant feeding are addressed because much of this core information is applicable to all infants with diseases and/or conditions.

Chapter 6, "Normal Nutrition After Infancy," focuses on normal, healthy children during their growth years. Information is provided on calcium and iron sources, feeding concerns, and exercise guidelines.

Chapter 7, "Food Hypersensitivities," deals with the diagnosis and nutrition management of infants and children with food hypersensitivities. This chapter contains the essentials about food challenges, elimination diets, and label reading. Links to other resources for the most common types of food sensitivities, such as milk and soy, are provided.

Chapter 8, "Weight Management," addresses obesity and eating disorders. The first section includes essential information about identification and treatment of obesity and includes bariatric surgery considerations. Essential details about the various types of eating disorders and their treatment challenges are included in the second part.

Chapter 9, "Inborn Errors of Metabolism," addresses newborn screening for inborn errors of metabolism (IEMs). This chapter provides principles and practical considerations in nutrition support of IEMs affecting amino acid, nitrogen, carbohydrate, and fatty acid oxidation metabolism. Sample formula calculations for diet prescriptions are included, which can help the registered dietitian new to this field.

Chapter 10, "Developmental Disabilities," addresses some of the common nutritional concerns and unique nutritional challenges of infants and children with disabilities. Topics such as assessment issues, drug–nutrient interactions, seizures, and ketogenic diet are addressed, along with nutritional considerations for children with autism and attention deficit and attention hyperactivity disorders.

Chapter 11, "Pulmonary Diseases," includes all key nutritional concerns of cystic fibrosis, bronchopulmonary dysplasia, and asthma. Some important considerations include the vitamin and mineral needs and pancreatic enzyme therapy during cystic fibrosis, growth in infants with bronchopulmonary dysplasia, and asthma management.

Chapter 12, "Gastrointestinal Disorders," encompasses an array of common gastrointestinal problems, such as diarrhea, constipation, and lactose intolerance, as well as complex disorders, such as celiac disease and liver transplant. Practical tips on oral rehydration and foods high in fiber are provided.

Chapter 13, "Kidney Disease," addresses the unique nutrition issues of the infant or child before and during dialysis and after kidney transplant. Key principles of food intake evaluation, growth, and kidney function at various ages are essential to adequately caring for the infant or child with chronic kidney disease.

Chapter 14, "Cardiology," addresses the impact of congenital heart disease on the growth and nutritional status of infants and children. Issues such as extracorporeal membrane oxygenation, cardiomyopathy, chylothorax, and hyperlipidemias as well as ways to increase the caloric density of food for these stressed infants and children are addressed.

Chapter 15, "Diabetes," stresses the impact of diabetes on the infant/child and family. Issues such as meal composition and timing, blood sugar, and insulin management are addressed. Guidelines for managing pregnancy, dyslipidemias, and weight control are provided as well as practical tips on treating hypoglycemia and use of the glycemic index.

Chapter 16, "HIV and AIDS," provides details on the goals and strategies of nutritional management of the pediatric patient with HIV infection and AIDS. The use of highly active antiretroviral therapy and other therapies are reviewed.

Chapter 17, "Oncology and Sickle Cell Disease," addresses the more common types of cancers (such as leukemia) in infants and children and their treatment challenges. The chapter also describes hematologic conditions such as sickle cell disease and covers key aspects of nutrition support during cancer treatment, use of integrative medicine, and food safety. Unique topics such as graft versus host disease and bone marrow transplant and their nutrition issues are included.

Chapter 18, "Nutrition in Burns," addresses the metabolic changes and physiologic challenges of providing adequate nutrition to the infant or child in this stressed state. Evaluation of fluid and energy requirements is emphasized. Special formulas, such as the Parkland formula modified for children, and the use of nutrition support modalities used for rehabilitation postburn are detailed.

Chapter 19, "Enteral Nutrition," and Chapter 20, "Parenteral Nutrition," contain the details needed to manage the nutritional status for all infants and children who cannot subsist and grow adequately on an oral diet. Use of enteral and/or parenteral nutrition may be short term or for longer periods of time and requires considerable knowledge of many factors by nutrition practitioners managing infants and children in the hospital, rehabilitation center, home, and other setting.

Chapter 21, "Botanicals," defines the nomenclature for herbs and phytomedicines. Key issues include the use of approved botanicals in pediatric practice and how to calculate the proper dose for medicinal herbs. An overview of commonly used medicinal herbs in pediatrics is provided.

The practice of pediatric nutrition with infants, young children, and adolescents in all settings, such as community, outpatient, and inpatient settings, continues to grow in complexity. Clinical expertise must be balanced with an awareness of the importance of human contact and social development. It is hoped that readers of this first edition of the *Essentials of Pediatric Nutrition* will have the tools and resources needed to assess, monitor, and determine appropriate interventions aimed at maximal nutrition status and growth. Because infants and children have unique nutritional needs and physiology, advanced study in pediatric nutrition by health practitioners is vital for exemplary health care. This text contains essential and unique nutritional information that pediatric practitioners can use and apply in their individual settings for each infant or child.

Acknowledgments

Thank you to the staff at Jones & Bartlett Learning and our copyeditors for their fine work. Thank you also to all of our authors for being contributors to this book and for sharing your expertise with us. A special thanks to the nutrition volunteers, Aparna Kohli and Meg Steffey Shrier, who worked with Patt.

Contributors

Phyllis B. Acosta, MS, MPH, DrPH
Nutrition Consultant
Southeastern Region Genetics Group, Emory University
Atlanta, Georgia

Susan Akers, RD, LD
Pediatric Dietitian
MetroHealth Medical Center
Cleveland, Ohio

Diane M. Anderson, PhD, RD
Associate Professor of Pediatrics
Baylor College of Medicine
Houston, Texas

Jennifer Autodore, MA, RD, CSP, LDN
Pediatric Clinical Dietitian
Children's Hospital of Philadelphia
Philadelphia, Pennsylvania

Jenni Beary, MA, RD, CSP, LDN
Pediatric Clinical Dietitian
Children's Hospital of Philadelphia
Philadelphia, Pennsylvania

Susan Bessler, MS, RD, CSO
Clinical Pediatric Dietitian
Children's Hospital and Research Center Oakland
Oakland, California

Lynn Christie, MS, RD, LD
Research Project Manager Dietician
Department of Pediatric Allergy and Immunology
Arkansas Children's Hospital
Little Rock, Arkansas

Wm. Cameron Chumlea, PhD
Fels Professor
Lifespan Health Research Center
Departments of Community Health and Pediatrics
Boonshoft School of Medicine
Wright State University
Dayton, Ohio

Harriet H. Cloud, MS, BS
Owner, Nutrition Matters
Birmingham, Alabama

Janice Hovasi Cox, MS, RD, CSP
Neonatal/Pediatric Dietitian
The Children's Hospital at Bronson
Kalamazoo, Michigan

Amanda Croll, RD, LDN
Pediatric Clinical Dietitian
Children's Hospital of Philadelphia
Philadelphia, Pennsylvania

Shannon Despino, RD, LDN
Clinical Dietitian Consultant
Scottsdale, Arizona

Marìa Duarte-Gardea, PhD, RD
Chair, Department of Public Health Services
The University of Texas at El Paso
El Paso, Texas

Sharon Feucht, MS, RD, CSP
Nutritionist
Center on Human Development and Disability
University of Washington
Seattle, Washington

Michele Morath Gottschlich, PhD, RD, CNSD
Director
Nutrition Services
Shriners Hospital for Children
Cincinnati, Ohio

Sharon Groh-Wargo, PhD, RD, LD
Associate Professor and Senior Nutritionist
Case Western Reserve University
School of Medicine at MetroHealth Medical Center
Cleveland, Ohio

Laurie Anne Higgins, MS, RD, LDN, CDE
Coordinator of Pediatric Nutrition Education and Research
Pediatric, Adolescent, and Young Adult Section
Joslin Diabetes Center
Boston, Massachusetts

Laura V. Hudspeth, MS, RD
Infant and Pediatric Clinical Dietitian
University of Alabama at Birmingham
Birmingham, Alabama

Kathryn Hunt, BS, RD, CD
Clinical Pediatric Oncology Dietitian
Seattle Children's Hospital
Seattle, Washington

Susan Konek, MA, RD, CSP, CNSD, LDN
Director of Clinical Nutrition
The Children's Hospital of Philadelphia
Philadelphia, Pennsylvania

Haley W. Lacey, MD, RD, LD
Clinical Dietitian
Children's Health System of Alabama
Birmingham, Alabama

Michael LaMonte, PhD, MPH
Assistant Professor
Department of Social and Preventive Medicine
University at Buffalo, The State University of New York
Buffalo, New York

Betty Lucas, MPH, RD
Nutritionist
Center on Human Development and Disability
University of Washington
Seattle, Washington

Paula Charuhas Macris, MS, RD, FADA, CSO, CD
Nutrition Education Coordinator and Pediatric Nutrition Specialist
Seattle Cancer Care Alliance
Seattle, Washington

Theresa Mayes, RD
Clinical Dietitian
Shriners Hospital for Children
Cincinnati, Ohio

Ingrida Mara Melbardis, RD, CSP
Pediatric Dietitian
The Children's Hospital at Bronson
Kalamazoo, Michigan

Monica Nagle, RD, CNSD, LDN
Pediatric Clinical Dietitian
Children's Hospital of Philadelphia
Philadelphia, Pennsylvania

Beth Ogata, MS, RD, CSP
Nutritionist
Center on Human Development and Disability
University of Washington
Seattle, Washington

Linda A. Phelan, RD, CSR, LD
Pediatric Renal and NICU Dietitian
Oregon Health and Science University
Doernbecher Children's Hospital
Portland, Oregon

Erin Redding, RD, LDN
Nutrition Specialist
New England Dairy and Food Council
Boston, Massachusetts

Jill Rockwell, RD, CNSD
Clinical Dietitian
Children's Medical Center of Dallas
Dallas, Texas

Melanie Savoca, MS, RD, LDN
Pediatric Clinical Dietitian
Children's Hospital of Philadelphia
Philadelphia, Pennsylvania

Lisa Simone Sharda, MA, RD
Pediatric Clinical Dietitian
Children's Memorial Hospital
Chicago, Illinois

Bonnie A. Spear, PhD, RD
Professor of Pediatrics
University of Alabama at Birmingham
Birmingham, Alabama

Alyce Thomas, RD
Prenatal Nutrition Consultant
St. Joseph's Regional Medical Center
Paterson, New Jersey

John Westerdahl, PhD, MPH, RD, CNS
Director
Bragg Health Institute
Santa Barbara, California

Sarah Weston, RD, LDN
Clinical Dietitian for Gastroenterology
Children's Hospital of Philadelphia
Philadelphia, Pennsylvania

CHAPTER 1

Prenatal Nutrition

Alyce Thomas and María Duarte-Gardea

Introduction

Infant care does not begin on the day a baby is born; it is a journey that takes place before conception. The health and nutritional status of the mother prior to and during pregnancy are the major determinants to a successful outcome. Preconception care, which includes nutrition, physical activity, and behavioral interventions, is an important adjunct to the health care of all women in their reproductive years. As preconception care becomes the norm and not the exception to routine medical care, women will seek to enter prenatal care early in their pregnancy. Any delay in accessing prenatal care may result in an increase in negative outcomes. Important components of preconception and prenatal care are nutrition counseling for normal pregnancy with medical nutrition therapy (when needed), and they should be incorporated into the health care of all women.

Preconception

Despite having the highest per capita healthcare costs in the world, the United States ranks 29th in infant mortality rate.[1] The primary reason for this high infant mortality rate is the number of preterm births when compared to other nations. One of the contributing factors to the poor pregnancy outcome in the United States is the date when a woman enters prenatal care. If prenatal care does not begin until late in the first trimester or in the second or third trimester, the delay may result in serious health consequences for the mother and her infant. To reduce the risks associated with delayed prenatal care, the focus must be on improving the woman's health prior to conception. Because more than half of all pregnancies are unplanned or unintended, preconception care should be incorporated into the routine primary medical care of every woman of childbearing age.[2,3] Ideally, the medical care for adolescent girls would transition from the pediatrician to the family physician, which would ensure continuous medical care.

The goal of preconception care is for every woman to receive services that will enable her to achieve optimal health before pregnancy. This includes health care for women between pregnancies.[4] The Centers for Disease Control and Prevention (CDC) has identified 4 goals and 10 recommendations to improve health and pregnancy outcomes in the United States (http://www.cdc.gov/mmwr/pdf/rr/rr5506.pdf).[5] Nutrition is emphasized as one of the eight areas for risk screening.[6,7] Two of the CDC-selected preconception risk factors for adverse pregnancy outcomes that are directly affected by a woman's nutritional health are diabetes and obesity. Two other conditions, hypertension and polycystic ovary syndrome, are not listed in the CDC's preconception healthcare recommendations, but they may also affect perinatal outcome.

Diabetes

Women with pregestational diabetes are at increased risk for poor perinatal outcomes such as retinopathy and cardiovascular disease.[8,9] Congenital anomalies and increased risk of stillbirth and miscarriage are among the complications associated with hyperglycemia during pregnancy. Conception should be delayed until optimal glycemic levels are achieved. The risk of perinatal complications decreases in women with pregestational diabetes if their glycosylated hemoglobin levels are as close to normal as possible without significant hypoglycemia.[8,10] Preconception counseling to all women with diabetes is essential to reduce the risk of malformations associated with unplanned pregnancies and poor metabolic control.[8,9] Effective contraception methods should be used at all times until good metabolic control is achieved.[9]

The overall goals of nutrition therapy for women with preexisting diabetes are to achieve and maintain blood glucose levels in the normal range through dietary and lifestyle modifications to decrease the risk of perinatal complications.[8] Evidence-based nutrition recommendations for type 1 and type 2 diabetes can be found online at the American Dietetic Association's Evidence Analysis Library and the American Diabetes Association's position statement on nutrition recommendations.[11,12]

Women with previous gestational diabetes mellitus (GDM) are at risk of developing type 2 diabetes mellitus later in life or GDM in subsequent pregnancies.[10] Six to 8 weeks after delivery, a 75-gram oral glucose tolerance test (OGTT) should be performed on all women with GDM. GDM women should be screened every year if the fasting glucose or 2-hour postprandial on the postpartum OGTT was elevated.[10]

Obesity

Obesity is a risk factor for cardiovascular disease, diabetes, and other health problems.[13,14] Obesity also affects the outcome of pregnancy in the mother and her fetus. A higher prevalence of gestational diabetes, impaired glucose tolerance, hypertension, thromboembolism, preeclampsia, sleep apnea, cesarean section, preterm delivery, and postpartum weight retention are associated with maternal obesity.[15,16] Fetal complications include macrosomia, congenital anomalies, shoulder dystocia, and childhood obesity.[15–17] Ideally, women should delay conception until they have achieved a normal weight to improve their pregnancy outcome.[15,17,18]

Assessment includes determining the degree of obesity and health status by evaluating the BMI, waist circumference, and overall medical risk. (Also see Chapter 3 on nutrition assessment and Chapter 8 on weight management.) Management involves weight loss, maintenance, and control of other risk factors. The goals for weight loss and management include: (1) to reduce body weight, (2) to maintain lower body weight, and (3) to prevent further weight gain.

Hypertension

Hypertensive disorders during pregnancy are a leading cause of maternal mortality and are associated with an increased risk of preterm birth and intrauterine growth retardation.[19] A woman's blood pressure should be evaluated prior to conception in order to define its status, assess its severity, determine the presence of organ damage, and plan treatment strategies.[20] Certain medications, such as angiotensin II receptor blockers (ARBs) and angiotensin converting enzyme (ACE) inhibitors, are contraindicated in pregnancy and should be discontinued before the woman plans to conceive.[19] Methyldopa and beta blockers are safe to use during pregnancy.[19,20]

The incidence of hypertension in pregnant teenagers is increasing, which is related to higher rates of obesity among adolescents. Pregnant teenagers are more at risk of developing preeclampsia than women in the 20- to 30-year age group, and preeclampsia is most common among young primiparas.[21]

The American Dietetic Association's evidence-based nutrition practice guidelines for hypertension recommend a comprehensive program in the management of elevated blood pressure, which includes medical nutrition therapy, weight reduction, and physical activity.[22] A comprehensive program can prevent target organ damage and improve cardiovascular outcomes.[19,20,22,23] The DASH (Dietary Approaches to Stop Hypertension) dietary pattern has been shown to reduce systolic blood pressure by 8–14 mm Hg.[22–24] Lowering the daily sodium intake to less than 2300 mg also helps to lower blood pressure.[22–24]

Polycystic Ovary Syndrome

Polycystic ovary syndrome (PCOS) is an endocrine condition that affects about 1 in every 10 women.[25] It is associated with various metabolic dysfunctions, including menstrual irregularities, infertility, hyperandrogenism, hypertension, insulin resistance, and hyperinsulinemia.[25,26] Women with PCOS are at increased risk of developing cardiovascular disease, type 2 diabetes, and the metabolic syndrome.[25] Although most women with PCOS tend to be overweight, it is also seen in normal weight women with excessive abdominal fat distribution.[27]

Treatment for PCOS consists of dietary and lifestyle changes, including physical activity, weight management, behavior modification, and medication, if necessary. Insulin sensitivity has been shown to improve with weight loss.[28] Dietary patterns that emphasize unrefined carbohydrates with moderate protein and unsaturated fats are often used.[25–30] Dietary fats, especially saturated and trans fats, may play a role in insulin resistance by increasing inflammation. A diet high in trans fats may increase the risk of ovulatory infertility.[31]

Metformin is commonly used in the treatment of PCOS to decrease insulin resistance, reduce hyperandrogenism, and increase ovulation, and it may prevent the development of GDM.[25] Orlistat coupled with calorie restriction may also decrease insulin resistance and weight in women with PCOS.[32]

Lifestyle Factors

Other modifiable risk factors have been identified that when addressed in the preconception period will help to improve pregnancy outcome. These risk factors include alcohol, folate deficiency, maternal phenylketonuria, and smoking.

Alcohol

Prenatal exposure to alcohol use during pregnancy is the leading cause of preventable birth defects and developmental disabilities.[33,34] Risks to the fetus include spontaneous abortions, intrauterine growth restriction, central nervous system and facial malformations, and mental retardation. *Fetal alcohol spectrum disorders* (FASD) is a term that describes a range of effects that can occur in the fetus due to alcohol exposure in utero. Fetal alcohol syndrome (FAS) is the most commonly known of the disorders. There is no safe level of alcohol consumption during pregnancy, thus women who are pregnant or who may become pregnant should abstain from alcohol use.[35]

Folate Deficiency

Folate has been shown to protect against neural tube defects (NTDs), which include spina bifida and anencephaly.[36] All women of reproductive age are advised to take 400 mcg of folic acid daily through fortified foods and/or supplements.

Maternal Phenylketonuria

Phenylketonuria (PKU) is a metabolic disorder characterized by mental retardation, microcephaly, low birth weight, and congenital heart defects.[37,38] Women who were diagnosed with PKU as infants and enter pregnancy with elevated phenylalanine levels are at increased risk of delivering infants with congenital anomalies. Because the most critical period of pregnancy is in the first 10 weeks after conception, a phenylalanine-restricted diet is recommended for PKU women throughout their reproductive years.

Smoking

Women who smoke are at increased risk for heart disease, certain types of cancers, and lung disease.[39] Smoking during pregnancy has an adverse effect on both the woman and the fetus. Maternal effects include spontaneous abortion, premature rupture of the membranes, placenta previa, placenta abruption, and preterm delivery. Fetal effects associated with tobacco include intrauterine growth restriction, low birth weight, and sudden infant death syndrome. The CDC recommends cessation of smoking before pregnancy.[39]

Pregnancy

Pregnancy is a time of increased energy and nutrient needs for a woman to support fetal growth and development, as well as her own. The length of gestation and the prepregnancy weight of the mother are two of the most influential factors affecting prenatal outcome.

Weight Issues in Pregnancy

Prepregnancy weight and weight gain are important aspects in pregnancy because both are associated with maternal outcomes, mode of delivery, preterm birth, birth weight, and postpartum weight retention. The Institute of Medicine (IOM) provides guidelines for weight gain during pregnancy according to the prepregnancy BMI. These guidelines seek to improve maternal and infant outcomes.

Weight Gain Recommendations

Recommendations for weight gain during pregnancy should be individualized according to the prepregnancy BMI to improve pregnancy outcome, avoid excessive maternal postpartum weight retention, and reduce the risk of adult chronic disease in the child.[40]

Recommendations of total and weekly weight gain for the second and third trimesters for each BMI are displayed in **Table 1-1**. The recommended total weight gain for the first trimester is 0.5–2 kg, or 1.1–4.4 pounds, depending on the prepregnancy BMI.[41,42]

Overweight and Obesity

The incidence of obesity is high among black women, black Mexican American, and white women of childbearing age.[43] In addition, the risk of GDM is higher among women who are overweight and obese.[44] Other complications associated with maternal overweight and obesity are hypertension, preeclampsia, cesarean section, preterm delivery, labor induction, postpartum hemorrhage, macrosomia, and neonatal hypoglycemia.[45–51] Multiple maternal and infant detrimental effects are associated with maternal overweight and obesity. Thus, to ameliorate these adverse outcomes, all overweight and obese women of reproductive age should receive counseling on the roles of diet and physical activity in reproductive

TABLE 1-1 Total and Mean Weight Gain Recommendations During Pregnancy

	Underweight (< 18.5)	Normal (18.5–24.9)	Overweight (25–29.9)	Obese (> 29.9)
Total				
Kg	12.5–18	11.5–16	7–11.5	5–9
Lb	28–40	25–35	15–25	11–20
Weekly Gain for Second and Third Trimesters				
Mean, Kg	0.51	0.4	0.28	0.22
Range, Kg	(0.44–0.58)	(0.35–0.50)	(0.23–0.33)	(0.17–0.27)
Mean, Lb	1	1	0.6	0.5
Range, Lb	(1–1.3)	(0.8–1)	(0.5–0.7)	(0.4–0.6)

Source: Adapted from Institute of Medicine. *Weight Gain During Pregnancy: Reexamining the Guidelines.* Report brief. Washington, DC: National Academies Press; 2009. Reprinted with permission from the National Academies Press, Copyright 2009, National Academy of Sciences.

health prior to pregnancy, during pregnancy, and in the interconceptional period.[52]

Multiple Gestation

Multiple births have risen in the United States, primarily due to the increasing use of assisted reproductive technologies (ART). Newborns conceived through ART are at higher risk for prematurity, low birth weight, and perinatal mortality. Women who conceive through ART are more likely to develop preeclampsia and gestational diabetes and experience preterm birth, or vacuum or forceps delivery. The most common antenatal complications include preterm premature rupture of membranes, hemorrhage, and anemia.[53–56] Triplet and quadruplet pregnancies often have higher risks than twin pregnancies for most maternal and neonatal complications. Maternal anthropometric, nutritional, and previous reproductive factors may be particularly important in reducing these excess risks and improving outcomes in multiple births.[57] Most infants of multiple gestation are preterm births (37 weeks gestation) and are among the low-birth-weight (2500 g) and very-low-birth-weight (1500 g) infant populations. Weight gain recommendations for twin pregnancies include a range of maternal weight gain of 37–54 pounds for the normal BMI category, 31–50 pounds for overweight women, and 25–42 pounds for obese women, with a suggested rate gain of 1.5 pounds per week during the second and third trimesters.[41]

Gastrointestinal Discomforts

Nausea and Vomiting

Symptoms of nausea and vomiting in pregnancy (NVP) constitute a frequent and often highly unpleasant syndrome during early gestation. Nausea and/or vomiting often occur in pregnant women during the first trimester.[58] Commonly referred to as "morning sickness," NVP may occur at any time during the day or night. Nausea, a frequent discomfort of early pregnancy, can last well into the second trimester and varies greatly in its severity. NVP symptoms in multigravidas may last beyond the first trimester with each additional pregnancy.[59]

Management of NVP depends on the severity of the symptoms. Dietary modifications may resolve mild cases. First trimester nausea may improve by consuming small amounts of liquid or food at frequent intervals and avoiding fried, spicy, and high-fat foods. Some pregnant women may tolerate foods high in carbohydrates, such as crackers, rather than high-protein or high-fat foods.[40] Some women respond by avoiding cooking odors, getting out of bed slowly in the morning, and drinking small amounts of liquids between meals.[60–62] A multivitamin and a vitamin B_6 supplement should be consumed early in the pregnancy-planning process. Eating ginger may help as a nonpharmacologic option.[63]

Hyperemesis gravidarum (HG), or severe nausea and vomiting, is a high-risk condition usually requiring hospital admission, antiemetic medications, rehydration, correction of electrolytes, and nutritional support. Some women may lose considerable weight and may require hospitalization with parenteral nutrition. Excessive weight loss should be prevented.[62,63]

Heartburn

Heartburn is a common symptom in pregnancy and may be caused by the effects of pregnancy hormones on the lower esophageal sphincter and gastric clearance. Interventions that may relieve symptoms include advice on diet and lifestyle, antacids, antihistamines, and proton pump inhibitors.[64] Practical approaches that may ease heartburn in pregnancy include avoiding lying down immediately after eating; sleeping with the head slightly elevated to avoid acid reflux; consuming small, frequent meals; and avoiding known irritants, such as caffeine, chocolate, or highly seasoned foods.[40]

Ptyalism

Ptyalism is of unknown origin and is usually defined as an excessive secretion of saliva. It is common in women with nausea and vomiting who might have difficulty swallowing their saliva.[65] Dietary alterations to overcome ptyalism include the use of chewing gum or lozenges and restricting fluids. Ptyalism during pregnancy may resolve at 35 to 36 weeks gestation or it may last until after delivery.[66]

Constipation

Constipation is common during pregnancy and occurs most frequently during the third trimester as the weight of the uterus puts pressure on the rectum, which may also result in hemorrhoids. Increased consumption of liquids (six to eight glasses daily) in combination with high-fiber foods and regular physical activity are recommended to alleviate constipation. A diet containing high-fiber foods such as whole grains, legumes, fruits, and vegetables is helpful to achieve the DRI for fiber of 28 grams per day.[67]

Diarrhea

Diarrhea during pregnancy may be the result of foodborne infections, irritable bowel syndrome, or other causes. Acute diarrhea may lead to severe dehydration that can result in the loss of important electrolytes from the body. Symptoms of dehydration include excessive thirst, dry mouth, scant or no urine or dark yellow urine, decreased tears, severe weakness or lethargy, and dizziness. Fluids are the most effective treatment for preventing dehydration in pregnant women. Consumption of liquids, such as oral rehydration fluids, juice, or water, can help pregnant women reduce the risk of becoming dehydrated. Medical attention should be required when diarrhea is not resolved within 24 hours. Diarrhea with bloody stools, fever, or severe abdominal pain requires immediate medical attention.

Eating Disorders

The eating disorders (EDs) anorexia nervosa, bulimia nervosa, and those not otherwise specified have profound effects on the overall well-being of women and their children. Women with past histories of ED are likely to have some ED behaviors and/or concerns about weight gain during pregnancy.[68] Complications associated with eating disorders during pregnancy include miscarriage, premature labor, low birth weight, stillbirth or fetal death, and delayed fetal growth. See Chapter 8 on eating disorders.

Physical Activity

Physical activity is recommended for most pregnant women who do not have medical or obstetric risks. The recommendation for normal-risk pregnant women is 30 minutes or more of moderate-intensity physical activity on most, if not all, days of the week. Activities with a high risk of abdominal trauma should be avoided. Physical activity is contraindicated in conditions such as restrictive lung disease, incompetent cervix, multiple gestation, premature labor, rupture of membranes, and placenta previa.[69] It is important to evaluate the overall health of pregnant women, including obstetric and medical risks, before prescribing an exercise program. Additional factors to take into consideration are prepregnancy BMI, weight gain goals, dietary intake, and history of physical activity.

Nutrient Recommendations

The quality of the diet during pregnancy has a profound impact on fetal and maternal outcomes. A well-balanced diet providing recommended calories and optimal nutrients throughout pregnancy should promote normal fetal growth and development and desired maternal outcomes. Conversely, maternal malnutrition, especially during the first trimester, a crucial period of fetal development, may predispose the infant to chronic diseases in adult years. Chronic diseases such as coronary heart disease, hypertension, and type 2 diabetes may originate in impaired intrauterine growth and development.[70,71]

The dietary reference intakes (DRIs), the recommended dietary allowances (RDAs), adequate intake (AI), tolerable upper intake level (UL), and estimated average requirement (EAR) serve as a guide to prevent nutritional deficiencies and to promote optimal health benefits. Recommended levels of energy and nutrient intakes vary for adults, children, and women who are pregnant or breastfeeding.[67,72] (See Appendix F.)

Energy

The energy allowance for pregnancy can be estimated by dividing the gross energy cost (80,000 kcal) by the approximate duration (250 days following the first month), yielding an average value of 300 kcal per day in addition to the allowance for nonpregnant females.[67,72] Caloric requirements for pregnant adolescents (14–18 years) and adult women (19–50 years) can be calculated by using the estimated energy requirements (EER) formula.[67] **Table 1-2** displays EER formulas to determine energy requirements for normal prepregnancy BMI for each trimester. The DRIs for total energy indicate that for healthful birth outcomes pregnant women should consume an extra 340 kcal/day in the second trimester and 452 kcal/day in the third trimester.

The formulas displayed in Table 1-2 are not applicable to overweight and obese women. An estimate of the caloric requirement for overweight and obese women can be obtained by using an adjusted body weight in the Harris Benedict formula and adding 150–300 kcal for the second and third trimesters.[67,72] (See **Table 1-3**.)

A simple method to determine caloric needs during pregnancy for normal weight women is to estimate a daily need of 30 kcal per kilogram prepregnancy weight per day during the first trimester and then add 300 kcal during the second and third trimesters. In underweight women, these caloric prescriptions would need to be increased. Regardless of the method used to estimate caloric level, weight gain pattern, goals, and appetite are used along with frequent monitoring to make the necessary caloric adjustments.

TABLE 1-2 Estimated Energy Requirements for Normal Prepregnancy BMI

First Trimester [EER + 0]	EER = 354 − (6.91 × A) + PA × (9.36 × Wt + 726 × Ht)
Second Trimester [EER + 340]	EER = 354 − (6.91 × A) + PA × (9.36 × Wt + 726 × Ht) + 340
Third Trimester [EER + 452]	EER = 354 − (6.91 × A) + PA × (9.36 × Wt + 726 × Ht) + 452

Abbreviations: A = age; PA = physical activity coefficient: sedentary (1.0), low activity (1.12), active (1.27), very active (1.45); Wt = weight in kilograms; Ht = height in meters.

Source: Data from Institute of Medicine. *Dietary Reference Intakes for Energy, Carbohydrates, Fiber, Fat, Fatty Acids, Cholesterol, Protein and Amino Acids (Macronutrients).* Washington, DC: National Academies Press; 2002.

TABLE 1-3 Energy Requirements for Overweight and Obese Prepregnancy BMI

Energy = [655 + (9.6 × AdBWt kg) + (1.8 × Ht cm) – (4.7 × A)] × PA + (150 – 300) kcal

Abbreviations: AdBWt = Adjusted Body Weight: [(Actual Body Wt – Desirable Body Wt) × 0.25] + Desirable Body Wt.

Macronutrients

In addition to providing the RDA or AI for carbohydrates, proteins, and fat, the DRIs for macronutrients also provide a range of daily macronutrient distribution. The Acceptable Macronutrient Distribution Range (AMDR) is the range of intake for a particular energy source that is associated with reduced risk of chronic disease while providing intakes of essential nutrients. The AMDR for pregnancy is the same as for all healthy adults: 45–65% of kcal from carbohydrates, 10–35% of kcal from protein, and 20–35% of kcal from fat.[67]

Carbohydrates and Nutritive Sweeteners

The major types of carbohydrates in the diet are starch, a complex carbohydrate, and simple sugars, such as glucose, fructose, sucrose, and lactose. To assure provision of glucose to the fetal brain (approximately 33 g/day), as well as to supply the glucose fuel requirement for the mother's brain, the RDA for pregnancy for ages 14 and older is 175 g of carbohydrate per day.

Carbohydrate-containing foods have been ranked according to their effect on blood glucose levels compared with a reference food (either glucose or white bread). This concept is known as the glycemic index (GI), and it classifies foods as low (< 55), medium (56–69), or high (> 70) GI foods. Foods with low GI scores (e.g., oatmeal, bran cereal) contain slowly digested carbohydrates, which produce only small fluctuations in blood glucose and insulin levels. Foods with high GI scores (e.g., sweetened beverages, sugar) contain rapidly digested carbohydrates, which produce a rapid rise and fall in the blood glucose level.[73] High glycemic foods may affect pregnancy outcomes. However, the concept of GI foods is controversial and is not currently recommended.[67]

Fiber

Fiber is composed of complex carbohydrates and can be classified as insoluble or soluble. Insoluble fibers, such as cellulose, hemicellulose, and lignin, increase water-holding capacity, thus increasing fecal volume and decreasing gastric transit time. Soluble fibers, such as gums and pectins, form gels, resulting in slowed gastrointestinal transit time and slowed or decreased nutrient absorption. Soluble fibers also bind other nutrients, such as cholesterol and minerals, decreasing their absorption. Foods high in insoluble fiber include wheat bran, whole grains, seeds, and the skins of fruits and vegetables. Foods containing high levels of soluble fiber include oats, legumes, barley, and some fruits and vegetables. Adequate fiber is needed to prevent constipation and for normal bowel health.

Nonnutritive Sweeteners

The Food and Drug Administration (FDA) has approved five nonnutritive sweeteners: saccharin, aspartame, acesulfame potassium (or acesulfame K), sucralose, and neotame. The use of aspartame within FDA guidelines appears to be safe during pregnancy. Aspartame (Equal or Nutrasweet) is the methyl ester dipeptide of the natural amino acids L-aspartic acid and L-phenylalanine. Women with PKU must restrict their phenylalanine intake, and thus must avoid aspartame.

Acesulfame potassium (Sweet One or Sunette) and sucralose (Splenda) are considered safe for use during pregnancy. Saccharin (Sweet'N Low) crosses the placenta and may remain in fetal tissue because of the slow fetal clearance. Careful use of saccharin is advised during pregnancy. Neotame®, a derivative of the dipeptide composed of the amino acids aspartic acid and phenylalanine, is readily eliminated from the body. It is considered safe for the general population, including pregnant and lactating women, children, and people with diabetes. Although no specific recommendations have been made regarding their use during pregnancy, moderation of ingestion of nonnutritive sweeteners may be appropriate.[74]

Dietary Fat

Dietary fat provides energy and is essential for the absorption and transport of fat-soluble vitamins. Besides having an impact on weight gain, dietary fat also plays an important role in the modulation of lipid profile. Essential fatty acids (EFA) are required in the human diet. Two closely related families of EFA are omega-3 and omega-6 fatty acids. The major fatty acids of the omega-6 series are linoleic (18:2n-6), γ-linolenic (18:3n-6), and arachidonic (20:4n-6) acids. The AMDR of fat for pregnant women is 20–35% of total energy, the same as for nonpregnant women. The AI of omega-6 linoleic acid is 13 g/d and for omega-3, ∝-linolenic acid is 1.4 g/d.[72]

Protein

Pregnant women have additional protein requirements to support the expansion of maternal tissue and fetal growth.

Protein intake has a significant influence on birth weight. A high-protein diet may be more detrimental than inadequate protein. It appears that moderate protein intake is optimal during pregnancy.[75] The current RDA of 71 g of protein for pregnant women is 25 g more than the requirement for nonpregnant women. The additional 25 g is based on 1.1 g/kg/day using prepregnant weight. See Appendix Table F-1 for the DRIs for macronutrients for pregnant women.

Micronutrients

Certain vitamins and minerals are of particular significance during pregnancy. The main cause of many deficiencies is the quality of the diet. Women who avoid meat and/or milk are also at higher risk of micronutrient depletion during pregnancy and lactation. In certain dietary patterns high in unrefined grains and legumes, the amount of nutrients consumed may be adequate, but dietary constituents, such as phytates and polyphenols, will limit micronutrient absorption.

Several micronutrient deficiencies are well known as contributors to abnormal prenatal development and/or pregnancy outcome. These include magnesium, iron, folate, and vitamin D deficiencies. Less well recognized for their importance are deficiencies of B vitamins (and subsequently elevated plasma homocysteine concentrations).[76] See **Table 1-4** for the RDAs and adequate intakes for micronutrients for pregnant and nonpregnant adolescents and women.

Magnesium

Magnesium may be effective in the management of eclampsia and preeclampsia, arrhythmia, severe asthma, and migraine.[77] The RDA of 360–400 mg of magnesium in pregnancy is an increase of 40 mg over nonpregnant requirements.[72]

Iron

The requirement for iron is significantly increased during pregnancy due to increased iron utilization by the developing fetus and placenta as well as blood volume expansion. Iron deficiency during pregnancy leads to maternal anemia, defined as a hematocrit less than 32% or a hemoglobin less than 11 g/dL. Iron supplementation at a dose of 30 mg/day should be started after 12 weeks of gestation, when iron requirements begin to increase.[78] The DRI for iron during pregnancy is 27 mg/day.[72]

Folate

A deficiency of folate during the first days after conception may result in low birth weight, premature birth, and/or neural tube defects (NTDs) and elevated homocysteine levels, which may be a predictor of poor pregnancy outcomes.[76,79] Folate is found naturally in food; folic acid, the synthetic form of folate, is found in supplements and fortified foods. Folic acid is 100% absorbed when consumed, whereas folate is only partially absorbed. Folic acid is added to breakfast cereals and many other foods with the purpose of preventing NTDs. The DRI for folate during pregnancy is 600 µg/day.[72]

Vitamin D

Vitamin D is essential for skeletal health, and a prolonged deficiency will result in infant rickets and adult osteomalacia. Serum 25(OH)D (25-hydroxyvitamin D) concentration is a useful indicator of vitamin D nutritional status.[77] The AI for vitamin D is the same as for nonpregnant women.

B Vitamins

B vitamins such as thiamine, riboflavin, niacin, biotin, pantothenic acid, vitamin B_6, folate, and vitamin B_{12} participate in many metabolic pathways, including those involved in energy metabolism. Poor maternal vitamin B status may be a major cause of homocysteinemia and poor pregnancy outcomes.

Comorbidities During Pregnancy

Pregnant women experiencing diabetes, hypertension, and preeclampsia require individualized dietary modification that will help to reduce the risks associated with these conditions.

Diabetes

The risk of developing gestational diabetes (GDM) has increased in the last 10 years, primarily among women who are overweight or obese.[44] GDM is defined as glucose intolerance occurring during pregnancy.[80,81] Women at risk for GDM typically have a previous history of GDM, may exhibit obesity, have a strong family history of diabetes, or belong to an ethnic group with a high prevalence of diabetes. GDM is associated with fetal macrosomia, large-for-gestational-age infants, and an increased risk of a difficult labor and delivery.[82,83] Intensive treatment of hyperglycemia in women with GDM lessens the risk of adverse outcomes by reducing the risk of fetal macrosomia and providing the best outcome for normal or large-for-gestational-age infants.[84,85]

Nutrition management consists of specifying the appropriate amount of carbohydrates that will help the patient gain the recommended amount of weight, while achieving normoglycemia and preventing ketonuria. The recommendation of a minimum of 175 g of carbohydrates per day is the same as for pregnant women without GDM.[86] Carbohydrates are less tolerated at breakfast than at other meals and should be adjusted based on monitoring weight, blood glucose, and ketones.[87] For optimal glucose control, carbohydrates should be distributed throughout the day in three meals and three snacks.

The amount of protein, fat, and vitamins and minerals should be based on the DRI for pregnant women. Vitamin and mineral supplementation should be encouraged when

TABLE 1-4 Recommended Dietary Allowances and Adequate Intakes for Micronutrients

	Nonpregnant		Pregnant	
Micronutrient	Females 13–18 yr	Females 19–50 yr	Females 13–18 yr	Females 19–50 yr
Thiamine (mg/day)[a]	1.0	1.1	1.4	1.4
Riboflavin (mg/day)[a,c]	1.0	1.1	1.4	1.4
Niacin (mg/day)[a]	14	14	18	18
Biotin (μg/day)[b]	25	30	30	30
Pantothenic acid (mg/day)[b]	5	5	6	6
Vitamin B_6 (mg/day)[a]	1.2	1.3	1.9	1.9
Folate (μg/day)[a,d]	400	400	600	600
Vitamin B_{12} (μg/day)[a]	2.4	2.4	2.6	2.6
Choline (mg/day)[b]	400	425	450	450
Vitamin C (mg/day)[a]	65	75	80	85
Vitamin A (μg/day)[a,e]	700	700	750	770
Vitamin D (μg/day)[b,f]	5	5	5	5
Vitamin E (mg/day)[a,g]	15	15	15	15
Vitamin K (μg/day)[b]	75	90	75	90
Sodium (mg/day)[b]	1500	1500	1500	1500
Chloride (mg/day)[b]	2300	2300	2300	2300
Potassium (mg/day)[b]	4700	4700	4700	4700
Calcium (mg/day)[b]	1300	1000	1300	1000
Phosphorus (mg/day)[a]	1250	700	1250	700
Magnesium (mg/day)[a]	360	310	400	350
Iron (mg/day)[a]	15	18	27	27
Zinc (mg/day)[a]	9	8	12	11
Iodine (μg/day)[a]	150	150	220	220
Selenium (μg/day)[a]	55	55	60	60
Copper (μg/day)[a]	890	900	1000	1000
Manganese (mg/day)[b]	1.6	1.8	2.0	2.0
Fluoride (mg/day)[b]	3	3	3	3
Chromium (μg/day)[b]	24	25	29	30
Molybdenum (μg/day)[a]	43	45	50	50

[a]Recommended dietary allowance (RDA)

[b]Adequate intake (AI)

[c]Niacin recommendations are expressed as niacin equivalents (NE).

[d]Folate recommendations are expressed as dietary folate equivalents (DEF).

[e]Vitamin A recommendations are expressed as retinol activity equivalents (RAE).

[f]Vitamin D recommendations are expressed as cholecalciferol and assume absence of adequate exposure to sunlight.

[g]Vitamin E recommendations are expressed as α-tocoferol.

DRIs are not met through dietary intake. Most women with GDM return to normal glucose levels in the postpartum period. Postpartum counseling should highlight the importance of attaining a normal BMI and regular physical activity in an effort to reduce the lifetime risk of GDM in subsequent pregnancies or the risk of type 2 diabetes.[88]

Hypertension and Preeclampsia

Gestational hypertension and preeclampsia are more common in overweight and obese pregnant women. Gestational hypertension is defined as a systolic blood pressure of at least 140 mm Hg or a diastolic blood pressure of at least 90 mm Hg.[52] Many women with gestational hypertension diagnosed before 30 weeks gestation develop preeclampsia. Risk factors include preeclampsia in a previous pregnancy, maternal age younger than 20 years or older than 40 years, obesity, insulin resistance, diabetes, and genetic factors.[40,89]

The cause of preeclampsia is unknown, but may be related to an inadequate placental blood supply, possibly due to maternal hypertension, which causes placental oxidative stress and the release of placental factors into maternal circulation that trigger an inflammatory response. Subclinical inflammation is more common in obese individuals, hence obese women may enter pregnancy with preexisting inflammation that enhances their risk for preeclampsia.[52,90]

The incidence of preeclampsia is greater in twins than in single births.[91] Preeclampsia is associated with preterm delivery, low-birth-weight infants, neonatal death, maternal morbidity and mortality, and an increased risk of developing cardiovascular disease later in life.[92–94] A diet consisting of a high intake of vegetables, plant foods, and vegetable oils may decrease the risk of preeclampsia.[90]

Food Safety

Seafood

Nearly all fish and shellfish contain traces of mercury. Mercury occurs naturally in the environment, but it also can be released into the air through industrial pollution that may accumulate in oceans, thus exposing fish to this contaminant.[95] Mercury in seafood products readily crosses the placental barrier and has the potential to damage the developing fetal nervous system.[95,96] The FDA and the Environmental Protection Agency (EPA) recommend that pregnant women, women of childbearing age, and young children avoid eating shark, swordfish, mackerel, and tilefish.[97] The recommendation is to consume up to 12 ounces (two average meals) a week of a variety of fish and shellfish that are lower in mercury,[98] such as shrimp, canned light tuna, salmon, pollock, and catfish. Another recommendation is to check local advisories concerning the safety of fish caught by family and friends in local lakes, rivers, and coastal areas.

Listeriosis

Listeriosis is a serious infection caused by consuming food contaminated with the pathogen *Listeria monocytogenes*, a gram-positive anaerobe that grows at temperatures as low as 3°C (37°F) and can multiply in refrigerated foods.[99] Pregnant women, the elderly, and adults with weakened immune systems are susceptible to listeriosis.[100] Symptoms of listeriosis include influenza-like symptoms, persistent fever, and gastrointestinal symptoms, such as nausea, vomiting, and diarrhea. The onset time to gastrointestinal symptoms is probably greater than 12 hours; the onset time to the serious forms of listeriosis may range from a few days to 3 weeks.

The manifestations of listeriosis include septicemia, meningitis (or meningoencephalitis), encephalitis, and intrauterine or cervical infections in pregnant women, which may result in spontaneous abortion or stillbirth.[101] Listeriosis is diagnosed by culturing the organism from blood, cerebrospinal fluid, or stool. The FDA recommends all pregnant women avoid the following foods to prevent listeriosis:[99]

- Hot dogs or luncheon meats (including deli meats such as ham, turkey, salami) unless reheated until steaming hot.
- Soft cheeses, such as feta and brie, unless made with pasteurized milk.
- Refrigerated pâtés or meat spreads. Canned and shelf-stable versions are safe.
- Refrigerated smoked seafood unless cooked (as in a casserole). Canned and shelf-stable versions can be eaten safely.
- Unpasteurized milk, eggs, or juice, or foods made from these foods.

Post-Delivery Issues

Proper nutrition also plays an important role after delivery. Obtaining the recommended types and amounts of nutrients after delivery can help women alleviate symptoms associated with postpartum depression.

Depression

Perinatal depression refers to major and minor episodes during pregnancy (antenatal) or within the first 12 months after delivery (postpartum or postnatal). The term *maternal depression* has been used interchangeably with perinatal depression. Signs and symptoms for perinatal depression are similar to those for the disease in the general population: depressed mood, loss of interest or pleasure, feelings of guilt or low self-worth, disturbed sleep or appetite, low energy, and poor concentration. Many factors have been associated with depression. One biological factor given increasing consideration is inadequate nutrition. Women are particularly vulnerable to the adverse effects of poor nutrition on mood because pregnancy and lactation increase nutrient requirements. Depletion of nutrient reserves throughout pregnancy and a lack of recovery postpartum may increase a woman's risk for maternal depression.[102] Deficiencies in nutrients such as folate, vitamin B_6, vitamin B_{12}, vitamin D, calcium, iron, zinc, and omega-3 fatty acids may contribute to postpartum depression.[102,103]

Breastfeeding

The DRIs for lactation are similar to the dietary recommendations for pregnancy for macronutrients and most micronutrients. Nutrients required in greater amounts during lactation compared to pregnant women are: vitamin A (1300 μg/day), vitamin C (120 mg/day), riboflavin (1.6 mg/day), vitamin B_6 (2.0 mg/day), vitamin B_{12} (2.6 μg/day), choline (550 mg/day), copper (1300 mg/day), iodine (290 μg/day), selenium (70 μg/day), zinc (12 mg/day), and potassium (5100 mg/day).

Breastfeeding should always be promoted.[104] Breastfeeding provides multiple benefits to the infant and mother. Benefits for the infant include optimal nutrition, enhanced immune system, protection against allergies and intolerances, promotion of correct development of the jaw and teeth, and reduced risk for chronic disease. Advantages of breastfeeding for the mother include increased energy expenditure, which may lead to faster return to prepregnancy weight, and decreased risk for chronic diseases, such as type 2 diabetes, and postpartum depression.[105] The longer a woman breastfeeds, the lower the risk of metabolic syndrome. Lactation may also have persistent favorable effects on women's cardiometabolic health.[105]

Lifestyle Interventions

Lifestyle interventions aimed at the prevention of overweight and chronic disease in the perinatal and postpartum periods are important to prolong a state of optimal health. Nutrition education plays an important role in the modification of eating habits. For women with GDM, dietary modifications, including lowering fat and carbohydrate intake, in combination with physical activity, can reduce the risk of developing GDM in subsequent pregnancies.[106]

Case Study

Nutrition Assessment of Pregnant Adolescent

Patient history: A 17-year-old female with history of irregular periods who has gained 20 pounds in the last 6 months. She also has noticed having heavy acne and sprouting hair on her chest and face. She reports fatigue, depression, and alopecia. The pediatrician has diagnosed her as having PCOS. She is a senior in high school and does not participate in gym classes. She usually does homework after school or is on the Internet or watches TV during the evening.

Family history: Mother has type 2 diabetes.

Food/nutrition-related history: Skips breakfast and occasionally eats lunch at the school cafeteria, but mostly eats a hamburger, French fries, and a soda at the fast-food restaurant located two blocks from the school. Dinner is usually a large meal consisting of a meat, starch, and salad. Her average fiber intake is 16 g/day, and sodium intake is 4000 mg/day.

Anthropometric Measurements

Weight: 190 pounds (86.2 kg)

Height: 64 in (1.63 m)

BMI: 32.5 kg/m^2

Estimated energy needs: Mifflin-St. Jeor's method BMR = 10 × weight (kg) + 6.25 × height (cm) − 5 × age (years) − 161

Estimated protein needs: 15–30% of total calories

Laboratory data: (normal values in parentheses)

Fasting insulin: 29 mIU/mL (1.8–24.6 mU/L)
Total testosterone: 58 ng/dL (20 ng/dL)
Luteinizing hormone (LH)/follicle stimulating hormone (FSH) ratio: 3.5:1 ↑ (1:1)
Prolactin, thyroid stimulating hormone (TSH), and liver function test: Normal
Total cholesterol: 230 mg/dL (< 170 mg/dL)
LDL cholesterol: 150 mg/dL (< 110 mg/dL)
HDL cholesterol: 33 mg/dL (≥ 35 mg/dL)
Fasting glucose: 120 mg/dL (59–96 mg/dL)

Nutrition Diagnoses

1. Inappropriate eating choices related to (RT) lack of variety of foods and consumption of large meals
2. Excessive caloric intake from fat RT frequent consumption of high-fat foods
3. Excessive caloric intake from high glycemic index carbohydrates RT frequent consumption of carbonated and sweetened beverages
4. Consumption of lower fiber and high sodium intake as evidenced by consumption of lower than recommended fiber intake and consumption of higher than recommended sodium intake
5. Inadequate meal pattern RT skipping breakfast
6. Continuous risk of weight gain RT lack of physical activity

Nutrition Interventions

Planning

1. Teach the basis of healthy eating including the following topics: importance of eating a variety of foods, meal planning, portion size, low-fat cooking methods, and food record keeping.

2. Plan consumption of three meals and three snacks a day to reduce body weight and improve hormone, lipid, and glucose profile.
3. Plan the following daily macronutrient distribution:
   - *Protein:* 15–30% of total calories (e.g., lean meats, egg substitute, low-fat dairy products, legumes, nuts, soy products like tofu, soymilk, and soynuts)
   - *Carbohydrates:* 35–40% calories from low GI carbohydrates (e.g., whole grain cereals, legumes)
   - *Fat:* 35–45% of total daily calories, including sources of:

     Polyunsaturated fats (PUFAs): Corn, soybean, safflower, and cottonseed oils

     Monounsaturated fats (MUFAs): Olive oil, canola oil, peanuts, avocados, and olives

     Omega-3 fatty acids: Fatty types of fish, flaxseed, canola and olive oils, nuts

     Saturated fat: No more than 5% total calories from saturated fat

     Trans fats: Avoid consumption (e.g., fast foods, partially hydrogenated vegetable oil, commercial baked goods, chips, crackers, vegetable shortening)
   - *Fiber:* 25 g of insoluble fiber (e.g., wheat bran, whole grains, cabbage, carrots) and soluble fiber (e.g., oat bran, oatmeal, beans, peas, citrus fruits, vegetables), increasing fiber intake gradually and adding 8 cups of water per day
4. Plan to address the following micronutrients:
   - *Sodium:* Reduce sodium intake to 2300 mg/day (e.g., avoid canned soups, baked goods, soy sauce, seasoned salts, processed foods, monosodium glutamate [MSG])
   - *Magnesium:* Include dietary sources of magnesium (e.g., whole grains, legumes, vegetables, seeds and nuts, dairy products, meats)
   - *Vitamin D:* Include dietary sources of vitamin D (e.g., salmon, tuna fish, orange juice, fortified dairy products)
5. Recommend moderate to vigorous physical activity for 60–90 minutes daily. Initiate with 10 minutes, adding gradual increments of 5–10 minutes per day.

Implementation

1. Comprehensive nutrition education:
   - Instruct on healthy eating practices, including variety and low-fat cooking methods.
   - Review cooking methods conducive to healthy meals.
   - Review portion size.
   - Review how to read food labels.
   - Instruct on meal planning to include three meals and three snacks, emphasizing the importance of eating breakfast.
   - Include low-GI and high-calcium foods.
   - Instruct on avoidance of high-GI carbohydrates, sweetened beverages, unhealthy fats, and salty products.
   - Instruct on reducing fat, salt, and sodium when eating out.
   - Provide patient education related to lifestyle modification.
   - Provide patient education related to diabetes prevention.
2. Nutritional supplements:
   - Offer a chromium picolinate and biotin supplement as adjunctive therapy to improve glucose control and lipid profile.

Nutrition Monitoring and Evaluation

- Evaluate meal patterns of three meals and three snacks a day and its effect on weight loss goals (nutrition-related behavioral and environmental outcomes and nutrition-related patient/client-centered outcome).
- Assess intake of low-GI carbohydrates, fiber, protein, fat, sodium, and magnesium at follow-up clinic visits (food and nutrient intake outcomes).

Questions for the Reader

1. What is the patient's estimated energy needs based on her initial assessment?
2. What is the patient's estimated carbohydrate intake based on her initial assessment?
3. What is the purpose of including low-GI carbohydrates?
4. Why is it important to distribute total calories in three meals and three snacks throughout the day?
5. Write three possible Problem, Etiology, Signs/Symptoms (PES) statements.
6. What will you do during the follow-up visit 2 months later:
   a. If the patient has not lost any weight?
   b. If the patient has not changed her eating habits?
   c. If the patient has not engaged in physical activity?
   d. If the fasting glucose level continues to be elevated?
   e. If the total-cholesterol and LDL-cholesterol levels continue to be elevated?

REFERENCES

1. MacDorman MF, Mathews TJ. Recent trends in infant mortality in the United States. *NCHS Data Brief.* 2008;9:1–8. Available at: http://www.cdc.gov/nchs/data/databriefs/db09.pdf. Accessed January 26, 2010.
2. Centers for Disease Control and Prevention. *Proceedings of the Preconception Health and Health Care Clinical, Public Health, and Consumer Workgroup Meetings.* Atlanta, GA: CDC; 2006.
3. Finer LB, Henshaw SK. Disparities in rates of unintended pregnancy in the United States, 1994–2001. *Perspect Sex Reprod Health.* 2006;38(2):90–96.
4. Lu MC, Kotelchuck M, Culhane JF, et al. Preconception care between pregnancies: the content of internatal care. *Matern Child Health J.* 2006;10:S107–S122.
5. CDC/ATATSDR Preconception Care Work Group and the Select Panel on Preconception Care, Recommendations to improve preconception health and health care—United States. *MMWR.* 2006;55(RR-6). Available at: http://www.cdc.gov/mmwr/pdf/rr/rr5506.pdf. Accessed June 18, 2011.
6. American Academy of Pediatrics, American College of Obstetricians and Gynecologists. *Guidelines for Perinatal Care.* 6th ed. Elk Grove, IL: American Academy of Pediatrics; 2007.
7. American College of Obstetricians and Gynecologists. ACOG Committee opinion no. 313. The importance of preconception care in the continuum of women's health care. *Obstet Gynecol.* 2005;106(3):665–666.
8. Kitzmiller JL, Block JM, Brown FM, et al. Managing preexisting diabetes for pregnancy: summary of evidence and consensus recommendations for care. *Diabetes Care.* 2008;31(5):1060–1079.
9. American Diabetes Association. Preconception care of women with diabetes. *Diabetes Care.* 2004;27(Suppl 1):S76–S78.
10. American Diabetes Association. Standards of medical care in diabetes—2010. *Diabetes Care.* 2010;33(Suppl 1):S11–S61.
11. American Dietetic Association. Diabetes 1 and 2 evidence analysis project. Evidence Analysis Library. Available at: http://www.adaevidencelibrary.com. Accessed December 18, 2009.
12. American Diabetes Association. Nutrition recommendations and interventions for diabetes. *Diabetes Care.* 2008;31(Suppl 1): S61–S78.
13. National Heart, Lung and Blood Institute. *Clinical Guidelines on the Identification, Evaluation and Treatment of Overweight and Obesity in Adults: Evidence Report.* Washington, DC: National Heart, Lung and Blood Institute. NIH Publication. No. 98-4083; 1998.
14. National Heart, Lung and Blood Institute. *The Practical Guide. Identification, Evaluation, and Treatment of Overweight and Obesity in Adults.* Washington, DC: National Institutes of Health. NIH Publication No. 00-4084; 2000.
15. Galtier F, Raingeard I, Renard E, et al. Optimizing the outcome of pregnancy in obese women: from pregestational to long-term management. *Diabetes Metab.* 2008;34:19–25.
16. Zhong Y, Cahill AG, Macones GA, et al. The association between prepregnancy maternal body mass index and preterm delivery. *Am J Perinatol.* 2009. Available at: DOI 10.1055/s-0029-1241736. Accessed December 20, 2009.
17. Walters MR, Smith Taylor J. Maternal obesity: consequences and prevention strategies. *Nurs Womens Health.* 2009;13(6): 487–495.
18. Rasmussen KM, Catalano PM, Yaktine AL. New guidelines for weight gain during pregnancy: what obstetrician/gynecologists should know. *Curr Op Obstet Gynecol.* 2009;21:521–526.
19. Roberts JM, Pearson G, Cutler J, Lindheimer M. Summary of the NHLBI working group on research on hypertension during pregnancy. *Hypertens.* 2003;41:437–445.
20. National Heart, Lung and Blood Institute. *The Seventh Report of the Joint National Committee on Prevention, Detection, Evaluation, and Treatment of High Blood Pressure.* Washington, DC: NHLBI; 2004.
21. Alton I. Nutrition-related special concerns of adolescent pregnancy. In: Story M, Stang J, eds. *Nutrition and the Pregnant Adolescent: A Practical Reference Guide.* Minneapolis, MN: Center for Leadership, Education and Training in Maternal and Child Nutrition. University of Minnesota; 2000:89–112.
22. American Dietetic Association. Hypertension evidence analysis project. Evidence Analysis Library. Available at: http://www.adaevidencelibrary.com. Accessed December 21, 2009.
23. Sacks FM, Svetkey LP, Vollmer WM, et al. Effects on blood pressure of reduced dietary sodium and the Dietary Approaches to Stop Hypertension (DASH) diet. *N Engl J Med.* 2001;344:3–10.
24. Appel LJ, Moore TJ, Obarzanek E, et al. A clinical trial of the effects of dietary patterns on blood pressure. *N Engl J Med.* 1997;336(16):1117–1124.
25. Glueck CJ, Pranikoff J, Aregawi D, Wang P. Prevention of gestational diabetes by metformin plus diet in patients with polycystic ovary syndrome. *Fertil Steri.* 2008;89(3):625–634.
26. Jeanes YM, Barr S, Smith K, Hart KH. Dietary management of women with polycystic ovary syndrome in the United Kingdom: the role of dietitians. *J Hum Nutr Diet.* 2009;22:551–558.
27. Moran LJ, Brinkworth GD, Norman RJ. Dietary therapy in polycystic ovary syndrome. *Semin Reprod Med.* 2008;26(1):85–92.
28. Franks S, Robinson S, Willis DS. Nutrition, insulin and polycystic syndrome. *J Reprod Fertil.* 1996;1:47–53.
29. American Dietetic Association. Case problem: dietary recommendations to combat obesity, insulin resistance, and other concerns related to polycystic ovary syndrome. *J Am Diet Assoc.* 2000;100(8):955–960.
30. Marsh K, Brand-Miller J. The optimal diet for women with polycystic ovary syndrome. *Br J Nutr.* 2005;94:154–165.
31. Charvarro JE, Rich-Edwards JW, Rosner BA, Willett WC. Dietary fatty acid intakes and the risk of ovulatory infertility. *Am J Clin Nutr.* 2007;85:231–237.
32. Panidis D, Farmakiotis D, Rousso D, et al. Obesity, weight loss, and the polycystic ovary syndrome: effect of treatment with diet and orlistat for 24 weeks on insulin resistance and androgen levels. *Am Soc Reprod Med.* 2008;89(4):899–906.
33. Centers for Disease Control and Prevention. Alcohol use among pregnant and nonpregnant women of childbearing age—United States, 1991–2005. *MMWR.* 2009;58(19):529–532.
34. Floyd RL, Jack BW, Cefalo R, et al. The clinical content of preconception care: alcohol, tobacco, and illicit drug exposure. *Am J Obstet Gynecol.* 2008;199(6 Suppl 2):S333–S339.
35. Office of the Surgeon General. U.S. Surgeon General releases advisory on alcohol use in pregnancy. News release. February 2005. Available at: http://surgeongeneral.gov/pressreleases/sg/02222005.html. Accessed March 13, 2010.

36. Gardiner PM, Nelson L, Shellhass CS, et al. The clinical content of preconception care: nutrition and dietary supplements. *Am J Obstet Gynecol.* 2008;199(6 Suppl 2):S345–S356.
37. Rouse B, Azen C. Effect of high maternal blood phenylalanine on offspring congenital anomalies and developmental outcome at ages 4 and 6 years: the importance of strict dietary control preconception and throughout pregnancy. *J Pediatr.* 2004;144: 235–239.
38. Matalon KM, Acosta PB, Azen C. Role of nutrition in pregnancy with phenylketonuria and birth defects. *Pediatrics.* 2003;112(6):1534–1536.
39. Centers for Disease Control and Prevention. Smoking prevalence among women of reproductive age—United States, 2006. *MMWR.* 2008;57(31):849–852.
40. Kaiser LL, Allen L. Position of the American Dietetic Association: nutrition and lifestyle for healthy pregnancy outcome. *J Am Diet Assoc.* 2002;102:1479–1490.
41. Institute of Medicine. Weight gain during pregnancy: reexamining the guidelines. Available at: http://www.nap.edu/openbook.php?record_id=12584&page=254. Accessed December 1, 2009.
42. Institute of Medicine. *Weight Gain During Pregnancy: Reexamining the Guidelines.* Report brief. Washington, DC: The National Academies Press; 2009.
43. Krummel DA. Postpartum weight control. *J Am Diet Assoc.* 2007;107:37–40.
44. Chu SY, Callaghan WM, Kim C, et al. Maternal obesity and risk of gestational diabetes mellitus. *Diabetes Care.* 2007;30:2070–2076.
45. Baeten JM, Bukusi EA, Lambe M. Pregnancy complications and outcomes among overweight and obese nulliparous women. *Am J Public Health.* 2001;91:436–440.
46. Glazar NL, Hendrickson AF, Schellenbaum GD, Mueller BA. Weight change and the risk of gestational diabetes in obese women. *Epidemiol.* 2004;15:733–737.
47. Pirkola J, Puta A, Bloigu A, et al. Prepregnancy overweight and gestational diabetes as determinants of subsequent diabetes and hypertension after 20 years follow-up. *J Clin Endocrinol Metab.* 2009;94:2464–2470.
48. Doherty DA, Magann EF, Francis J, et al. Prepregnancy body mass index and pregnancy outcomes. *Int J Gynaecol Obstet.* 2006;95:242–247.
49. Driul L, Cacciaguerra G, Citossi A, et al. Prepregnancy body mass index and adverse pregnancy outcomes. *Arch Gynecol Obstet.* 2008;278:23–26.
50. Cnattingius S, Bergstrom R, Lipworth L, Kramer MS. Prepregnancy weight and the risk of adverse pregnancy outcomes. *N Engl J Med.* 1998;338:147–152.
51. Edwards LE, Dickes WF, Alton IR, Hakanson EY. Pregnancy in the massively obese: course, outcome, and obesity prognosis of the infant. *Am J Obstet Gynecol.* 1978;131:479–483.
52. Position of the American Dietetic Association and American Society for Nutrition: obesity, reproduction, and pregnancy outcomes. *J Am Diet Assoc.* 2009;109:918–927.
53. Ellings JM, Newman RB, Hulsey TC, et al. Reduction in very low birth weight deliveries and perinatal mortality in a specialized, multidisciplinary twin clinic. *Obstet Gynecol.* 1993;81:387–391.
54. Gardner MO, Goldenberg RL, Cliver SP, et al. The origin and outcome of preterm twin pregnancies. *Obstet Gynecol.* 1995;85: 553–557.
55. Albrecht JL, Tomich PG. The maternal and neonatal outcome of triplet gestations. *Am J Obstet Gynecol.* 1996;174:1551–1556.
56. Peaceman AM, Dooley SL, Tamura RK. Antepartum management of triplet gestations. *Am J Obstet Gynecol.* 1992;167:1117–1120.
57. Luke B, Brown MB. Maternal morbidity and infant death in twin vs triplet and quadruplet pregnancies. *Am J Obstet Gynecol.* 2008;198:401.e1–e10.
58. Kolasa KM, Weismiller DG. Nutrition during pregnancy. *Am Fam Physician.* 1997;56:205–212.
59. Chan RL, Olshan AF, Savitz DA, et al. Maternal influences on nausea and vomiting in early pregnancy. *Matern Child Health J.* 2009.
60. O'Brien B, Naber S. Nausea and vomiting during pregnancy: Effects on the quality of women's lives. *Birth.* 1992;19:138–143.
61. Chandra K, Magee L, Einarson A, Koren G. Nausea and vomiting in pregnancy: results of a survey that identified interventions used by women to alleviate their symptoms. *J Psychosom Obstet Gynaecol.* 2003;24:71–75.
62. Nelson-Piercy C. Treatment of nausea and vomiting in pregnancy: When should it be treated and what can be safely taken. *Drug Safety.* 1998;19(2):155–164.
63. American College of Obstetrics and Gynecology practice bulletin. Nausea and vomiting of pregnancy. *Obstet Gynecol.* 2004;103:803–814.
64. Feizo MS, Poursharif B, Korst LM, et al. Symptoms and pregnancy outcomes associated with extreme weight loss among women with hyperemesis gravidarum. *J Womens Health (Larchmt).* 2009;18(12):1981–1987.
65. Erick M. Ptyalism gravidarum: an unpleasant reality [letter to the editors]. *J Am Diet Assoc.* 1998;98:129.
66. Dowswell T, Neilson JP. Interventions for heartburn in pregnancy. Cochrane Database Syst Rev. 2008 Oct 8;(4):CD007065.
67. Institute of Medicine. *Dietary Reference Intakes for Energy, Carbohydrates, Fiber, Fat, Fatty Acids, Cholesterol, Protein and Amino Acids (Macronutrients).* Washington, DC: National Academies Press; 2002.
68. Micali N, Treasure J, Simonoff E. Eating disorders symptoms in pregnancy: a longitudinal study of women with recent and past eating disorders and obesity. *J Psychosom Res.* 2007;63:297–303
69. American College of Obstetricians and Gynecologists Committee. Opinion no. 267: exercise during pregnancy and the postpartum period. *Obstet Gynecol.* 2002;99:171–173.
70. Godfrey KM, Barker DJ. Fetal nutrition and adult disease. *Am J Clin Nutr.* 2000;71(5 Suppl):1344S–1352S.
71. Godfrey KM, Barker DJ. Fetal programming and adult health. *Public Health Nutr.* 2001;4(2B):611–624.
72. Institute of Medicine, National Academy of Sciences. *Dietary Reference Intakes for Energy, Carbohydrate, Fiber, Fat, Fatty Acids, Cholesterol and Amino Acids.* Washington, DC: National Academies Press; 2005.
73. Foster-Powell K, Holt SH, Brand-Miller JC. International table of glycemic index and glycemic load values. *Am J Clin Nutr.* 2002;76:55–56.
74. Position of the American Dietetic Association: use of nutritive and nonnutritive sweeteners. *J Am Diet Assoc.* 2004;104:255–275.
75. Sloan NL, Lederman SA, Leighton J, et al. The effect of prenatal dietary protein intake on birth weight. *Nutr Res.* 2001;21:129–139.
76. Allen LH. Multiple micronutrients in pregnancy and lactation. *Am J Clin Nutr.* 2005;81:1206S–1212S.

77. Linus Pauling Institute Micronutrient Information Center. Magnesium. Available at: http://lpi.oregonstate.edu/infocenter. Accessed December 28, 2009.
78. Institute of Medicine. *Nutrition During Pregnancy. Weight Gain and Nutrient Supplements.* Washington, DC: National Academies Press; 1990.
79. Institute of Medicine. *Dietary Reference Intakes for Thiamin, Riboflavin, Niacin, Vitamin B_6, Folate, Vitamin B_{12}, Pantothenic Acid, Biotin, and Choline.* Washington, DC: National Academies Press; 2000.
80. Hadar E, Oats J, Hod M. Towards new diagnostic criteria for diagnosing GDM: the HAPO study. *Perinat Med.* 2009;37(5):447–9.
81. Position of the American Diabetes Association: gestational diabetes mellitus. *Diabetes Care.* 2004;27:S88–S90.
82. American College of Obstetricians and Gynecologists. Gestational diabetes. ACOG Practice Bulletin No. 30. *Obstet Gynecol.* 2001;98:525–538.
83. Casey BM, Lucas MJ, McIntire DD, Leveno KJ. Pregnancy outcomes in women with gestational diabetes compared with the general obstetric population. *Obstet Gynecol.* 1997;90:869–873.
84. Franz MJ, Bantle JP, Beebe CA, et al. Evidence-based nutrition principles and recommendations for the treatment and prevention of diabetes and related complications [technical review]. *Diabetes Care.* 2002;25:148–198.
85. Garcia-Patterson A, Corcoy R, Balsells M, et al. In pregnancies with gestational diabetes mellitus and intensive therapy, perinatal outcome is worse in small-for-gestational-age newborns. *Am J Obstet Gynecol.* 1998;179:481–485.
86. Thomas AM, Gutierrez YM. *American Dietetic Association Guide to Gestational Diabetes Mellitus.* Chicago IL: American Dietetic Association; 2005.
87. Peterson CH, Jovanovic-Peterson L. Percentage of carbohydrate and glycemic response to breakfast, lunch and dinner in women with gestational diabetes. *Diabetes.* 1991;40:S172–S174.
88. American Dietetic Association. Evidence analysis library. Gestational diabetes. Available at: http://www.adaevidencelibrary.com/topic.cfm?cat=1399. Accessed December 17, 2009.
89. Cedergren MI. Maternal morbid obesity and the pregnancy outcome. *Obstet Gynecol.* 2004;103:219–224.
90. Brantsæter AL, Haugen M, Samuelsen SO, et al. A dietary pattern characterized by high intake of vegetables, fruits, and vegetable oils is associated with reduced risk of preeclampsia in nulliparous pregnant Norwegian women. *J Nutr.* 2009 June; 139: 1162–1168.
91. Kametras NA, McAuliffe F, Krampl E, et al. Maternal cardiac function in twin pregnancy. *Obstet Gynecol.* 2003;102:806–815.
92. Sibai BM, Lindheimer M, Hauth J, et al. Risk factors for pre-eclampsia, abruption placentae and adverse neonatal outcomes among women with chronic hypertension. *N Eng J Med.* 1998;339:667–671.
93. Churchill D, Perry IJ, Beevers DG. Ambulatory blood pressure in pregnancy and fetal growth. *Lancet.* 1997;349:7–10.
94. Nijdam ME, Timmerman MR, Franx A, et al. Cardiovascular risk factor assessment after pre-eclampsia in primary care. *BMC Fam Pract.* 2009;8(10):77.
95. Chan HM, Egeland GM. Fish consumption, mercury exposure and heart disease. *Nutrition Reviews.* 2004;62:68–72.
96. Dey PM, Gochfeld M, Reuhl KR. Developmental methylmercury administration alters cerebellar PSA-NCAM expression and Golgi sialytransferase activity. *Brain Res.* 1999;845:139–151.
97. Environmental Protection Agency. Fish advisories. What you need to know about mercury in fish and shellfish. Available at: http://www.epa.gov/fishadvisories/advice. Accessed December 13, 2009.
98. Evans E. The FDA recommendations on fish intake during pregnancy. *J Obstet Gynecol Neonat Nurs.* 2002;31:541–546.
99. Food and Drug Administration. Foodborne pathogenic microorganisms and natural toxins handbook. *Listeria monocytogenes.* Available at: http://www.fda.gov/Food/FoodSafety/FoodborneIllness/default.htm. Accessed December 17, 2009.
100. Lungu B, Ricke SC, Johnson MG. Growth, survival, proliferation and pathogenesis of *Listeria monocytogenes* under low oxygen or anaerobic conditions: a review. *Anaerobe.* 2009;15:7–17.
101. Posfay-Barbe KM, Wald ER. Listeriosis. *Semin Fetal Neonatal Med.* 2009;14:228–233.
102. Leung BM, Kaplan BJ. Perinatal depression: prevalence, risks, and the nutrition link—a review of the literature. *J Am Diet Assoc.* 2009;109(9):1566–1575.
103. Logan AC. Omega-3 fatty acids and major depression: a primer for the mental health professional. *Lipids Health Dis.* 2004;3:25.
104. James DC, Lessen R. Position of the American Dietetic Association: promoting and supporting breastfeeding. *J Am Diet Assoc.* 2009;109:1926–1942.
105. Gunderson EP, Jacobs DR, Chiang V, et al. Duration of lactation and incidence of the metabolic syndrome in women of reproductive age according to gestational diabetes mellitus status: a 20-year prospective study in CARDIA—The Coronary Artery Risk Development in Young Adults Study. *Diabetes.* 2010;59(2):495–504.
106. Moses RG, Shand JL, Tapsell LC. The recurrence of gestational diabetes: could dietary differences in fat intake be an explanation? *Diabetes Care.* 1977;20:1647–1650.

CHAPTER 2

Physical Growth

Wm. Cameron Chumlea and Michael LaMonte

What Is Growth?

Physical growth is the increase in the mass of body tissues that occurs in genetically determined rates, patterns, and ages as a healthy infant grows into an adult. Good nutrition and exercise are necessary for optimal growth and maturation, and most normal, healthy children grow and mature with few, if any, problems. However, the obesity epidemic affects and is interrelated with the growth and maturation of children and has potential consequences for both the current and future health of affected children.[1,2]

Measurement of Growth

Accurate and reliable measures of body size present a broad description of a child's growth status. The most useful measures are recumbent length from birth to 3 years of age, stature after age 3 years, head circumference from birth to age 3 years (see **Figure 2-1**, **Figure 2-2**, and **Figure 2-3**, respectively), and weight at every age.[3] Descriptions and protocols for these measurements are available in video formats from the Centers for Disease Control and Prevention (CDC)/National Center for Health Statistics (NCHS)[4,5] (http://www.cdc.gov/growthcharts) and the World Health Organization (WHO)[6] (http://www.who.int/childgrowth/training/en). These media demonstrate standardized measurement techniques similar to those in the *Anthropometric Standardization Reference Manual*.[3]

Whereas recumbent length and stature describe linear growth, weight is a measure of the mass of all body tissues. Weight indexed for stature can describe levels of overweight or obesity, but this measure of adiposity is most accurate when applied to groups rather than individuals. The body mass index (BMI) is the most common stature-standardized weight indicator of overweight or obesity in children.[7] BMI is computed as weight divided by stature squared, with all measures in the metric system ($kg/m^2 \times 10{,}000$). Additional measures related to body fatness are limb and trunk circumferences and skinfold thicknesses. Midarm circumference is an index of the underlying fat and muscle tissue; abdominal circumference is an indicator of abdominal fatness;[8] and skinfolds are a measure of subcutaneous adipose tissue thickness. Two common skinfold sites are the triceps on the back of the arm over the triceps muscle and the subscapular just below the scapula. Large values for BMI, midarm and abdominal circumferences, and triceps and subscapular skinfolds are positively correlated with total and percent body fat in children.[9,10]

It is important to assess a child's level of fatness, because obesity is the most prevalent health problem of childhood. Today, a big child, one who exceeds expected stature and weight standards for a given age, is likely overweight or obese rather than just healthy. It is also important to measure bone mineral content and bone mineral density in children in order to identify those with low levels (due to low calcium and protein intakes) who are at risk for osteopenia and osteoporosis in adulthood.[11,12] Measuring a child's body composition can identify risk factors for some chronic adult diseases at an early point in time when treatment may be most effective.

Periods and Patterns of Growth

A child's growth pattern can be divided into four periods: infancy from birth to 2 years of age; the preschool years, from about 3 to 6 years of age; the middle childhood years, from about 7 to 10 years of age; and adolescence, from about 11 to 18 years of age. A child's growth and size are related to his or her level of maturity and also reflect his or her genetic potential. At the same age, early-maturing children are taller and heavier than late-maturing children, and tall parents tend to have tall children and short parents tend to have short children. Weight has a strong genetic component that explains familial aspects of obesity, but epigenetic and environmental factors also affect the development of obesity.

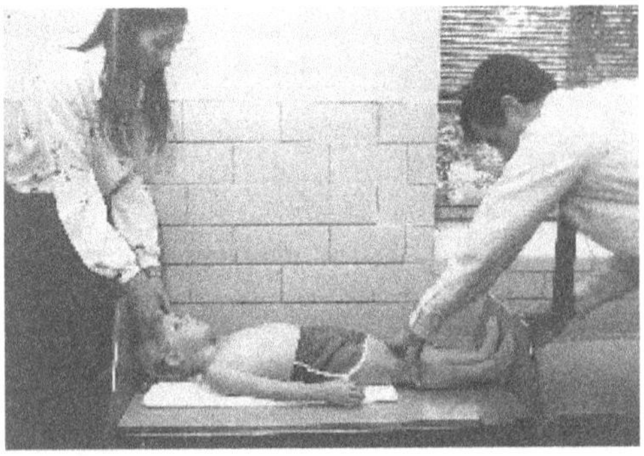

FIGURE 2-1 Measurement of Recumbent Length

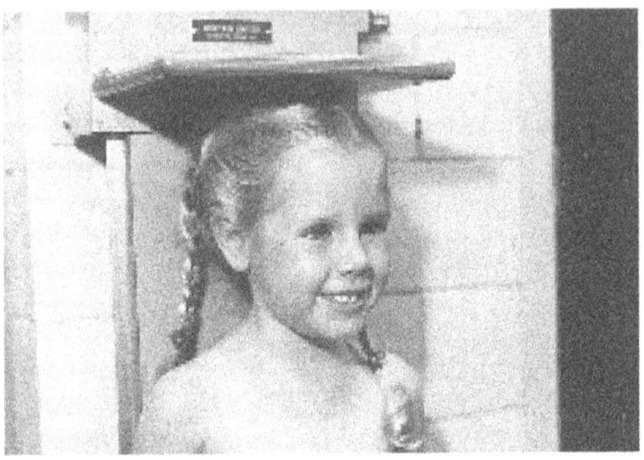

FIGURE 2-2 Measurement of Stature

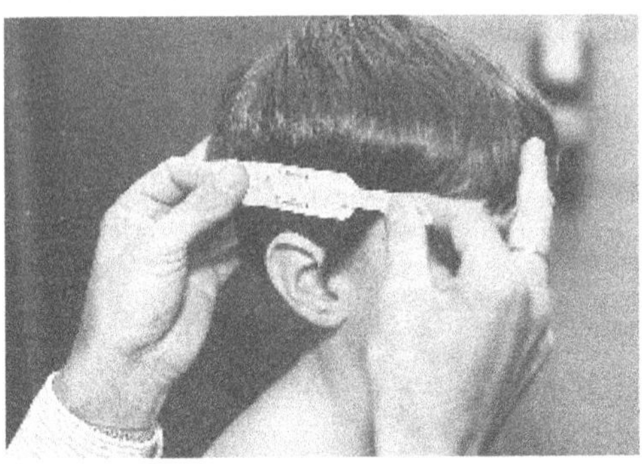

FIGURE 2-3 Measurement of Head Circumference

Infancy

Infancy is distinguished by a very rapid growth period. Body size and dimensions increase faster than at any other time in postnatal life. Many healthy infants lose weight shortly after birth, but regain their birth weight after about a week.[13] Most normal infants double their birth weight by about 5 months and triple it by 1 year of age. During the first year of life, weight, on average, increases 200%, body length 55%, and head circumference 40%. Similar changes occur in the trunk, arms, and legs. Between 1 and 2 years of age, the average infant grows about 12 cm (4.7 inches) in length and gains about 2.5 kg (5.5 pounds) in weight.

An infant's head is disproportionately large compared with the dimensions of other body parts. At birth, its diameter exceeds that of the chest, and its length is about a quarter of the body's total length. Head circumference increases from an average of about 35–36 cm at birth to an average of about 45–46 cm at 1 year of age. Measures of head circumference reflect brain growth, and the brain doubles its birth weight by 1 year of age.

Preschoolers

During the preschool years, the rate of growth slows, and it stabilizes by about 4 to 5 years of age. At 4 years of age, the average increase in stature and weight is about 6–8 cm (2.4-3.1 inches) and about 2–4 kg (4.4–8.8 pounds), respectively, per year. Head circumference remains an important measure during the preschool years because the brain more than triples its birth weight by 6 years of age. Sex differences in size and weight during the preschool years are slight, but the pattern of more adipose tissue in girls than boys appears by age 6 years. This is also a critical period for the development of overweight and onset of obesity in boys and girls, and the risk increases for subsequent obesity later in childhood and adulthood.

Middle Childhood

During middle childhood, children grow at a steady rate. The average child at age 7 years grows about 5–6 cm (2–2.4 inches) per year in stature and about 2 kg (4.4 pounds) per year in weight, but the increase in weight is about 4 kg (8.8 pounds) per year by age 10 years. The legs grow at a greater rate than the trunk during middle childhood, so that although the trunk accounts for about 55% of total stature at age 7 years, it accounts for only about 45% by 10 years of age. During this period, the increasing maturity of the average girl causes her to grow more per year in stature and weight than the average boy, which contributes, in part, to the larger size of girls at the start of adolescence. At 7 years of age, boys are, on average, only about 2 cm (0.8 inch) taller than girls, but there is little difference in weight. By 10 years of age, the average girl is 1 cm (0.4 inch) taller, 1 kg (2.2 pounds) heavier, and the thickness of subcutaneous adipose tissue is about 25% greater than that of the average boy.

Adolescence

Adolescence starts before puberty and spans the years until growth and maturation are mostly completed, which is around 16 to 18 years of age in girls and 18 to 20 years of age in boys. A final increase in body size, shape, and weight transforms a child into an adult. Most girls have their pubescent growth spurts between 11 and 14 years of age and, on average, are taller than boys the same age. Boys, on average, enter their pubescent growth spurts about 2 years after girls, so they have an additional 2 years of prepubertal growth. In addition, the pubescent growth spurt lasts for a longer time in boys than girls, and the related amount of growth is larger in boys. The average peak height velocity (i.e., the maximum rate of growth in stature during the growth spurt) ranges in boys about 9.5–10.5 cm (3.7–4.1 inches) per year, whereas in girls the maximum velocity is about 8.5–9.0 cm (3.3–3.5 inches) per year. During adolescence, girls add more body fat than boys, and boys develop more skeletal muscle tissue than girls. These differences result in the sex difference in adult body shape and, to a large extent, the increased physical ability and performance of the average boy.[14]

Assessing Growth Status

Recumbent length, stature, weight, head circumference, and BMI are used to describe a child's growth status. These measures should be collected at regular intervals and plotted on growth charts (see Appendix B).[15] Infants should be assessed about every 3 months for well-baby visits and annually thereafter. Growth charts present an assessment or comparison of the stature or length, weight, head circumference, and BMI of an infant, child, or adolescent with the percentile distribution of other children at the same ages. The CDC/NCHS and the WHO each produce growth charts, both of which are recommended for use with U.S. children.[3,5] Copies of these charts can be downloaded from the CDC (http://www.cdc.gov/growthcharts) and WHO (http://www.who.int/childgrowth) websites.

Plotting a child's growth values on the CDC or WHO growth chart indicates that at this time and for this age the child has a normal value (between the 15th and 85th percentiles), representing 70% of the population, or that additional information is needed to determine the validity of a possibly unusual value (below the 15th or above the 85th percentiles), representing 30% of the population. Additional health information is needed to determine the reason for a child's unusual percentile value location. The WHO charts are also available as z-score charts, where zero represents the mean and a positive or negative z-score is one standard deviation above or below the mean. These charts can be of greater clinical use to healthcare providers than the percentile charts for some children.[3]

BMI Charts

To help address the pediatric obesity epidemic, the CDC and WHO sets of growth charts from 2 to 20 years of age now contain charts to plot a child's BMI (see Appendix B for the CDC charts and http://www.who.int/growthref for the WHO charts), a useful, recommended index of overweight and obesity.[6] The CDC classifies overweight in children as a BMI for age greater than the 95th percentile and obesity as greater than the 97th percentile. The WHO BMI charts are like the CDC charts, but the WHO defines overweight in children as a BMI for age between the 85th and 95th percentiles and obesity as above the 95th percentile.

Case Study

Demonstrating the Use of the CDC Growth Charts

A boy is observed for a regular checkup at 10, 11, and 12 years of age. At each visit, his weight and stature are measured and plotted on the CDC growth chart (see **Figure 2-4**). His weight at 10 years was 37 kg, at 11 was 45 kg, and at 12 years was 54 kg. His stature was 143 cm at 10 years, 150 cm at 11 years, and 156 cm at 12 years. Plotting these values on his growth chart indicates that this boy had a weight at the 75th percentile at 10 years of age, but his weight has progressed to the 90th percentile by 12 years of age. His stature was at the 75th percentile at 10 years of age also, and it has risen slightly above the 75th percentile at 11 and 12 years of age. Based on these data, it is reasonable to assume that this boy, whose weight and stature were within normal values at age 10 years, is possibly entering his adolescent growth spurt early. However, no corresponding increase in stature accompanies his increase in weight, which limits this assumption.

To clarify these data, his BMI was calculated and plotted on the CDC BMI growth chart (see **Figure 2-5**). At age 10 years, his BMI was 18 at the 75th percentile, which would be normal, but by age 12, his BMI had increased to 22 at the 90th percentile. The additional BMI plotted data lend support to the reasonable possibility that this boy has progressed from a normal weight to either a potential overweight category based on the CDC criteria or to an overweight category based on the WHO category. This change from a normal weight to overweight places this boy by 12 years of age at risk for obesity in adolescence and later in adulthood. Dietary intervention along with increased physical activity should be considered as possible treatments after further health information is obtained.

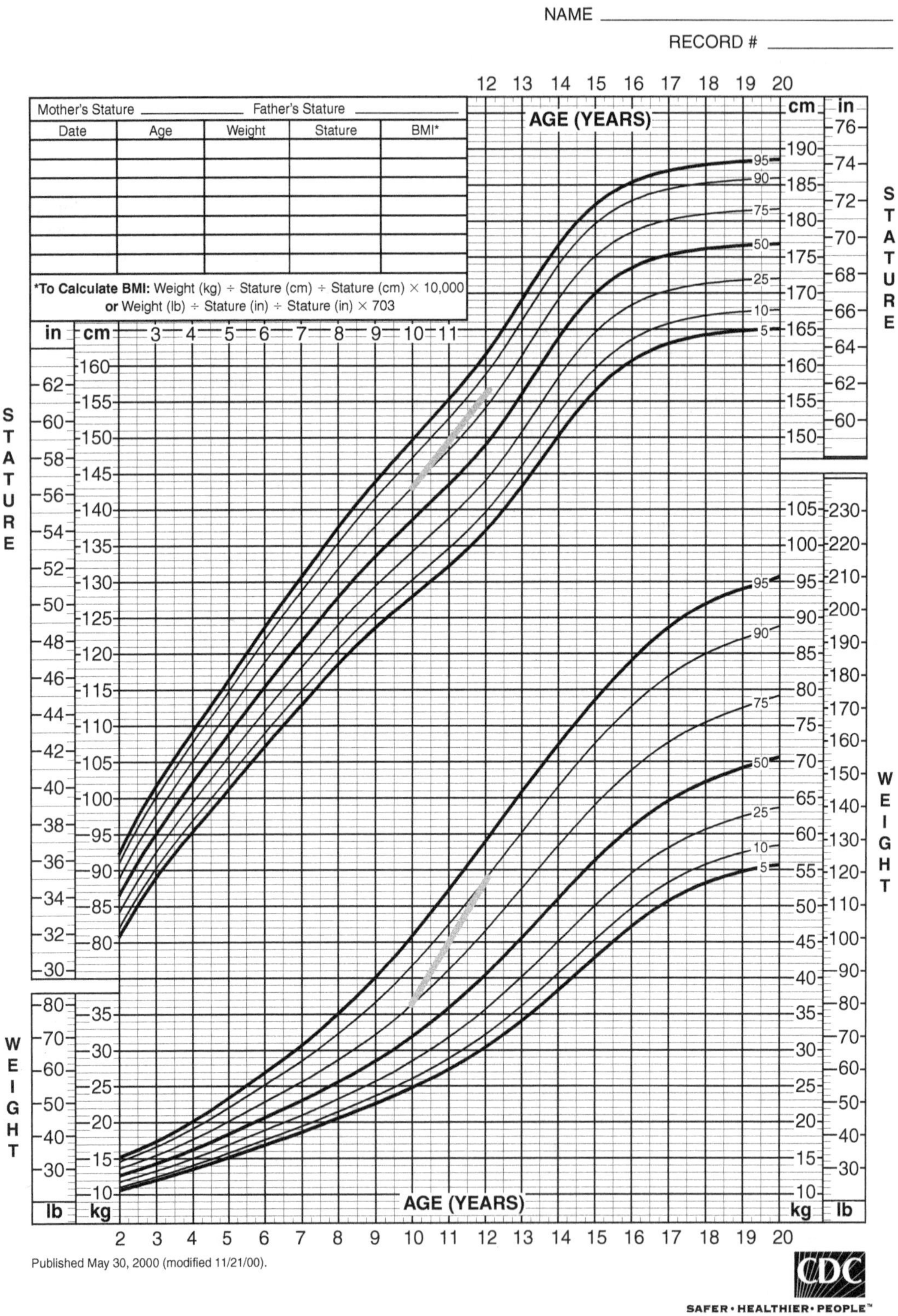

FIGURE 2-4 Plots of Weight and Stature for a Boy at 10, 11, and 12 Years of Age on the CDC Growth Chart

Source: Developed by the National Center for Health Statistics in collaboration with the National Center for Chronic Disease Prevention and Health Promotion (2000). Available at: http://www.cdc.gov/growthcharts.

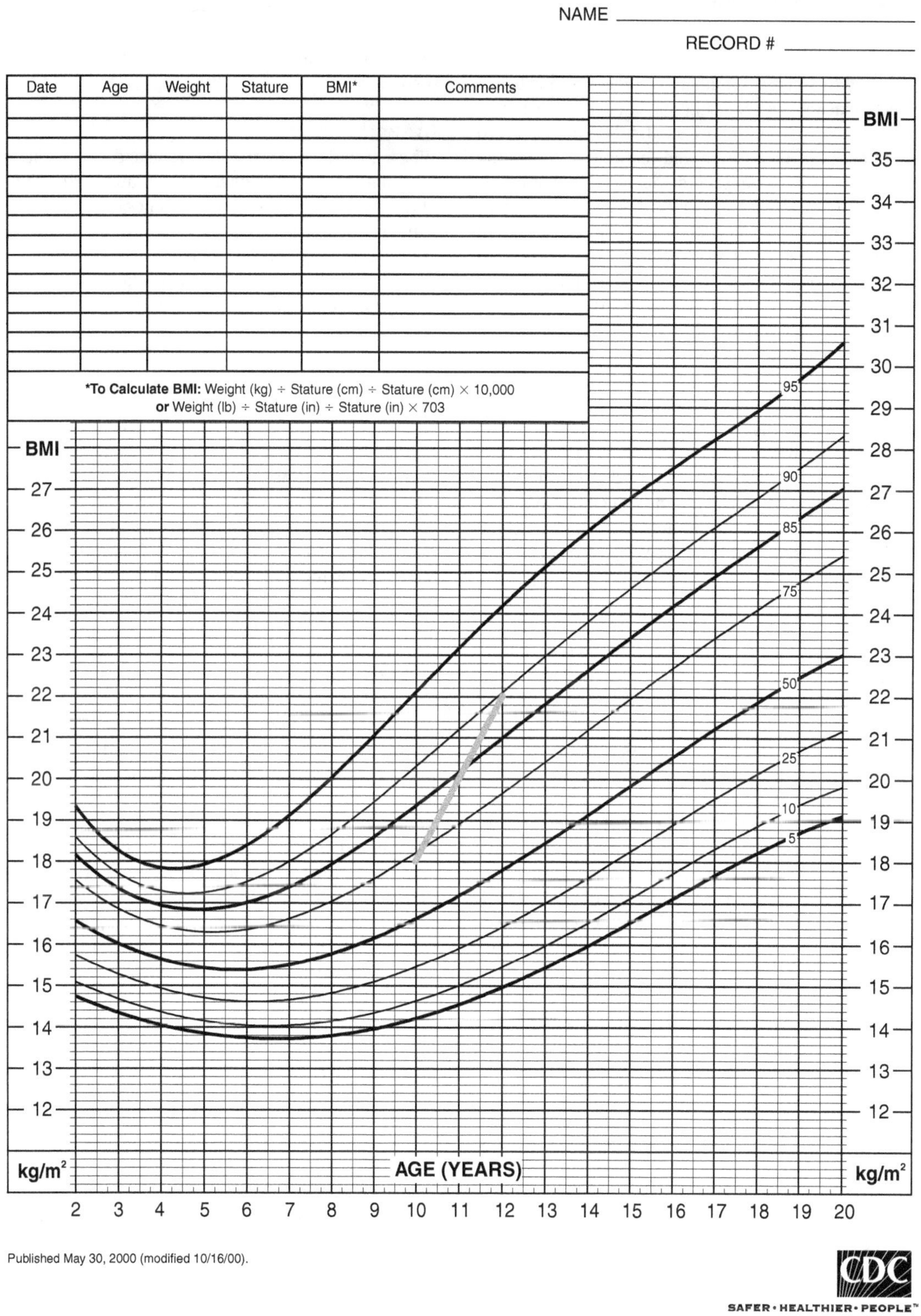

FIGURE 2-5 Plots of BMI for a Boy at 10, 11, and 12 Years of Age on the CDC BMI Growth Chart

Source: Developed by the National Center for Health Statistics in collaboration with the National Center for Chronic Disease Prevention and Health Promotion (2000). Available at: http://www.cdc.gov/growthcharts.

Race/Ethnicity

There are growth and maturational differences among black, white, and Mexican American children, but in most instances these differences, on average, are small.[4,13,16] There are also small differences in the growth and maturation of healthy Chinese American and Japanese American children or American children of other racial or ethnic groups compared with that of the white, black, and Mexican American children represented on the current CDC growth charts, and this is also the case for the WHO growth charts. Similar race/ethnicity differences are reported by clinicians in other countries who also use the CDC and WHO charts. In addition, when a child reaches puberty and progresses through his or her adolescent growth spurt, the individuality of that child creates large percentile differences during these adolescent years compared to earlier positions that usually dissipate with maturity. The percentile position on the growth chart of that infant or child is, in part, a function of the differences in his or her genetic background as compared to that of the children used to construct these growth charts, and these individual disparities occur regardless of the set of growth charts used.

Comparing the CDC and WHO Growth Charts

The 2000 CDC growth charts represent national data from the largest sample of U.S. children ever assembled for this purpose, and they are the best national data of their kind available today. The WHO growth charts reflect the growth of breastfed infants for the first few months of life, and there are well-reported growth differences between breastfed and formula-fed infants and the potential subsequent health effects.[14,15] After infancy, the diet and nutrition of the children represented on the WHO charts, which maybe above average in quality because they were selected from urban middle class families, may be similar to that of the U.S. children on the CDC growth charts. If the mother can successfully breastfeed her infant for a longer period of time (up to 6 months or more), then the WHO charts in most cases provide the best growth reference. Otherwise, it is difficult, on an individual basis, to provide an "ironclad" justification for the use of the CDC over the WHO growth charts for the majority of infants and children in the United States.

Premature Growth

It is important to account for the gestational age of premature infants or those small at birth when plotting their growth on the current CDC/NCHS growth charts.[13] The amount of prematurity is subtracted from an infant's chronologic age (e.g., for an infant with a gestational age of 28 weeks, this is a correction of 12 weeks or 3 months of chronological age). Current growth charts for preterm low-birth-weight infants are discussed in Chapter 4. After about 2.5 years of age, it is frequently no longer necessary to make the adjustment for most healthy children who were premature.

Growth Velocity

When growth is measured at repeated visits, the amount of change in a measurement or the rate of growth per unit of time can be quantified. Increment growth reference data supplement the status growth charts by indicating if a child's rate of growth is normal or unusual. The WHO has developed increment (or rate) charts with percentiles reflecting the tempo of growth for children between 1 and 5 years of age.

Maturation

The central nervous system integrates the activities of the endocrine system, coordinating growth and sexual maturation. Before puberty, the central nervous system inhibits hormone production, but this inhibition decreases near puberty when the sex hormones reach adult concentrations. Endocrine and adrenal androgens influence growth, sexual maturation, and the development of secondary sex characteristics. The reproductive system matures at puberty, making sexual reproduction possible. Puberty is identified in girls by the onset of menstruation or menarche, but there is no similar marker in boys. The ages of individual children at the onset and completion of growth and sexual maturation are highly variable.

The progression of sexual maturation is assessed using Tanner stages as indicators (see Appendix C). Breast buds in girls (Tanner stage B-2) and genital enlargement in boys (Tanner stage G-2) indicate the onset of sexual maturation, which is followed by the appearance of pubic hair (Tanner stage PH-2) in both sexes. For girls, the 25th to 75th percentiles for the age at onset of sexual maturation, Tanner stage B-2, range from 8.5 to 10.5 years in blacks, 8.6 to 11.2 years in Mexican Americans, and 9.5 to 11 years for whites. The 25th to the 75th percentiles for the age at onset of sexual maturation, Tanner stage G-2 for boys, range from 7.5 to 10.9 years in blacks, 8.9 to 11.7 years in Mexican Americans, and 8.6 to 11.4 years whites. The onset of sexual maturation is significantly earlier in black girls and boys than in white and Mexican American girls and boys.[17]

The sequence of Tanner stages between paired indicators is concordant for about 60% of healthy children. However, about 30% of healthy children are discordant (i.e., they enter or are in a stage for one indicator and at the same time they enter or are in earlier or later stages for the other indicator), and this discordance affects their growth. Boys whose pubic hair stages are more advanced than their genital stages and girls whose breast development stages are more advanced than their pubic hair stages are heavier and have higher BMI percentiles than concordant children.

Children with the opposite discordance have lesser weights and BMI percentiles than concordant children. This variation in weight and BMI among healthy concordant and discordant children is greater than that among early and late maturing children.

A girl attains menarche, or starts to menstruate, about 2 years after her breasts start to grow and about 12 to 18 months after her peak height velocity. Girls who attain menarche before 10.5 to 11.0 years are relatively "early" and those who attain menarche after 13.75 years are relatively "late." Peak height velocity (age at most rapid growth in stature) occurs in girls about a year or two before it does in boys, but the sex difference in age between sexual maturity stages can be less than half a year.[18]

Body Composition

Muscle, adipose tissue, and bone are the primary body tissues that change during growth. These tissues are frequently quantified using a model that divides the body into fat and fat-free components based on assumptions that the densities of fat and lean tissues are constant.[19] The density of fat varies little at any age, but the density of lean tissue varies depending on its hydration and the relative proportions of muscle and bone, which vary among children based on age, gender, race, level of maturation, exercise, and nutritional status.[20] Accurate body composition estimates are calculated from measures of body density, bone density, and the volume of total body water in a model that accounts for differences among growing children in their levels of fatness, muscle mass, age, ethnicity, and sex.[21] Dual energy x-ray absorptiometry (DXA) is the most accurate, precise, and easiest method for estimating body composition in infants and children. Data on the body composition of children and adolescents are available, including fat-free mass (FFM), total body fat (TBF), and percent body fat (%BF), but body composition references for infants and very young children remain limited.[22] Reference averages for FFM and %BF estimates from bioelectrical impedance available from teenagers in the NHANES III are presented in **Figure 2-6** and **Figure 2-7**, respectively. There are differences in average values between white, black, and Mexican American children for FFM and %BF.

Muscle Growth

Lean body mass (LBM) is metabolically active and is composed of muscle tissue, the internal organs, and the skeleton. LBM contains a small amount of fat; in contrast, FFM is LBM without any fat. Growth in FFM and LBM is primarily due to an increase in skeletal muscle mass, which is the largest single tissue component of the body, the major constituent of which is body water. At birth, 25% of body weight is skeletal muscle, and this increases to about 50% of body weight at adulthood. FFM, LBM, and skeletal muscle mass are positively associated with stature (i.e., a tall child has a greater amount at the same level of maturity). Skeletal muscle mass increases in boys and girls during childhood and is roughly equal between them until about 13 to 14 years of age. In girls, muscle continues to grow into adolescence but stops around 16 years of age. In boys, skeletal muscle grows rapidly after 13 years of age and well into late adolescence. This growth period in boys is about twice as long as in girls, and, as a result, boys have much more skeletal muscle as girls, which is located primarily in the shoulders and arms. At maturity, boys have greater absolute amounts of FFM or LBM than girls, irrespective of stature.

Growth of Body Fat

Body fat stores energy. In children, the majority of the body's fat is subcutaneous, but adipose tissue is also deposited in the visceral parts of the body. From infancy up to adolescence, the growth of body fat, or adipose tissue, is fairly steady in boys and girls. Adipose tissue thickness on the arms, legs, and trunk increases during childhood in both sexes but slightly more so in girls so that by the onset of puberty girls have about 25% more body fat than boys. Body fatness continues to increase during adolescence in girls but in boys decreases after about 13 years of age because the underlying skeletal muscle and bone grow at a greater rate at this time. Both sexes deposit adipose tissue on the torso, but adolescent girls add adipose tissue to breasts, buttocks, thighs, and across the back of the arms, which accentuates the adult sex differences in body shape. The majority of total body fat growth among obese children is subcutaneous, but internal adipose tissue deposition similar to that of middle-aged adults is now appearing in obese children.[23]

Skeletal Growth

Skeletal growth is a continuous process. The bones of the legs and the vertebrae are the major locations of growth in stature, which reflects growth in bone length. Bone growth is steady until the adolescent growth spurt, but slows afterward. By about 18 years of age for girls and around 20 to 22 years of age for boys, the epiphyses or growth plates at the ends of long bones have fused to the shaft, or diaphysis, and the skeleton is mature. Assessment of skeletal maturation from radiographs of the hand/wrist or knee is an index of a child's biological age known as *skeletal age.* The skeleton is the body's reserve of calcium, and an important aspect of skeletal growth is the building of this calcium reserve. The importance of this reserve for children is that those who end growth with a low bone mass (i.e., a low calcium reserve) are at an increased risk for developing adult osteopenia and possible osteoporosis. Peak bone mass is the maximum mineral mass attained by the skeleton. This

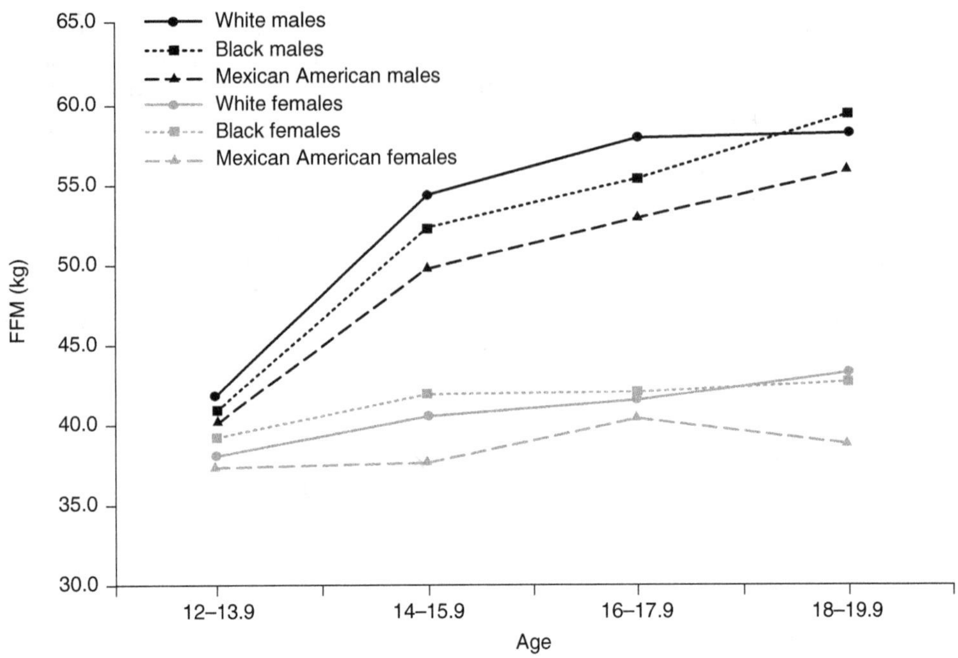

FIGURE 2-6 Means for Fat-Free Mass for U.S. Children, 12 to 19 Years of Age, from NHANES III

Source: From Chumlea WC, Guo SS, Kuczmarski RJ, Flegal KM, Johnson CL, Heymsfield SB, Lukaski H, Friedl K, Hubbard VS. Body composition estimates from NHANES III bioelectrical impedance data. *Int J Obes Relat Metab Disord.* 2002: 1596–1609.

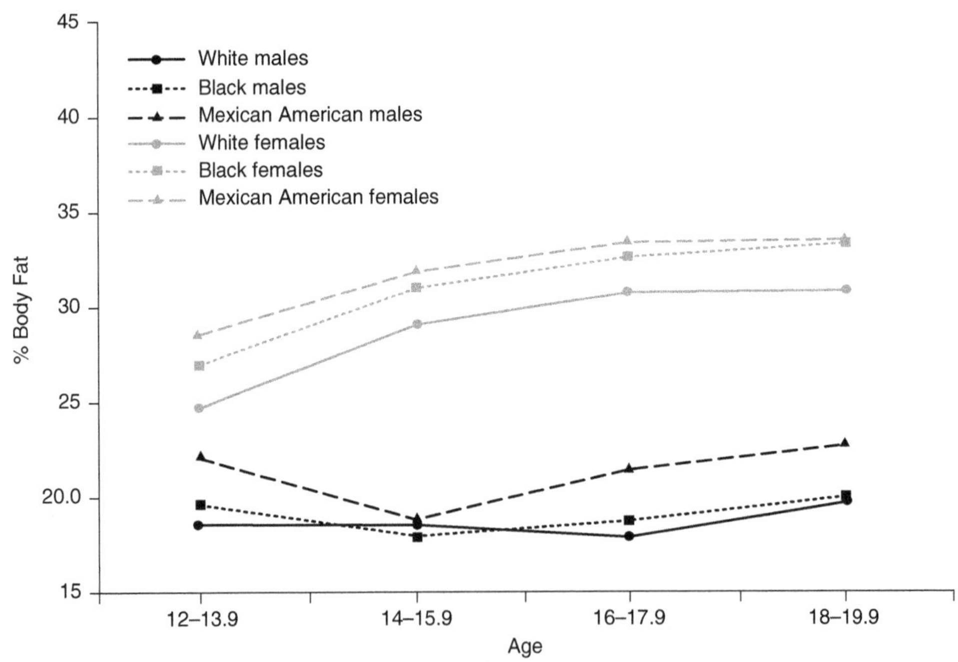

FIGURE 2-7 Means for Percent Body Fat for U.S. Children, 12 to 19 Years of Age, from NHANES III

Source: From Chumlea WC, Guo SS, Kuczmarski RJ, Flegal KM, Johnson CL, Heymsfield SB, Lukaski H, Friedl K, Hubbard VS. Body composition estimates from NHANES III bioelectrical impedance data. *Int J Obes Relat Metab Disord.* 2002: 1596–1609.

peak occurs in the late-middle part of the third decade of life, but by maturity the majority of peak bone mass has been reached.

Limited reference data for bone mineral content and density are now available for children at many ages.[2,24] These data and the use of DXA along with calcium supplementation provide mechanisms for monitoring the growth of the skeleton and affecting its calcium content. This information can help children with low bone mass and density and low calcium intake attain their peak bone mass and reduce the prevalence of osteoporosis in their future.

Special Children

Assessing the growth status of children with Down's syndrome, cerebral palsy, contractures, braces, mental retardation, and the like is difficult. If the child can stand, standard methods can be used. If the child is nonambulatory, then recumbent methods are recommended. Reference data from the CDC need to be interpolated depending upon the condition of the child in question. (See also Chapter 10.) Several websites provide useful information about measuring handicapped children. Accurate records are important, and the CDC growth charts can be used.

REFERENCES

1. Dietz WH, Franks AL, Marks JS. The obesity problem. *N Engl J Med.* 1998;338(16):1157; author reply 1158.
2. Troiano RP, Flegal KM, Kuczmarski RJ, et al. Overweight prevalence and trends for children and adolescents. The National Health and Nutrition Examination Surveys, 1963 to 1991. *Arch Pediatr Adolesc Med.* 1995;149(10):1085–1091.
3. Lohman TG, Roche AF, Martorell R. *Anthropometric Standardization Reference Manual.* Champaign, IL: Human Kinetics; 1988.
4. National Centers for Health Statistics, Centers for Disease Control and Prevention. *Analytic and Reporting Guidelines: The Third National Health and Nutrition Examination Survey (1988–1994)* [CD-ROM]. Washington, DC: National Centers for Health Statistics; 1997.
5. U.S. Department of Health and Human Services. *National Health and Nutrition Examination Survey III. Anthropometric Procedures* [videotape]. Washington, DC: U.S. Department of Health and Human Services, Public Health Services; 1996.
6. de Onis M, Onyangoa AW, Van den Broeck J, et al. Measurement and standardization protocols for anthropometry used in the construction of a new international growth reference. *Food Nutr Bull.* 2004;25(1):S27–S36.
7. Guo SS, Wu W, Chumlea WC, Roche AF. Predicting overweight and obesity in adulthood from body mass index values in childhood and adolescence. *Am J Clin Nutr.* 2002;76:653–658.
8. Goran MI, Gower BA. Relation between visceral fat and disease risk in children and adolescents. *Am J Clin Nutr.* 1999;70(1 Part 2): 149S–156S.
9. Roche AF, Siervogel RM, Chumlea WC, Webb P. Grading of body fatness from limited anthropometric data. *Am J Clin Nutr.* 1981;34:2831–2838.
10. Liem ET, De Lucia Rolfe E, L'Abee C, et al. Measuring abdominal adiposity in 6- to 7-year-old children. *Eur J Clin Nutr.* 2009;63(7):835–841.
11. Sakuragi S, Abhayaratna K, Gravenmaker KJ, et al. Influence of adiposity and physical activity on arterial stiffness in healthy children: the lifestyle of our kids study. *Hypertension.* 2009;53(4):611–616.
12. Matkovic V, Jelic T, Wardlaw GM, et al. Timing of peak bone mass in Caucasian females and its implication for the prevention of osteoporosis. Inference from a cross-sectional model. *J Clin Invest.* 1994;93(2):799–808.
13. Moore WM, Roche AF. *Pediatric Anthropometry.* 3rd ed. Columbus, OH: Ross Laboratories; 1987.
14. Beunen G. Muscular strength development in children and adolescents. In: Froberg K, Lammert O, Hansen H, Blimkie C, eds. *Exercise and Fitness—Benefits and Risks.* Denmark: Odense University Press; 1997:192–207.
15. Kuczmarski RJ, Ogden CL, Grummer-Strawn LM, et al. CDC growth charts: United States. *Adv Data.* 2000;314:1–27.
16. Whitaker RC, Wright JA, Pepe MS, et al. Predicting obesity in young adulthood from childhood and parental obesity. *N Engl J Med.* 1997;337(13):869–873.
17. Sun SS, Schubert CM, Chumlea WC, et al. National estimates of the timing of sexual maturation and racial differences among U.S. children. *Pediatrics.* 2002;110:911–919.
18. Chumlea WC, Schubert CM, Roche AF, et al. Age at menarche and racial comparisons in U.S. girls. *Pediatrics.* 2003;111(1):110–113.
19. Siri W. Body composition from fluid spaces and density analysis of methods. In: Brozek J, Henschel A, eds. *Techniques for Measuring Body Composition.* Washington, DC: National Academies Press; 1961:223–244.
20. Lohman TG. Applicability of body composition techniques and constants for children and youths. *Exerc Sport Sci Rev.* 1986;14:325–357.
21. Guo SS, Chumlea WC, Roche AF, Siervogel RM. Age- and maturity-related changes in body composition during adolescence into adulthood: the Fels Longitudinal Study. *Int J Obes Relat Metab Disord.* 1997;21:1167–1175.
22. Chumlea WC, Guo SS, Kuczmarski RJ, et al. Body composition estimates from NHANES III bioelectrical impedance data. *Int J Obes Relat Metab Disord.* 2002:1596–1609.
23. Brambilla P, Bedogni G, Moreno LA, et al. Crossvalidation of anthropometry against magnetic resonance imaging for the assessment of visceral and subcutaneous adipose tissue in children. *Int J Obes (Lond).* 2006;30(1):23–30.
24. Maynard LM, Guo SS, Chumlea WC, et al. Total body and regional bone mineral content and area bone mineral density in children aged 8 to 18 years: the Fels Longitudinal Study. *Am J Clin Nutr.* 1998;68:1111–1117.

CHAPTER 3

Assessment Basics

Susan Bessler

Introduction

The nutrition assessment identifies nutritionally depleted or at-risk infants and children, provides essential information for developing achievable nutritional care plans, and serves as a mechanism for evaluating the effectiveness of nutritional care.

Screening

Well-designed nutritional screening is effective in identifying children who are at an elevated nutritional risk and therefore may require a more comprehensive nutritional assessment.[1-5] Nutritional screenings can also predict outcomes in specific diagnoses.[6] The information gathered for screening includes indices of nutritional status routinely collected during scheduled healthcare appointments or upon admission to a healthcare facility.[7,8]

Nutritional screening protocols must be adapted to the needs of the specific population served and the staff and facility resources.[9] The success of the program depends on the coordinated efforts of the multidisciplinary team in completing assigned responsibilities.[1,10]

Key issues to be resolved when planning a nutritional screening program include designation of team member responsibilities, selection of nutritional parameters to be screened, timing of the screening, determination of how the data will be analyzed, and determination of the intended action once the data have been evaluated. Family-administered screening instruments that have the child's primary caretaker report data have been developed for use in the community setting.[11] The routine collection of lab values depends on the needs of the population and the laboratory support available. Once the nutritional data have been obtained, the child is assessed for nutrition risk and the appropriate referral or action plan is made. **Exhibit 3-1** is an example of a hospital screening form that weighs the criteria and dictates the next appropriate step in the care plan. Ideally, the data selected for the nutrition screen are objective (reproducible regardless of who is completing the screen), specific (identifying patients truly at risk), and sensitive (identifying all at-risk patients).[12] The nutrition screening process generally takes place at or soon after a clinic visit or hospital admission. Periodic rescreening should be done in settings such as extended care facilities for long-term patients to monitor changes in nutritional risk status.[13]

Nutritional Assessment

The assessment of a child's nutritional status is based on pertinent information collected from the child's medical history, anthropometric data, laboratory data, physical findings, and dietary interview.

Medical History

Approximately 10–15% of children in the United States have special healthcare needs.[14] These children may be at risk for associated nutrition sequelae, such as overweight, feeding problems, and chronic constipation. A child's medical history should include a review of social history, growth, acute or chronic illnesses, history of preexisting nutrient deficiencies, history of surgical or diagnostic procedures, and history of relevant therapies such as chemotherapy or radiation.[15] Medications should be reviewed for possible drug–nutrient interactions.

Anthropometric Data

Age-appropriate growth is the hallmark of adequate nutrition. Anthropometric data, as described in Chapter 2, should be obtained and BMI determined.

Weight, Height, and Head Circumference

Monitoring growth through measurement of weight, length/height, and head circumference (in children 3 years of age or younger) is a routine practice in most pediatric healthcare systems. These data are plotted on growth charts (see Appendix B) according to age and sex.

EXHIBIT 3-1 Sample Assessment Form

Admitting Diagnosis

[ ] Group 1 (8 points): New DM, CF, Inborn Errors of Metabolism, SBS, Iron Deficiency, Burns, Decubitus, IBD, FTT, Nutritional Rickets, Eating Disorder, Ketogenic Diet

[ ] Group 2 (4 points): CP, CHD, Liver Disease, Renal Disease, BPD, Bowel Surgery, Immunodeficiency, Obesity with Comorbidity, Chylothorax, Major Trauma

[ ] Group 3—Higher Risk Oncology (4 points): Relapsed ALL, AML, Bone Marrow Transplant, Solid Tumor Grade III or higher

[ ] Group 4 (0 points): All other diagnoses

Anthropometrics

wt:______ kg:______% ht:______ cm:______%

wt/ht:______ % *or* BMI (kg/m^2):________ %

[ ] Wt/ht or BMI <= 5% (8 points)

Diet Order

[ ] NPO (1 point) [ ] Modified/Special Diet (3 points)

[ ] Tube Feeding * (5 points) [ ] Food Allergies (1 point)

[ ] TPN * (5 points) [ ] Mechanical Feeding Problems (1 point)

[ ] Other (0 points)

Additional Information

[ ] Age <= 3 years old (1 point)

[ ] Admitted > 1 week ago (1 point)

Conclusion

[ ] Patient at high nutritional risk. Registered dietitian will provide further assessment and care planing within 48 hours of admission (8 or more points).

[ ] Patient at lower nutritional risk. Registered dietitian to monitor per standards and rescreen within the week. Contact registered dietitian for further assessment if status changes (less than 8 points).

* All patients receiving enteral or parenteral support will be assessed by the registered dietitian within 72 hours of initial nutrition support order.

Abbreviations: DM, diabetes mellitus; CF, cystic fibrosis; SBS, short bowel syndrome; IBD, irritable bowel syndrome; FTT, failure to thrive; CP, cerebral palsy; CHD, congenital heart defect; BPD, bronchopulmonary dysplasia; ALL, acute lymphocytic leukemia; AML, acute myelocytic leukemia; TPN, total parenteral nutrition.

Source: Courtesy of the Clinical Nutrition Service, Children's Hospital Oakland, Oakland, California.

Upper Arm and Skinfold Measurements

Upper arm measurements and skinfold measurements (which include those on the triceps, biceps, subscapular area, and abdomen) are used to predict and monitor body fat and muscle stores, clarify other anthropometric findings, and, in some settings, predict morbidity and mortality.[16] The upper arm measurements most commonly evaluated include triceps skinfold (TSF), midarm circumference (MAC), and midarm muscle circumference (MAMC). MAMC is calculated using the following equation

$$\text{MAMC (cm)} = \text{MAC (cm)} - (0.314 \times \text{TSF [mm]})$$

The standards most commonly used for ages 1 through 75 are those revised by Frisancho et al.[17,18] Standards for children younger than 1 year of age have been published based on data from children in the United States[19] and England.[20,21] Mid-upper-arm-circumference (MUAC) standards are based on data from the NHANES I and II data (see Appendix C). MUAC standards for height can be used when age is unknown.[22] Skinfold measurements can be monitored over time using a child as his or her own control.

Although useful, these measurements have limitations. Caution must be used in comparing a child to the reference data. The data published by Frisancho et al.[17] include measurements for a solely white population; therefore, use with other ethnic populations that may have different body compositions may be erroneous.[23–26] Even within the same reference population (i.e., ethnicity), mean body composition measurements can change over time.[20] Accurate skinfold measurements require both precise instruments that need to be checked and calibrated frequently and trained anthropometrists. These measurements can be challenging to obtain and reproduce,[27] especially in an obese or active child.

Body Mass Index

BMI was discussed in Chapter 2. Mean BMI decreases from age 1 year to ages 4 to 6 years, at which point it increases. Children who rebound from this trough at earlier ages are at a higher risk for obesity later in life.[18,28] A child at greater than the 85th percentile is considered overweight, and one at greater than the 95th percentile is considered obese. BMI can also be used to determine appropriate therapy to address the obesity.[29] BMI doesn't consistently quantify adiposity in an individual, however. Two children with similar BMIs may have different proportions of fat and muscle mass.[30] Also, BMI may underpredict adiposity in some children with disease states.[31]

Other Considerations

See Chapters 4 and 10 for information on obtaining and interpreting anthropometric indices in premature infants and children with developmental disorders. Children with delayed or precocious growth should have a bone age assessment done. For the older child, data relating to the stage of sexual maturity can alter assessment findings.[32,33] See Chapter 2 and Appendix C for the Tanner stages.

Laboratory Measurements

Some laboratory measurements of nutritional status are collected routinely as part of a normal healthcare evaluation. Others are performed when the diagnosis, medical history, or nutritional history indicates nutritional risk. Appendix E lists laboratory norms based on age categories for selected tests of nutritional status.[34] The interpretation of laboratory findings must take into consideration the present and past medical status of the child. Many biochemical indices of nutritional status for normal individuals are altered by acute or chronic disease.

Serum Proteins

Albumin is the serum protein most commonly measured for assessment of nutritional status because it is inexpensive and readily available. However, due to a relatively long half-life of approximately 2 weeks and reduced degradation during periods of low protein intake, diagnosis of nutritional depletion can be missed or delayed if based solely on serum albumin levels. Likewise, serum albumin level serves as a relatively late indicator of nutritional repletion. Serum albumin may be decreased during malnutrition due to inadequate availability of precursors.[35] Albumin can also be depressed during infection, trauma, enteropathy, liver disease, or renal disease and elevated in dehydration and for other reasons.[35,36] Serum proteins with shorter half-lives, such as pre-albumin, more rapidly assess response to nutritional therapy; though, like serum albumin, they may also be low during stress, sepsis, and acute illnesses secondary to fluid shifts and preferential synthesis of acute phase proteins.[35-38] Measurement of the acute phase protein C-reactive protein (CRP) may help determine whether a low serum protein level is caused by stress or nutritional deficiency.[39]

Iron Status

Iron deficiency anemia is a common pediatric nutritional problem in the United States[40] and is routinely assessed in the inpatient and community settings. Hemoglobin and/or hematocrit measurements are commonly used to assess iron nutrition. However, they are decreased only during later stages of iron deficiency and may be decreased for reasons other than iron deficiency, such as during acute or chronic infections or hereditary defects in red blood cell production (e.g., thalassemia major, sickle cell disease).[41,42] Serum ferritin level is highly correlated with total body stores of iron and is the most sensitive index of iron status among healthy individuals. An elevated free erythrocyte protoporphyrin level and a decreased serum iron/total iron-binding capacity ratio and transferrin saturation occur when iron stores are depleted. These biochemical findings are present before changes in hemoglobin and red blood cell morphology. With the exception of serum ferritin level, which rises, laboratory indicators for iron deficiency decrease during infection and chronic inflammation.[43,44]

Immunologic Function

Protein-energy malnutrition as well as subclinical deficiencies of one or more nutrients can impair immune response and increase risk for infection. The measurement of functional parameters of the immune system can, therefore, be useful to assess nutritional status. Among the immunologic indexes that are associated with nutritional status are levels of T-lymphocytes and leukocyte terminal deoxynucleotidyl transferase, appearance of delayed cutaneous hypersensitivity, and total lymphocyte count. These tests vary in sensitivity for detecting nutritional depletion.[45] The total lymphocyte count (TLC) is the index of immune function most readily available for hospitalized patients. This value can be calculated from white blood cell (WBC) counts as follows:

$$\text{WBC/mm}^3 \times \%\ \text{lymphocytes} = \text{TLC/mm}^3$$

Values less than 1500 are associated with nutritional depletion. In infants younger than 3 months of age, values of less than 2500 may be abnormal.[46] Independent of nutritional status, values of immunologic function may be altered during trauma, chemotherapy, immunosuppressant drug therapy and for other reasons.[45]

Clinical Evaluation

Examination and evaluation of general appearance and specific systems is an essential part of the nutritional assessment. Severe nutritional deprivation is usually easily detectable. Milder, nonspecific signs of malnutrition are more commonly observed but may be harder to detect. The presence of a suspected clinical deficiency is often reflected in the diet history and should be further supported by biochemical evaluation.[45,47] **Table 3-1** lists clinical signs associated with nutrient deficiencies and specifies laboratory findings recommended to substantiate the diagnosis

Diet Evaluation

The thorough collection of dietary data should include the quantity and quality of foods, psychosocial factors impacting food selection and intake, and clinical/physical factors related to nutritional status. Specific factors include:[47,48]

- Food-related factors
  - Chronological feeding history from birth or onset of nutritional problem
  - Current nutrient intake
  - Feeding skills
  - History of prescribed or self-imposed diets or outcome
  - Food allergies or intolerances
- Psychosocial factors
  - Family history and dynamics
  - Socioeconomic status including use of supplemental food programs

TABLE 3-1 Clinical Signs and Laboratory Findings in the Malnourished Child and Adult

Clinical Sign	Suspect Nutrient	Supportive Objective Findings
Epithelial		
Skin		
Xerosis, dry scaling	Essential fatty acids	Triene/tetraene ratio > 0.4
Hyperkeratosis, plaques around hair follicles	Vitamin A	↓Plasma retinol
Ecchymoses, petechiae	Vitamin K	Prolonged prothrombin time
	Vitamin C	↓Serum ascorbic acid
Hair		
Easily plucked, dyspigmented, lackluster	Protein-calorie	↓Total protein
		↓Albumin
Nails		↓Transferrin
Thin, spoon-shaped	Iron	↓Serum Fe
		↓TIBC
Mucosal		
Mouth, lips, and tongue	B vitamins	
Angular stomatitis (inflammation at corners of mouth)	B_2 (riboflavin)	↓RBC glutathione reductase
Cheilosis (reddened lips with fissures at angles)	B_2	See above
	B_6 (pyridoxine)	↓Plasma pyridoxal phosphate†
Glossitis (inflammation of tongue)	B_6	See above
	B_2	See above
	B_3 (niacin)	↓Plasma tryptophan
Magenta tongue	B_2	↓Urinary N-methyl nicotinamide†
Edema of tongue, tongue fissures	B_3	See above
Gums		See above
Spongy, bleeding	Vitamin C	↓Plasma ascorbic acid
Ocular		
Pale conjunctivae secondary to anemia	Iron	↓Serum Fe, ↑TIBC, ↓serum folic acid, or ↓RBC folic acid
	Folic acid	
	Vitamin B_{12}	↓Serum B_{12}
	Copper	↓Serum copper
Bitot's spots (grayish, yellow, or white foamy spots on the whites of the eye)	Vitamin A	↓Plasma retinol
Conjunctival or corneal xerosis, keratomalacia (softening of part or all of cornea)	Vitamin A	↓Plasma retinol
Musculoskeletal		
Craniotabes (thinning of the inner table of the skull); palpable enlargement of costochondral junctions ("rachitic rosary"); thickening of wrists and ankles	Vitamin D	↓25-OH-vit D ↓Alkaline phosphatase ± ↓Ca, ↓PO_4 Long bone films
Scurvy (tenderness of extremities, hemorrhages under periosteum of long bones; enlargement of costochondral junction; cessation of osteogenesis of long bones)	Vitamin C	↓Serum ascorbic acid Long bone films
Skeletal lesions	Copper	↓Serum copper X-ray film changes similar to scurvy because copper is also essential for normal collagen formation
Muscle wasting, prominence of body skeleton, poor muscle tone	Protein-calorie	↓Serum proteins ↓Arm muscle circumference

TABLE 3-1 *(Continued)*

Clinical Sign	Suspect Nutrient	Supportive Objective Findings
General		
Edema	Protein	↓Serum proteins
Pallor 2° to anemia	Vitamin E (in premature infants)	↓Serum vitamin E ↑Peroxide hemolysis
	Iron	Evidence of hemolysis on blood smear
	Folic acid	↓Serum Fe, ↑TIBC ↓Serum folic acid
	Vitamin B_{12}	Macrocytosis on RBC smear ↓Serum B_{12}
	Copper	Macrocytosis on RBC smear ↓Serum copper
Internal systems		
Nervous		
Mental confusion	Protein	↓Total protein, ↓albumin, ↓transferrin
	Vitamin B_1 (thiamine)	↓RBC transketolase
Cardiovascular	Vitamin B_1	Same as above
Beriberi (enlarged heart, congestive heart failure, tachycardia)		
Tachycardia 2° to anemia	Iron Folic acid B_{12} Copper Vitamin E (in premature infants)	See above
Gastrointestinal		
Hepatomegaly	Protein-calorie	↓Total protein, ↓albumin, ↓transferrin
Glandular		
Thyroid enlargement	Iodine	↓Total serum iodine: inorganic, PBI*

*Bio Science Laboratories, 7600 Tyrone Avenue, Van Nuys, CA 91405

Abbreviations: Fe, iron; PBI, protein-bound iodine; RBC, red blood cells; TIBC, total iron binding capacity.

Source: Reprinted with permission from Kerner A, *Manual of Pediatric Parenteral Nutrition*, pp. 22–23, © 1983, Wiley Medical.

- Patient's self-perception of nutritional status and/or caretaker's perception of child's nutritional status
- Religious or cultural beliefs impacting food intake
- Clinical/physical factors
  - Vitamin, mineral, herbal supplements and medication
  - Stooling habits and characteristics
  - Activity
  - Sleep patterns

See **Exhibit 3-2** for a sample dietary interview worksheet.

Complementary and Alternative Medicine

Families whose children have an acute or chronic condition may augment routine medical treatment with complementary and alternative medicine (CAM). Information on a family's past or present use of a CAM is important; however, they may not readily volunteer this information. Specific questions, such as those outlined in **Exhibit 3-3**, may be useful in eliciting this information.[49] See Chapter 21 for further information on botanicals.

Collection of Current Intake Data

The diet history can be comprehensive or specific. Several approaches to quantifying nutrient intake data include the following:

- A *diet history* is designed to determine the pattern of usual food intake. This type of history requires a detailed interview by a trained nutritionist.[50,51] This method yields higher estimated values than the 24-hour recall and diet record.
- A *24-hour recall* provides an estimate of nutrient intake based on the individual's recollection of food consumed over the previous day.

EXHIBIT 3-2 Dietary Interview Summary Portion of a Nutrition Clinic Evaluation

NUTRITION CLINIC EVALUATION

Date of Visit: ______________________________ Age: ______________

Diagnosis: ______________________________ Onset: ______________

Concomitant Conditions: ______________________________

______________________________ Ref. Phys. ______________________________

Problem: ______________________________

____

____

Concerns of Parents or Patient: ______________________________

____

____

Nutrition History: ______________________________

____

____

Recent Nutrition History: ______________________________

____

____

Formula: Kind ______________ Amount ______________ Cal. Density ______________

Food Intake: ______________________________

____

____

Food Summary (no. of servings/day):

Meat ____________ Milk ____________ Fr/Veg ____________ Grains ____________

____

____

Fever/Vomiting: ______________________________ Elimination: ______________________________

Appetite: ______________________________

Feeding Ability/Concerns: ______________________________

____

____

____

Vitamin Mineral Supp: ______________________________

Activity level 1–8, 8 high ______________________________

____

Social Setting in Regard to Meal Prep: ______________________________

____

____

Social History: ______________________________

____

____

Pertinent Family Medical/Weight History: ______________________________

____

____

____

EXHIBIT 3-3 Sample Questions to Elicit Information on Use of Complementary and Alternative Medicine

1. Is your child receiving any herbal preparations? If yes:
   - What is the name (if known)?
   - For what purpose is it given?
   - How is it administered (tea, tincture, fluid extract, tablet, or capsule)?
   - How much? How often?
   - Is it prescribed/recommended? Where is it purchased?
   - How is it tolerated? Any side effects noted?
2. Is your child receiving any additional vitamins or minerals? (If yes, the bulleted questions apply)
3. Are there any foods or vitamins you specifically avoid for your child?
4. Who are the people involved in your child's health care (caretakers and health providers)?
5. Do you have any questions regarding complementary or alternative health care?

- *Three-day to 7-day food records* provide prospective food intake data. These are recorded by the parent, child, or other caregiver (and requires literacy) and are returned to the nutritionist for analysis.
- In inpatient facilities, *nutrient intake analyses (calorie counts)* are frequently ordered to assess a child's food intake.
- *Food frequencies* estimate the frequency and amount of specific foods eaten.

Dietary Intake Evaluation

Estimated intakes of specific nutrients are calculated using values derived from food composition tables or computerized nutrient analysis programs. The calculated intake is evaluated for adequacy by comparing it with the *dietary reference intakes* (DRIs).[52] The DRIs are the most commonly used reference allowances in the United States.[53–58] They are based on contemporary studies that address not only preventing classical nutritional deficiencies, but also reducing the risk of chronic diseases, promoting optimal health, and preventing nutrient toxicities.[58] The DRIs actually refer to at least six types of reference values: recommended dietary allowances (RDAs), adequate intakes (AIs), estimated average requirements (EARs), estimated energy requirements (EERs), acceptable macronutrient distribution range (AMDR), and tolerable upper limit (UL). The RDA is the dietary intake level that is sufficient to meet the nutrient requirements of nearly all healthy persons and includes a wide margin of safety above amounts required to prevent deficiency.[59] Therefore, a healthy child whose estimated intake for a nutrient falls below the RDA may not have a nutritional deficiency or even a nutritional risk unless this intake is substantially below the RDA for a sufficient length of time. When assessing the adequacy of diets for infants and children with acute or chronic disease, potential alterations in nutrient requirements should be considered. In cases where sufficient scientific evidence is not available to estimate an average requirement, *AIs* should be used as a goal for intake where no RDAs exist. The *EAR* is the intake value that is estimated to meet the requirement defined by a specified indicator of adequacy in 50% of an age- and gender-specified group. The *EER* is the dietary energy intake predicted to allow for a level of physical activity consistent with normal health and development. The *AMDR* is the range of macronutrient intakes for a particular energy source that are associated with reduced risk of chronic disease while providing adequate intakes of essential nutrients. The *UL* is the maximum level of daily nutrient intake that is unlikely to pose risks of adverse health effects to almost all of the individuals in a life stage and/or gender group.

Calculation of Energy Requirements

Accurate prediction of energy requirements is important for the healthy child and is magnified in situations such as when treating the obese or failure-to-thrive (FTT) child or implementing enteral or parenteral nutrition support in the acute or chronically ill child.[60] Energy needs can be estimated by using the DRIs[52] (see **Table 3-2** and Appendix F); however, these are based on populations of normal healthy subjects and may not be applicable to all children, such as those with altered activity related to clinical status.

In children with illnesses and concomitant malnutrition, energy expenditure may be most accurately predicted by the use of indirect calorimetry.[61] An equation to estimate energy requirements for children between 3 and 18 years of age who are overweight is shown in Appendix F.

Definition of Terms

Total energy expenditure (TEE) consists of the energy required to meet the basal metabolic rate (BMR), diet-induced thermogenesis, activity, and growth.[62] BMR assumes the following basal conditions:[63]

- Fasting (at least 10–12 hours after the last meal)
- Awake and resting in a lying position (measurements are taken shortly after awakening)
- Normal body and ambient temperature
- Absence of psychological or physical stress

Diet-induced thermogenesis, also referred to as the *specific dynamic action of food,* is the energy necessary for digestion, transport, and storage of nutrients. It accounts for 5–10% of daily energy expenditure.[64] *Resting energy expenditure* (REE)

TABLE 3-2 Equations for Predicting Energy Requirements of Children

Origin	Energy Determination	Gender	Age	Equation
Institute of Medicine[52]	Total energy requirement	Both Genders	0–3 mo	89 × wt + 75
			4–6 mo	89 × wt − 44
			7–12 mo	89 × wt − 78
			13–36 mo	89 × wt − 80
		Males	3–8 y	108.5 − 61.9 × age + PA × (26.7 × wt + 903 × ht [m])
			9–18 y	113.5 − 61.9 × age + PA × (26.7 × wt + 903 × ht [m]) PA = 1.0 for sedentary 1.13 for low active 1.26 for active 1.42 for very active
		Females	3–8 y	155.3 − 30.8 × age + PA × (10 × w + 934 × ht [m])
			9–18 y	160.3 − 30.8 × age + PA × (10 × w + 934 × ht [m]) PA = 1.0 for sedentary 1.16 for low active 1.31 for active 1.56 for very active
Harris-Benedict[65]	BMR	Male	Unspecified	66.47 + 13.75 W + 5.0 H − 6.76 A
		Female		655.1 + 9.56 W + 1.85 H − 4.68 A
World Health Organization (WHO)[62]	REE	Male	0–3 y	60.9 W − 54
			3–10 y	22.7 W + 495
		Female	0–3 y	61 W − 51
			3–10 y	22.5 W + 499
Schofield[66]	REE	Male	< 3 y	0.17 W + 15.17 H − 617.6
			3–10 y	19.6 W + 1.30 H + 414.9
			10–18 y	16.3 W + 1.37 H + 515.5
		Female	< 3 y	16.25 W + 10.23 H − 413.5
			3–10 y	16.97 W + 1.62 H + 371.2
			10–18 y	8.365 W + 4.65 H + 200.0
Altman and Dittmer[67]	REE	Male	3–16 y	19.56 W + 506.16
		Female		18.67 W + 578.64
Maffeis et al.[68]	REE	Male	6–10 y	1287 + 28.6 W + 23.6 H − 69.1 A
		Female		1552 + 35.8 W + 15.6 H − 36.3 A

Abbreviations: Unless otherwise specified, W = weight in kilograms; A = age in years; H = height in centimeters; REE, resting energy expenditure; BEE, basal energy expenditure.

is the energy expenditure of an individual at rest and in conditions of thermal neutrality. REE may include the thermal effect of a previous meal. BMR and REE usually differ by less than 10%.[63]

Standardized Equations

Equations have been developed to predict the BMR and REE of infants and children. A sampling of these equations is provided in Table 3-2.[52,65–68] BMR and REE estimates using standard calculations are based on the assumption that the individual is free of pathology and fever that affect energy expenditure; therefore, applying these equations to the ill pediatric patient requires an additional stress factor. **Table 3-3** highlights a sampling of current findings regarding potential alterations in energy expenditure with different disease states.[69–85] Regular reevaluation of energy needs

TABLE 3-3 Potential Changes in Energy Expenditure Associated with Different Diagnoses

Diagnosis	Research	Population	Potential Stress Factor
Closed head injury Postinjury day 1–14	Phillips et al. (1987)[69]	2–17 years	Measured energy expenditure averaged 1.3 times Harris and Benedict's predicted value on postoperative days 1–14.
	Redmond et al. (2006)[70]	0–24 years	Caloric needs are ~ BEE × 1.0–1.2 (for paralyzed patients).
	Havalad et al. (2006)[71]	6–16 years	Energy expenditure in children with severe head injury cannot be estimated accurately by standard equations.
Sickle cell anemia	Williams et al. (2002)[72]	5–11 years	Measured REE was 15% greater than predicted REE.
Inflammatory bowel disease	Kushner et al. (1991)[73]	19–40 years	No significant increase in energy needs.
Cancer	Barale and Charuhas (1999)[74]	Unspecified	Supports adding 60–80% BEE to calculated BEE.
Allogeneic stem cell transplantation Week 3 post transplant	Duggan et al. (2003)[75]	3–15 years	Measured REE was 0.90–0.95 predicted REE.
End stage liver disease	Greer et al. (2003)[76]	0–2 years	Children with end stage liver disease had a 27% higher mean REE.
Extrahepatic biliary atresia	Pierro et al. (1989)[77]	2–73 months	Energy expenditure was 29% higher than normal.
Spastic quadriplegic cerebral palsy	Stallings et al. (1996)[78]	2–18 years	Nonbasal energy expenditure was minimal.
Burns	Mayes et al. (1996)[79]	0.5–10 years mean 30% BSA burns	Supports application of a factor 30% REE.
Postsurgery	Powis et al. (1998)[80]	0–3 years major abdominal surgery	No increase in metabolic rate after major abdominal operations.
	Jones et al. (1993)[81]	0–4 months various surgeries	Mean increase of 15% REE following surgery.
Congenital heart defects	Barton et al. (1994)[82]	Less than 6 months severe congenital heart disease	Needs 40% greater than RDA for age.
HIV	Alfaro et al. (1995)[83]	4 months–4 years	Perinatally infected children without secondary infections are not hypermetabolic.
	Henderson et al. (1998)[84]	2 years–11 years	Measured energy expenditure was ~ 120% predicted REE (WHO equation).
Fevers	Dubois (1954)[85]	NA	REE increases 13% for each degree Centigrade of fever (7.2% for each degree Fahrenheit).

Abbreviations: REE, resting energy expenditure; BEE, basal energy expenditure.

should be completed as clinical status changes. Caution must be taken not to overfeed a critically ill child, because excess nutritional delivery can potentially increase pulmonary and hepatic pathophysiology.[86]

The final factor in determining energy needs is activity. A child's activity level can be established by determining the amounts of time spent performing various types of activities and calculating an activity factor based on a 24-hour time period. Activity factors of 1.3 are associated with sedentary lifestyles, whereas activity factors equal to or greater than 2.0 represent lifestyles high in physical activity. Children under normal unconstrained conditions are considered to be active if their activity factors range from 1.7 to 2.0 × REE. Light activities such as seated or standing activities, golf, and house cleaning use REE × 1.5 to 2.5. Moderate to heavy activities such as playing basketball or soccer use REE × 5.0 to 7.0. **Table 3-4** demonstrates the calculation of an activity factor and the total energy expenditure (TEE).

TABLE 3-4 Example of Calculation for Total Energy Expenditure in an 11-Year-Old Boy*

Activity Type	REE Multiple	Duration (h)	Weighted REE Factor
Resting	1.0	9	9
Very light	1.5	8	12
Light	2.5	4	10
Moderate	5.0	2	10
Heavy	7.0	1	7
TOTALS		24	48

Activity factor = weighted REE ÷ hours
= 48 ÷ 24
= 2.0

Total energy expenditure:

Gender	Age (yr)	Wt (kg)	REE† (kcal/d)	×	Activity Factor	=	TEE (kcal/d)
Male	11	35	1190	×	2.0	=	2382

*Hypothetical activity pattern

†Calculated from Allman and Dittmer equation in Table 3-2

Individual variation in true energy expenditure may exist largely due to differences in lean body mass. The person with the higher lean body mass will have the higher energy expenditure.[87] These standardized formulas may not be accurate in predicting individual energy needs for children with FTT, obesity, and some acute or chronic illnesses.[61,64,71,88,89]

Indirect Calorimetry

Indirect calorimetry is used to predict the energy needs for those whose energy needs are elusive, such as patients who are FTT, obese, or critically ill on nutrition support and those who are unable to be weaned from a ventilator. Indirect calorimetry measures oxygen consumption (VO_2) and carbon dioxide production (VCO_2). Most indirect calorimeters are open-circuit systems in which the patient breathes room air or air supplied from a mechanical ventilator and expires into a gas sampling system that eventually vents the expired air back into the room.[90] Indirect calorimetry provides two pieces of information: REE and a measure of substrate utilization as reflected in the respiratory quotient (RQ).[91]

The following abbreviated Weir equation calculates REE:[92]

$$\text{REE (kcal/min)} = 3.94 \times VO_2 + 1.11 \times VCO_2$$

Measured REE may need additional activity or stress added to accurately predict total energy needs. Also, measured REE does not account for anabolism or growth.[87] Growth in a sick or traumatized child may be inhibited, and applying growth factors may result in overfeeding.

Indirect calorimetry can also evaluate how the body is using fuel as reflected by the RQ. RQ is the ratio of carbon dioxide produced to oxygen consumed (VCO_2/VO_2). Glucose oxidation is associated with an RQ of 1.0, fat oxidation with an RQ of 0.7, and protein metabolism with an RQ of 0.8. Alcohol or ketone metabolism may reduce the RQ to 0.67, whereas overfeeding with lipogenesis may increase the RQ to 1.3. Knowledge of inefficient substrate utilization and subsequent reduction of RQ through alteration of energy substrates can be medically advantageous.[92–94]

Data Evaluation and Plan

The assessment and periodic reassessment of nutritional status is based on the careful evaluation of all gathered information. Interrelationships among the child's health status, feeding abilities, eating habits, anthropometric data, and laboratory findings need to be considered.[95–97] The nutritional care plan is developed to correct nutritional problems or to reduce nutritional risks identified through the assessment. Basic information included in the medical and dietary histories provides a foundation for designing a plan that is reasonable and achievable within a given setting. The following are examples of nutritional pathologies requiring a detailed assessment and care plan.

Protein-Energy Malnutrition

The identification of the presence and severity of protein-energy malnutrition (PEM) among children in hospitals and clinics is a valuable function of nutritional assessment. An estimated 20–40% of hospitalized pediatric patients may have PEM.[98] **Table 3-5** outlines anthropometric indices developed by Gomez and Waterlow to quantify the severity of chronic and acute PEM. Children may present with one or both forms of PEM. Acute, but not chronic, PEM may increase morbidity and increase length of hospital stay.[98]

Marasmus and Kwashiorkor

Marasmus and kwashiorkor are two classifications of severe, acute PEM. Marasmus develops over a period of weeks or months and is characterized by a wasted appearance due to diminished subcutaneous fat. Infants and children with marasmus have normal or low levels of serum albumin and other transport proteins and no evidence of edema. Liver size is normal.[95,96]

Conversely, kwashiorkor develops acutely, often in conjunction with an infection. Levels of serum albumin, other transport proteins, and lymphocytes are reduced. Edema is present and there may be subcutaneous fat stores that mask muscle wasting. Dermatitis and hair changes are usually present. In severe cases, fatty infiltration of the liver occurs.[96–98]

Marasmic kwashiorkor is the classification used to describe the presence of symptoms of kwashiorkor in a child with a weight for height less than 70% of standard or weight for age less than 60% of standard. This condition often develops following acute stress and is associated with high mortality.[98]

Failure to Thrive

Failure to thrive (FTT) refers to the failure of weight gain and, in more severe cases, linear growth and head circumference.[99] FTT has been classified as organic or nonorganic depending on the presence or absence of a medical diagnosis, although most children may have mixed etiologies. Additionally, many cases of FTT are idiopathic. Successful treatment of FTT is dependent on a comprehensive work-up. A detailed growth chart with plots at several ages is useful because it identifies the age at which a child's growth began to deviate from the norm and therefore provides diagnostic clues as to the causes. The following criteria are commonly used to identify growth failure:

- Growth below a specified percentile on the growth chart:
  - Weight-for-age plotting less than the third or fifth percentile on the Centers for Disease Control and Prevention (CDC) growth charts
  - Weight-for-length/height plotting less than the third or fifth percentile
- Poor growth velocity
  - Decreased growth velocity, with weight falling more than two major percentiles over 3 to 6 months
  - Decrease of more than two standard deviations on the growth chart over a 3- to 6-month period

Standard Deviation

The standard deviation (SD) score, or Z score, is useful in expressing how far a child's weight and length/height fall from the median, or 50th percentile, on the reference growth charts for children of the same age and sex.[100] It is calculated as follows:

$$\text{Z score} = \frac{\text{measurement value} - \text{median for age value of reference population}}{\text{standard deviation for age of reference population}}$$

Categorizing growth according to progressive decrements in SD scores (22.0, 23.0, 24.0) can be used to describe the

TABLE 3-5 Anthropometric Indexes Associated with Protein-Energy Malnutrition

		Degree of PEM			
Type of PEM	**Anthropometric Index**	**Normal**	**Mild**	**Moderate**	**Severe**
Chronic (stunting)	Height for age as % standard*	95	90–94	85–89	< 85
Acute (wasting)	Weight for age as % standard*	90	75–89	60–74	< 60
	Weight for height as % standard*	90	80–89	70–79	< 70
	Arm circumference/head circumference ratio†	> 0.31	0.28–0.31	0.25–0.28	< 0.25

*Original data for determining degree of PEM used the 50th percentile of Boston growth data as standard. The 50th percentile on CDC growth charts is now commonly used as the standard with these assessments.

†Ratio has been found to correlate with weight for age in children 3 months to 4 years of age.

Sources: Adapted with permission from Gomez F, Galvan R, Frenk S, Munoz JC, Chavez R, Vasquez J. Mortality in second and third degree malnutrition. *J Trop Pediatr.* 1956;2:77; and Waterlow JC. Classification and definition of protein-calorie malnutrition. *Br Med J.* 1972;3:566–569.

relative severity of undernutrition. Percentiles and equivalent SD scores for weight for age, length/height for age, and weight for length/height can be calculated easily using computer software developed by the CDC and the World Health Organization (WHO).[101] An SD of zero is equivalent to the 50th percentile; 21.65 SD corresponds to the fifth percentile cutoff used by the National Nutrition Surveillance System. A recommended cutoff point of 22.0 SD below the 2000 CDC growth chart median weight for age, length/height for age, and weight for length/height should be used to discriminate between well-nourished and poorly nourished children.[102] When compared over time, a positive change in SD indicates growth, whereas a negative change indicates a slowing of the growth rate.

Further work up of FTT is largely dependent on the child's age. In the newborn period, the assessment will likely focus on the success of breastfeeding and bottle feeding, including formula type, procurement, mixing, volume, and feeding tolerance. For a baby who is anorexic or who has significant vomiting or diarrhea, the nutrition assessment will focus on identifying causes and treatment for these pathologies. Medical diagnoses associated with FTT should be considered depending on the presence or absence of supporting factors. Some of these diagnoses include celiac disease, cystic fibrosis, cerebral palsy, and cardiac disease. A thorough diet history is paramount. Laboratory tests should be used to confirm the diagnosis or monitor treatment, although the results alone rarely identify the etiology of FTT.[103]

REFERENCES

1. Shapiro LR. Streamlining and implementing nutritional assessment. The dietary approach. *J Am Diet Assoc.* 1979;75:230–237.
2. Hunt DR, Maslovitz A, Rowlands BJ, Brooks B. A simple nutrition screening procedure for hospital patients. *J Am Diet Assoc.* 1985;85:332–335.
3. Christensen KS, Gstundtner KM. Hospital-wide screening improves basis for nutrition intervention. *J Am Diet Assoc.* 1985;85:704–706.
4. DeHoog S. Identifying patients at nutritional risk and determining clinical productivity; essentials for an effective nutrition care program. *J Am Diet Assoc.* 1985;85:1620–1622.
5. Hedberg AM, Garcia N, Trejus IJ, et al. Nutrition risk screening: development of a standardized protocol using dietetic technicians. *J Am Diet Assoc.* 1988;88:1553–1556.
6. Mezoff A, Gamm L, Konek S, et al. Validation of a nutritional screen in children with respiratory syncytial virus admitted to an intensive care complex. *Pediatrics.* 1996;97:543–546.
7. Fomon SJ. *Nutritional Disorders of Children.* Rockville, MD: U.S. Department of Health and Human Services, Education and Welfare; 1976. PHS publication no. (HAS) 75-5612.
8. Christakis G. Nutritional assessment in health programs. *Am J Public Health.* 1973;63(Suppl):1–56.
9. The Joint Commission. *Comprehensive Accreditation Manual for Hospitals (CAMH): The Official Handbook.* Oakbrook Terrace, IL: TJC; 2011.
10. Kamath SK, Lawler M, Smith AE, et al. Hospital malnutrition: a 33 hospital screening study. *J Am Diet Assoc.* 1986;86:203–206.
11. Campbell MC, Kelsey KS. The PEACH survey: a nutrition screening tool for use in early intervention programs. *J Am Diet Assoc.* 1994;94:1156–1158.
12. Chima CS, Diet-Seher C, Kushner-Benson S. Nutrition risk screening in acute care: a survey of practice. *Nutr Clin Pract.* 2008;23:417–423.
13. Noel MB, Wojnarosk SM. Nutrition screening for long-term care patients. *J Am Diet Assoc.* 1987;87:1557–1558.
14. Baer MT, Farnan S, Mauer AM. Children with special health care needs. In: Shorbaugh CO, ed. *Call to Action: Better Nutrition for Mothers, Children, and Families.* Washington, DC: National Center for Education in Maternal and Child Health; 1991:191–208.
15. Klawittler BM. Nutrition assessment of infants and children. In: Williams CD, ed. *Pediatric Manual of Clinical Dietetics.* Chicago, IL: American Dietetic Association; 1998:19–34.
16. Alam N, Wojtyniak B, Rahaman MM. Anthropometric indicators and risk of death. *Am J Clin Nutr.* 1989;49:884–888.
17. Frisancho AR. New norms of upper limb fat and muscle areas for assessment of nutritional status. *Am J Clin Nutr.* 1981;34:2540–2545.
18. National Center for Health Statistics. Plan and operation of the Health and Nutrition Examination Survey, United States, 1971–73. *Vital Health Stat.* 1973;1(10a and 10b):1–53.
19. Ryan AS, Martinez GA. Physical growth of infants 7–12 months of age: results from a national survey. *Am J Phys Anthropol.* 1987;73:449–457.
20. Paul AA, Cole TJ, Ahmed EA, Whithead RG. The need for revised standards for skinfold thickness in infancy. *Arch Dis Child.* 1998;78:354–358.
21. Tanner JM, Whitehouse RH. Revised standards for triceps and subscapular skinfolds in British children. *Arch Dis Child.* 1975;50:142–145.
22. The development of MUAC-for-age reference data recommended by a WHO expert committee. *WHO Bull.* 1997;75:11–18.
23. Cronk CE, Roche AF. Race and sex-specific reference data for triceps and subscapular skinfolds and weight/stature^2. *Am J Clin Nutr.* 1982;35:347–354.
24. Owen GM, Lubin AH. Anthropometric differences between black and white preschool children. *Am J Dis Child.* 1973;126:168–169.
25. Ryan AS, Martinez GA, Baumgartner RN, et al. Median skinfold thickness distributions and fat-wave patterns in Mexican-American children from the Hispanic Health and Nutrition Examination Survey (HHANES 1982–1984). *Am J Clin Nutr.* 1990;51:925S–935S.
26. Ryan AS, Martinez GA, Roche AF. An evaluation of the associations between socioeconomic status and the growth of Mexican-American children. Data from the Hispanic Health and Nutrition Examination Survey (HHANES 1982–1984). *Am J Clin Nutr.* 1990;51:944S–952S.

27. Bray GA, Greenway FL, Molitech ME. Use of anthropometric measures to assess weight loss. *Am J Clin Nutr.* 1978;31:769–773.
28. Rolland-Cachera MF, Deheeger M, Bellisle F, et al. Obesity rebound in children: a simple indicator for predicting obesity. *Am J Clin Nutr.* 1984;39:129–135.
29. Spear B, Barlow S, Ervin C, et al. Recommendations for treatment of child and adolescent overweight and obesity. *Pediatrics.* 2007;120:S254–S288.
30. Pietrobeloi A, Faith MS, Allison DB, et al. Body mass index as a measure of adiposity among children and adolescents; a validation study. *J Pediatr.* 1998;132:204–210.
31. Warner JT, Cowan FJ, Dunstan FDJ, Gregory JW. The validity of body mass index for the assessment of adiposity in children with disease states. *Ann Human Bio.* 1997;24:209–215.
32. Hannan WJ, Wrate RM, Cowen SJ, Freman CPL. Body mass index as an estimate of body fat. *Int J Eating Disord.* 1995;18:91–97.
33. Tanner JM. Issues and advances in adolescent growth and development. *J Adolesc Health Care.* 1987;8:470–478.
34. Behrman RE, Vaughan VC, eds. *Nelson Textbook of Medicine.* 13th ed. Philadelphia, PA: WB Saunders; 1987.
35. Russell MS. Serum proteins and nitrogen balance: evaluating response to nutrition support. *Dietetics in Nutrition Support Newsletter.* 1995;17:3–7.
36. Dowliko J, Nomplegsi DJ. The role of albumin in human physiology and pathophysiology. Part III albumin and disease states. *J Parenter Enter Nutr.* 1991:15:477–487.
37. Golden MHN. Transport proteins as indices of protein status. *Am J Clin Nutr.* 1982;35:1159–1165.
38. Yoder MC, Anderson DC, Gopalakrishna GS, et al. Comparison of serum fibronectin, prealbumin and albumin concentrations during nutritional repletion in protein-calorie malnourished infants. *J Pediatr Gastroenterol Nutr.* 1987;6:84–88.
39. Joyce DL, Waites KB. Clinical applications of C-reactive protein in pediatrics. *Pediatr Infect Dis J.* 1997;16:735–747.
40. Expert Scientific Working Group. Summary of a report on assessment of the iron nutritional status of the United States population. *Am J Clin Nutr.* 1985;42:1318–1330.
41. Centers for Disease Control and Prevention. Recommendations to prevent and control iron deficiency in the United States. *MMWR.* 1983;47(RR-3):1–25.
42. Dallman RR, Yip R, Johnson C. Prevalence and causes of anemia in the United States, 1976–1980. *Am J Clin Nutr.* 1984;39:437–445.
43. Yip R, Johnson C, Dallman PR. Age-related changes in laboratory values used in the diagnosis of anemia and iron deficiency. *Am J Clin Nutr.* 1984;39:427–436.
44. Yip R, Dallman PR. The roles of inflammation and iron deficiency as causes of anemia. *Am J Clin Nutr.* 1988;48:1295–1300.
45. Puri S, Chandra RK. Nutritional regulation of host resistance and predictive value of immunologic tests in assessment of outcome. *Pediatr Clin North Am.* 1985;32:499–515.
46. Hattner JT, Kerner JA Jr. Nutritional assessment of the pediatric patient. In: Kerner JA Jr., ed. *Manual of Pediatric Parenteral Nutrition.* New York: John Wiley & Sons; 1983:19–60.
47. Christakis G. Nutritional assessment in health programs. *Am J Public Health.* 1973;63(Suppl):1–56.
48. Pipes PL, Bumbalo J, Glass RP. Collecting and assessing food intake information. In: Pipes P, ed. *Nutrition in Infancy and Childhood.* St. Louis, MO: Times Mirror Mosby; 1989:58–85.
49. Eisenberg DM. Advising patients who seek alternative medical therapies. *Ann Intern Med.* 1997;127;61–69.
50. Burke BS. The dietary history as a tool in research. *J Am Diet Assoc.* 1947;23:1041.
51. Frank GC, Hollatz AT, Webber LS, Berenson GSS. Effect of interviewer recording practices on nutrient intake—Bogalusa Heart Study. *J Am Diet Assoc.* 1984;84:1432–1439.
52. Institute of Medicine, Food and Nutrition Board. *Dietary Reference Intakes for Energy, Carbohydrate, Fiber, Fat, Fatty Acids, Cholesterol, Protein and Amino Acids.* Prepub ed. Washington, DC: National Academies Press; 2005.
53. Institute of Medicine, Food and Nutrition Board. *Dietary Reference Intakes: Dietary Reference Intakes for Vitamin A, Vitamin K, Arsenic, Boron, Chromium, Copper, Iodine, Iron, Manganese, Molybdenum, Nickel, Silicon, Vanadium, and Zinc.* Washington, DC: National Academies Press; 2000.
54. Institute of Medicine, Food and Nutrition Board. *Dietary Reference Intakes for Vitamin C, Vitamin E, Selenium, and Carotenoids.* Washington, DC: National Academies Press; 2000.
55. Institute of Medicine, Food and Nutrition Board. *Dietary Reference Intakes for Calcium, Phosphorus, Magnesium, Vitamin D, and Fluoride.* Washington, DC: National Academies Press; 1997.
56. Institute of Medicine, Food and Nutrition Board. *Dietary Reference Intakes for Thiamine, Riboflavin, Niacin, Vitamin* B_6, Folate, Vitamin B_{12}, Pantothenic Acid, Biotin, and Choline. Washington, DC: National Academies Press; 2000.
57. Institute of Medicine, Food and Nutrition Board. *Dietary Reference Intakes for Sodium, Potassium, and Water.* Washington, DC: National Academies Press; 2004.
58. Yates AA, Schlicker SA, Suitor CW. Dietary reference intakes: the new basis for recommendations for calcium and related nutrients, B vitamins, and choline. *J Am Diet Assoc.* 1998;98:699–706.
59. Guthrie HA. The 1985 Dietary Allowance Committee; an overview. *J Am Diet Assoc.* 1985;85:1646–1648.
60. Garrel DR, Jobin N, De Jorge LHM. Should we still use the Harris and Benedict equations? *Nutr Clin Prac.* 1996;11:99–103.
61. Kaplan AS, Zemal BS, Neiswender KM, Stallings VA. Resting energy expenditure in clinical pediatrics: measured versus prediction equations. *J Pediatr.* 1995;127:200–205.
62. World Health Organization. *Energy and Protein Requirements.* Report of a joint FAO/WHO/UNU Expert Consultation. Geneva: World Health Organization; 1985. WHO Technical Report Series no. 724.
63. Bursztein S, Elwyn DH, Askanazi J, Kinney JM. The theoretical framework of indirect calorimetry and energy balance. *Energy Metabolism, Indirect Calorimetry and Nutrition.* Baltimore, MD: Williams & Wilkins; 1989:27–83.
64. Pencharz PB, Azcue MP. Measuring resting energy expenditure in clinical practice. *J Pediatr.* 1995;127:269–271.
65. Harris JA, Benedict FG. *A Biometric Study of Basal Metabolism in Men.* Washington, DC: Carnegie Institute of Washington; 1919. Publication no. 279.
66. Schofield WN. Predicting basal metabolic rate, new standards and review of previous work. *Hum Nutr Clin Nutr.*1985;39c(1s):5–42.
67. Altman P, Dittmer D, eds. *Metabolism.* Bethesda, MD: Federation of American Societies for Experimental Biology; 1968.
68. Maffeis C, Schutz Y, Micciolo R, et al. Resting metabolic rate in six- to ten-year-old obese and nonobese children. *J Pediatr.* 1993;122:556–562.

69. Phillips R, Ott K, Young B. Nutritional support and measured energy expenditure of the child and adolescent with head injury. *J Neuro Surg.* 1987;67:846–851.
70. Redmond C, Lipp J. Traumatic brain injury in the pediatric population. *Nutr Clin Pract.* 2006;21:450–461
71. Havalad S, Quaid MA, Sapiega V. Energy expenditure in children with severe head injury: lack of agreement between measured and estimated energy expenditure. *Nutr Clin Pract.* 2006;21:175–181.
72. Williams R, Olivi S, Mackert P, et al. Comparison of energy prediction equations with measured resting energy expenditure in children with sickle cell anemia. *J Am Diet Assoc.* 2002;102:956–961.
73. Kushner RF, Schoeller DA. Resting and total energy expenditure in patients with inflammatory bowel disease. *Am J Clin Nutr.* 1991;53:161–165.
74. Barale K, Charuhas P. Oncology and marrow transplantation. In: Samour PQ, King K, eds. *Handbook of Pediatric Nutrition.* Gaithersburg, MD: Aspen; 1999:480.
75. Duggan C, Bechard L, Donovan K, et al. Changes in resting energy expenditure among children undergoing allogeneic stem cell transplantation. *Am J Clin Nutr.* 2003;78(1):104–109.
76. Greer R, Lehnert M, Lewindon P, et al. Body composition and components of energy expenditure in children with end-stage liver disease. *J Pediatr Gastroenterol Nutr.* 2003;36(3):358–361.
77. Pierro A, Koletzko B, Carnielli V, et al. Resting energy expenditure is increased in infants and children with extrahepatic biliary atresia. *J Ped Surg.* 1989;24:534–538.
78. Stallings VA, Zemol BS, Davies JC, et al. Energy expenditure of children and adolescents with severe disabilities; a cerebral palsy model. *Am J Clin Nutr.* 1996;64:627–634.
79. Mayes TM, Gottschlich MM, Khoury J, Warren GD. Evaluation of predicted and measured energy requirements in burned children. *J Amer Diet Assoc.* 1996;96:24–29.
80. Powis MR, Smith K, Renii M, et al. Effect of major abdominal operations on energy and protein metabolism in infants and children. *J Ped Surg.* 1998;33:49–53.
81. Jones MO, Pierro P, Hammond P, Lloyd DA. The metabolic response to operative stress in infants. *J Ped Surg.*1993; 28:1258–1262.
82. Barton JS, Hindmarsh PC, Scrimseour CM, et al. Energy expenditure in congenital heart disease. *Arch Dis Child.* 1994;70:5–9.
83. Alfaro MP, Siegel RM, Baker RC, Heubi JE. Resting energy expenditure and body composition in pediatric HIV infection. *Pediatr AIDS HIV Infect.* 1995;6(6):276–280.
84. Henderson RA, Talusan K, Hutton N, et al. Resting energy expenditure and body composition in children with HIV infection. *J Acquir Immune Defic Syndr Hum Retrovirol.* 1998;19:150–157.
85. Dubois EF. Energy metabolism. *Ann Rev Physiol.* 1954;16: 125–134.
86. Chwals WJ. Overfeeding the critically ill child: fact or fantasy? *New Horizons.* 1994;2:147–155.
87. Subcommittee on the Tenth Edition of the RDAs, Food and Nutrition Board, National Research Council. *Recommended Dietary Allowances.* 10th ed. Washington, DC: National Academies Press; 1989.
88. Coss-Bu JA, Jefferson LS, Walding D, et al. Resting energy expenditure in children in a pediatric intensive care unit; comparison of Harris-Benedict and Talbot predictions with indirect calorimetry values. *Am J Clin Nutr.* 1998;67:74–80.
89. Bandini LG, Morelli JA, Must A, Dietz WH. Accuracy of standardized equations for predicting metabolic rate in premenarchal girls. *Am J Clin Nutr.* 1995;62:711–714.
90. Matarese LE. Indirect calorimetry: technical aspects. *J Am Diet Assoc.* 1997;97:s154–s160.
91. Porter C, Cohen NH. Indirect calorimetry in critically ill patients. Role of the clinical dietitian in interpreting results. *Am J Diet Assoc.* 1996;96:49–57.
92. Weir JB. New methods for calculating metabolic rate with special reference to protein metabolism. *J Physiol.* 1949;109:1–9.
93. Bursztein S, Elwyn DH, Askanazi J, Kinney JM. The theoretical framework of indirect calorimetry and energy balance. In: Elwyn DH, Askanazi J, Kinney JM, Bursztein S, eds. *Energy Metabolism, Indirect Calorimetry and Nutrition.* Baltimore, MD: Williams and Wilkins; 1989:27–83.
94. Ireton-Jones CS, Turner WW Jr. The use of respiratory quotient to determine the efficacy of nutrition support systems. *J Am Diet Assoc.* 1987;87:180–183.
95. Waterlow JC. Classification and definition of protein-calorie malnutrition. *Br Med J.* 1972;3:566–569.
96. Mclaren DS, Read WWC. Classification of nutritional status in early childhood. *Lancet.* 1972;2:146–148.
97. Waterlow JC. Note on the assessment and classification of protein-energy malnutrition in children. *Lancet.* 1973;2:87–89.
98. Pollack MM, Ruttimann UE, Wiley JS. Nutritional depletions in critically ill children; associations with physiologic instability and increased quantity of care. *J Parenter Enter Nutr.* 1985;9:309–313.
99. Leung AKC, Robson LM, Fagan JE. Assessment of the child with failure to thrive. *Am Fam Physician.* 1993;48(8):1432–1438.
100. Waterlow JC, Buzina R, Keller W, et al. The presentation and use of height and weight data for comparing the nutritional status of groups of children under the age of ten years. *Bull WHO.* 1977;55:486–498.
101. Centers for Disease Control and Prevention. *Epi Info, Version 3.5.1.* Available at: http://www.cdc.gov/epiinfo. Accessed January 18, 2010.
102. WHO Working Group. Use and interpretation of anthropometric indicators of nutritional status. *Bull WHO.* 1986;64:929–941.
103. Sills RH. Failure to thrive. The role of clinical and laboratory evaluation. *Am J Dis Child.* 1978;132:967–969.

CHAPTER 4

Premature Infant Nutrition

Diane M. Anderson

Introduction

Premature infants are defined as infants born before 37 weeks gestation.[1] The physiologic immaturity of premature infants renders them susceptible to a number of problems, including glucose instability, poor temperature control, and necrotizing enterocolitis (NEC), that may imperil their nutrition and growth (see **Table 4-1**). Low birth weight (LBW) refers to infants with a birth weight of 1500–2500 g (3.3–5.5 pounds); very low birth weight (VLBW) refers to infants between 1000–1500 g (2.2–3.3 pounds), and extremely low birth weight (ELBW) refers to infants who weigh less than 1000 g (less than 2.2 pounds).[1] Note that infants can be LBW but be full term due to poor intrauterine growth.

Assessment of intrauterine growth is determined by plotting the infant's birth weight by gestational age on various charts. On the Lubchenco, Fenton, or Olsen growth chart, small-for-gestational-age (SGA) infants have a birth weight of less than the 10th percentile.[2–4] Large-for-gestational-age (LGA) infants have a birth weight greater than the 90th percentile.[2,3,5] Appropriate-for-gestational-age (AGA) infants are between the 10th and 90th percentiles (see Appendix A). On the Fenton and Olsen charts, SGA and LGA can also be defined as two standard deviations from the mean birth weight (approximately the 3rd and the 97th percentiles, respectively).[3,4,6] The Fenton chart can be downloaded from http://members.shaw.ca/growthchart. **Table 4-2** lists the etiologies for SGA. Some of the factors associated with LGA infants include infant of diabetic mom, Beckwith's syndrome, high gestational weight gain, genetic predisposition, and multiparity. These assessments are used to anticipate medical and nutritional problems and management needs of the infant (see **Table 4-3**). For example, an infant born at 34 weeks gestation whose birth weight is 1200 g is premature because the gestational age is less than 37 weeks. On the intrauterine growth charts, the infant is SGA because birth weight is less than the 10th percentile, or less than two standard deviations from the mean birth weight.[2–4]

SGA infants are further classified by their body length and head circumference as symmetrically or asymmetrically growth restricted.[6] The symmetrically SGA infant's birth weight, head circumference, and body length are all classified as small, whereas the asymmetrically SGA infant has a low body weight but an appropriate head circumference and body length. Infants who experience asymmetrical growth restriction usually stand a better chance for catch-up growth.[7] The potential for catch-up growth is determined by the etiology of the poor fetal growth.[7]

Catch-up growth for premature infants continues until adulthood for weight and length.[8,9] Head circumference catch-up is limited to the first 6 to 12 months of life.[10,11] A suboptimal head circumference measurement at 8 months of age may result in decreased intellectual quotients, impaired cognitive functioning skills, and behavior problems at school age.[12] Many premature infants remain smaller than infants born with normal birth weight or at term gestation.[9,10]

Premature infants represent a heterogeneous group for nutrition management. Intrauterine growth establishes nutritional status at birth, and gestational age determines the nutrient needs and feeding modality employed. As the infant matures, postnatal nutrient needs and the feeding modality will vary. The infant's clinical condition can also change acutely and alter nutrition care. Due to these factors, their nutrition management requires daily decision making regarding what to feed, what volume and nutrient density to provide, and how to administer nourishment. Optimal growth and development is the goal. The intrauterine growth rate and weight gain composition without metabolic complications is the goal for premature infant nutrition.[13]

AGA premature infants frequently become SGA before hospital discharge. These infants are growing at the intrauterine growth rate of 15 g/kg/day but their weight curve

TABLE 4-1 Premature Infant's Risk Factors for Nutritional Deficiencies

1. Decreased nutrient stores
   - Premature infants are born before anticipated quantities of nutrients are deposited.
   - Low stores include glycogen, fat, protein, fat-soluble vitamins, calcium, phosphorus, magnesium, and trace minerals.
2. Rapid growth
   - Depletes small body nutrient stores.
   - With rapid growth, energy and nutrient needs will be increased.
3. Immature physiological systems
   - Digestion and absorption capabilities are decreased due to low concentrations of lactase, pancreatic lipase, and bile salts.
   - Gastrointestinal motility and stomach capacity are decreased, which limits gastric emptying and feeding volume.
   - A coordinated suck, swallow, and breathing is not developed until 32–34 weeks gestation.
   - Hepatic enzymes are deceased, which may make specific amino acids conditionally essential (cysteine) or toxic (phenylalanine), due to the inability to synthesize or degrade.
   - Immature renal function limits the infant's ability to control fluid, electrolytes, and acid/base status.
4. Cold stress results in energy expenditure for heat production instead of growth.
5. Illnesses
   - Respiratory distress syndrome will decrease gastrointestinal motility. Trophic feedings or small volume feedings will frequently be introduced.
   - Patent ductus arteriosus often requires fluid restriction, which limits caloric and nutrient intake. If the infant is treated with indomethacin, the infant will be made NPO.
   - Necrotizing enterocolitis forces nutrition management to parenteral nutrition for bowel rest. With refeeding, human milk is used but an elemental infant formula may be indicated. Some infants may develop short-gut syndrome as a complication and require extensive nutritional management for malabsorption.
   - Bronchopulmonary dysplasia can lead to an increased energy demand with fluid restriction. Nutrient-dense milks are often utilized. Chronic diuretic use will create electrolyte depletion.
   - Hyperbilirubinemia may be treated by phototherapy, which may increase the infant's insensible water loss and fluid requirement. If exchange transfusion is needed, introduction of enteral feedings will be delayed. Necrotizing enterocolitis has been reported as a complication of exchange transfusion therapy.
   - Sepsis may result in withholding all enteral fluids until it is established that the infant is stable.

Sources: Data from Schanler RJ, Anderson D. The low birth weight infant. Inpatient care. In: Duggan C, Watkins JB, Walker WA (eds). *Nutrition in Pediatrics: Basic Science Clinical Applications*, 4th ed. Hamilton, Ontario, Canada: BC Decker; 2008:377–394; Anderson DM. Nutritional assessment and therapeutic interventions for the preterm infant. *Clin Peri.* 2002;29:313–326; and Cloherty JP, Eichenwald EC, Stark AR. *Manual of Neonatal* Care, 6th ed. Philadelphia: Wolters Kluwer/Lippincott Williams & Wilkins; 2008.

has fallen below the 10th percentile for their postmenstrual age.[14] Additional energy and protein may be needed above what the American Academy of Pediatrics (AAP) suggests as a means to prevent extrauterine growth restriction (EUGR).[15] However, others report that ELBW infants do not require more energy or nutrients except for protein because excess energy intake may lead to increased adipose tissue.[16] An increase in protein intake of 4.6 g/kg may be needed for those infants who are not meeting the AAP guideline of 3.5–4 g/kg of enteral protein intake.[16]

Parenteral Nutrition

Parenteral nutrition (PN) is often indicated and initiated in the first few days of life to allow the premature infant to adapt to the extrauterine environment and to supplement enteral feedings. Enteral feedings are often advanced slowly, because premature infants have decreased enteral feeding tolerance and small gastric capacities. Premature infants are at risk for NEC, and enteral feedings will be advanced cautiously.[13] For the VLBW infant, PN should be initiated within the first 24 hours of life.[17,18] **Table 4-4** and **Table 4-5** offer suggested guidelines for parenteral administration of specific nutrients. **Table 4-6** briefly describes a protocol for PN management.

For the premature infant who is not fluid restricted, adequate nutrition can be provided by a peripheral line.[19] A central venous catheter is required for the infant who requires prolonged PN, has limited venous access, is fluid restricted, or has an increased nutrient demand that cannot be met by peripheral nutrition. Peripheral inserted central

TABLE 4-2 Etiologic Factors for SGA Births

• Normal variation	• High altitude
• Pregnancy-induced hypertension	• Maternal age < 16 years or > 40 years
• Chronic hypertension	• Multiple gestation
• Chronic renal disease	• Congenital malformations
• Diabetes with vascular complications	• Chromosomal abnormalities
• Intrauterine infection	• Placental insufficiency
• Poor gestation weight gain	• Twin-to-twin transfusion
• Cigarette smoking	• Placental and cord defects
• Drug or alcohol abuse	• Short interpregnancy interval

Sources: Data from Lee KG. Identifying the high-risk newborn and evaluating gestational age, prematurity, postmaturity, large-for-gestational-age, and small-for-gestational age infants. In: Cloherty JP, Eichenwald EC, Stark AR (eds). *Manual of Neonatal Care*, 6th ed. Philadelphia: Wolters Kluwer/Lippincott Williams & Wilkins; 2008:41–58; Kliegman RM. Intrauterine growth restriction. In: Martin RJ, Fanaroff AA, Walsh MC (eds). *Fanaroff and Martin's Neonatal-Perinatal Medicine Diseases of the Fetus and Infant*, 8th ed. Philadelphia: Mosby Elsevier; 2006:271–306; and Institute of Medicine and National Research Council. *Weight Gain During Pregnancy: Reexamining the Guidelines*. Washington, DC: The National Academies Press; 2009.

TABLE 4-3 Anticipated Problems for SGA and LGA Infants

Problems	Issues
Small for Gestational Age	
Hypoglycemia	Caused by Low glycogen stores Decreased gluconeogenesis Decreased glycogenolysis Abnormal counter-regulatory hormones Hyperinsulinemia
Increased energy demand	Caused by Increased growth rate Increased energy cost of growth
Heat loss	Caused by Large surface area Decreased subcutaneous fat
Large for Gestational Age	
Birth trauma	Shoulder dystocia, fractured clavicle, depressed skull fracture, brachial plexus injury, facial paralysis
Hypoglycemia	Caused by hyperinsulinism

Sources: Data from Lee KG. Identifying the high-risk newborn and evaluating gestational age, prematurity, postmaturity, large-for-gestational-age, and small-for-gestational age infants. In: Cloherty JP, Eichenwald EC, Stark AR (eds). *Manual of Neonatal Care*, 6th ed. Philadelphia: Wolters Kluwer/Lippincott Williams & Wilkins; 2008:41–58; and Kliegman RM. Intrauterine growth restriction. In: Martin RJ, Fanaroff AA, Walsh MC (eds). *Fanaroff and Martin's Neonatal-Perinatal Medicine Diseases of the Fetus and Infant*, 8th ed. Philadelphia: Mosby Elsevier; 2006:271–306.

venous catheters (PICC) are frequently used with premature infants because the PICC line can be placed at an infant's bedside.[19] A tunneled central venous catheter must be placed surgically under anesthesia and is used when a PICC line cannot be inserted.

Management Concerns

Fluid management is very individualized for the preterm infant. Insensible water losses will be high, and the infant's renal function and neuroendocrine control will be immature.[20] Fluid volume may be limited to prevent or treat patent ductus arteriosus (PDA) and bronchopulmonary dysplasia (BPD).[21,22] **Table 4-7** provides laboratory parameters that should be observed in guiding PN therapy. Insensible fluid losses are high for many reasons.[20,21] These losses can be decreased by the use of humidified incubators, plastic shields, and plastic wraps or clothing.

Preterm infants have a limited ability to hydrolyze triglycerides. Elevated serum triglyceride levels are more frequently found with decreasing gestational age, infection, surgical stress, and malnutrition and with the SGA infant.[13,23] Serum triglyceride levels should be kept under 200 mg/dL.[13] Intralipid should be administered at a maximum of 3 g/kg over a 24-hour infusion.[13,23]

Several amino acid parenteral solutions are formulated for the pediatric patient.[24] These solutions contain a larger percentage of total nitrogen as essential amino acids and branch chain amino acids, and they have a balanced pattern of nonessential amino acids instead of a single amino acid concentration.[24] The use of a pediatric amino acid solution results in plasma amino acid levels that are similar to the breastfed infant and improved weight gain and nitrogen balance.[25] The addition of cystine to TrophAmine (Kendall McGraw Laboratories), one of the pediatric amino acid solutions, may also improve nitrogen balance.[26]

Transition to Enteral Feedings

Weaning to enteral feedings is often a slow process that is needed to facilitate feeding tolerance and prevent the development of NEC.[13,27] Enteral feedings are gradually increased in volume and strength as parenteral fluids are decreased at a similar volume. Parenteral fluids are discontinued at approximately 100–120 mL/kg/day of enteral feedings.

TABLE 4-4 Parenteral Nutrition Guidelines: Energy, Protein, and Minerals per Day

Nutrient	Unit/kg
Energy (kcal)	90–100
Glucose (mg/kg/min)	6–12
Fat (g)	1-3
Protein (g)	2.7-3.5
Sodium (mEq)	2–4
Potassium (mEq)	1.5–2
Chloride (mEq)	2–4
Calcium (mg)	60–80
Phosphorus (mg)	39–67
Magnesium (mg)	4.3–7.2
Zinc (μg)	400
Copper (μg)	20
Chromium (μg)	0.2
Manganese (μg)	1
Selenium (μg)	2.0
Molybdenum (μg)	0.25
Iodide (μg)	1

Sources: Data from American Academy of Pediatrics Committee on Nutrition. Nutritional needs of preterm infants. In: Kleinman RE (ed). *Pediatric Nutrition Handbook*, 6th ed. Elk Grove Village, IL: American Academy of Pediatrics; 2009:79–112; and American Academy of Pediatrics, Committee on Nutrition. Parenteral Nutrition. In: Kleinman RE (ed). *Pediatric Nutrition Handbook*, 6th ed. Elk Grove Village, IL: American Academy of Pediatrics; 2009:519–540.

TABLE 4-5 Parenteral Vitamin Guidelines per Day

Vitamin	Dose/kg	Maximum Dose per Day*
Vitamin A (IU)	920	2300
Vitamin E (IU)	2.8	7
Vitamin K (μg)	80	200
Vitamin D (IU)	160	400
Vitamin C (mg)	32	80
Thiamine (mg)	0.48	1.2
Riboflavin (mg)	0.56	1.4
Niacin (mg)	6.8	17
Vitamin B_6 (mg)	0.4	1
Folate (μg)	56	140
Vitamin B_{12} (μg)	0.4	1
Biotin (μg)	8	20
Pantothenic acid (mg)	2	5

*Preterm infants receive 40% of the daily dose MVI Pediatric (INFUVITE Pediatric) per kg until the maximum daily dose is achieved at 2.5 kg.
Sources: Data from American Academy of Pediatrics Committee on Nutrition. Nutritional needs of preterm infants. In: Kleinman RE (ed). *Pediatric Nutrition Handbook*, 6th ed. Elk Grove Village, IL: American Academy of Pediatrics; 2009:79–112; and Greene HL, Hambidge KM, Schanler R, Tsang RC. Guidelines for the use of vitamins, trace elements, calcium, magnesium, and phosphorus in infants and children receiving total parenteral nutrition: report of the Subcommittee on Pediatric Parenteral Nutrient Requirements from the Committee on Clinical Practice Issues of the American Society for Clinical Nutrition. *Am J Clin Nutr*. 1988;48:1324–1342.

Enteral Nutrition

Enteral feedings should always be introduced and advanced slowly.[24] Infants with cardiovascular instability, which can present as severe acidosis, hypotension, or hypoxemia,[24] may not be fed. Trophic feedings are advocated for the first week of life to facilitate gut development and are not associated with increasing the incidence of NEC.[13,28] Trophic feedings are small volumes of feedings (1 mL/kg or more) given to nourish the gut but not serve as a major source of nutrition. Benefits of trophic feedings are listed in **Table 4-8**. These feedings can consist of human milk or premature infant formula provided at 10–20 mL/kg/day for 3 to 7 days.[24] When the infant's condition stabilizes, feedings are advanced.[24]

The use of human milk has been linked to a decreased incidence of NEC.[29] Donor breastmilk is frequently used to supplement the mother's own milk for her infant to provide this protection.[30] The type of milk selected depends on individual factors and can sometimes involve complex decisions. **Table 4-9** lists factors that must be considered. Whatever milk is chosen, it should provide appropriate amounts of energy, protein, minerals, and vitamins (see **Table 4-10**). The goal is to promote growth and to prepare the infant for hospital discharge. In **Table 4-11**, selected nutrients are compared for 150 mL of milk, which is the average volume of intake for a premature infant on full enteral feedings. Fortified human milk or premature infant formulas will meet the needs of most premature infants.

The premature infant's vitamin needs will be met by the use of powdered bovine-fortified human milk or premature infant formula; no additional supplementation is indicated.[13] Commercial donor milk fortifiers are not vitamin fortified, so multiple vitamin supplementation is recommended. Iron needs will be met by the consumption of 120 kcal/kg of an iron-fortified premature infant formula.[13] For the infant receiving human milk, iron supplementation can be initiated at 2–4 mg/kg/day once full-volume feedings have been

TABLE 4-6 Parenteral Nutrition Progression

	DOL to Begin	Beginning Quantity	Increase	Maximum or Goal	Considerations
Fluid (mL/kg/day)	1	80–100	10–20	140–160	• Fluid needs will vary by birth weight, gestational age, postnatal age, and environmental conditions. • The ELBW neonate may require 200 mL/kg/day to maintain normal hydration the first week of life. • Fluids should be provided to keep the infant in normal hydration status. Refer to Table 4-7 for monitoring guidelines.
Glucose (mg/kg/min)	1	4.5–6	1–2	11–12	• Begin on DOL 1 to prevent hypoglycemia. • Decrease glucose load for hyperglycemia. Glucose homeostasis will usually improve in 1–2 days. • Insulin infusions should be used with caution. Insulin usage may result in unstable blood glucose levels, hypoglycemia, and acidosis.
Protein (g/kg/day)	1	1–3	—	2.7–3.5	• Advance protein to meet needs. There is no documentation that gradual protein advancement is needed.
Lipids (g/kg/day)	1	1–2	1	3	• Provide over an 18–24 hour period. • The 20% intralipid is preferred over the 10% emulsion. Serum levels of cholesterol, triglycerides, and phospholipids are lower with use of the 20% emulsion.
Sodium chloride (mEq/kg/day)	2–3	1–3	—	2–4	• Allow diuresis to occur the first few days of life to decrease extracellular blood volume. • Start sodium to prevent hyponatremia.
Potassium (mEq/kg/day)	2	1.5–2	—	2–3	• Add potassium after urine flow is established and serum potassium level is normal. • Check for hyperkalemia because the ELBW infant has a decreased glomerular filtration rate, acidosis, and the release of nitrogen and potassium secondary to negative balance.
Magnesium (mg/kg/day)	1	4.3–7.2	—	4.3–7.2	• Remove from parenteral nutrition when mother has received magnesium.
Vitamins and trace minerals	1				

Abbreviations: DOL, day of life; ELBW, extremely low birth weight.

Parenteral nutrition progression may be slowed with fluid and electrolyte imbalance, glucose imbalance, renal failure, the anticipation of enteral feedings, or the initiation and tolerance of enteral feedings.

Sources: Data from American Academy of Pediatrics Committee on Nutrition. Nutritional needs of preterm infants. In: Kleinman RE (ed). *Pediatric Nutrition Handbook*, 6th ed. Elk Grove Village, IL: American Academy of Pediatrics; 2009:79–112; Schanler RJ, Anderson D. The low birth weight infant. Inpatient care. In: Duggan C, Watkins JB, Walker WA (eds). *Nutrition in Pediatrics: Basic Science Clinical Applications*, 4th ed. Hamilton, Ontario, Canada: BC Decker; 2008:377–394; Thureen PJ, Melara D, Fennessey PV, et al. Effect of low versus high intravenous amino acid intake on very low birth weight infants in the early neonatal period. *Pediatr Res.* 2003;53:24–32; and Doherty EG, Simmons CF. Fluid and electrolyte management. In: Cloherty JP, Eichenwald EC, Stark AR (eds). *Manual of Neonatal Care*, 6th ed. Philadelphia: Wolters Kluwer/Lippincott Williams & Wilkins; 2008:100–113.

achieved or after 2 weeks of age.[13] The fortifiers vary in their iron content, and extra iron supplements should be limited to those that have low iron content. When erythropoietin therapy is employed, iron supplementation at 6 mg/kg/day is recommended to facilitate red cell production.[13]

Pharmacological dosage of vitamin E (50–100 mg/kg/day) for premature infants to prevent retinopathy of prematurity, BPD, or intraventricular hemorrhage is not recommended.[13] Complications associated with its pharmacological dosing include NEC, sepsis, intraventricular hemorrhage, and death.[31]

TABLE 4-7 Fluid and Electrolyte Monitoring Parameters

Fluid intake	80–150 ml/kg*
Urine output	1–3 mL/kg/hour
Daily body weights	10–15% maximum total weight loss
Serum sodium	134–146 mmol/L
Serum potassium	3–7 mmol/L
Serum chloride	97–110 mmol/L
Serum creatinine	0.3–1 mg/dL
Blood urea nitrogen	3–25 mg/dL
Urine specific gravity	1.008–1.012

*The critically ill premature infant has highly variable fluid needs. This range represents the usual volume of fluid administered. To prevent over- or underhydration, fluids should be provided so as to keep the other monitoring parameters within normal levels.

Sources: Data from Pesce MA. Reference ranges for laboratory test and procedures. In: Kliegman RM, Behrman RE, Jenson HB, Stanton BF (eds). *Nelson Textbook of Pediatrics*, 18th ed. Philadelphia, PA: Saunders Elsevier; 2007:2943–2949; and Dell KM, Davis ID. Fluid, electrolyte, and acid base homeostasis. In: Martin RJ, Fanaroff AA, Walsh MC (eds). *Fanaroff and Martin's Neonatal-Perinatal Medicine Diseases of the Fetus and Infant*, 8th ed. Philadelphia: Mosby Elsevier; 2006:695–712.

To prevent BPD in the ELBW infant, vitamin A supplementation has been suggested due to its role in cell differentiation and tissue repair.[32] However, physicians must decide whether to use vitamin A supplementation in their nurseries.[13]

Osteopenia, or poor bone mineralization, is commonly reported for premature infants with poor calcium and phosphorus intake, and this is in addition to their poor nutrient stores at birth.[33] Risk factors include prolonged PN and/or diets of unfortified human milk. A diet of fortified human milk or premature infant formula will meet the infant's needs.[34] Vitamin D intake at 200–400 IU per day with the calcium- and phosphorus-enriched premature formula is adequate.[35] Chronic diuretic use can increase urinary calcium losses.[33]

Premature infants are at risk for trace mineral deficiency due to their poor nutrient stores at birth, rapid growth, and dependence on adequate nutrient intake. With use of PN, premature infant formula, or fortified human milk, deficiencies should be uncommon.[36] Infants who have excessive losses via an ileostomy drainage or high urine output related to renal failure may need two to three times the recommended guidelines for zinc.[24,37]

Two long-chain polyunsaturated fatty acids, docosahexaenoic acid, and arachidonic acid, are present in human milk and have been added to infant formulas. This addition to the premature infant's diet has resulted in mixed results for physical growth, visual function, and neurodevelopment.[38]

The feeding method employed will depend on the infant's gestational age and clinical condition and the nursery staff's experience.[13] **Table 4-12** describes the various feeding methods, and **Table 4-13** provides feeding guidelines. Due to the infant's constantly changing clinical condition and development, several methods will be used. Both continuous and bolus infusions are used with gavage feedings.[13] Transpyloric feedings require the use of continuous infusion to prevent an osmotic load presented to the intestine and dumping from occurring.[24] The delivery of nutrients to the infant is decreased with continuous infusions as human milk fat and fat additives and minerals in the human milk fortifier adhere to or precipitate in the delivery system.[39] A bolus feeding or a feeding given over 30 to 120 minutes on a pump can decrease the nutrient loss.[24,39]

TABLE 4-8 Benefits of Trophic Feedings

- Feeding
  - Improved feeding tolerance
  - Achieve full feedings sooner
  - Achieve full PO sooner
- Gastrointestinal
  - Increased plasma gastrin
  - Decreased intestinal transit time
  - More mature intestinal motor pattern
  - Increased calcium, copper, and phosphorus retention
- Clinical
  - Decreased serum bilirubin and days of phototherapy
  - Decreased incidence of cholestasis
  - Lower serum alkaline phosphatase activity levels
- Decreased length of stay

Sources: Data from American Academy of Pediatrics Committee on Nutrition. Nutritional needs of preterm infants. In: Kleinman RE (ed). *Pediatric Nutrition Handbook*, 6th ed. Elk Grove Village, IL: American Academy of Pediatrics; 2009:79–112; Schanler RJ, Anderson D. The low birth weight infant. Inpatient care. In: Duggan C, Watkins JB, Walker WA (eds). *Nutrition in Pediatrics: Basic Science Clinical Applications*, 4th ed. Hamilton, Ontario, Canada: BC Decker; 2008:377–394; Dunn L, Hulman S, Weiner J, Kliegman R. Beneficial effects of early hypocaloric enteral feeding on neonatal gastrointestinal function: preliminary report of a randomized trial. *J Pediatr.* 1988;112:622–629; Ziegler EE, Thureen PJ, Carlson SJ. Aggressive nutrition of the very low birthweight infant. *Clin Peri.* 2002;29:225–244; and Schanler RJ, Shulman RJ, Lau C, et al. Feeding strategies for premature infants: randomized trial of gastrointestinal priming and tube-feeding method. *Pediatrics.* 1999;103:434–439.

Breastfeeding

Mothers who want to breastfeed their premature infants must usually express their milk. Steps to encourage moms to continue breastfeeding or expressing their milk are listed in **Table 4-14**. Kangaroo care (skin-to-skin contact between the parent and the infant) will facilitate parent–infant bonding and has been linked to a longer period of lactation by the mother who delivers prematurely.[40]

TABLE 4-9 Milk and Formula Selection Indications and Concerns

Milk	Indications	Concerns
Human milk	• Nutrients are readily absorbed. • Anti-infective factors are present. • Decreased incidence of NEC and sepsis. • Nutrient composition is unique. • Maternal–infant attachment enhanced. • Maternal emotional support by family and healthcare team is indicated to facilitate lactation. • Quicker achievement of full enteral feedings versus premature infant formula. • Slower weight gain, but earlier discharge has been demonstrated on fortified human milk feedings versus premature infant formula.	• Milk from mothers who deliver prematurely will often contain a higher protein concentration than that found in the milk from mothers who deliver at term. This elevated protein concentration decreased by 28 days of lactation and may not meet the protein needs of the rapidly growing premature infant. • The concentration of protein, calcium, phosphorous, and sodium is too low to meet the needs of many premature infants. To increase nutrient density, human milk fortifiers should be added to the milk. • Iron supplementation at 2–4 mg/kg is needed for those infants receiving the low iron–containing fortifier. For those who are provided the fortifier with iron, no iron supplementation is needed. • Milk volume production may be inadequate to nourish the infant.
Formulas for premature infants	• Glucose polymers comprise 50–60% of the carbohydrate calories, which decreases the lactose load presented to the premature infant for digestion. Glucose polymers also decrease the osmolality of the formula. • Lactose comprises 40–50% of the carbohydrate calories. • Medium chain triglycerides (MCTs) are 40–50% of the fat calories. MCTs do not require pancreatic lipase or bile salts for digestion and absorption. • Protein is at a higher concentration than that incorporated into standard infant formula to meet the increased protein needs of the preterm infant. • The protein is a 60/40 or 100/0 whey/casein ratio as compared with the 18/82 ratio found in bovine milk. This whey predominance prevents the elevation of plasma phenylalanine and tyrosine levels. • Calcium and phosphorous are two to three times the concentration found in standard infant formulas. These levels will maintain normal serum calcium and phosphorous levels, prevent osteopenia, and promote calcium and phosphorous accretion at the fetal rate. • Sodium, potassium, and chloride concentrations are greater than in standard infant formulas to meet the increased electrolyte needs of the premature infant. • Vitamins, trace minerals, and additional minerals are incorporated into these formulas at high concentration to meet the infant's increased nutrient need while facilitating a limited volume intake. • Iron-fortified formulas are available, which eliminates the need for iron supplementation. • Formula osmolality is within the physiologic range at 235–300 mOsm/kg water for the 20–24 kcal/ounce, which facilitates formula tolerances and decreases the risk of NEC. • A 30 kcal/ounce formula is available for the infant who needs fluid restriction to support growth, such as the infant with BPD. The osmolality is 325 mOsm/kg water. • Premature formulas can be used until the infant reaches 2.5–3.6 kg, depending on the formula vitamin concentration and volume intake.	• Feeding volumes should be advanced slowly with the very-low-birth weight infant. • Vitamin and iron supplements are not indicated for the infant receiving iron-fortified premature infant formula.

(continues)

TABLE 4-9 *(Continued)*

Milk	Indications	Concerns
Premature discharge formulas (transition formulas)	• Designed for the premature infant at discharge. The infant should weigh at least 1.8 kg when this formula is provided. • Formula should be initiated at least 3 days prior to discharge to document formula tolerance and weight gain. • Formulas have a nutrient composition between the concentrated premature formulas and the standard infant formulas. • Glucose polymers comprise 50–60% of the carbohydrate calories, and lactose comprises 40–50%. • Medium Chain Triglycerides (MCTs) are 20–25% of the fat calories. • The protein is either a 60/40 or 50/50 whey/casein ratio. • Improved bone mineral concentration and greater weight and length gains were documented with premature infants fed a transition formula for the first 9 months of life.	• Indications for this formula are not clearly defined. There is no consensus as to which premature infants should receive this formula nor the length of time they should remain on this formula. One suggestion is that the premature infant should remain on this formula until weight for length is between the 25th and 50th percentiles. • Transitional formulas can be provided up to 1 year of corrected age if needed. The greatest effect is during the first 3 to 6 months of corrected age. • Formulas are iron fortified and vitamin dense such that nutrient supplementation may not be needed. To meet the term infant guideline of 400 IU/day for vitamin D, a vitamin D supplement may be needed. • Formulas are available as a powder and can be concentrated to meet the needs of the infant with bronchopulmonary dysplasia. This formula can be provided in the nursery and in the home setting.
Standard infant formulas	• Can be used at discharge for larger premature infants who can gain 20–30 g/day while consuming at least 180 mL/kg/day of this formula.	• Nutrient content is inadequate for the premature infant during the neonatal period. • During the early neonatal period, these formulas may not be tolerated well. Lactose is the sole carbohydrate source, and only long chain fatty acids are incorporated into these formulas.
Elemental infant formula	• Infants who are recovering or suffering from gastrointestinal disorders can benefit from elemental infant formula. • Casein hydrolysates and amino acid formulas are available. • MCTs are a component of some of these formulas. • Glucose or glucose and sucrose are the carbohydrate sources.	• Nutrient content is inadequate for the premature infant, with special reference to calcium and phosphorus levels. • The time to switch to a premature formula must always be considered to improve nutrient intake. Depending on the infant's feeding history, the formulas can be switched or the premature infant formula can be provided as one feed per day and advanced by one additional feed per day as tolerated.
Soy formulas		• These formulas are not indicated for premature infants. • The premature infant is at risk for osteopenia. The phytates in the formula bind phosphorous and make it unavailable for absorption. The aluminum content may also interfere with appropriate bone growth. • The amino acid profile may be inappropriate for the premature infant. • Decreased weight gain and length growth have been reported when soy formulas were fed to premature infants.

Sources: Data from American Academy of Pediatrics Committee on Nutrition. Nutritional needs of preterm infants. In: Kleinman RE, ed. *Pediatric Nutrition Handbook*, 6th ed. Elk Grove Village, IL: American Academy of Pediatrics; 2009:79–112; Schanler RJ, Anderson D. The low birth weight infant. Inpatient care. In: Duggan C, Watkins JB, Walker WA (eds). *Nutrition in Pediatrics: Basic Science Clinical Applications*, 4th ed. Hamilton, Ontario, Canada: BC Decker; 2008:377–394; American Academy of Pediatrics Committee on Nutrition. Failure to thrive. In: Kleinman RE (ed). *Pediatric Nutrition Handbook*, 6th ed. Elk Grove Village, IL: American Academy of Pediatrics; 2009:601–636; Abbott Nutrition. Our products. Available at: www.abbottnutrition.com/Our-Products/Our-Products.aspx. Accessed March 15, 2010; MeadJohnson Nutrition. Healthcare Professional Resource Center Product Information. Available at: http://www.mjn.com/app/iwp/hcp2/content2.do?dm=mj&id=/HCP_Home2/ProductInformation&iwpst=MJN&ls=0&csred=1&r=3456090752. Accessed March 15, 2010; and American Academy of Pediatrics, Bhatia J, Greer F, Committee on Nutrition. Use of soy protein-based formulas in infant feeding. *Pediatrics*. 2008;121:1062–1068.

TABLE 4-10 Enteral Nutrient Guidelines per kg/day

Nutrient	Amount	Nutrient	Amount
Energy (kcal)	105–130	Molybdenum (μg)	0.3
Protein (g)	3.5–4	Iodine (μg)	10–60
Carbohydrate (g)	10– 14	Vitamin A (IU)	700–1500
Fat (g)	5–7	Vitamin D (IU)	150–400*
Sodium (mEq)	2–3	Vitamin E (IU)	6–12
Potassium (mEq)	2–3	Vitamin K (μg)	8–10
Chloride (mEq)	2–3	Vitamin C (mg)	18–24
Calcium (mg)	100–220	Thiamine (μg)	180–240
Phosphorus (mg)	60–140	Riboflavin (μg)	250–360
Magnesium (mg)	7.9–15	Niacin (mg)	3.6–4.8
Iron (mg)	2–4	Vitamin B_6 (μg)	150–210
Zinc (μg)	1000–3000	Folate (μg)	25–50
Copper (μg)	120–150	Vitamin B_{12} (μg)	0.3
Chromium (μg)	0.1–2.25	Biotin (μg)	3.6–6
Manganese (μg)	0.7–7.5	Pantothenic acid (mg)	1.2–1.7
Selenium (μg)	1.3–4.5		

*Maximum of 400 IU/day

Source: Data from American Academy of Pediatrics Committee on Nutrition. Nutritional needs of preterm infants. In: Kleinman RE (ed). *Pediatric Nutrition Handbook*, 6th ed. Elk Grove Village, IL: American Academy of Pediatrics; 2009:79–112.

TABLE 4-11 Milk Comparison for the Premature Infant at 150 mL/kg

Guideline (per kg)	EBM + HMF 24 kcal/oz (powder bovine)	EBM + HMF 24 kcal/oz (liquid donor milk)	Premature Infant Formula 24 kcal/oz	Premature Discharge Formula 22 kcal/oz
105–130 kcal	120	120	120	110
3.5–4 g protein	2.9–3	2.9	3.6–4	3.1–3.2
100–220 mg calcium	169–209	203	197–219	117–132
2–4 mg iron	0.5–2.3	0.2	2.2	2
1–3 mg zinc	1.38–1.8	0.99	1.56–1.8	1.33–1.38
150–400 IU vitamin D	180–225	39	183–288	77–88

Abbreviations: EBM, expressed breast milk; HMF, human milk fortifier; term human milk nutrient concentrations used for calculations.

Sources: Data from American Academy of Pediatrics Committee on Nutrition. Nutritional needs of preterm infants. In: Kleinman RE (ed). *Pediatric Nutrition Handbook*, 6th ed. Elk Grove Village, IL: American Academy of Pediatrics; 2009:79–112; Abbott Nutrition. Our products. Available at: http:// www.abbottnutrition.com/Our-Products/Our-Products.aspx. Accessed March 15, 2010; MeadJohnson Nutrition. Healthcare Professional Resource Center Product Information. Available at: http://www.mjn.com/app/iwp/hcp2/content2.do?dm=mj&id=/HCP_Home2/ProductInformation&iwpst=MJN&ls=0&csred=1&r=3456090752. Accessed March 15, 2010; Gerber. Start healthy stay healthy resource center. Gerber infant nutritional products. Available at: http://medical.gerber.com/products. Accessed March 15, 2010; and Prolact + H^2MF™ *Nutrient Values*. Prolacta Bioscience MKT-0164 Rev-1. 2009.

TABLE 4-12 Methods of Feeding

Type	Considerations
Breast/bottle	Most physiological methods. Infant at least 32 to 34 weeks gestation. Infant medically stable. Infant's respiratory rate less than 60 breaths per minute.
Gavage	Supplement to breast/bottle feedings. Suggested for infants less than 32 weeks gestation. Use for intubated infant. Use for neurologically impaired neonate.
Transpyloric	Employ when gavage feedings not tolerated. Use when the infant is at risk for milk aspiration. Use for the infant with decreased gut motility. Use for the infant with anatomic abnormality of the gastrointestinal tract. Infant intubated. Tube is placed under guided fluoroscopy. Complications include dumping syndrome, nutrient malabsorption, and perforation of intestine. Continuous infusions indicated.
Gastrostomy	Gastrointestinal malformation. Infant neurologically impaired.

Sources: Data from American Academy of Pediatrics Committee on Nutrition. Nutritional needs of preterm infants. In: Kleinman RE (ed). *Pediatric Nutrition Handbook*, 6th ed. Elk Grove Village, IL: American Academy of Pediatrics; 2009:79–112; Schanler RJ, Anderson D. The low birth weight infant. Inpatient care. In: Duggan C, Watkins JB, Walker WA (eds). *Nutrition in Pediatrics: Basic Science Clinical Applications*, 4th ed. Hamilton, Ontario, Canada: BC Decker; 2008:377–394; Sapsford A. Enteral nutrition. In: Pediatric Nutrition Practice Group, Groh-Wargo S, Thompson M, Cox JH (eds). *ADA Pocket Guide to Neonatal Nutrition*. Chicago: American Dietetic Association; 2009:64–103; and Ellard D, Anderson DM. Nutrition. In: Cloherty JP, Eichenwald EC, Stark AR (eds). *Manual of Neonatal Care*, 6th ed. Philadelphia: Wolters Kluwer/ Lippincott Williams & Wilkins; 2008:114–136.

TABLE 4-13 Feeding Guidelines

Trophic feedings*	Provide to infants < 1250 g BW Give for 3 days 10–20 mL/kg/day Human milk or 20 kcal/oz premature infant formula Bolus feedings
Feeds initiation and advancement	< 1250 g BW 10–20 mL/kg/day 1250–1500 g BW 20 mL/kg/day 1500–2000 g BW Initiate at 20 mL/kg/day and advance by 20–40 ml/kg/day 2000–2500 g BW Initiate at 20–30 mL/kg/day and advance by 20–40 mL/kg/day to ab libitum (ab lib) depending on clinical status of infant > 2500 g BW Start at 50 mL/kg/day or ab lib with minimum and advance by 20–40 mL/kg/day
Milk selection	< 1800–2000 g BW or < 34 weeks PMA • Human milk; fortify with four packs human milk fortifier/100 mL milk when 100 mL/kg feeds achieved. • Liquid donor milk fortifier added at 40–100 mL/kg/day of human milk • Premature infant formula ≥ 2000 g BW or ≥ 34 weeks PMA • Human milk • Standard infant formula

*Trophic feedings should begin on day 1 or 2 for the medically stable infant. The infant should have a physiologic range blood pressure while receiving 5 µg/kg/min or less of dopamine.

Abbreviations: BW, birthweight; PMA, postmenstrual age.

Source: Data from Clinical Review Committee Nutriton, Metabolic Management Nutrition. In: Anderson DM, Eichenwald EC, Chan SW, et al. (eds). *Guidelines for Acute Care of the Neonate*, 17th ed. Houston, TX: Section of Neonatology Department of Pediatrics, Baylor College of Medicine; 2009:97–108.

Nutrition Assessment

Nutrition assessment is a continual process for the premature infant. Dietary considerations, anthropometric measurements, feeding tolerance, and laboratory indices will need to be monitored.

Dietary Considerations

Daily assessment is necessary to determine the need for changing the feeding volume, solution strength, or feeding method. Intake is evaluated against nutrient guidelines, and the feeding technique should be advanced to the most physiological method possible for the infant. Breast or bottle feedings are introduced as the infant's coordination of sucking, swallowing, and breathing is developed at 32 to 34 weeks gestation.[13] The number of oral feedings should be increased per day as the infant demonstrates the ability to feed effectively. Feedings are frequently limited to 20 minutes per feeding period to prevent fatigue and excessive energy expenditure.[41] Enteral feedings may be limited to once a day until the infant demonstrates successful feeding.

TABLE 4-14 Steps to Support Lactating Women

1. Instruction
   - Methods of milk expression
   - Sterilization of expression equipment
   - Storage and transport of milk
   - Diet for lactation
   - Tips for relaxation
2. Tips to help with let down prior to expression
   - Showering
   - Hand massaging of the breasts
   - Applying warm washcloths to the breasts
   - Consuming warm beverages
   - Visiting the infant
   - Talking to the infant's nurse by phone
   - Placing the infant's picture on the pump
3. Nursery staff and nursery support
   - Availability of lactation consultant for mothers and staff
   - Education of nursery staff on milk expression and breastfeeding
   - Electric pump and pumping room conveniently available to the nursery
   - Electric pumps available for rental and hand pumps for purchase
   - Mother's milk used to feed the infant whenever it is available
   - Help mother with the initiation of nursing
   - Promote kangaroo care for skin-to-skin contact
4. Initiation of breastfeeding
   - Wake baby up
   - Express a little milk prior to nursing so nipple is easier to grasp by the small infant
   - Position infant so mother and infant are stomach to stomach
   - Allow mother to room in with baby prior to discharge to establish breastfeeding pattern

Sources: Data from American Academy of Pediatrics Committee on Nutrition. Nutritional needs of preterm infants. In: Kleinman RE (ed). *Pediatric Nutrition Handbook*, 6th ed. Elk Grove Village, IL: American Academy of Pediatrics; 2009:79–112; Hurst NM, Valentine CJ, Renfro L, et al. Skin-to-skin holding in the neonatal intensive care unit influences maternal milk volume. *J Peri.* 1997;17:213–217; and Hurst NM, Myatt A, Schanler RJ. Growth and development of a hospital-based lactation program and mother's own milk bank. *JOGNN.* 1998;27:503–510.

Growth Measurements

Anthropometric measurements are difficult to perform on premature infants. However, the new high-humidity hybrid incubators contain bed scales that enable infants to be weighed without removing them from their humidity- and temperature-controlled environment.[22]

Weekly weights, lengths, and head circumferences are plotted on intrauterine growth charts to track longitudinal growth and to assess whether the infant is growing at the intrauterine growth rate. Most premature infants will parallel their birth curve and demonstrate catch-up growth later in life. Initial weight loss that reflects the loss of extracellular fluid ranges from 10–15% of birth weight during the first week of life.[42] After regaining birth weight, the weight gain goal is 15–20 g/kg/day for infants who weigh less than 2000 g.[24,43] When the infant weighs 2 kg or more, a weight gain of 20–30 g/day is appropriate.[24,43] Head circumferences and length measurements should increase by 0.7–1.0 cm/wk.[24]

Daily weights and weekly lengths and head circumferences can be plotted on postnatal premature infant growth charts.[14] These charts demonstrate how the infant is growing compared to other premature infants. These charts profile the initial weight loss seen with infants at week 1 of life. The goal is for the infant to stay on his or her growth curve or demonstrate greater growth.

Weights will be influenced by many factors, including the use of different scales and the infant's hydration status. Weights should be taken at the same time each day. Alterations in the head circumference measurement will occur from birth to week 1 of life due to head molding or edema. Length board measurements should be used to obtain accurate length measurements. Skinfolds and mid-arm circumference measurements are generally not employed for routine clinical care, and the standards for such measurements are limited.[14,44,45]

When a series of daily or weekly measurements indicates inadequate growth, a search must be made for the cause. **Table 4-15** lists areas to check.

Assessment of Feeding Tolerance

Feeding intolerance and clinical compromise are common for the premature infant, so constant surveillance is required to detect early signs of feeding intolerance, sepsis, or NEC.[43] Feeding may need to be held due to signs of illness, including persistent apnea, bradycardia, temperature instability, or lethargy.

Gastric residuals are often present and may be due to immature intestinal motor activity.[43] During trophic feedings, residuals may be acceptable if the infant is clinically stable.[46] With bolus feedings, a residual up to 50% of the feeding volume or 1.5 times the hourly rate for continuous feeding is often accepted.[24] Undigested formula may indicate that the feeding volume is too large, that the infant does not tolerate this formula, that the infant has poor gastrointestinal motility, or that the infant has NEC or intestinal obstruction. Residuals containing bile may indicate that feeding tubes have moved into the intestine and are common when the infant is fed transpylorically.[43] Bile

TABLE 4-15 Possible Etiologies for Inadequate Weight Gain

1. Nutrient calculations are incorrect.
2. Parenteral nutrition is not optimized.
3. Infant just achieved full enteral feedings meeting guidelines.
4. Infant is not receiving ordered diet.
   - Intravenous fluid administration has been interrupted to give blood or drugs, or the intravenous line has become infiltrated.
   - Infant is unable to consume what is ordered by bottle, and no gavage supplements were provided.
   - Feedings were held because the infant's respiratory rate increased or body temperature instability developed.
   - Feedings were held for clinical tests.
5. Infant does not tolerate given formula.
6. Calculated nutrient guidelines are inadequate for the infant due to illness.
7. Infant is cold stressed.
8. Infant has outgrown previous diet order.
9. Nutrition solution was not prepared correctly.
10. Incorrect formula was provided to infant.
11. Human milk issues
    - Continuous infusion will lead to fat separation in feeding syringe. Switch to bolus feedings or put over a pump for 30 to 90 minutes.
    - Ensure correct number of fortifier packets were added to milk.
    - Ensure infant is not receiving only the foremilk, which is low in fat.
12. Metabolic issues
    - Acidosis
    - Electrolyte abnormality
13. Low hemoglobin
14. Ostomy output

Sources: Data from Anderson DM. Nutritional assessment and therapeutic interventions for the preterm infant. *Clin Peri.* 2002;29:313–326; and Anderson DM. Nutrition for premature infants. In: Samour PQ, King K (eds). *Handbook of Pediatric Nutrition*, 3rd ed. Burlington, MA: Jones & Bartlett Learning; 2005:53–74.

also may indicate intestinal obstruction.[43] Residuals are not a consistent marker of feeding intolerance or NEC, but they should be noted in relation to other clinical parameters.[24]

The tonicity of the abdomen should be observed. Increases in abdominal girth will occur with air swallowing, feeding intolerance, infrequent stooling, or NEC. When the abdomen is distended and/or tender, an evaluation to rule out bowel obstruction is done.[47] A workup for sepsis and NEC may be considered.

Blood in the stool or residual is a concern and should be evaluated. Blood may be a sign of illness, feeding-tube irritation of the intestine, anal fissure, or swallowed blood during delivery.

Assessing Nutrient Adequacy and Tolerance

The specific clinical signs of nutrient deficiency/toxicity and the associated laboratory values should be assessed regularly or when a vitamin/mineral deficiency is suspected.[48] Acceptable standards for laboratory values are difficult to establish because premature infants differ by their physical maturity, and other factors. For example, serum proteins will vary by the infant's hepatic maturity and energy and protein intake. Blood urea nitrogen may be helpful to monitor for the premature infant fed human milk to determine protein supplementation needs.[49,50]

During the first week of life, serum electrolytes, glucose, creatinine, and urea nitrogen are monitored daily, or more frequently when values are abnormal. As these blood parameters stabilize, they can be checked when clinically indicated.[24] Serum electrolytes are assessed for those infants receiving diuretics or those with a history of abnormal values until values are normal. Additional parameters monitored when PN is being administered include serum triglycerides to check lipid tolerance, direct bilirubin to detect cholestasis, and serum alanine aminotransferase (ALT) and serum glutamic-pyruvic transaminase to evaluate hepatic function.[24] Serum calcium, phosphorus, and alkaline phosphatase levels may be monitored to detect osteopenia in the premature infant.[24] Hematocrit and hemoglobin levels are checked, as needed.[24]

Discharge Concerns

The premature infant is ready for discharge from the hospital when body temperature can be maintained, breastfeeding or bottle-feeding supports growth, and cardiorespiratory function is mature and stable.[51] Most important, the caretaker must be ready to care for the high-risk infant.

The infant should be evaluated for participation in the Special Supplemental Nutrition Program for Women, Infants, and Children (WIC), early intervention programs, and a developmental follow-up program for premature infants. The follow-up program should monitor the infant's growth and development, offer aid with chronic illness management, provide early detection of problems, make referrals to specialized services as indicated, and give the parents support and guidance in caring for their prematurely born infant.[11] A primary care physician must be identified to provide well-baby and sick care.[51]

Most infants will be discharged home on human milk, standard infant formula, or preterm discharge (transition) formula. The breastfed infant should receive a daily multiple vitamin containing 400 IU of vitamin D and a 2 mg/kg iron supplement.[13,52] Breastfed premature infants may need additional nutrients to grow well. The infant formula-fed with iron will not require additional iron supplementation. Infants receiving the premature discharge formula may require extra vitamins, and the premature infant receiving term formula should receive a multivitamin until 3 kg of body weight is achieved.[13] Infants with a birth weight less than 1800 grams should be evaluated for use of preterm discharge formula and remain on the discharge formula until weight for length is at the 25th percentile or greater.[7] Infants suffering from BPD may need a nutrient-dense formula. The premature discharge formulas can be concentrated easily to 24 or 27 kcal/oz.

Conclusion

Although premature infants begin life in a compromised nutritional state, nutrition and medical therapies continue to evolve that enhance the infant's potential for optimal growth and development.[13] Daily nutrition evaluation of the premature infant is necessary to ensure that appropriate nutrition therapy can be provided.

Case Study

Nutrition Assessment of Preterm Infant

Patient history: A 980-gram female infant was born at 27 weeks gestation and classified as an appropriate for gestational age premature infant on a premature growth chart. Length was 36 cm, and head circumference was 25 cm. Today, the patient is 21 days old or 30 weeks postmenstrual age (PMA). Patient had respiratory distress syndrome, which required intubation and surfactant therapy. Patient is now on room air.

Nutrition history: Patient was on parenteral nutrition, but is now on total enteral feedings of human milk from her mother at 160 mL/kg.

Anthropometrics

Weight: 1085 g

Length: 38 cm

Head circumference: 27 cm

Nutrition Problem

Nutrient intake is inadequate for the premature infant.

Nutrition Interventions

As discussed on team rounds, human milk fortifier will be added to human milk to provide 24 kcal/oz milk. At 160 mL/kg, the infant will receive 128 kcal/kg and 3 g protein/kg. The fortifier will bring the nutrient content up to meet the guidelines for prematurity.

Nutrition Monitoring and Evaluation

The infant's weekly rate of weight, head circumference, and length will be calculated and measurements recorded on the Fenton Growth Chart.

Questions for the Reader

1. How did weight, length, and head circumference plot at birth and at 3 weeks or 30 weeks gestation on the Lubchenco growth chart?
2. What are the kilocalorie and protein goals per kg for this infant?
3. What milk is recommended for the premature infant?
4. What would the feed volume be per feed for feeding every 3 hours at 160 mL/kg?
5. Write one PES.
6. Calculate energy and protein intakes on fortified human milk with powdered bovine fortifier at 160 mL/kg.
7. What should be monitored on a weekly basis in this infant before discharge?

REFERENCES

1. American Academy of Pediatrics, American College of Obstetricians and Gynecologists. *Guidelines for Perinatal Care,* 6th ed. Elk Grove, IL: American Academy of Pediatrics; 2007.
2. Battaglia FC, Lubchenco LO. A practical classification of newborn infants by weight and gestational age. *J Pediatr.* 1967;71:159–163.
3. Fenton TR. A new growth chart for preterm babies: Babson and Benda's chart updated with recent data and a new format. *BMC Pediatrics.* 2003;3:13.
4. Olsen IE, Groveman SA, Lawson ML, et al. New intrauterine growth curves based on United States data. *Pediatrics.* 2010;125:e214–e224.
5. Cloherty JP, Eichenwald EC, Stark A, eds. *Manual of Neonatal Care,* 6th ed. Philadelphia: Wolters Kluwer/Lippincott Williams & Wilkins; 2008.
6. Lee KG. Identifying the high-risk newborn and evaluating gestational age, prematurity, postmaturity, large-for-gestational-age, and small-for-gestational-age infants. In: Cloherty JP, Eichenwald EC, Stark AR, eds. *Manual of Neonatal Care,* 6th ed. Philadelphia: Wolters Kluwer/Lippincott Williams & Wilkins; 2008:41–58.
7. American Academy of Pediatrics Committee on Nutrition. Failure to thrive. In: Kleinman RE, ed. *Pediatric Nutrition Handbook,* 6th ed. Elk Grove Village, IL: American Academy of Pediatrics; 2009:601–636.
8. Hack M. Young adult outcomes of very-low-birth-weight children. *Semin Fetal Neonat Med.* 2006;11:127–137.
9. Hack M, Schluchter M, Cartar L, et al. Growth of very low birth weight infants to age 20 years. *Pediatrics.* 2003;112:e30–e38. Available at: http://www.pediatrics.org/cgi/content/full/112/1/e30. Accessed August 8, 2010.
10. Farooqi A, Hagglof B, Sedin G, et al. Growth in 10- to 12-year-old children born at 23 to 25 weeks' gestation in the 1990s: a Swedish national prospective follow-up study. *Pediatrics.* 2006;118:e1452–e1465.
11. Wilson-Costello DE, Hack M. Follow-up for high risk neonates. In: Martin RJ, Fanaroff AA, Walsh MC, eds. *Fanaroff and Martin's Neonatal-Perinatal Medicine Diseases of the Fetus and Infant,* 8th ed. Philadelphia: Mosby Elsevier; 2006:1035–1044.
12. Hack M, Breslau N, Weissman B, et al. Effect of very low birth weight and subnormal head size on cognitive abilities at school age. *N Engl J Med.* 991;325:231–237.
13. American Academy of Pediatrics Committee on Nutrition. Nutritional needs of preterm infants. In: Kleinman RE, ed. *Pediatric Nutrition Handbook,* 6th ed. Elk Grove Village, IL: American Academy of Pediatrics; 2009:79–112.
14. Ehrenkranz RA, Younes N, Lemons JA, et al. Longitudinal growth of hospitalized very low birth weight infants. *Pediatrics.* 1999;104:280–289.
15. Tsang RC, Uauy R, Koletzko B, Zlotkin SH, eds. *Nutrition of the Preterm Infant. Scientific Basis and Practical Guidelines,* 2nd ed. Cincinnati, OH: Digital Educational Publishing; 2005.
16. Agostoni C, Buonocoe G, Carnielli VP, et al. Enteral nutrient supply for preterm infants: commentary from the European Society of Paediatric Gastroenterology, Hepatology and Nutrition Committee on Nutrition. *J Pediatr Gastroenterol Nutr.* 2010;50:85–91.
17. Thureen PJ, Melara D, Fennessey PV, et al. Effect of low versus high intravenous amino acid intake on very low birth weight infants in the early neonatal period. *Pediatr Res.* 2003;53:24–32.
18. Te Braake FWJ, Van Den Akker CHP, Wattimena DJL, et al. Amino acid administration to premature infants directly after birth. *J Pediatr.* 2005;147:457–461.
19. Carlson SJ. Parenteral nutrition. In: Pediatric Nutrition Practice Group, Groh-Wargo S, Thompson M, Cox JH, eds. *ADA Pocket Guide to Neonatal Nutrition.* Chicago, IL: American Dietetic Association; 2009:29–63.
20. Doherty EG, Simmons CF. Fluid and electrolyte management. In: Cloherty JP, Eichenwald EC, Stark AR, eds. *Manual of Neonatal Care,* 6th ed. Philadelphia: Wolters Kluwer/Lippincott Williams & Wilkins; 2008:100–113.
21. Stephens BE, Gargus RA, Walden RV, et al. Fluid regimens in the first week of life may increase risk of patent ductus arteriosus in extremely low birth weight infants. *J Perinatol.* 2008;28:123–128.
22. Kim SM, Lee EY, Chen J, et al. Improved care and growth outcomes by using hybrid humidified incubators in very preterm infants. *Pediatrics.* 2010;125:e137–e145.
23. Putet G. Lipid metabolism of the micropremie. *Clin Perinatol.* 2000;27:57–69.
24. Schanler RJ, Anderson D. The low birth weight infant. Inpatient care. In: Duggan C, Watkins JB, Walker WA, eds. *Nutrition in Pediatrics: Basic Science Clinical Applications,* 4th ed. Hamilton, Ontario, Canada: BC Decker; 2008:377–394.
25. Helms RA, Christensen ML, Mauer EC, et al. Comparison of pediatric versus standard amino acid formulation in preterm neonates requiring parenteral nutrition. *J Pediatr.* 1987;110:466–472.
26. Rivera A, Bell EF, Stegink LD, Ziegler EE. Plasma amino acid profiles during the first three days of life in infants with respiratory distress syndrome: effect of parenteral amino acid supplementation. *J Pediatr.* 1989;115:464–468.
27. American Academy of Pediatrics Committee on Nutrition. Parenteral nutrition. In: Kleinman RE, ed. *Pediatric Nutrition Handbook,* 6th ed. Elk Grove Village, IL: American Academy of Pediatrics; 2009:519–540.
28. Dunn L, Hulman S, Weiner J, Kliegman R. Beneficial effects of early hypocaloric enteral feeding on neonatal gastrointestinal function: preliminary report of a randomized trial. *J Pediatr.* 1988;112:622–629.
29. Schanler RJ, Shulman RJ, Lau C. Feeding strategies for premature infants: beneficial outcomes of feeding fortified human milk versus preterm formula. *Pediatrics.* 1999;103:1150–1157.
30. Morales Y, Schanler RJ. Human milk and clinical outcomes in VLBW infants: how compelling is the evidence of benefit? *Sem Perinatol.* 2007;31:83–88.
31. Institute of Medicine. *Dietary Reference Intakes for Vitamin C, Vitamin E, Selenium, and Carotenoids.* Washington, DC: National Academies Press; 2000.
32. Tyson JE, Wright LL, Oh W, et al. Vitamin A supplementation for extremely-low-birth-weight infants. *N Eng J Med.* 1999;340:1962–1968.
33. Mitchell SM, Rogers S, Hicks PD, et al. High frequencies of elevated alkaline phosphatase activity and rickets exist in extremely low birth weight infants despite current nutritional support. *BMC Pediatr.* 2009;9:47. doi:10.1186/1471-2431-9-47.

34. Kliegman RM. Intrauterine growth restriction. In: Martin RJ, Fanaroff AA, Walsh MC, eds. *Fanaroff and Martin's Neonatal-Perinatal Medicine Diseases of the Fetus and Infant,* 8th ed. Philadelphia: Mosby/Elsevier; 2006:271–306.
35. Koo WWK, Krug-Wispe S, Neylan M, et al. Effect of three levels of vitamin D intake in preterm infants receiving high mineral containing milk. *J Pediatr Gastroenterol Nutr.* 1995;21:182–189.
36. Rao R, Geoergieff M. Microminerals. In: Tsang RC, Uauy R, Koletzlo B, Zlotkin SH, eds. *Nutrition of the Preterm Infant: Scientific Basis and Practical Guidelines.* Cincinnati, OH: Digital Educational Publishing; 2005:277–310.
37. Shulman RJ. Zinc and copper balance studies in infants receiving total parenteral nutrition. *Am J Clin Nutr.* 1989;49:879–883.
38. Heird WC, Lapillonne A. The role of essential fatty acids in development. *Annu Rev Nutr.* 2005;25:549–571.
39. Rogers S, Hicks PD, Hamzo M, et al. Continuous feedings of fortified human milk lead to nutrient losses of fat, calcium and phosphorous. *Nutrients.* 2010;2:230–240. doi:10.3390/nu2030240.
40. Hurst NM, Valentine CJ, Renfro L, et al. Skin-to-skin holding in the neonatal intensive care unit influences maternal milk volume. *J Perinatol.* 1997;17:213–217.
41. Kalhan SC, Price PT. Nutrition and selected disorders of the gastrointestinal tract. In: Klaus MH, Fanaroff AA, eds. *Care of the High-Risk Neonate,* 5th ed. Philadelphia: W. B. Saunders; 2001:147–194.
42. Dell KM, Davis ID. Fluid, electrolyte, and acid base homeostasis. In: Martin RJ, Fanaroff AA, Walsh MC, eds. *Fanaroff and Martin's Neonatal-Perinatal Medicine Diseases of the Fetus and Infant,* 8th ed. Philadelphia: Mosby Elsevier; 2006:695–712.
43. Anderson DM. Nutritional assessment and therapeutic interventions for the preterm infant. *Clin Peri.* 2002;29:313–326.
44. Vaucher YE, Harrison GG, Udall JN, Morrow G. Skinfold thickness in North American infants 24–41 weeks gestation. *Hum Biol.* 1984;56:713–731.
45. Sasanow SR, Georgieff MK, Pereira GR. Mid-arm circumference and mid-arm/head circumference ratios: standard curves for anthropometric assessment of the neonatal nutritional status. *J Pediatr.* 1986;109:311–315.
46. Metabolic Management Committee. Nutrition. In: Anderson DM, Eichenwald EC, Chan SW, et al., eds. *Guidelines for Acute Care of the Neonate,* 17th ed. Houston, TX: Section of Neonatology Department of Pediatrics, Baylor College of Medicine; 2009: 97–108.
47. Premji SS, Paes B, Jacobson K, et al. Evidence-based feeding guidelines for very low-birth-weight infants. *Adv Neonat Care.* 2002;2:5–18.
48. Moyer-Mileur LJ. Anthropometric and laboratory assessment of very low birth weight infants: the most helpful measurements and why. *Sem Perinatol.* 2007;31:96–103.
49. Ridout E, Melara D, Rottinghaus S, et al. Blood urea nitrogen concentration as a marker of amino-acid intolerance in neonates with birthweight less than 1250 g. *J Perinatol.* 2005;25:130–133.
50. Arslanoglu S, Moro GE, Ziegler EE. Preterm infants fed fortified human milk receive less protein than they need. *J Perinatol.* 2009;29:489–492.
51. American Academy of Pediatrics Committee on Fetus and Newborn. Hospital discharge of the high-risk neonate. *Pediatrics.* 2008;122:1119–1126.
52. American Academy of Pediatrics, Wagner CL, Greer FR, Section on Breastfeeding and Committee on Nutrition. Prevention of rickets and vitamin D deficiency in infants, children, and adolescents. *Pediatrics.* 2008;122:1142–1152.

CHAPTER 5

Infant Nutrition

Susan Akers and Sharon Groh-Wargo

Introduction

This chapter addresses the current recommended feeding practices for healthy, full-term infants and common feeding problems encountered during the first year of life.

Nutrition Issues at Birth

All states in the United States encourage parents to have their newborn infants tested for congenital disorders within 48 hours of life. Actual test procedures and the various disorders screened are state specific. Most states screen for a core panel of 29 disorders, with the additional potential for 25 others.[1]

The goal of newborn screening is to identify congenital disorders such as inborn errors of metabolism, endocrine disorders, and perinatally acquired infectious diseases before symptoms occur. Some of these disorders, such as phenyl ketonuria, are treatable with alterations in nutrition. (See Chapter 9 for nutrition management of inborn errors of metabolism.)

Nutrient Needs

Newborn infants are born with a relatively poor vitamin K status. Therefore, a one-time intramuscular injection of 0.5–1 mg vitamin K is recommended for all newborn infants at birth.[2] Most newborns can obtain all necessary nutrient requirements from human milk or infant formula alone except for vitamin D. As the infant reaches 4 to 6 months, nutrient needs become greater than human milk or formula alone can provide. Solid foods become necessary for adequate satiety. Supplemental iron and fluoride also may become necessary. During infancy, distribution of calories is generally recommended to be 40–50% fat and 7–11% protein, with the remaining calories from carbohydrates.[3] Fluid needs are estimated at 700 mL per day for 0- to 6-month-old infants and 800 mL per day for 7- to 12-month-old infants.[4] Average estimated daily energy requirements (kcal/kg) based on reference body weights for 0 to 6 months (6 kg) and 7 to 12 months (9 kg) of age are 90 kcal/kg and 80 kcal/kg, respectively, with a range of 80–110 kcal/kg. Specific energy needs can be estimated with the equations in **Exhibit 5-1**.[3] Mean daily protein needs are estimated at 1.5 g protein/kg for 0- to 6-month-old and 1.2 g protein/kg for 7- to 12-month-old infants. DRIs are available online at http://www.nap.edu (see Appendix F).

Breastfeeding

Breastfeeding is the recommended method of feeding for virtually all infants.[2,5] Both the American Academy of Pediatrics (AAP)[6] and the American Dietetic Association (ADA)[7] promote breastfeeding as the best source of infant nutrition.

Nutritional and health advantages commonly listed for human milk and breastfeeding include:

- Superior nutritional composition[5–8]
- Provision of immunologic and enzymatic components[5,6]
- Health benefits for mothers[5,6]
- Lower cost and increased convenience[6]
- Enhanced maternal–infant bonding[5]
- Decreased incidence of respiratory and gastrointestinal infections[6,9]
- Leaner body composition for infants at 1 year of age[10]
- Decreased incidence of atopic dermatitis[11]
- Controversial benefits of decreased risk for obesity in adulthood[12,13] and improved cognitive development[8]

Human milk is not a uniform body of fluids but a secretion of the mammary gland with changing composition.[5] The composition of human milk varies from individual to individual and also with stage of lactation, time of day, time into feeding, and maternal diet[14] (see **Table 5-1**). The four stages of human milk expression are colostrum, transitional milk, mature milk, and extended lactation, each containing its own significant biochemical components and properties:

- Colostrum is the milk produced during the first several days following delivery. It is lower in fat and energy than mature milk but higher in protein, fat-soluble vitamins, minerals, and electrolytes.[5] This early stage of lactation also provides a rich source of antibodies.[7] Colostrum has an 80:20 ratio of casein to whey, which decreases to about 55:45 in mature human milk.[5]

- Transition milk begins approximately 7 to 14 days postpartum, when the concentration of immunoglobulins and total proteins decreases and the amount of lactose, fat, and total calories increases.[5]
- The third phase, beginning at about 2 weeks postpartum, referred to as mature milk and detailed in Table 5-1, continues throughout lactation until about 7 to 8 months.[5]
- Extended lactation (7 months to 2 years) results in milk different from colostrum, transitional, and mature human milk. Its carbohydrate, protein, and fat content remains relatively stable, but concentrations of vitamins and minerals (such as calcium and zinc) continue to decrease gradually over time until weaning off breast milk.[5,15]

The nutritional requirements during lactation are high, exceeding those in both pregnancy and the nonpregnant state, and are designed to meet the additional demands of lactation without compromising the mother's nutrient stores.[14] The DRIs for the lactation period can be found online at http://www.nap.edu. In general, the recommendations for breastfeeding women during lactation include a well-balanced diet and an additional 300–400 calories, which includes 25 grams of protein per day for milk production. For mothers not motivated to eat a well-balanced diet or for those avoiding primary food groups, continuation of a prenatal vitamin and possibly calcium supplementation are recommended. Energy requirements are greater if weight gain during pregnancy was low, weight during lactation falls below standards for height and age, and/or more than one infant is being nursed. Iron supplementation of the mother should be continued postpartum in order to replenish iron stores depleted by pregnancy.[16] Most breastfeeding women experience increased thirst.

TABLE 5-1 Composition of Mature Human Milk and Cow Milk

Nutrient (per liter)	Human Milk	Cow Milk
Macronutrients		
Energy (kcal)	650–700	627
Protein (g)	9	32
Carbohydrate (g)	67–70	46
Fat (g)	35	35
Vitamins		
Retinol (mg)	0.3–0.6	Variable
Carotenoids (mg)	0.2–0.6	N/A
Vitamin D (μg)	0.33	—*
Vitamin E (mg)	3–8	0.4
Vitamin K (μg)	2–3	1–4
Vitamin C (mg)	100	30
Thiamine (μg)	200	388
Riboflavin (μg)	400–600	914
Vitamin B_6 (μg)	90–310	554
Vitamin B_{12} (μg)	0.5–1	4.3
Nicotinic acid (μg)	1800–6000	1667
Folic acid (μg)	80–140	60
Pantothenic acid (μg)	2000–2500	3251
Biotin (μg)	5–9	47
Minerals		
Calcium (mg)	200–250	1150
Phosphorus (mg)	120–140	910
Magnesium (mg)	30–35	96
Iron (mg)	0.3–0.9	0.5
Zinc (μg)	1000–3000	4
Manganese (μg)	3	40
Copper (μg)	200–400	30
Chromium (μg)	0.5	< 5
Selenium (μg)	7–33	Variable
Fluoride (μg)	4–15	45
Sodium (mg)	120–250	515
Potassium (mg)	400–550	1400
Chloride (mg)	400–450	970
Other Composition Data		
Protein source	60–70% whey; 30–40% casein	18% whey; 82% casein
% calories protein	6–7	20
Carbohydrate source	Lactose	Lactose
% calories carbohydrate	43	30
Fat source	Human	Butterfat
% calories fat	50	50
Potential renal solute load (mOsm/L)	93	308
Osmolality (mOsm/kg H_2O)	290–300	275

*Vitamin D added.

Abbreviation: N/A, not available.

Sources: Data from Lawrence RA, Lawrence RM. *Breastfeeding: A Guide for the Medical Profession*, 6th ed. St. Louis, MO: Mosby; 2005; American Academy of Pediatrics, American College of Obstetricians and Gynecologists. *Breastfeeding Handbook for Physicians.* 2006; Fomon SJ. *Nutrition of Normal Infants*. St. Louis, MO: Mosby; 1993; and Jensen RG. *Handbook of Milk Composition*. New York: Academic Press; 1995.

EXHIBIT 5-1 Equations for Calculating Energy Needs of Infants

0–3 months: (89 × weight [kg] − 100) + 175 kcal
4–6 months: (89 × weight [kg] − 100) + 56 kcal
7–12 months: (89 × weight [kg] − 100) + 22 kcal

Source: Data from Institute of Medicine. *Dietary Reference Intakes for Energy, Carbohydrate, Fiber, Fat, Fatty Acids, Cholesterol, Protein, and Amino Acids (Macronutrients)*. Washington, DC: National Academies Press; 2005.

This should naturally result in additional intake of fluids. Regular exercise and weight loss up to 2 kg per month should not affect milk production.[17]

In summary, the composition of breast milk remains stable even with significant variability in women's diets. Except in cases of chronic deficiency, the quantity and quality of breast milk can support growth and promote the health of infants even when the mother's supply of nutrients is somewhat limited.[11] However, maternal diet can affect milk composition in the following ways:

- Fatty acid composition mirrors maternal intake.[8,14]
- Vitamin content is reduced in maternal deficiency and increases with supplementation.
- Mineral content is generally unaffected by maternal intake except for selenium and iodine.[5]
- Colic symptoms may appear in babies whose mothers drink a lot of cow's milk, due to transmission of allergens in the milk.[18]
- Caffeine, nicotine, and alcohol will pass into milk and may cause adverse effects in the baby when maternal consumption is high.[5,19,20]
- Medications, both prescription and over-the-counter, and environmental contaminants may pass into milk.[2,5,6]

Successful lactation is greatly influenced by the mother's motivation and confidence and by the support she receives from others. Infant suckling stimulates the release of hormones: prolactin, which is responsible for milk production, and oxytocin, which is responsible for milk release, from the pituitary.[21] In order to establish and sustain lactation, the baby needs to have access to the breast on demand. The more a mother nurses, the more milk she will produce. The following list offers some tips for ensuring breastfeeding success:

- *Initial breastfeeding:* This should take place as soon after delivery as possible, ideally within the first hour of life.
- *Positioning:* The mother should find a comfortable position either lying down or sitting up. Pillows can support the baby's body and the mother's back and arms. She should change the position of the baby with every feeding during the first few weeks so that pressure on the mother's nipple is rotated. The mother should use one hand to support and guide her breast and the other hand around the baby's back, cupping the infant's bottom to provide support.
- *Latching on:* The mother can stimulate the rooting reflex by touching the baby's closest cheek. When the mouth is open wide, she pulls the baby close. Be sure that most of the mother's areola is in the baby's mouth, the baby's lower lip is turned out, and the tongue is under the mother's nipple. Rapid sucking, followed by slower, rhythmic sucking and swallowing, will stimulate the milk ejection reflex (MER), or the actual release of milk. Signs that let-down has occurred include rapid swallowing by the infant, tingling in the breast, tightening in the uterus, milk around the baby's mouth, or milk dripping from the other breast. The mother can insert her finger in the side of the baby's mouth to break the suction before moving the baby off the breast.
- *Timing:* During the first few weeks, the baby should be nursed 8 to 12 times a day, or about every 2 to 3 hours. The feedings will become less frequent after breastfeeding is established. It is more important to completely empty the first breast and get adequate hind milk than it is to breastfeed from both sides. Alternating breasts from feeding to feeding establishes good milk supply on both sides. The baby should dictate the duration of feeding.
- *Assessing adequacy (or "How do I know if my baby is getting enough?"):* A newborn who is receiving adequate fluid and calories will (1) have at least six to eight thoroughly wet diapers a day (or only four to five heavy wet diapers if they are disposable); (2) have a bowel movement with most feedings; (3) nurse 8 to 12 times a day; (4) seem satisfied after nursing; and (5) gain approximately 1 oz each day in the first 3 months of life.[5,21,22]

A number of situations arise during the early weeks of breastfeeding that, if unanticipated and poorly managed, can jeopardize a successful nursing experience. Some of the most common complaints include sore nipples, engorgement, jaundice, and poor milk supply. Online or local support can help with these problems. Moms returning to work or school after their babies are born can continue to breastfeed by:

- Arranging to go to the baby or having the baby brought to them
- Pumping and saving the milk in a refrigerator for use within 48 hours or a freezer for up to 3 months
- Discontinuing the feeding(s) when they are away but continuing to nurse at other times

There are several good sources that discuss these alternatives, as well as issues related to milk storage.[5,21–24]

Infant Formulas

Breast milk composition is the gold standard by which infant formulas are modeled. However, when breastfeeding is not chosen, is unsuccessful, or is stopped before 1 year of age, bottle-feeding with a commercially prepared iron-fortified infant formula is the recommended alternative.[2] The infant formula market continues to expand and offers a wide variety of products.

Types of Formulas

Formulas are grouped by the following categories: standard, soy, protein hydrolysate, elemental or amino acid, and follow-up formulas. See **Table 5-2** for an overview of infant formula products. Formulas for premature infants or children older than 1 year old are discussed in Chapters 4 and 6.

The most common human milk substitute is standard infant formula. These formulas are made from cow's milk by removing the butterfat, adding vegetable oils, and decreasing the protein. Standard formulas vary in their ratio of casein to whey. Approximately 40–50% of energy provided by standard infant formula comes from fat.[2] The addition of arachidonic acid (ARA) and docosahexaenoic acid (DHA) to infant formulas is recognized as safe.

Although the incidence of primary lactose intolerance remains rare in infancy, the infant formula market does include lactose-free products. The only indications for using a lactose-free formula are galactosemia, primary lactase deficiency, and relief of temporary or secondary lactose intolerance following gastroenteritis.[25]

Prebiotics, probiotics, and mixtures of pre- and probiotics are now being added to infant formulas. Oligosaccharides function as prebiotics and are the third most abundant component of human milk.[26] There are fewer concerns about potential adverse effects of probiotic-supplemented products when they are fed to infants older than 5 months due to their more mature immune response, an established intestinal colonization, and exposure to a variety of organisms from the environment.[27]

Cow's milk–based formulas thickened with added rice starch are available for infants with gastroesophageal reflux (GER).[25] An added rice starch formula intended to help babies sleep longer is also available (http://www.mjn.com). (Also see Chapter 12.) Standard formulas are marketed as iron fortified (12 mg/quart) and low iron (1 mg/quart). Only the iron-fortified formulas meet the iron requirements of infancy; the AAP has discouraged the use of low-iron formulas.[28]

Soy formulas can be useful for infants with galactosemia, with congenital lactase deficiency, or who are born to families practicing vegetarianism.[25] Soy formulas should not be used for infants with cow's milk protein (CMP) allergy. About 10–14% of infants with CMP allergy will also have a soy allergy.[29,30] Infants with CMP allergy or those with CMP-induced enteropathy or enterocolitis should be fed protein hydrolysates or amino acid–based formulas.

Soy formulas contain methionine-, carnitine-, and taurine-fortified soy protein isolate. The protein content of soy formula is higher than that of standard formula because the biologic value of soy protein is lower than cow's milk protein. Soy formulas contain a blend of vegetable oils and most are supplemented with ARA and DHA. All soy formulas are lactose-free, and some are also sucrose-free or corn-free. Soy phytates and fiber oligosaccharides contained in soy formulas interfere with the absorption of calcium, phosphorous, zinc, and iron and, as a result, calcium and phosphorous levels in soy formulas are 20% higher than cow's milk–based formulas. They also are fortified with zinc and iron.[28,29] Overall, soy formulas are adequate for promoting normal growth and development when fed to full-term, healthy infants. Soy formulas are not recommended for premature infants.[31]

Indications for using hydrolyzed protein formulas include CMP allergy, soy allergy, or significant nutritional challenges related to a variety of gastrointestinal or liver diseases.[25,30] Both partially hydrolyzed and extensively hydrolyzed formulas are available. Extensively hydrolyzed formulas contain only peptides that have a low molecular weight and are considered truly hypoallergenic.[30] Hydrolyzed formulas should be used during the first year of life for infants who are at risk for atopic disease when exclusive breastfeeding for 4 to 6 months is not possible or for infants who are formula fed.[30] Sources of carbohydrate and fat vary among the protein hydrolysate formulas and should be considered when they are fed for indications other than protein allergy or hypersensitivity. Extensively hydrolyzed formulas are significantly more expensive than milk- or soy-based formulas.

Infants with severe protein hypersensitivity and persistence of symptoms on other formulas can be switched to nonallergenic, amino acid–based formulas.[25]Amino acid–based formulas are extremely expensive and difficult for families to obtain. WIC participants in some states can obtain these formulas; other families must pay out of pocket or fight for insurance coverage.

"Follow-up formulas" are designed for older infants and toddlers who are taking solid foods but not enough to meet all essential nutrients needed for optimal growth and development.[25] These formulas offer no clearly established superiority over traditional formulas or breast milk for infants, but they may be appropriate as a beverage for a toddler whose diet is consistently poor.[2] In general, follow-up formulas cost less than standard infant formula but more than cow's milk and are higher in iron than cow's milk.

Evaporated milk preparations for infants should not be used due to their inadequate nutrient composition.[2] Although not recommended, a home-prepared formula from evaporated milk is probably preferable to using unmodified cows' milk when commercial formula or breast milk is temporarily unavailable. The usual recipe is one can of evaporated whole milk (13 oz), 19.5 oz of water, and 3 tablespoons of sugar or corn syrup.[32]

TABLE 5-2 Summary of Formula Products for Infants and Young Toddlers

Product Names	Manufacturer	Comments on Composition[#]	Forms Available[§]				
			P	LC	RTF	H	ALL
Milk-Based: For healthy full term infants when breast milk not available							
Enfamil Premium Triple Health Guard	Mead Johnson	Prebiotic; Nucleotides					✓
Nestle Good Start Gentle Plus	Gerber		✓	✓	✓		
Nestle Good Start Protect Plus	Gerber	Probiotic	✓				
Nestle Good Start Nourish Plus	Gerber	No DHA/ARA	✓				
Similac Advance Early Shield	Abbott Nutrition	Prebiotic; carotenoids; nucleotides					✓
Similac Organic	Abbott Nutrition	Certified USDA organic; nucleotides	✓		✓	✓	
Store Brand Standard	PBM Products*	Nucleotides	✓				
Store Brand Organic	PBM Products*	Certified USDA organic; nucleotides	✓				
Store Brand Prebiotic	PBM Products*	Prebiotic; nucleotides	✓				
Store Brand Probiotic	PBM Products*	Probiotic	✓				
Milk-Based Low/No Lactose: Perceived sensitivity to lactose; fussiness; gas							
Enfamil Gentlease	Mead Johnson	Partially hydrolyzed protein; reduced lactose	✓				
Similac Sensitive	Abbott Nutrition	Lactose free; nucleotides					✓
Store Brand Sensitivity	PBM Products*	Lactose free; nucleotides	✓				
Store Brand Gentle	PBM Products*	Partially hydrolyzed protein; reduced lactose	✓				
Milk-Based Added Rice Starch: Frequent spit-up							
Enfamil A.R	Mead Johnson		✓		✓	✓	
Similac Sensitive RS	Abbott Nutrition	Lactose free	✓		✓		
Store Brand Added Rice Starch	PBM Products*		✓				
Soy-Based: Galactosemia; lactose free for primary or secondary lactose intolerance; vegetarian family							
Good Start Soy Plus	Gerber		✓	✓	✓		
Isomil Advance	Abbott Nutrition						✓
Isomil DF	Abbott Nutrition	Added dietary fiber to firm loose/watery stools			✓		
Prosobee	Mead Johnson						✓
Store Brand Soy	PBM Products*		✓				
Store Brand Organic Soy	PBM Products*	Certified USDA organic	✓				
Protein Hydrolysate: hypoallergenic; extensively hydrolyted protein for allergy to cow milk							
Alimentum	Abbott Nutrition		✓		✓	✓	
Nutramigen	Mead Johnson						✓
Nutramigen with Enflora LGG	Mead Johnson	Probiotic	✓				
Pregestimil	Mead Johnson		✓			✓	
Amino Acid–Based: nonallergenic; elemental formula for severe cow milk protein allergy							
EleCare	Abbott Nutrition	33% MCT	✓				
Neocate Infant	Nutricia	5% MCT; No DNA or ARA	✓				
Neocate Infant with DNA and ARA	Nutricia	33% MCT	✓				
Nutramigen AA	Mead Johnson	0% MCT	✓				

(continues)

TABLE 5-2 *(Continued)*

Product Names	Manufacturer	Comments on Composition[#]	Forms Available[§]				
			P	LC	RTF	H	ALL
Follow-up: complete nutrition for older infants and toddlers							
Enfagrow Premium Next Step	Mead Johnson	10–36 months	✓		✓		
Enfagrow Premium Next Step Soy	Mead Johnson	10–36 months	✓				
Go and Grow Milk-Based	Abbott Nutrition	9–24 months	✓				
Go and Grow Soy-Based	Abbott Nutrition	9–24 months	✓				
Good Start Gentle Plus 2	Gerber	9–24 months	✓				
Good Start Protect Plus 2	Gerber	9–24 months; Probiotic added	✓				
Good Start Soy Plus 2	Gerber	9–24 months	✓				
Store Brand Follow-up	PBM Products*	9 months and older	✓				

#Products contain DHA and ARA unless otherwise noted

*Store brands include: CVS/pharmacy; Walgreens; Wegmans; AAFES; Publix; Target; PathMark; Sam's Club; NEX; VyVee; Shopko; Walmart; RiteAid; Topco; ToysRus; Safeway; Giant Eagle; Weis; Food Lion; Price Chopper; Meijer; BJ's; Winn Dixie; Western Family; Drug Mart; Kroger; Ralphs; Fry's; QFC; Dillons; Smith's; King Soopers; FredMeyer; Food4Less; Roundy's; SuperValu; Albertsons; Jewel-Osco; Cub Foods; ACME; Bigg's; Shaw's Star; Amway

§P = powder; LC = liquid concentrate; RTF = ready to feed; H = ready to feed for hospital use.

Sources: Table data retrieved from manufacturers' websites (accessed January 10, 2010): Abbott Nutrition, http://abbottnutrition.com; Gerber, http://www.gerber.com; Mead Johnson, http://www.mjn.com; Nutricia, http://www.nutriciahealthcare.com; WalMart Store Brand, http://www.pbmproducts.com (detailed nutritional information on WalMart Store Brand at http://www.parentschoicemedical.com).

Evaporated milk formula has all of the same disadvantages as unmodified cow's milk: poorly digested fat; low concentration of essential fatty acids, iron, zinc, and vitamins E and C; and excessive amounts of protein, sodium, potassium, chloride, and phosphorous. A multivitamin supplement is recommended, and additional iron is needed unless the infant takes sufficient quantities of appropriate solid foods. After 6 months of age, supplemental fluoride is prescribed unless the water used in formula preparation is fluoridated.[2]

Goat's milk is not recommended. If fed to infants, goat's milk must be supplemented with folic acid.[2] Cow's milk is not recommended until 1 year of age.[2] Soy (e.g., Silk), rice (e.g., Rice Dream), and almond (e.g., Blue Diamond Almond Breeze) "milks" are not nutritionally adequate for infants and should not be fed during the first year of life.[2]

Infant Formula Preparation and Feedings

Infant formulas come packaged in three ways: ready-to-feed, concentrated liquid, and powder. Ready-to-feed formulas provide sterile feedings of known caloric concentration for those who like the convenience. Ready-to-feed formulas do not contain fluoride. Concentrated liquid formulas are readily available and mix easily by combining with water in a 1:1 ratio. Powder is ideal if only a small amount of formula is desired, and it may be the least expensive form of formula. Powder formula is generally prepared by mixing one level scoop of powder with 2 ounces of water. It is important to use the scoop provided in the can of powder because scoop sizes vary across different formula powders.

The source of water is important to consider. Both powder and concentrated liquid formula can be the source of fluoride for the infant if reconstituted with fluoridated water. This is especially important when the infant reaches 6 months of life and needs a source of dietary fluoride. Infant formula should be mixed with cold tap water that's brought to a boil and then boiled for 1 minute and cooled.[33] Boiling longer than 1 minute may concentrate the minerals in the water to an undesirable degree.[2] For most infants older than 3 months of age, the water does not need to be boiled, and the formula can be prepared with tap water.[34] Bottled waters, including distilled and spring water, cannot be assumed to be sterile unless specifically labeled as such.[35] Bottled "nursery" water is sold near infant formula in many stores and is often labeled as sterile.

Hands should be washed thoroughly before mixing and feeding the formula. All equipment used in preparing and storing the formula should be clean and the formula should be fed from clean bottles and nipples. Bottles made of polycarbonate plastic contain bisphenol A, an environmental toxin. Infants may experience low-dose exposure to bisphenol A due to leaching from the bottle, especially if the plastic is scratched or worn.

Most prepared formulas can be kept in the refrigerator for 24 to 48 hours; however, it is safest to consume formula within 24 hours. Open cans of powder have a 30-day shelf life. Powder formulas are not sterile and may contain the bacterium *Enterobacter sakazakii*.[36] Safe handling practices are especially important for reconstituting powders for very young infants. Mixing the smallest batch of formula practical and limiting storage periods decreases the time a potential pathogen has to proliferate.

Warming a bottle is best done by putting the unopened bottle in a bowl of warm water for 5 to 10 minutes prior to feeding.[2] Microwave heating is not advised. An update on infant formula for consumers entitled "FDA 101: Infant Formula" is available at http://www.fda.gov/ForConsumers/ConsumerUpdates/ucm048694.htm.

Good bottle-feeding technique includes holding the infant so that face-to-face contact is maximized and tilting the bottle so that the nipple is filled with milk. Bottles should never be propped, because this can cause dental caries.[34] Breast- or bottle-feeding in the supine position is associated with an increased risk of ear infections.[37] Infants should be fed in a semi-upright position. Sugar should not be added to the formula or sucrose-containing fluids placed in the bottle because this increases the risk of dental caries.[2,34] Adding solids, such as cereal, to the bottle also is not recommended.[34]

Most infants can finish a bottle in 15 to 30 minutes. If most feedings exceed this time frame, a pediatric feeding specialist should evaluate the infant to rule out any severe oral or motor delay or dysfunction. Other possible reasons for slow feeding include a nipple with a hole that is too small or clogged or a collapsed nipple. Burping is usually done midway through the feeding and at the end of the feeding. Partially used bottles should be discarded after the feeding and not saved for the next feeding time. Beginning at birth to 4 months of age, an infant will need to be fed 2 to 6 ounces per feeding and fed 8 to 12 times each day. By 12 months of age, the infant will be fed 7 to 8 ounces per feeding but only fed 3 to 4 times each day.[38]

Nutrient Supplements

A one-time intramuscular dose of vitamin K (0.5–1.0 mg) is needed at birth.[2] Additionally, vitamin D, iron, and fluoride need to be supplemented during infancy. **Table 5-3** provides the composition of selected infant vitamin and mineral drops.

Vitamin D has important extraskeletal effects, including protection against infection, and deficiency can result in rickets.[39–41] Thus, all newborn infants should be supplemented with 400 IU vitamin D per day within the first few days of life.[39] Supplementation should continue until at least 1 liter per day of vitamin D–fortified milk is consumed. Infants particularly at risk for vitamin D deficiency are those who live at higher latitudes (particularly above 40°), especially during the winter, and are dark skinned. Consideration should be given to supplementing these high-risk infants with up to 800 IU vitamin D per day.[40]

Full-term infants usually have adequate iron stores for the first 4 to 6 months of life.[2] Although the amount of iron in human milk is minimal, its bioavailability is quite high, approximately five times greater than cow's milk.[2] However, by 6 months of age exclusively breastfed infants require additional iron (1 mg/kg/day) either as a supplement or through the introduction of sufficient iron-fortified infant cereal and/or meat.[2,42,43] The AAP supports the use of iron-fortified formulas (12 mg iron/quart) as the preferred alternative to feeding infants if breastfeeding is not chosen.[2] Iron-fortified formula provides approximately 2 mg/kg per day of iron when fed at about 120 kcal/kg per day. Maintaining a good iron status decreases the risk of iron-deficiency anemia and its irreversible association with cognitive and motor impairments.[2]

A source of dietary fluoride is recommended for infants after 6 months of age. Commercial formulas do not contain fluoride unless mixed with fluoridated water. A daily supplement of 0.25 mg fluoride is recommended for infants older than 6 months of age who live in areas where tap or well water supplies contain less than 0.3 ppm of fluoride, who consume ready-to-feed formula or formula reconstituted with nonfluoridated bottled water, or who are exclusively breastfed.[2]

Diets of breastfeeding mothers should be assessed for adequacy of vitamin B_{12} if the mother is following an animal protein–restricted diet, especially those who comply with vegan guidelines.[2] When the mother takes a limited diet in any nutrient, supplementation is indicated for both the mother and infant.

Solid Food

During infancy, the most important source of nutrition for growth and development is breast milk or infant formulas. During the second half of infancy, the addition of infant cereal and solid foods benefits the infant nutritionally and developmentally. Complementary feedings allow infants to be exposed to an array of flavors and food textures that can initiate lifelong healthy eating habits. There is no nutritional benefit to adding solids to an infant's diet until at least the fourth month of life or, ideally, closer to 6 months of age.[2]

Infants who are exclusively breastfed may benefit from the addition of complementary foods earlier than those who are formula fed.[2] Around 6 months of age, breastfed infants may be at risk for iron deficiency anemia and can benefit from an additional iron source such as iron-fortified cereals or meats. When considering the introduction of complementary foods, caregivers should consider the individual readiness of the infant along with the following potential concerns:

- Energy requirements and growth of the infant
- Iron and zinc status of the infant and foods being introduced

TABLE 5-3 Composition of Selected Infant Vitamin and Mineral Drops (1 mL)

Product	Brand Name and Manufacturer	Vitamin D (IU)	Vitamin C (mg)	Vitamin A (IU)	Iron (mg)	Fluoride (mg)
Tri-Vitamin	Tri-Vi-Sol (Mead Johnson)	400	35	1500		
Tri-Vitamin with Iron	Tri-Vi-Sol with Iron (Mead Johnson)	400	35	1500	10	
Vitamin D	D-Vi-Sol (Mead Johnson)	400				
Iron	Fer-In-Sol (Mead Johnson)				15	
Fluoride	Luride* (Colgate)					0.5

*Prescription required

Sources: Table data retrieved from manufacturers' websites (accessed July 31, 2011): Mead Johnson, http://www.mjn.com; Colgate, http:// www.colgate.com.

- Risk of infectious morbidity for the infant (mainly in underdeveloped countries where sanitation is a concern)
- Potential risk of atopic disease if there is a personal or family history of intolerance
- Long-term impact on neurocognitive development and behavior

Readiness to start solid foods generally occurs during the first 4 to 6 months of life. Observations of individual physical and psychological developments are better determinants of readiness for starting complementary foods than age alone. All infants develop at different rates, and caregivers should respect this unique trait and level of comfort with initiating spoon-feeding and new textures. Awareness of the infant's hunger and satiety cues with spoon-feeding are just as important as feeding cues during breast- and bottle-feeding. Infants who turn away during a feeding are usually indicating that they are satisfied and want the feeding to stop. "Infants have the innate ability to self regulate their energy intake."[44] This self-regulating instinct can be affected by factors such as coercive feeding, overly restrictive feeding, or the feeding environment in general. Encouraging infants to establish a healthy self-confidence with regard to satiety and hunger is one of the most important aspects of infant feeding. Feedings should transition from exclusive liquids at birth, with breast milk or iron-fortified formulas, to a well-balanced diet of table foods shared by the family at 1 year of age.

Physical readiness includes gross motor development as well as oral motor development. Prior to 4 months of age, infants have poor head control and are uncoordinated with lip closure. Additionally, infants possess an extrusion reflex that permits them to swallow only liquid foods easily.[45] During this phase, infants have limited or no interest in oral feeding other than breast- or bottle-feeding. Around 4 to 6 months of age, infants learn oral and gross motor skills that aid in accepting solid foods. At this age, oral motor skills evolve from the reflexive suck to the ability to swallow nonliquid foods and to transfer contents from the front of the tongue to the back of the mouth. Gross motor development includes sitting independently and maintaining balance while using hands to reach and grasp for objects.[42] Head control is improved, and infants are ready to sit in high chairs and grasp pieces of food. Infants will begin to turn toward food or watch others eating, but still lack the hand-to-mouth coordination necessary to feed themselves.[46]

Independent eating behaviors usually begin during the fourth month of life.[47] By 6 months, infants are able to indicate a desire for food by opening their mouth, leaning forward to indicate hunger, and turning away to show disinterest or satiety. Until an infant can express these feelings, feeding of solids will probably represent a type of forced feeding, potentially leading to overfeeding and risk of obesity and/or general anxiety toward eating.

In addition to determining the quantity of feedings, infants should be encouraged to develop more independence with feeding in the following ways:

- Self-feeding of soft finger foods
- Sipping from a cup by 6 to 8 months of age[47]
- Holding the bottle or cup independently
- Controlling the timing of feeds in an effort to promote self-regulation of hunger and satiety[48]

A variety of foods should be experienced throughout infancy. The introduction of unfamiliar foods allows the infant to gain experience with various tastes and textures, promoting successful weaning to the family diet. Caregivers who find it difficult to give freedom or control to infants with self-feeding often promote frustration and insecurity with regards to eating. Food refusal and failure to thrive often result from this negative feeding environment.

As solid foods displace breast milk or formula in the diet, vitamin and mineral intake are also affected. Foods selected for the infant feeding should be nutrient-dense items. Introducing meats between 4 and 6 months may help prevent a deficiency of iron or zinc,[2] especially for exclusively breast-fed infants. Introduction of solids should not mislead caregivers into thinking consumption of breast milk or infant formula is any less significant. Optimal volumes of breast milk and/or iron-fortified infant formula are still essential to meet the majority of the infant's nutrient needs.

For more information on infant foods and infant feeding, go to http://www.gerber.com, http://www.heinzbaby.com, http://www.beechnut.com, or http://www.healthychildren.org (an AAP-sponsored site).

The infant's first food is usually infant rice cereal thinned to a semi-liquid consistency with breast milk or infant formula. This is customary because rice allergy is unlikely in infancy.[42] Resistance to the initial spoon-feeding is common because infants are not familiar with the spoon. Holding the infant in one's arms, rather than sitting him or her in a high chair, may relieve some of the initial apprehension. Each new food item introduced to the infant's diet should be fed for 2 to 3 days while examining the infant for symptoms of intolerance. Signs of potential intolerance include skin rashes, vomiting, diarrhea, and wheezing. In the absence of such symptoms, the quantity, frequency, and consistency of the food item can be increased, and a second food can be presented. See **Table 5-4** for further recommendations on the progression of solid foods. Once a variety of single ingredients have been introduced and tolerated, a combination of these ingredients can be offered.

A gag reflex of varying degrees is apparent until 7 to 9 months of age. At this time, most infants are beginning to chew and tolerate smooth to chunky foods, and a normal

TABLE 5-4 Guidelines for Progression of Solid Foods

Age in Months	Feeding Skills	Oral Motor Skills	Types of Food	Suggested Activities
Birth–4		Rooting reflex Sucking reflex Swallowing reflex Extrusion reflex	Breast milk Infant formula	Breast-feeding Bottle-feeding
5	Able to grasp objects voluntarily Learning to reach mouth with hands	Disappearance of extrusion reflex		Possible introduction of thinned cereal
6	Sits with balance while using hands Ready for high chair	Transfers food from front of tongue to back Closes lips around spoon	Infant cereal Strained fruit Strained vegetables	Prepare cereal with formula or breast milk to a semi-liquid texture Use spoon Feed from a dish Advance to ⅓–½ cup cereal before adding fruits and vegetables
7	Improved grasp Drinks from cup with help	Mashes food with lateral movements of jaw Learns side-to-side or "rotary" chewing	Infant cereal Strained to junior texture of fruits, vegetables, and meats	Thicken texture to lumpier texture Sit child in high chair with feet supported Introduce cup
8–10	Holds bottle without help Drinks from cup without spilling Decreases fluid intake and increases solids Coordinates hand-to-mouth movement	Swallows with closed mouth	Soft, mashed, or minced table foods	Begin finger foods Do not add salt, sugar, or fats to foods Present soft foods in chunks ready for finger feeding
10–12	Feeds self with fingers and spoon Holds cup without help	Tooth eruption Improved ability to bite and chew	Soft, chopped table foods	Provide meals in pattern similar to rest of family Use cup at meals

Sources: Data from Fomon SJ. *Nutrition of Normal Infants*. St. Louis, MO: Mosby; 1993; Butte N, Cobb K, Duyer J, et al. The start healthy feeding guidelines for infants and toddlers. *J Amer Diet Assoc*. 2004;104:442–484; and Hinton S, Kerwin D. *Maternal and Child Nutrition*. Chapel Hill, NC: Health Sciences Consortium Corporation; 1981.

TABLE 5-5 Nutrient Composition of Selected Commercial Baby Food Products

Food		Amount	Calories	Protein	Carbohydrates	Fat	Sodium	Sugar	Fiber
Instant Cereal	Single grain rice	¼ cup	60	1	12	0.5	0	17	0
Stage 1 Vegetable	Carrots G	1 pack	25	< 1	5	0	80	4	1
	Carrots H	1 jar	50	1	9	1	25	6	3
Stage 1 Fruit	Bananas G	1 pack	60	< 1	15	0	5	12	1
	Bananas H	½ bowl	65	1	15	0	1.5	11	1
Stage 2 Vegetable	Garden Vegetable G	1 pack	40	2	7	0.5	35	3	2
	Mixed Vegetable H	1 jar	50	3	10	0.3	22	1	2
Stage 2 Fruit	Apple Berry G	1 pack	50	0	12	0	0	10	1
	Apple Berry H	1 jar	90	0	23	0	6	19	2
Stage 2 Dinner	Sweet Potato Turkey G	1 jar	80	2	16	1	50	9	2
	Sweet Potato Turkey H	1 jar	90	4	20	0.3	35	4	2
Graduate	Chicken and Pasta G	1 tray	110	9	16			3	3
Stage 3 Dinner	Chicken Cass. Veg w/Rice H	1 tray	180	8	35	6	40	5	3

Abbreviations: G, Gerber; H, Heinz.

Sources: Table data retrieved from manufacturers' websites (accessed January 10, 2010): Gerber, http://www.gerber.com; Heinz, http://www.heinzbaby.com.

gag reflex is developing. Choking, however, indicates that the infant is not ready for the transition to solid foods. It is not unusual for caregivers to be overly cautious about this natural gag reflex and mistake it for choking. Providers must be attentive to situations where infant feeding and solid texture progression is being delayed due to caregiver anxiety. Infants will pick up on this anxiety around feeding and begin to develop insecurity with regards to the feeding environment.

Many commercial baby food products are on the market today. Virtually all are prepared without added sodium and many without added sugar. Juices are generally enriched with vitamin C; cereals are enriched with iron, thiamine, riboflavin, niacin, calcium, and phosphorus. Products advertised as "first foods" are single-ingredient foods. "Dinners," baked goods, desserts, "graduates," "junior foods," and some cereals contain a combination of ingredients. Textures from strained to chunky are available, along with foods designed for teething. Baby food manufacturers use various descriptors to identify the different textures. Words such as "stage," "first," "second," or "graduate" can tell a parent or caregiver approximately when in infancy the baby might be ready to handle the texture of the food. Commercial baby foods are a time-efficient means of providing an infant with solids and, if chosen wisely, can supply a nutrient-dense diet. Certain items will provide more nutrients than seemingly comparable choices. For example, plain meats contain from 220–250% of the protein and up to 200% of the iron of "meat dinners." The nutrient contents of selected commercial baby foods are listed in **Table 5-5**. See also http://www.nal.usda.gov/fnic/foodcomp/search for the nutrient analysis of commercial baby foods.

Home-prepared baby foods are an alternative to commercially prepared foods. They are more economical and allow greater flexibility in altering food consistency but can be more time consuming to prepare. Homegrown foods should not be prepared if the lead concentration of soil in residential areas is excessive or if good food-handling techniques aren't used.[49] These precautions can help to prevent nutrient deficiencies, foodborne illness, and lead toxicity.

Families should start with single-ingredient foods and then progress to multiple-ingredient foods and spices after the infant has shown tolerance without adverse reaction. It is important to avoid excessive sodium, sugar, and additives commonly found in some table foods. Infant diets should have variety and include nutrient-dense foods. Foods should be easy to hold, vary in texture and temperature, and contain a balance of all the food groups. The diets of family members and caregivers play a significant role in influencing the types of foods infants are eating.

The final phase of infant feeding, between the 10th and 12th months, includes increasing independence with self-feeding. The caregiver and child interactions around eating help establish healthy eating relationships that will extend into childhood and adulthood.

Overweight Issues

Initial risk factors for infants and children becoming overweight or obese appear to develop sooner than anticipated. Prior to conception, mothers can already have risk factors for unhealthy weight gain in their children. Mothers who are overweight themselves, smoke, or gain excessive weight during pregnancy have a greater risk of having an infant and/or child who will be overweight.[50] Infants put to breast learn very early on how to self-regulate their intake of nutrition to meet individual satiety. Formula-fed infants are often given standard amounts of formula, and parents and caregivers are not as attentive to feeding cues. This subtle difference in feeding environment may be enough to teach self-regulation with eating for years to come.

The greatest risk factor for overweight or obesity in infancy or childhood is having an overweight parent. The earlier an infant or child is identified as overweight, the more likely he or she is to be overweight for life.

The following goals have been established for infant feeding to prevent childhood overweight or obesity:[51]

- Breastfeed exclusively for 6 months.
- Avoid sweet beverages.
- Respect infant self-regulation during feeding (breast-, formula-, or solid-food feedings).
- Avoid using food for comfort.

Dental Caries

Baby bottle tooth decay (BBTD) is an oral health disorder characterized by rampant dental caries associated with inappropriate infant feeding practices The disorder affects the primary teeth of infants and young children, particularly those who are permitted to fall asleep with a bottle filled with juice or other fermentable liquid.[2] Nursing caries, similar to tooth decay caused by BBTD from formulas, also can occur with prolonged or inappropriate breastfeeding at naptime or too frequently throughout the day.

The American Academy of Pediatric Dentistry (AAPD) recommends the cessation of ad lib breast- or bottle-feeding with the initial eruption of teeth. Providing liquids concentrated in mono- and disaccharides, such as juices and sweetened beverages, is the leading cause of BBTD.[2] Infants who refuse cold foods or grimace when chewing should be examined for BBTD. Infants with BBTD will have tooth discoloration varying from yellow to black. Preventive measures include the following:

- Feeding only infant formula or water from a bottle
- Cleaning the infant's teeth and gums with a damp washcloth or gauze pad after each feeding
- Avoiding juices in the first year; if given, offer it in a cup rather than a bottle
- Filling bedtime bottles with water, if necessary

The greater the exposure to sugary rich foods and beverages, the more likely an infant is to develop tooth decay.

Cow's Milk

During the first 12 months of life, infants should be provided breast milk or iron-fortified infant formulas.[2] Very early introduction of cow's milk increases the risk of developing allergy to milk protein and potentially other foods as well. Resistance to allergy increases with gastrointestinal maturity,[2,52] so that at 6 months of age small amounts of foods containing cow's milk protein can be introduced into the infant's diet with a reduced risk of developing allergy.

Risks of iron deficiency anemia[53] and other micronutrient deficiencies are a problem when cow's milk replaces breast milk or formula before 12 months of age. Occult loss of blood from the gastrointestinal tract is associated with the introduction of cow's milk in both early and later infancy. Cow's milk is also a poor source of vitamin C, vitamin E, and essential fatty acids.

Lastly, the additional protein and electrolytes in cow's milk increases the renal solute load and places the infant at risk for dehydration during periods of vomiting, diarrhea, or exposure to dry heat in winter or to the sun in the summer. Thus, it is best to delay the introduction of cow's milk until the infant is 1 year old. When the infant's diet is changed to cow's milk after the first year, it should be whole cow's milk, as opposed to 2% or skim milk, to provide essential fat and calories.

Water and Fruit Juices

Additional water is not necessary during the first year if infants are receiving adequate amounts of breast milk or formula to sustain adequate weight gain. Even in hot months infants can obtain adequate amounts of free water from breast milk or iron-fortified formula. The only exception to this rule is if the caregiver observes the infant having a reduction in urine output or if the urine appears to be dark in color.[2] Juices should be avoided during the first 6 months of life. Juices will put the infant at risk of displacing nutrient-dense breast milk or formula with high-sugar and low-nutrient juices.

If an infant is experiencing harder stools, small amounts of juice can be tried on an as-needed basis only. The carbohydrate source in fruit juice is primarily from a combination of fructose, glucose, and sorbitol. See **Table 5-6** for the

TABLE 5-6 Carbohydrate Sources in Select Juices (g/100 g of food) (mOsm/kg H_2O)

Juice	Fructose	Glucose	Sucrose	Sorbitol	Osmolality
Apple	6.0	2.4	2.5	0.5	638
Pear	6.6	2.0	3.7	2.2	764
White grape	7.5	7.1	0.6		1030

Values may vary depending on the dilution of the juice and type of fruit used. *Sources:* Data from Fomon SJ. *Nutrition of Normal Infants*. St. Louis, MO: Mosby; 1993; Smith MM, Davis M, Chasalow FI, et al. Carbohydrate absorption from fruit juice in young children. *Pediatrics.* 1995;95:340–344; and Hyams JS, Etienne NL, Leichtner AM, et al. Carbohydrate malabsorption following fruit juice ingestion in young children. *Pediatrics.* 1988;82:64–68.

carbohydrate sources in various fruit juices.[54] Infants may better absorb and have greater tolerance to juices containing fructose when found in combination with sucrose and glucose.[54,55] Fruit juices containing these sugars appear to have beneficial effects similar to those of fiber for infants with constipation.

Excessive juice intake puts infants and children at risk for dental caries, failure to thrive, short stature, and obesity later in the preschool years.[56] If an infant has poor weight gain, it is very important to obtain a thorough diet history with specific inquiry into juice or water consumption. If juice is included, only 100% juice should be used, and volumes should not exceed 4 to 6 ounces a day for children up to 6 years old.[2]

Feeding Intolerances and Other Problems

Formula intolerance, constipation, acute diarrhea, and food refusal are common feeding problems encountered during infancy. These problems can usually be resolved through simple measures. If ignored, the problems may become exacerbated and cause detrimental effects to an infant's nutritional status and growth.

The incidence of allergy in infants and children appears to range between 1% and 8%, depending on the patient's age and the specific allergen.[2] Most infants and children appear to outgrow their food allergy as they go through the toddler years; however, some reactions can be severe or even life threatening and never outgrown. Intolerance to lactose must not be confused with milk protein allergy. Lactose intolerance is not common in infancy and has an enzymatic etiology, whereas milk allergy is based on immunologic mechanisms. Gastrointestinal disturbance is common to both disorders. Diarrhea is frequently observed in both, but vomiting is exclusive to milk allergy. In addition to gastrointestinal symptoms, dermatologic, respiratory, and possibly systemic reactions, such as anaphylactic shock (although this is rare), may occur in milk allergy.[57]

Milk allergy is usually identified in the first 4 months of infancy. This onset is due to the immaturity of both the gastrointestinal tract and the immune system.[58] Infants at "high risk" are those with at least one parent with food allergies or siblings with allergies. It is not possible to prevent allergies if a child is predisposed to them. See Chapter 7 for further details about food allergies.

Constipation

Constipation is defined by timing and consistency of the stool compared with the usual number of bowel movements. An infant is constipated when there is no bowel movement for several days or if defecation is extremely dry, hard, or painful.[59] "Normal" stooling patterns vary from infant to infant and with differences in dietary intake.

After passing meconium, usually within the first 24 hours of life, the number of stools gradually decreases from over four times a day to one to two a day by the end of the first year.[60] Infants being breastfed or receiving hydrolyzed protein formulas typically experience between 1 and 12 bowel movements a day.[60] Infants fed soy-based formulas tend to have more stools, which are hard and firm.[61]

Stool color also varies with the protein source in milk or formula. Breast milk–fed infants typically have stools that look loose to pasty and are yellowish in color. Constipation is rare in breastfed infants; however, infants may have days when they do not have a bowel movement due to enhanced absorption of nutrients from breast milk. Formulas with soy, whey, or casein hydrolyzed protein sources may produce stools that range from yellow to green or brownish in color.[60] Behaviors during infant stooling that might alarm parents or caregivers include flushing, grunting, and change in stool color with change in diet.[59] These behaviors are actually normal and should decrease over time.

Treating nonanatomic constipation requires dietary intervention. Five measures can be taken in the following sequence:

1. Verify constipation through family interview.
2. Ensure proper diet, including free fluid intake versus fluid losses.
3. Ensure accurate preparation of formula if infant is bottle-fed.
4. Feed an additional 2 ounces of water after each feeding.
5. Provide 2 ounces of pear or apple juice per day.

If there is no relief after following these recommendations and the infant appears to be in pain or cramping, a physician should be notified.

The most recent change in infant formulas is the addition of prebiotics that attempt to mimic the complex mixture of oligosaccharides present in human breast milk. The potential benefits of using an infant formula with prebiotics include softer stools, increased stool frequency, and reduction in infection rates and atopic dermatitis.

Regardless of which formula infants are being fed, parents should be discouraged from "formula jumping." This only causes confusion for the infant and the professional attempting to distinguish between a "fussy" infant and a true intolerance or allergic finding.

Diarrhea

Acute infantile diarrhea is defined as the sudden onset of increased stool frequency, volume, and water content with greater than three stools in a 24-hour period.[62] Acute diarrhea can result from a variety of causes (e.g., viral infection, excessive juice intake, antibiotic-associated diarrhea), but it occurs most often in areas where there is poor sanitation and limited availability of clean water supplies. Persistent diarrhea is defined as lasting greater than 14 days. Infants with persistent diarrhea are usually malnourished and have repetitive cycles of infection and malabsorption.

Diarrhea lasting more than 4 days or resulting in greater than 10% dehydration may require intravenous fluid therapy. However, bottle-fed infants suffering from mild to moderate diarrhea can be rehydrated with an oral rehydration solution for 4 to 6 hours (see **Table 5-7**).

After dehydration status is assessed and resolved, reintroduction of age-appropriate foods and liquids should occur as soon as possible. Beverages such as juice, broth, or sport drinks should not be provided because their high osmolality may induce osmotic diarrhea, exacerbating the initial problem.[60] Continued breastfeeding is beneficial if being breastfed. Lactose-free formulas could be considered in infants who are malnourished or have severe dehydration with persistent diarrhea.[62]

Reflux

Gastroesophageal reflux (GER), or chalasia, affects many infants. GER is otherwise referred to as regurgitation or spitting up or the presence of gastric contents in the esophagus. When complications arise from recurrent reflux, the condition is called GERD, or gastroesophageal reflux disease.[63] All infants experience some degree of GER. Mild GER may be treated with modifications in feeding positions and dietary regimens. More severe GERD requires a physician's assessment.

Feeding the infant in an upright position may prevent GER. In this position, gravity aids in gastric emptying. A truly upright position is most reliable in preventing GER.[64] Regardless of the presence of GER, infants should sleep in supine position in order to reduce the risk of sudden infant death syndrome (SIDS).[63]

Thickening formula with cereal is a routine practice in preventing GER. However, it does not decrease the number of esophageal reflux episodes. Adding cereal to the formula increases the caloric concentration of formula, alters the protein:carbohydrate:fat ratio, interferes with breastfeeding, and possibly delays gastric emptying.

Milk protein intolerance can cause reflux or vomiting in infants. If the feeding regimens suggested in this section do not improve symptoms, switching to an alternate protein source may be warranted.

Inadequate Food Intake

The two important feeding milestones during infancy are self-feeding and the development of a positive relationship with food and eating. If these do not occur, a spiral effect of food refusal and poor nutrient intake can ensue. Food refusal can occur in infancy because of physical or emotional stress. This is more typically classified as organic, indicating a medical or functional etiology caused by environmental influences. Illness and an unfavorable atmosphere for feeding are typical contributors to food refusal. The consequence of this problem is failure to thrive (FTT).

Food refusal originating from excessive or deficient stimulation is more difficult to discern. Commotion and overly aggressive or restrictive caregivers can cause development of negative associations with feeding. Routine negative interactions at mealtime can keep an infant from wanting to explore and advance with the normal self-feeding progression. As the stages of eating advance from liquid

TABLE 5-7 Nutrient Comparisons of Clear Liquids and Rehydration Solutions

Product	Na (mEq/L)	K (mEq/L)	Cl (mEq/L)	Sugar (g/L)	Starch (g/L)	Osmolality (mOsm/L)
Cola	1.7	0.1–0.6	—	53–58.5	—	750
Apple Juice	4.6	26	1.1	39.5	—	747
Gatorade	20–23	2.5–3	23	25–28	—	330–365
Chicken Broth	250	8	—	—	—	500
Enfalyte	50	25	45	25	—	167
Pedialyte	45	20	35	25	—	270

Sources: Data from Swedberg J, Steiner J. Oral rehydration therapy in diarrhea: not just for Third World children. *Postgrad Med.* 1983;74:335–341; and Synder J. Oral rehydration therapy for acute diarrhea. *Semin Pediatr Gastroenterol Nutr.* 1990;1:8; and from product information provided by Abbott Nutrition and Mead Johnson Nutritionals.

and dependence as a newborn to table foods as a toddler, parents need to be attuned to their child's developmental transition with eating.[65] The caregiver may restrict the infant's exploration of food and/or rush through a meal, disrupting the feeding pace. Concerned that the infant is feeding poorly or losing weight, caregivers become tense. This tension only exacerbates the reluctance to feed.

The most effective means of treating feeding disorders after identification is to increase appropriate behavior and decrease maladaptive behavior between the infant and caregiver and between the infant and the feeding experience. As infants get closer to their first birthday, their interest in self-feeding and encouragement of self-regulation with food intake should be promoted.

Case Study

Nutrition Assessment of Breastfed Infant

Patient History

BA is a 6-month-old girl born at term to a healthy, 26-year-old mother with no family history of allergy. The baby is being seen today for WIC recertification. BA's anthropometric measurements are 7.1 kg (weight), 65 cm (length), and 42.25 cm (head circumference). Mother puts the baby to breast five to six times per day using one breast at each feeding. Each feeding lasts about 15 minutes. BA is this mother's first baby, and the mother reports that the baby "is a good breastfeeder"—she latches well with audible sucking and visible swallowing—and she burps easily with minimal spitting up. The baby has three or more very soft, yellow stools each day. In the last few weeks, the mother has noticed that the baby seems less satisfied after feeding. The baby had been sleeping through the night but now occasionally wakes early for a feeding. The baby gets a daily 1 mL dose of Tri-vi-sol, an infant vitamin drop. The WIC dietitian notices that BA has good head control and puts her hands in her mouth.

Recommendations

Anticipatory guidance is offered so the parents know what to expect. This includes:

- Obtain a high chair if one is not currently available.
- Provide opportunities for the infant to eat with others.
- Add more solid food variety in the next 1 to 2 months, starting with stage one meats followed by fruits and vegetables.
- Advance texture as tolerated. Wait 2 to 3 days between new foods to assess for a possible allergic reaction.
- Offer finger foods (dry cereal or toast; small tender pieces of meat, vegetables, or fruits; noodles; etc.) as tolerated, around 8 or 9 months.
- Assess for anemia at 9 to 15 months.
- Offer cup feeding as tolerated at 9 to 12 months.
- Delay juice and cow's milk until 12 months.
- Continue the vitamin D supplement until the baby consumes 1 liter or quart per day of vitamin D-fortified milk.

Questions for the Reader

1. Plot BA's length, weight, head circumference, and weight-for-length on a CDC growth chart. What percentiles is she in?
2. Using the Nutrition Care process, does BA have a nutritional diagnosis?
3. What interventions are needed at this WIC visit? What food and/or nutrient supplements would you recommend for BA?

REFERENCES

1. Newborn Screening Authoring Committee. Newborn screening expands: recommendations for pediatricians and medical homes—implications for the system. *Pediatrics.* 2008;121:192–207.
2. Kleinman R. *Pediatric Nutrition Handbook,* 6th ed. Elk Grove Village, IL: American Academy of Pediatrics; 2009.
3. Institute of Medicine. *Dietary Reference Intakes for Energy, Carbohydrate, Fiber, Fat, Fatty Acids, Cholesterol, Protein, and Amino Acids (Macronutrients).* Washington, DC: National Academies Press; 2005.
4. Institute of Medicine. *Dietary Reference Intakes for Water, Potassium, Sodium, Chloride, and Sulfate.* Washington, DC: National Academies Press; 2005.
5. Lawrence RA, Lawrence RM. *Breastfeeding: A Guide for the Medical Profession,* 6th ed. St. Louis, MO: Mosby; 2005.
6. American Academy of Pediatrics. Breastfeeding and the use of human milk. *Pediatrics.* 2005;115:496–506.
7. Position of the American Dietetic Association: promoting and supporting breast-feeding. *J Am Diet Assoc.* 2009;109:1926–1942.
8. Heird W. The role of polyunsaturated fatty acids in term and preterm infants and breast-feeding mothers. *Pediatr Clin North Am.* 2001;48:173–188.
9. Scariati PD, Grummer-Strawn LM, Fein SB. A longitudinal analysis of infant morbidity and the extent of breast-feeding in the United States [Abstract]. *Pediatrics.* 1997;99(6):5.

10. Dewey KG, Heinig MJ, Nommsen LA, et al. Breast-fed infants are leaner than formula-fed infants at 1 year of age: the DARLING study. *Am J Clin Nutr.* 1993;57:140–145.
11. Gdalevich M, Mimouni D, David M, Mimouni M. Breast-feeding and the onset of atopic dermatitis in childhood: a systemic review and meta-analysis of prospective studies. *J Am Acad Dermatol.* 2001;45:520–527.
12. Gillman M. Breast-feeding and obesity. *J Pediatr.* 2002;141: 749–750.
13. American Academy of Pediatrics, Committee on Nutrition. Prevention of pediatric overweight and obesity. *Pediatrics.* 2003;112:424–430.
14. Picciano MF. Representative values for constituents of human milk. *Pediatr Clin North Am.* 2001;48:263–264.
15. Karra MV, Udipi SA, Kirksey A, Roepke JLB. Changes in specific nutrients in breast milk during extended lactation. *Am J Clin Nutr.* 1986;43:495–503.
16. Institute of Medicine. *Nutrition During Lactation.* Washington, DC: National Academy of Sciences; 1991.
17. Jensen RG. *Handbook of Milk Composition.* San Diego, CA: Academic Press; 1995.
18. Hill DJ, Roy N, Heine RG, et al. Effect of a low-allergen maternal diet on colic among breastfed infants: a randomized, controlled trial. *Pediatrics.* 2005;116:e709–e715.
19. Berlin CM, Denson HM, Daniel CH, Ward RM. Deposition of dietary caffeine in milk, saliva, and plasma of lactating women. *Pediatrics.* 1984;73:59–63.
20. Luck W, Nau H. Nicotine and cotinine concentrations in serum and urine of infants exposed via passive smoking or milk from smoking mothers. *J Pediatr.* 1985;107:816–820.
21. American Academy of Pediatrics, American College of Obstetricians and Gynecologists. *Breastfeeding Handbook for Physicians.* Elk Grove Village, IL: American Academy of Pediatrics; 2006.
22. Meek JY, ed. *New Mother's Guide to Breastfeeding.* New York: Bantam Books; 2002.
23. Fomon SJ. *Nutrition of Normal Infants.* St. Louis, MO: Mosby; 1993.
24. Jensen RG. *Handbook of Milk Composition.* New York: Academic Press; 1995.
25. O'Connor NR. Infant formula. *Am Fam Physician.* 2009;79(7):565–570.
26. Boehm G, Stahl B. Oligosaccharides from milk. *J Nutr.* 2007;137:847S–849S.
27. Agostoni C, Axelsson I, Braegger C, et al. Probiotic bacteria in dietetic products for infants: a commentary by the ESPGHAN Committee on Nutrition. *J Pediatr Gastroenterol Nutr.* 2004;38:365–374.
28. American Academy of Pediatrics, Committee on Nutrition. Iron fortification of infant formulas. *Pediatrics.* 1999;104:119–123.
29. Bhatia J, Greer F, Committee on Nutrition. Use of soy protein-based formulas in infant feeding. *Pediatrics.* 2008;121:1062–1068.
30. Zeiger RS, Sampson HA, Bock SA, et al. Soy allergy in infants and children with IgE-associated cow's milk allergy. *J Pediatr.* 1999;134:614–622.
31. Greer FR, Sicherer SH, Burks AW, Committee on Nutrition and Section on Allergy and Immunology. Effects of early nutritional interventions on the development of atopic disease in infants and children: the role of maternal dietary restriction, breastfeeding, timing of introduction of complementary foods, and hydrolyzed formulas. *Pediatrics.* 2008;121:183–191.
32. Fomon SJ, Filer LJ, Anderson TA, Ziegler EE. Recommendations for feeding normal infants. *Pediatrics.* 1979;63:52–59.
33. U.S. Food and Drug Administration. FDA 101: infant formula. Available at: http://www.fda.gov/ForConsumers/ConsumerUpdates/ucm048694.htm. Accessed December 29, 2009.
34. Dietz WH, Stern L, eds. *American Academy of Pediatrics Guide to Your Child's Nutrition.* New York: Villard; 1999.
35. Teske S, Robbins S. Formula preparation and handling. In: Robbins ST, Beker LT, Pediatric Nutrition Practice Group, eds. *Infant Feedings: Guidelines for Preparation of Formula and Breastmilk in Health Care Facilities.* Chicago, IL: American Dietetic Association; 2004:31–67.
36. Centers for Disease Control and Prevention. *Enterobacter sakazakii* infections associated with the use of powdered infant formula. *MMWR.* 2002;51:297–300.
37. Tully SB, Bar-Halm Y, Bradley RL. Abnormal tympanography after supine bottle-feeding. *J Pediatr.* 1995;126:S105–S111.
38. Nevin-Folino NL, ed. *Pediatric Manual of Clinical Dietetics,* 2nd ed. Chicago: American Dietetic Association; 2003.
39. Wagner CL, Greer FR, Section on Breastfeeding and Committee on Nutrition. Prevention of rickets and vitamin D deficiency in infants, children, and adolescents. *Pediatrics.* 2008;122:1142–1152.
40. Misra M, Pacaud D, Petryk A, et al. Vitamin D deficiency in children and its management: review of current knowledge and recommendations. *Pediatrics.* 2008;122:398–417.
41. Holick MF. Vitamin D deficiency. *N Engl J Med.* 2007;357:266–281.
42. Fomon S. Feeding normal infants: rationale for recommendations. *J Am Diet Assoc.* 2001;101:1002–1005.
43. Butte N, Cobb K, Duyer J, et al. The start healthy feeding guidelines for infants and toddlers. *J Amer Diet Assoc.* 2004;104:442–484.
44. Fox MK, Devaney B, Reidy K, et al. Relationship between portion size and energy intake among infants and toddlers: evidence of self-regulations. *J Am Diet Assoc.* 2006;106:S77–S83.
45. Lipsitt L, Crook C, Booth C. The transitional infant: behavioral development and feeding. *Am J Clin Nutr.* 1985;41:485–496.
46. Cloud H. Feeding problems of the child with special health care needs. In: Ekvall SW, ed. *Pediatric Nutrition in Chronic Diseases and Developmental Disorders: Prevention, Assessment, and Treatment.* New York: Oxford University Press; 1993:203–218.
47. Chatoor I, Hirsch R, Persinger M. Facilitating internal regulation of eating: a treatment model of infantile anorexia. *Infants Young Child.* 1997;9(4):12–22.
48. Underwood B. Weaning practices in deprived environments: the weaning dilemma. *Pediatrics.* 1985;75(Suppl):194–198.
49. Shils ME, Olson JA, Shike M. *Modern Nutrition in Health and Disease,* 8th ed. Philadelphia, PA: Lea & Febiger; 1994.
50. Owen CG, Martin RM, Whincup PH, et al. Effect of infant feeding on risk of obesity across the life course: a quantitative review of published evidence. *Pediatrics.* 2005;115:1367–1377.
51. Murray R, Battista M. Managing the risk of childhood overweight and obesity in primary care practice. *Curr Probl Pediatr Adolesc Health Care.* 2009;39:145–166.
52. Tunnessen WW, Oski FA. Consequences of starting whole cow milk at 6 months of age. *J Pediatr.* 1987;111:813–816.

53. Walter T, DeAndraca I, Chadud P, et al. Iron deficiency anemia: adverse effects on infant psychomotor development. *Pediatrics.* 1989;84:7–17.
54. Fomon SJ. *Nutrition of Normal Infants.* St. Louis, MO: Mosby; 1993.
55. Hoekstra JH, van Kempen AA, Kneepkens CM. Apple juice malabsorption: fructose or sorbitol? *J Pediatr Gastroenterol Nutr.* 1993;16:39–42.
56. Levine AA. Excessive fruit juice consumption: how can something that causes failure to thrive be associated with obesity? [Selected summary]. *J Pediatr Gastroenterol Nutr.* 1997;25:554–555.
57. Wyllie R, Hyams JS. *Pediatric Gastrointestinal Diseases.* Philadelphia, PA: WB Saunders; 1993.
58. Walker A. Absorption of protein and protein fragments in the developing intestine: role in immunologic/allergic reactions. *Pediatrics.* 1985;75(Suppl):167.
59. Montgomery DF, Navarro F. Management of constipation and encopresis in children. *J Pediatr Health Care.* 2008;22:199–204.
60. Hyams J, Treem WR, Etienne NL, et al. Effects of infant formula on stool characteristics of young infants. *Pediatrics.* 1995;95:50–54.
61. Hillemier C. Gastroesophageal reflux. *Pediatr Clin North Am.* 1996;43(1):197–212.
62. Grimwood K, Forbes D. Acute and persistent diarrhea. *Pediatr Clin N Am.* 2009;56:1343–1361.
63. Vandenplas Y, Rudolph C, Lorenzo CD, et al. Pediatric gastroesophageal reflux clinical practice guidelines: joint recommendations of the North American Society of Pediatric Gastroenterology, Hepatology, and Nutrition and the European Society of Pediatric Gastroenterology, Hepatology, and Nutrition. *J Pediatr Gastroenterol Nutr.* 2009;49:498–547.
64. Orenstein S, Whitington P. Positioning for prevention of infant gastroesophageal reflux. *J Pediatr.* 1983;103:534–537.
65. Couch SC, Falciglia GA. Improving the diets of the young: considerations for intervention design. *J Am Diet Assoc.* 2006; 106:S10–S11.

CHAPTER 6

Normal Nutrition After Infancy

Betty Lucas, Beth Ogata, and Sharon Feucht

Introduction

From 1 year of age through adolescence, children experience changes in physical, cognitive, and social-emotional growth. The 1-year-old toddler is beginning to be more independent; the 18-year-old is also taking steps into the world, becoming more independent and self-sufficient. This chapter will focus on the nutritional needs and issues of normal, healthy children during these growing years.

Growth

After the rapid growth of infancy, physical growth slows during the preschool and school years. The elementary school years are the latent period prior to the pubertal growth spurt of adolescence. Children will have individual growth patterns, with spurts in height and weight followed by periods of little or no growth. These patterns usually correspond to similar changes in appetite and food intake. Parents and other caregivers need to realize that these changes are normal so they can avoid struggles over food and eating.

Developmental progress during the growing years influences many aspects of food and eating. The very young child prefers foods that can be picked up or don't have to be chased across the plate. Food jags may be more an expression of independence than of actual likes and dislikes. In older children, the influence of peers and the media will affect snack choices. Teenagers want foods that fit into their lifestyles, are quick and easy to fix, and are inexpensive. Understanding the developmental characteristics and milestones at any particular age will help parents and professionals to set realistic expectations, support eating behavior and food decisions that are developmentally appropriate, and avoid unnecessary conflicts.

Nutrient and Energy Needs

The primary factor in determining nutrient needs is usually a child's rate and stage of growth. Other factors include physical activity, body size, basal energy expenditure, and state of health. Actual needs vary and are based on individual characteristics. (See Chapter 3 and Appendix F for further details about the RDAs, DRIs, and AIs.)

Energy needs vary due to individual differences in basal metabolism, growth, physical activity, onset of puberty, and body size. The DRIs include equations for estimated energy requirements (EERs) for children who are not overweight and weight maintenance total energy expenditure (TEE) for children who are overweight. EER equations through age 2 years include allowances for age and weight. EER and TEE equations for children 3 years and older include allowances for age, sex, weight, height, and level of physical activity.[1] These references for energy intake in children and adolescents provide tools to assess energy intake and to develop nutrition care plans that incorporate the individual child's size, activity, and state of health.

Protein needs decrease as the growth rate slows after infancy and then increase at puberty. Total protein intake increases steadily until about 12 years of age in girls and 16 years of age in boys. Protein intakes usually exceed recommended needs. Some children and adolescents, however, may be at risk for protein malnutrition if energy is inadequate so that protein is used for energy. Examples include those with inadequate energy intakes (extreme use of low-fat diets, dieters and athletes in training who limit food), those who are strict vegetarians, and some with food allergies. Dietary evaluation of protein intake should include the growth rate, energy intake, and quality of the protein sources.

The nutrients most likely to be low or deficient in the diets of children and adolescents are calcium, vitamin D, magnesium, vitamin A, vitamin E, and vitamin C.[2–6] Certain populations of children, such as low-income, Native American, and other groups with limited food and health resources (e.g., the homeless), are more at risk for poor diet and nutrient deficiencies.

Calcium needs are determined by growth velocity, rates of absorption, and availability of other nutrients, such as phosphorus, vitamin D, and protein. Because of individual variability, a child receiving less than the recommended allowance of calcium is not necessarily at risk. Approximately 100 mg of calcium per day is retained as bone in the preschool years. This doubles or triples for adolescents during peak growth periods.[7] Adolescence is a critical period for optimal calcium retention to achieve peak bone mass, especially for females who are at risk for osteoporosis in later years. Calcium intake, however, often decreases during the teen years. An AI of 1300 mg of calcium per day for ages 9 to 18 years supports optimal bone mineralization.[8]

Those who consume none or only limited amounts of dairy products—the major source of calcium—may be at risk for calcium deficiency. Some adolescents may also receive less calcium than needed because of rapid growth, dieting, and substituting carbonated beverages for milk. In assessing calcium status, vitamin D intake should be considered because of its major role in calcium metabolism. For children with limited sunshine exposure, dietary intake is critical. Vitamin D–fortified milk is the primary food source of this nutrient; other dairy products are not usually made with fortified milk. **Table 6-1** contains a list of calcium food sources. Levels of physical activity also affect an individual's calcium needs for optimal bone development.[9]

Iron needs are determined by the rate of growth, iron stores, increasing blood volumes, and rate of absorption from food sources. Menstrual losses, as well as rapid growth, increase the need for iron in adolescent females. To reach adulthood with an adequate store of iron, recommended daily intakes are 7 mg for children ages 1 to 3 years, 10 mg

TABLE 6-1 Calcium Equivalents

1 cup milk* = approx. 300 mg calcium	1 cup (8 oz) yogurt†
	1 cup calcium-fortified orange juice
	1 cup calcium-fortified soy milk‡
	1 cup calcium-fortified rice milk or almond milk‡,§
¾ cup milk =	1 oz cheddar, jack, or Swiss cheese
⅔ cup milk =	1 oz mozzarella or American cheese
	2 oz canned sardines (with bones)
½ cup milk =	2 oz canned salmon (with bones)
	½ cup custard or milk pudding
	½ cup cooked greens (mustard, collards, kale)
¼ cup milk =	½ cup cottage cheese
	½ cup ice cream
	¾ cup dried beans, cooked or canned

*Some low-fat or skim milks and some low-fat yogurts have additional nonfat dry milk (NFDM) solids added. Some labels will read "fortified." Such products will contain more calcium than indicated here.

†Most commercially prepared yogurt does not contain vitamin D.

‡The amount of calcium varies; not all milks are fortified with calcium and/or vitamin D.

§Rice and almond milks (and other nut milks) have significantly less protein than cow's milk and soy milk.

for 4- to 8-year-olds, 11 mg for pubertal males, and 15 mg for pubertal females.[10]

Vitamin D is an important nutrient for its role in bone health and for other potential roles, including prevention of cancer, cardiovascular disease, and infectious diseases. All infants, children, and adolescents should have an intake of 400 IU per day of vitamin D.[11] Serum 25-hydroxyvitamin D (25[OH]D) levels are used to measure deficiency and insufficiency.

Except for children living in nonfluoridated areas, fluoride supplementation is not needed.[12] Vitamin D intake may need to be evaluated to determine if a vitamin D supplement is needed, especially in young children.[11] High-nutritional-risk groups that might benefit from supplementation include children and adolescents:

1. With anorexia, inadequate appetite, or who consume fad diets
2. With chronic disease (e.g., cystic fibrosis, inflammatory bowel disease, hepatic disease)
3. From deprived families or those who are abused or neglected
4. Using a dietary program to manage obesity
5. Who do not consume adequate amounts of dairy products
6. With failure to thrive

Children with food allergies, those who omit entire food groups, and those with limited food acceptances may need supplementation. No risk is involved if parents wish to give their children a standard pediatric multivitamin. Megadose levels of nutrients should be discouraged in order to prevent toxicity, especially of fat-soluble vitamins. The DRIs include tolerable upper intake levels (UL), which can be used to determine excessive levels of vitamins and minerals from supplemental sources.[8]

Use of other dietary supplements, including herbal preparations, are common. Although many supplements are harmless and may be beneficial, others may be dangerous and/or affect nutritional status. Evaluation of dietary intake should include questions about the use of supplements.[13] Botanicals are discussed in Chapter 21.

Food Intake Variability

Because appetite usually follows the rate of growth, food intake is not always smooth and consistent. Nutrient intake in healthy children varies. Children and adolescents often exhibit decreased intake of whole milk and eggs, greater use of low-fat and nonfat milk, more snacking, and more eating away from home.[2,5] Unfortunately, many children are overweight, and many do not meet the recommendations for fruit, vegetable, grain, and meat intake.[14]

Food intake and habits are determined by numerous factors. Major influences for children include the family, peers, media, and body image. Family food choices and eating-related behaviors influence the types of foods children will accept.[15] Eating habits and food likes and dislikes are formed in the early years and often continue into adulthood. Parents and siblings are primary models for young children to imitate. Mealtime atmosphere, both positive and negative, can influence how a child approaches and handles family meals. The positive effects of regular family meals can last into adulthood.[16]

Television is the primary media influence on children of all ages. The food items generally advertised to young audiences are sweetened cereals, fast food, snack foods, and candy—foods high in sugar, fat, and salt.[17] The commercial messages are not based on nutrition, but on an emotional/psychological appeal—fun, gives you energy, yummy taste. Younger children generally cannot discriminate between the regular program and commercial messages and frequently give more attention to the latter because of their fast, attention-getting pace. Screen time and low physical activity levels are related to overweight and obesity, and television viewing has been inversely associated with fruit and vegetable intake.[18–21]

As children move into the world, others influence their food choices. In preschool, the group snack time may encourage a child to try a new food. During school years, friends influence participation in the school lunch program. Peer pressure is particularly strong in adolescence as teenagers strive for more independence and eating becomes a more social activity.

Puberty is the period of greatest awareness of body image. It is normal for teens to be uncomfortable and dissatisfied with their changing bodies. The media and popular idols offer a standard that adolescents compare themselves with, no matter how unrealistic it may be. Even prepubertal school-age girls have become increasingly preoccupied with body image and "dieting." To change their body image, they may try restrictive diets that may put them at risk for poor nutritional status. The increasing prevalence of childhood overweight also has impacted the positive body image of growing children and adolescents.

Feeding the Young Child

Parents often become concerned when their toddler refuses some favorite foods and appears to be disinterested in eating. These periods (food jags) vary in intensity from child to child and may last a few days or years. At the same time, the child is practicing self-feeding skills. These changes and behaviors during the preschool years are a normal part of the development and maturation of young children.[22] When parents understand this, they are more likely to avoid struggles and negative feedback around food and eating.

Portion sizes for young children are small by adult standards. See http://www.mypyramid.gov for tips for families and children, including food groups and portion sizes. A long-standing rule of thumb is to initially offer 1 tablespoon of each food for every year of age for preschool children, with more provided according to appetite.

Most children eat four to six times a day. Snacks contribute significantly to the total day's nutrient intake and should be planned accordingly. Foods that make nutritious snacks are listed in **Table 6-2**. Foods chosen for snacks should be those least likely to promote dental caries. Parents of young children frequently become concerned about the adequacy of their children's intakes. **Table 6-3** offers nutrition solutions to these common, normal variations in eating behaviors.

Just as important as providing adequate nutrients to young children is supporting a positive feeding environment—both physically and emotionally—so that as they grow they acquire skills, develop positive attitudes, and have control over food decisions as appropriate for their developmental level.

TABLE 6-2 Foods that Make Nutritious Snacks

Protein Foods	Fruits#	Breads and Cereals#	Vegetables
Natural cheese	Apple wedges*	Whole-grain breads	Carrot sticks*
Milk	Bananas	Whole-grain, low-fat crackers	Celery*
Plain yogurt	Pears	Rice crackers	Green pepper strips*
Cooked turkey or beef	Berries	English muffins	Cucumber slices*
Unsalted nuts and seeds*	Melon	Bagels	Cabbage wedges*
Peanut butter*	Oranges and other citrus fruits	Tortillas	Tomatoes
Hard-cooked eggs	Grapes*	Pita bread	Jicama*
Cottage cheese	Unsweetened canned fruit	Popcorn*	Vegetable juices
Tuna	Unsweetened fruit juices		Cooked green beans
			Broccoli and cauliflower florets

*Foods that are hard, round, and do not easily dissolve can cause choking. Do not give to children under 3 years of age. (Peanut butter is more dangerous when eaten in chunks or spread thickly rather than thinly on crackers or bread.)

#Fruits, juices, and most cereal/bread products contain fermentable carbohydrate, which is a factor in the development of dental caries.

TABLE 6-3 Common Feeding Concerns in Young Children

Common Concerns	Possible Solutions
Refuses meats	• Offer small, bite-size pieces of moist, tender meat or poultry. • Incorporate into meatloaf, spaghetti sauce, stews, casseroles, burritos, or pizza. • Include legumes, eggs, and cheese. • Offer boneless fish (including canned tuna and salmon).
Drinks too little milk	• Offer cheeses and yogurt, including cheese in cooking (e.g., macaroni and cheese, cheese sauce, pizza). Use milk to cook hot cereals. Offer cream soups and milk-based puddings and custards. • Allow child to pour milk from a pitcher and use a straw. • Include powdered milk in cooking and baking (e.g., biscuits, muffins, pancakes, meatloaf, casseroles)
Drinks too much milk	• Offer water if thirsty between meals. • Limit milk to one serving with meals or offer at end of meal; offer water for seconds. • If bottle is still used, wean to cup.
Refuses vegetables and fruits	• If child refuses vegetables, offer more fruits, and vice versa. • Prepare vegetables that are tender but not overcooked. • Steam vegetable strips (or offer raw if appropriate) and allow child to eat with fingers. • Offer sauces and dips (e.g., cheese sauce for cooked vegetables, dip for raw vegetables, yogurt to dip fruit). • Include vegetables in soups and casseroles. • Add fresh or dried fruit to cereals. • Prepare fruit in a variety of ways (e.g., fresh, cooked, juice, in gelatin, as a salad). • Continue to offer a variety of fruits and vegetables.
Eats too many sweets	• Limit purchase and preparation of sweet foods in the home. • Avoid using as a bribe or reward. • Incorporate into meals instead of snacks for better dental health. • Reduce sugar by half in recipes for cookies, muffins, quick breads, and the like. • Work with staff of day care, preschools, and others to reduce use of sweets.

Children younger than age 4 are at greatest risk for choking on food. Foods most likely to cause choking are those that are round, hard, and do not readily dissolve in saliva, such as hot dogs, grapes, raw vegetables, popcorn, peanut butter, nuts, and hard candy. Other foods can also cause choking problems if too much is stuffed into the mouth, if the child is running while eating, or if the child is unsupervised.

Excessive fruit juice consumption should be avoided because it can lead to chronic diarrhea and failure to thrive.[23] Thus, fruit juice should be limited to 4 to 6 ounces per day for children 1 to 6 years of age and 8 to 12 ounces for children 7 to 18 years of age. Whole fruit should be encouraged to provide dietary fiber.[24]

Feeding Children 6 to 12 Years of Age

The years from 6 to 12 are a period of slow but steady growth, with increases in food intake as a result of appetite (see Table 6-2). Because children are in school, they may eat fewer times during the day, but after-school snacks usually are a routine. Skipping breakfast may begin in these years. With participation in organized sports and other activities, sitting down to a family meal may be less frequent.

Feeding Teenagers

Adolescence is a period of rapid growth. As teenagers achieve more independence and spend a greater amount of time away from home, they have additional variable intakes and irregular eating patterns. Skipping meals is greatest in this age group, and snacking is common. Although fast foods are popular with all segments of the population, they are very appealing to teenagers. Negative impacts of fast foods on the diets of adolescents will depend on how frequently they are eaten and the choices made. High fast-food consumption is associated with decreased intake of milk, fruits, and vegetables.

School Nutrition

Children and teens spend much of their time in school and many participate in events after school. Most children eat at least one meal daily in the school environment; others may consume two meals and a snack. School lunches, school wellness policies, and food sources outside the cafeteria all have received attention with the goal to maximize health.

Children usually participate in the school lunch program or bring a packed lunch from home. The National School

Lunch Program is administered by the U.S. Department of Agriculture (USDA). Federal guidelines are established so the lunch provides approximately one-third of the RDAs or AIs for students. Many schools also participate in the School Breakfast Program. Free and reduced-price meals are available for low-income children. Incorporating the U.S. Dietary Guidelines into child nutrition programs has resulted in menus with lower fat content and more fresh fruits, vegetables, and whole-grain products.[25]

Vending machines with sugary foods and drinks may be available to children and adolescents during the school day. Problems associated with increased soda consumption include risk of obesity, deficits in bone mass, and increased dental caries. Efforts should focus on improving food and beverage choices in school vending machines.

School wellness policies are required in institutions that participate in school meal programs. School districts set goals for nutrition education, physical activity, campus food provision, and other school-based activities to promote student wellness. School nutrition services should be integrated with a coordinated comprehensive school health program and school nutrition policy.[26]

Other Nutrition Issues

As children grow and develop, various nutrition-related issues or problems arise. These are not uncommon in otherwise healthy children, and they can be prevented or managed with minimal intervention.

Dental Caries

Dental caries remain a common oral health disease in the pediatric population. The increased use of dental sealants has been helpful in reducing dental caries.[27] Nutrition and oral health are closely related. Inadequate intake of energy and protein can delay tooth eruption, affect tooth size, and cause salivary gland dysfunction. Micronutrients (e.g., calcium, vitamin D, fluoride) are also critical to the development and maintenance of oral structures.[28,29] Poor oral health can negatively affect a child's nutritional status and has implications for overall health. Missing or decayed teeth may increase the risk of nutrient deficiency by preventing a child from eating certain foods. Pain or malformed teeth can contribute to problems with speech and communication, interfere with sleep, and negatively affect an individual's self-image.

Dental caries develop in the presence of carbohydrate, bacteria, and a susceptible tooth. The process of decay begins with the interaction of bacteria (*Streptococcus mutans*) and fermentable carbohydrate on the tooth surface. When the bacteria within the dental plaque (the gelatinous substance on the tooth surface) metabolize the carbohydrate, organic acids are produced. When the acid reduces the pH to 5.5 or less, demineralization of the tooth enamel occurs.[30] Individuals with high salivary counts of *S. mutans* appear to be at risk for caries.[31]

Sucrose is the most common carbohydrate recognized in the caries process. Even starch can easily be broken down into fermentable carbohydrate by salivary amylase. Many foods high in starch often contain sucrose or other sugars, which may make the food more cariogenic than sugar alone because starch is retained longer in the mouth. Honey is just as cariogenic as sucrose. The cariogenicity of specific foods depends not only on the type and amount of fermentable carbohydrate, but also on the retentiveness of foods to the tooth surface and the frequency of eating. All of these factors influence the length of time the teeth are exposed to an acidic environment, which leads to tooth decay.[30]

Some protein foods (e.g., nuts, hard cheeses) have a protective effect against caries.[32] Eating these foods at the same time as high-sugar foods prevents a reduction in plaque pH. Because children of all ages eat frequently, snacks should emphasize foods that are low in sucrose, are not sticky, and stimulate saliva flow (see Table 6-2). Desserts, when consumed, should be eaten with meals. School-age children and adolescents may benefit from chewing sugarless gum after snacks containing fermentable carbohydrate, because this may reduce caries.[33]

Good oral hygiene complements dietary efforts. In infancy, parents can clean the gums and teeth with a clean cloth. The toothbrush should be introduced in the toddler period. The key is to incorporate brushing and flossing as a regular, consistent routine, with parental supervision in the early years. If the water supply is not fluoridated, use of a fluoride supplement is recommended into the teen years. Topical fluoride applications are recommended based on assessment of caries risk. All children should see a primary dental care provider by 12 months of age or 6 months after the first tooth erupts.[34,35]

Children younger than 3 years of age are most likely to have early childhood caries (ECC). Rampant caries develop on the primary upper front teeth (incisors) and often on the cheek surface of primary upper first molars. Children from poor families are at highest risk for ECC, and a history of ECC may increase the risk for future caries in permanent teeth.[34]

The primary cause of ECC is prolonged exposure of the teeth to a sweetened liquid (formula, milk, juice, or sweetened beverages). This occurs most often when the child is routinely given a nursing bottle at bedtime or during naps. ECC occurs less often in breastfed infants.[36] Toddlers who hold their own bottles and have access to bottles or sippy cups with sweetened liquids anytime throughout the day are at high risk. Education is the primary strategy to prevent ECC. Parents should be counseled about the disorder early in infancy and encouraged to avoid putting a baby to sleep with a bottle. Juices and liquids other than milk or formula should be offered in a cup. In normal infants, weaning from the bottle should begin at about 1 year of age.

Iron Deficiency Anemia

Iron deficiency anemia is common in children between 1 and 2 years of age and in adolescent females.[37] Programs such as the Women, Infants and Children (WIC) food program have helped reduce the incidence of anemia. Unfortunately, some young children, especially those in low-income households, are at high risk for iron deficiency and may have poorer cognitive performance and delayed psychomotor development.[38,39] Iron-deficient children also are at risk for increased lead absorption when exposed to sources of lead.

Dietary factors, as well as growth and physiologic needs, play a role in development of anemia. Some toddlers consume a large volume of milk to the exclusion of solids; plain meats are often not well-accepted by preschool children because they require more chewing. For many of these children, most dietary iron comes from nonheme sources such as vegetables, grains, and cereals. Because the typical U.S. diet contains approximately 6 mg iron per 1000 calories, adolescents dieting to lose weight will have minimal iron intake.

Absorption of iron from food depends on several factors. One is the iron status of the individual; those with low iron stores will have a higher absorption rate. The absorption rate is higher for heme iron, which is found in meat, fish, and poultry, than for nonheme iron, which is found in vegetables and grains. Absorption of nonheme iron can be enhanced by increasing consumption of meat, fish, or poultry (MFP) and foods containing ascorbic acid.[40] Other foods or compounds can inhibit iron absorption. **Table 6-4** lists good iron sources as well as absorption enhancers and inhibitors. Simple but conscientious menu planning can help improve iron availability to children and teenagers.

Universal screening up to 2 years of age is recommended for communities and populations with significant levels of iron deficiency anemia or for infants whose diets put them at risk. Guidelines for treatment and follow-up of iron deficiency anemia are available.[37] A heme profile (hemoglobin or hematocrit) is usually used to screen for anemia; however, other tests are more sensitive and can provide more information about an individual's iron status. Hemoglobin, serum ferritin, and C-reactive protein should be used to screen for iron deficiency, based on risk.

TABLE 6-4 Food Sources of Iron

Food	Iron (mg)
Meat, Fish, and Poultry (1 oz)*	
Chicken liver	2.8
Beef liver	2.2
Turkey, roasted	1.7
Beef pot roast	1.3
Hamburger	1.1
Fresh pork, roasted	1.1
Ham	0.7
Chicken	0.6
Tuna, canned	0.5
Hot dog	0.3
Salmon	0.3
Fish stick	0.1
Cereals, Grains, Vegetables, and Fruits#	
Cooked cereals (½ cup)	0.7–1.3
Ready-to-eat cereals (¾ cup)	0.3–9.0
Whole-wheat bread, enriched	0.6–0.8
bread (1 slice)	1.3–3.0
Legumes, cooked (½ cup)	1.5–2.0
Greens (spinach, mustard, beet),	1.3
cooked (½ cup)	1.0–1.5
Green peas, cooked (½ cup)	1.0
Dried fruit (¼ cup)	0.5
Nuts, most kinds (2 Tbsp.)	0.9
Wheat germ (1 Tbsp.)	0.9
Molasses, light (1 Tbsp.)	0.9

Dietary Enhancers of Nonheme Iron Absorption	Dietary Inhibitors of Noneheme Iron Absorption
Meat, fish, poultry	Tea (tannic acid)
Ascorbic acid	Sequestering additives (such as EDTA used in fats and soft drinks to clarify and prevent rancidity)
Antacids	

*Heme iron sources (approximately 40% of the iron in these foods); well-absorbed.

#Nonheme sources; lower level of absorption; enhancers eaten at the same time will increase absorption.

Impact of Diet on School Performance and Behavior

What impact does a child's diet have on his or her school performance and behavior? Skipping breakfast affects classroom learning. Food additives, sugar, and allergies may cause hyperactivity in children. Although severe malnutrition early in life is known to negatively affect intellectual development, the impact of marginal malnutrition, skipping meals, or hunger has been more difficult to document. Generally, children function better when they eat breakfast. Thus, nutrition education and feeding programs should be targeted to children at risk so they might be better able to achieve in school.[41]

The impact of diet and nutrition on a child's behavior is a controversial topic. Although malnourished children and those experiencing iron deficiency anemia often demonstrate decreased attention and responsiveness, less interest in their environment, and reduced problem-solving ability, the effects of periodic hunger or "food insecurity" are less clear. Negative academic and psychosocial outcomes are associated with food insufficiency.[42]

Attention deficit hyperactivity disorder (ADHD) is a developmental disorder with specific criteria: inattention, impulsivity, hyperactivity, onset before 7 years of age, and duration of at least 6 months. The etiology of ADHD is not clear; however, some nutritional factors, including food additives, sugar, and food allergies, have been proposed as causes. Although treatment usually includes behavioral management, medication, and/or special education, various dietary treatments have been proposed.

The Feingold diet, popularized in the 1970s, theorized that artificial colorings and flavorings in the food supply caused hyperactivity. Treatment consisted of removing natural salicylates (found mostly in fruits) and some preservatives (BHA, BHT) from the child's diet. Some children with ADHD (usually preschoolers) may benefit from the diet. The Feingold diet plus elimination of foods that the parents believe are bothersome to their child (e.g., chocolate, sugar, caffeine) may improve behavior.[43] The modified Feingold diet, which includes fruits, has been evaluated favorably with regard to nutrient content and thus poses little risk for the child.[44] Families using the diet should receive nutritional counseling and should consider other helpful treatments for their child's ADHD.

Sugar (sucrose) is popularly believed to cause hyperactivity in children or behavior problems and delinquency in adolescents. This has not been proven. However, sugar consumption should be limited for a number of reasons, including improved oral health and promotion of better, more nutrient-dense diets. This can be reinforced with families, while helping them remain objective about a sugar–behavior relationship.

Stimulant medications such as methylphenidate (e.g., Ritalin, Concerta, Metadate, Focalin), dextroamphetamine (e.g., Dexedrine, Dextrostate), and mixed salts of a single-entity amphetamine (e.g., Adderall), are commonly used to treat ADHD.[45] They usually result in improvement of motor restlessness, increase attention span, and decrease irritability. Nonstimulant medications are sometimes prescribed for ADHD. Decreased energy intake is a factor in decreased growth rates for those receiving stimulant medication. Individuals who take stimulant medications should have their growth monitored regularly and the efficacy of the drug reassessed periodically.

Vegetarian Diets

Well-planned vegetarian diets are appropriate throughout the life cycle, including during childhood and adolescence.[46] By definition, a vegetarian diet does not contain meat, fish, or fowl or products containing these foods.[46] However, a range of vegetarian diet patterns is possible, including lacto-ovo vegetarians (consume grains, vegetables, fruits, legumes, seeds, nuts, dairy products, and eggs), lacto vegetarians (no eggs consumed), ovo vegetarians (no dairy consumed), and vegans (exclude all products of animal origin) as well as food patterns that include only raw food or other specific food types. The more restrictive vegetarian diets will most likely not meet the needs of growing children and adolescents.[47]

A vegetarian lifestyle can result in many positive health outcomes, including lower low-density lipoprotein cholesterol levels, lower blood pressure, lower rates of hypertension, and decreased risk of type 2 diabetes, However, vegans and other vegetarians may have lower intakes of vitamin B_{12}, calcium, vitamin D, zinc, and long-chain omega-3 fatty acids. Adequate intake of the these nutrients, as well as iron and riboflavin, must be assured.[46]

Families may choose to implement vegetarian food patterns throughout their child's development. Infants can be breastfed or receive soy formula (vegan) or cow's milk formula (lacto). Infants born prematurely should not receive soy formula (see Chapter 4). Solid foods should be introduced following recommended guidelines, based on developmental readiness. Depending on the type of vegetarian diet followed by the family, anticipatory guidance may include explanations of the need for offering foods with appropriate textures and that are dense in energy and nutrients. Children consuming a well-planned and not overly restrictive diet grow and develop as their peers.[47] Adolescents with vegetarian food patterns may need guidance to ensure they consume a variety of foods to meet their needs. This guidance may include use of vitamin and/or mineral supplements at appropriate levels.

Adolescent Pregnancy

The risk of complications for pregnant teens is higher than for any other age group. The nutritional status of the pregnant adolescent is influenced by both physiologic and environmental/social factors. Young pregnant teenagers are still growing, resulting in maternal–fetal competition for nutrients, and thus indicating increased nutrient needs in addition to pregnancy.[48,49] See Chapter 1 for further details about nutrition needs during pregnancy, breastfeeding, and the postpartum period.

Substance Abuse

Alcohol, tobacco, and marijuana are the most widely used illicit substances among teenagers. Abuse of inhalants and nonmedical use of prescription medications are also common.[50] Alcoholism in adolescence is a significant public health problem. Any negative effect on nutritional status will depend on the frequency and amount of drinking as well as usual food habits. Teenagers who consume alcohol may have decreased intakes of milk, fruits, and vegetables and have symptoms of poor nutrition (e.g., tiredness, bleeding gums, muscle weakness).[51] For the female who consumes alcohol and becomes pregnant, there is risk of fetal alcohol syndrome in her infant.

Smoking remains relatively popular among teenagers. Teens who smoke may have an increased need for some nutrients, such as ascorbic acid, and smoking during pregnancy can reduce infant birth weight. Smokeless (chewing) tobacco and water-pipe tobacco smoking are also popular with both school-age children and adolescents.[52,53] Regular tobacco use is related to periodontal disease, oral cancer, dependence, and hypertension.

The negative nutritional consequences of a substance user's habit will depend on factors such as lifestyle, available food, and money to buy food. During a nutrition evaluation, the areas of alcohol consumption, tobacco use, and illegal drug use should be explored. Nutrition education and counseling can focus on improving health and nutrition. Some teenagers may need a comprehensive treatment program that includes a nutrition component.

Exercise

Regular physical activity should be encouraged for all children because of its importance in maintaining a healthy body, enhancing psychological well-being, and preventing premature death.[54] Regular physical activity improves an individual's endurance, flexibility, and strength.[55] Benefits from physical activity include improved cardiorespiratory endurance, improved muscular fitness, favorable body composition, improved bone health, and improved cardiovascular and metabolic health biomarkers. Physical activity may reduce symptoms of anxiety and depression.[55] Exercise can be fun, it can help people make new friends, and it offers a way to spend quality family time.[56] Current physical activity recommendations for those ages 6 through 17 years of age are:[55]

- Children and adolescents should engage in 1 hour or more of physical activity every day.
- Most of the 1 hour or more a day should be either moderate-or vigorous-intensity aerobic physical activity.
- As part of their daily physical activity, children and adolescents should do vigorous-intensity activity at least 3 days per week. They also should do muscle-strengthening and bone-strengthening activity at least 3 days per week.

The 2008 Physical Activity Guidelines for Americans contain information regarding activities that will meet these recommendations and are appropriate for children.[55]

Many children and adolescents participate in competitive sports and are interested in the effects of nutrition on athletic performance. Adequate energy and fluid intake is needed to support growth and to meet the increased demands of physical activity. See **Table 6-5** for exercise levels with age, nutrition, fluid, and health assessment guidelines.[57–64] Children and adolescents who participate in sports may need to adjust their intakes before, during, and after an event (e.g., pregame snacks of foods with complex carbohydrates).

Performance-enhancing substances for athletic or other purposes should be strongly discouraged.[65] Parents, coaches, and other youth sports organizations should encourage the young athlete to consume whole, nutritious foods as part of a balanced diet in addition to participating in appropriate physical training.[65]

Health Promotion

Americans are increasingly interested in their health and the prevention of chronic diseases such as cardiovascular disease, cancer, obesity, type 2 diabetes, and hypertension. The use of low-fat dairy products and limiting of high-fat foods is appropriate for healthy, growing children older than 2 years of age. Recommendations for lipid screening and cardiovascular health in children by the American Academy of Pediatrics (AAP) are similar to the guidelines recommended by the National Cholesterol Education Program (NCEP) and the American Heart Association.[66–69] Everyone older than 2 years of age should follow a diet that includes no more than 30% of energy as fat (10% or less from saturated fat) and no more than 200–300 mg cholesterol per day. A balanced energy intake with sufficient physical activity to maintain a healthy weight should be promoted. The diet should include fruits, vegetables, fish, whole grains, and low-fat dairy products.

Heart Health

Low-fat milk should be used for children 12 to 24 months of age who are obese or who have a family history of obesity, dyslipidemia, or cardiovascular disease (CVD).[66] Cholesterol screening should be done for children (ages 2 years and older) at risk: those with a positive family history of dyslipidemia or premature (≤55 years of age for men and ≤65 for women) CVD. Other risk factors that might indicate a need for screening include family history of overweight, hypertension, cigarette smoking, or diabetes mellitus.

For children identified by screening, the NCEP intervention is dependent on low-density lipoprotein (LDL) cholesterol categories.[67] For those with an acceptable level (less than 110 mg/dL), the recommended dietary pattern (step-one diet) is suggested, with a repeat lipoprotein analysis in 5 years. Children with a borderline level of LDL cholesterol (110–129 mg/dL) would be provided with an individualized step-one diet and reevaluated in 1 year. Those with high LDL cholesterol levels (greater than 130 mg/dL) would initially be given the step-one diet and, if necessary, the step-two diet (further reduction to less than 7% saturated fat and less than 200 mg cholesterol per day).

TABLE 6-5 Exercise Levels with Age, Nutrition, Fluid, and Health Assessment Guidelines

Definitions	Examples (not inclusive)	Recommended Age	Nutrition Comments	Fluid Intake	Recommended Health Assessment
1. ROUTINE: The duration of the activity is less than 20 min, and it may or may not reach 60% of maximum heartbeat rate.	Recess play, casual walking, recreational noncontinual sport (i.e., T-ball, volleyball)	Minimum activity level for any age	Normal nutrition for age from MyPlate.	Normal for age.	Yearly routine exam from a pediatrician or physician for all ages of children.
2. HEALTH FITNESS: 60–80% of maximum heartbeat rate is achieved for greater than 20 min at least three times per week for a minimum of 6 months. The activity should involve muscular strength and flexibility.	Brisk walking, jogging, running, cycling, hiking, swimming, dancing	Preferred level for any age	Normal nutrition for age from MyPlate. If desired weight for height, possibly more calories.	Good hydration, especially in adverse weather. Normal requirements for age and replacement of lost fluid from activity.	Yearly routine exam from a pediatrician or physician for all ages of children. Education from a physician or health professional on healthy practices (diet, fluid, injury prevention, warm-up and cool-down techniques, etc.). Immediate attention from an appropriate health professional for an injury or insult.
3. COMPETITIVE SPORTS: An activity less than or equal to 6 months that consists of team involvement, preseason training, and competing either as a team member or individually at an intramural or interschool level.	Swimming, gymnastics, diving, volleyball, wrestling, sprinting, relay, football, soccer, basketball, tennis, field hockey, crosscountry	Junior high age and above	Nutrition assessment, recommendations, and education, preferably from a registered dietitian, for an individual's season intake to achieve weight and body composition for the sport. Recommendations will be dependent on type of activity, duration, and intensity.	Pre-event, event, and postevent (or prepractice and postpractice) hydration. Good hydration at other times. Electrolyte replacement may be needed if heavy sweating occurs or in adverse weather conditions.	Preparticipation assessment by a health team consisting of a physician, dietitian, nurse or nurse practitioner, and possibly a physical therapist. Examination as well as education should be given to students at this time. Immediate attention from an appropriate health professional for any injury or insult during the sports season.

(continues)

TABLE 6-5 *(Continued)*

Definitions	Examples (not inclusive)	Recommended Age	Nutrition Comments	Fluid Intake	Recommended Health Assessment
3a. Competitive under 6 months: Short endurance—intense activity that lasts for 20 min or less.	Same as 3	Junior high age and above	2 g pro/kg for growing athletes ≥1 g pro/kg for mature athletes.		
3b. Competitive under 6 months: Long endurance—activity, intense or nonintense, that lasts for longer than 20 min.	Same as 3	High school age and above	May need refueling with carbohydrate during the event if long in duration (more than 4 h).	Electrolyte replacement needs assessed and replacement given if necessary.	
4. COMPETITIVE SPORTS: Longer than 6 months. Same as Competitive, but usually involved at a personal level other than school.	Same as 3, but may include state or national competition	High school age and above	Same as 3.	Same as 3.	Same as 3. It is very important that a physician determine that the maturation age of the participant is appropriate for the sport.
4a. Competitive at least 6 months: Short endurance—same as 4.	Same as 3				
4b. Competitive at least 6 months: Long endurance—same as 4.	Same as 3				
5. PERFORMING: An activity that requires dedicated practice (several times a week) to perform with a group or individually a routine lasting anywhere from 5 min to 1 hr (or longer) in competition or performance.	Ballet, dance, or gymnastics	Junior high age and above as determined by a physician	Nutrition assessment, recommendations, and education provided, preferably by a registered dietitian due to the usually restricted intake to achieve desired weight for performance.	Normal hydration and replacement of lost fluids from practice or performance	Preparticipation assessment by a physician, dietitian, and possibly an orthopedist or physical therapist. Injury attention as in competitive sports.

6. MARCHING BAND: Involvement with a band that competes or performs in marching or choreographed performance. Includes preseason training as well as competition or performance.	High school marching or competing bands	Junior high age and above	Nutrition assessment, recommendations, and education, preferably from a registered dietitian, in a group setting, or individually if necessary.	Same as in 3a and 3b.	Same as in 2 or 3a and 3b. Nutrition attention by a registered dietitian if the participant is less than 85% or greater than 120% of desired weight for height.
7. SEASONAL: Intramural involvement with a team or individual activity, not based heavily on winning but just participation. Practice required. May or may not last longer than 20 min three or more times a week, but activity is not sustained longer than 2 or 3 months.	Soccer, softball, swimming lessons	All ages	Same as in 2.	Same as in 3a and 3b.	Preparticipation assessment by a pediatrician or physician, as in 2. Nutrition attention by a registered dietitian if the participant is less than 85% or greater than 120% of desired weight for height.

Sources: Luckstead SR. Cardiac risk factors and participation guidelines for youth sports. *Ped Clin North Am.* 2002;49:4; National Academy of Sciences. Institute of Medicine. Food and Nutrition Board. Dietary reference intakes: recommended intakes for energy, carbohydrate, fiber, fat, fatty acids, cholesterol, protein and amino acids. Available at: http://www.iom.edu/Global/News%20 Announcements/~/media/C5CD2DD7840544979A549EC47E56A02B. Accessed July 31, 2011; U.S. Department of Agriculture. MyPlate. Available at: http://www.choosemyplate.gov. Accessed July 31, 2011; Story M, Holt K, Sofka D, eds. *Bright Futures in Practice: Nutrition*, 2nd ed. Arlington, VA: National Center for Education in Maternal and Child Health; 2002: 203–211; American Academy of Pediatrics Committee on Sports Medicine and Fitness. Medical concerns in the female athlete. *Pediatrics*. 2000;106(3):610–613; Rogoi A. Effects of endurance training on maturation. *Consultant*. 1985;25:68–83; Bar-Or O, Barr S, Bergeron M, et al. Youth in sport: nutritional needs. Gatorade Sports Science Institute 1997;RT30(8):4. Available at: http://www.gssiweb.com. Accessed July 31, 2011.

Some experts do not believe that these recommendations are appropriate, especially for the young child.[70] Growth failure has been seen in some infants and toddlers whose parents, well intentioned but misguided, restricted their children's diet to prevent atherosclerosis, obesity, and poor eating habits.[71] Although there is little evidence that dietary intervention in the growing years will decrease serum cholesterol levels or modify other risk factors later in life, young children appear to be able to consume low-fat diets (less than 30% of energy as fat) without negatively influencing the level of energy or micronutrients consumed or affecting growth.[72–74] It seems appropriate to recommend a gradual transition to a diet meeting the NCEP guidelines for children older than 2 years of age.

Many adolescents are exceeding NCEP recommendations for total and saturated fat and cholesterol intakes. A higher percentage of black girls than white girls are not meeting recommendations.[75] Children in low-income families with food insufficiency often have higher cholesterol intakes than their peers from higher income, food-sufficient households. They were more likely to be overweight, consume less fruit, and watch more television than their peers from low-income, food-sufficient families.[76]

Bone Health

Prevention of osteoporosis begins with optimal calcium and vitamin D intake and maximal bone density in the growing years. However, many young people, especially adolescents, do not receive the recommended AI of 1300 mg of calcium. Those who consume limited amounts of dairy products are at risk for calcium deficiency. Some adolescents may also receive less calcium than needed because of rapid growth, dieting practices, and substituting carbonated beverages for milk. Nutrition education is important to improve these diet trends.

Fiber and Health

Children and adolescents do not consume enough fiber and whole-grain foods, similar to the adult population.[77] (See Appendix F.) The 2010 dietary guidelines recommend a more plant-based diet that emphasizes vegetables, beans and peas, fruits, whole grains, and nuts and seeds. Increasing dietary fiber can help prevent constipation, protect against coronary heart disease, and often results in greater intake of fruits and vegetables.

Education

Children first learn about food and nutrition from their families in their own homes. This begins in an informal manner, with parental attitudes, foods commonly served (e.g., potatoes or tortillas may be served daily; okra or bok choy may never be served), and family opinions about what foods are good nutritionally. Later, more formal nutrition education occurs in preschools, Head Start programs, day cares, schools, and clubs. Information is also assimilated from the media, advertising, written materials, the Internet, and peers.

A child's developmental level should be taken into account when teaching nutrition concepts. For example, Piaget's learning theory can be used to correlate developmental periods and cognitive characteristics with progress in feeding and nutrition.[78] Younger children do best with hands-on personal experience with food. A personal approach works well with children and adolescents, such as the use of computer software to examine their own dietary profiles. Social marketing strategies, such as television and the Internet, can be used to communicate health messages to "tweens" (9- to 13-year-olds).[79] Using theoretical concepts to design nutrition education programs and evaluating the effectiveness of these programs is necessary to have an impact on the target population.[80,81] The use of an ecological model may increase understanding of eating behaviors, especially among adolescents. The ecological model examines the influences of individual (e.g., biologic), social environmental (e.g., peers), physical environmental (e.g., school), and macrosystem or societal (e.g., marketing) factors on behaviors.[82] Lastly, nutrition education efforts for children should not overlook parents and the family as a whole.

Case Study

Nutrition Assessment of a School-Age Child

Patient History

A 6.5-year-old male (Ryan) was referred to the nutritionist due to lack of weight gain and slowed growth over the past year. At age 6 years, Ryan was diagnosed with attention deficit hyperactivity disorder (ADHD). Concerta (methylphenidate HCl) was prescribed. Current dose is 36 mg daily, but it has varied based on a balance between medication effectiveness and reduced appetite.

Food/Nutrition-Related History

Typical intake: Three meals and two snacks—estimated energy intake 1500 kcal/day

Early morning: Ryan wakes at 5:45 am. He prepares for school, takes his medication, and watches television for 30 minutes before the family leaves. Prior to starting before-school care 5 months earlier, Ryan ate breakfast at home: 3 packets instant oatmeal or 1.5 cups Cheerios or 2 eggs. Drank 10 ounces 2% milk and ate 1/2 cup fruit.

Breakfast: Offered at before-school care at 7:30 am, but Ryan is not hungry at this time—he may eat a few bites.

Lunch: Parents send lunch. Ryan consumes half a peanut butter and jelly sandwich and perhaps half a small bag of chips; he may eat a 4-ounce cup of applesauce. He drinks water. Family sends a juice box, but Ryan usually does not drink it. He prefers milk but does not like school milk.

Snack: Offered at after-school program; they report Ryan always eats the snack and drinks water.

5 pm: Family picks up from after-school program. Ryan is hungry and will finish some of his lunch (chips and applesauce).

6:30 pm: Eats 1.5 cups casserole, chili, or stew or 3 ounces chicken and 1 cup rice. Eats 1/4 cup vegetables; if green beans can eat 2 cups. Drinks 10 ounces milk.

7 pm: 4–5 times each week Ryan asks for a snack after dinner and will eat applesauce, cheese, or 1 piece of bologna.

A pediatric chewable vitamin, Flintstones Complete, is offered daily. For the past 4 months the family has offered L'il Critters Immune C plus Zinc and Echinacea daily.

Ryan is described as active by family.

Anthropometric Measurements

Weight: 21 kg

Height: 125 cm

BMI: 13.4

Previous growth: According to records from Ryan's primary care provider, for the previous 3 years height has been following the 95th percentile, weight plotted between the 50th and 75th percentiles, and BMI plotted between the 10th and 25th percentiles.

Estimated energy needs: Calculate EER (estimated energy requirement).

EER (boys 3 through 8 years) = $88.5 - 61.9 \times$ age [years] + PA ($26.7 \times$ wt [kg] + $903 \times$ ht [m]) + 20

$= 88.5 - 61.9(6.5) + 1.26(26.7 \times 21 + 903 \times 1.25) + 20$

$= 1835$

Calculate estimated protein needs based on the DRI: $0.95 \times$ wt [kg] = 21 grams

Medical tests: None indicated

Nutrition Diagnoses

Inadequate energy intake related to decreased appetite from use of Concerta, as evidenced by reported intake below EER and lack of weight gain during the past year.

Intervention Goals

1. Increase energy intake to initially meet EER.
2. Gain weight at a rate appropriate for age.

Nutrition Interventions

Energy intake: Offer breakfast at home before giving medication dose.

Monitoring and Evaluation

- Evaluate growth and weight gain in 3 months.
- Evaluate diet for energy intake in 3 months.

Questions for the Reader

1. What are the nutrition-related side effects, if any, from this medication?
2. What are Ryan's BMI, height, and weight percentiles on the growth chart?
3. How do current BMI, height, and weight compare to previous percentiles?
4. How does Ryan's actual energy intake compare to the calculated EER?
5. Is Ryan's intake above tolerable upper limits for any nutrient based on supplement use?
6. What will you do during the follow-up visit 3 months later if Ryan has not gained weight since the last contact?

REFERENCES

1. Food and Nutrition Board, Institute of Medicine, National Academy of Sciences. *Dietary Reference Intakes for Energy, Carbohydrate, Fiber, Fat, Fatty Acids, Cholesterol, Protein, and Amino Acids.* Washington, DC: National Academies Press; 2005.
2. U.S. Department of Agriculture, Agricultural Research Service. Food and nutrient intakes by children 1994–96, 1998. ARS Food Surveys Research Group. Available at: www.ars.usda.gov/SP2UserFiles/Place/12355000/pdf/scs_all.pdf. Accessed February 10, 2004.
3. Alaimo K, McDowell MA, Briefel RR, et al. Dietary intake of vitamins, minerals, and fiber of persons ages 2 months and over in the United States: third National Health and Nutrition Examination Survey, Phase I, 1988–1991. *Adv Data Vital Stat.* 1994;258. PHS 95-1250.
4. Suitor CW, Gleason PM. Using dietary reference intake–based methods to estimate the prevalence of inadequate nutrient intake among school-aged children. *J Am Diet Assoc.* 2002;102(4):530–536.
5. Moshfegh A, Goldman J, Cleveland L. *What We Eat in America, NHANES 2001–2002: Usual Nutrient Intakes from Food Compared to Dietary Reference Intakes.* Washington, DC: U.S. Department of Agriculture, Agricultural Research Service; 2005.
6. Moshfegh A, Goldman J, Ahuja J, et al. *What We Eat in America, NHANES 2005–2006: Usual Nutrient Intakes from Food and*

Water Compared to 1997 Dietary Reference Intakes for Vitamin D, Calcium, Phosphorus, and Magnesium. Washington, DC: U.S. Department of Agriculture, Agricultural Research Service; 2009.

7. Matkovic V, Fontana D, Tominac C. Factors that influence peak bone mass formation: a study of calcium balance and the inheritance of bone mass in adolescent females. *Am J Clin Nutr.* 1990;52:878–888.
8. Food and Nutrition Board, Institute of Medicine. *Dietary Reference Intakes: The essential guide to nutrient requirements.* Washington, DC: National Academies Press; 2006.
9. Anderson JJ. Calcium requirements during adolescence to maximize bone health. *Pediatrics.* 2001;20(2 Suppl):186S–191S.
10. Food and Nutrition Board, Institute of Medicine, National Academy of Sciences. *Dietary Reference Intakes: Vitamin A, Vitamin K, Arsenic, Boron, Chromium, Copper, Iodine, Iron, Manganese, Molybdenum, Nickel, Silicon, Vanadium, and Zinc.* Washington, DC: National Academies Press; 2001.
11. Wagner CL, Greer FR. Prevention of rickets and vitamin D deficiency in infants, children, and adolescents. *Pediatrics.* 2008; 122:1142–1152.
12. Feeding the child. In: Kleinman RE, ed. American Academy of Pediatrics, Committee on Nutrition. *Pediatric Nutrition Handbook,* 6th ed. Elk Grove Village, IL: American Academy of Pediatrics; 2009:155–156.
13. Lanski SL, Greenwald M, Perkins A, Simon HK. Herbal therapy use in a pediatric emergency department population: expect the unexpected. *Pediatrics.* 2003;111(5):981–985.
14. Munoz KA, Krebs-Smith SM, Ballard-Barbash R, et al. Food intakes of U.S. children and adolescents compared with recommendations. *Pediatrics.* 1997;100:323–329.
15. Galloway AT, Lee Y, Birch LL. Predictors and consequences of food neophobia and pickiness in young girls. *J Am Diet Assoc.* 2003;103(6):692–698.
16. Larson NI, Neumark-Sztainer D, Hannan PJ, Story M. Family meals during adolescence are associated with higher diet quality and healthful meal patterns during young adulthood. *J Am Diet Assoc.* 2007;107(9):1502–1510.
17. Bell RA, Cassady D, Culp J, Alcalay R. Frequency and types of foods advertised on Saturday morning and weekday afternoon English- and Spanish-language American television programs. *J Nutr Educ Behav.* 2009;41(6):406–413.
18. Laurson KR, Eisenmann JC, Welk GJ, et al. Combined influence of physical activity and screen time recommendations on childhood overweight. *Pediatrics.* 2008;153(2):209–214.
19. American Public Health Association. Policy statement 2003-17. Food marketing and advertising directed at children and adolescents: implications for overweight. Available at: http://www.apha.org/advocacy/policy/policysearch/default.htm?id=1255. Accessed August 9, 2010.
20. Boynton-Jarrett R, Thomas TN, Peterson KE, et al. Impact of television viewing patterns on fruit and vegetable consumption among adolescents. *Pediatrics.* 2003;112(6 Pt 1):1321–1326.
21. Harris JL, Bargh JA, Brownell KD. Priming effects of television food advertising on eating behavior. *Health Psychology.* 2009;28(4):404–413.
22. Wright CM, Parkinson KN, Shipton D, Drewett RF. How do toddler eating problems relate to their eating behavior, food preferences and growth? *Pediatrics.* 2007;120:e1069–e1075.
23. Smith MM, Lifshitz F. Excess fruit juice consumption as a contributing factor in nonorganic failure to thrive. *Pediatrics.* 1994;93:438–443.
24. Committee on Nutrition, American Academy of Pediatrics. The use and misuse of fruit juice in pediatrics. *Pediatrics.* 2001;107(5): 1210–1213. [Policy statement reaffirmed October 2006.]
25. U.S. Department of Agriculture, Food and Nutrition Service, Office of Analysis, Nutrition and Evaluation. School Nutrition Dietary Assessment Study-II Summary of Findings. Alexandria, VA: USDA; 2001:1–44.
26. Briggs M, Safaii S, Beall D. Position of the American Dietetic Association, Society for Nutrition Education, and American School Food Service Association—nutrition services: an essential component of comprehensive school health programs. *J Am Diet Assoc.* 2003;103:505–514.
27. Dye BA, Tan S, Smith V, et al. Trends in oral health status: United States, 1988–1994 and 1999–2004. *Vital Health Stat.* 2007;11(248):1–92.
28. Faine MP. Nutrition issues and oral health. In: *Proceedings from Promoting Oral Health of Children with Neurodevelopmental Disabilities and Other Special Health Care Needs.* May 4–5, 2001. Center on Human Development and Disability, University of Washington, Seattle, WA. Available at: http://www.mchoralhealth.org/PDFs/LEND2001.pdf. Accessed February 10, 2004.
29. Palmer CA. *Diet and Nutrition in Oral Health.* Upper Saddle River, NJ: Prentice Hall; 2003.
30. White-Graves MV, Schiller MR. History of foods in the caries process. *J Am Diet Assoc.* 1986;86:241–245.
31. Garcia-Closas R, Garcia-Closas M, Sera-Majem L. A cross-sectional study of dental caries, intake of confectionery and foods rich in starch and sugars, and salivary counts of *Steptococcus mutans* in children in Spain. *Am J Clin Nutr.* 1997;66:1257–1263.
32. Navia JM. Carbohydrates and dental health. Am *J Clin Nutr.* 1994;59(Suppl):719S–727S.
33. Makinen KK, Hujoel PP, Bennett CA, et al. A descriptive report of the effects of a 16-month xylitol chewing gum programme subsequent to a 40-month sucrose gum programme. *Caries Res.* 1998;32:107–112.
34. American Academy of Pediatric Dentistry. Policy on early childhood caries (ECC): classifications, consequences, and preventive strategies. 2003, revised 2008. Available at: http://www.aapd.org/media/Policies_Guidelines/P_ECCClassifications.pdf. Accessed November 1, 2009.
35. American Academy of Pediatrics, Section on Pediatric Dentistry. Oral health risk assessment timing and establishment of the dental home. *Pediatrics.* 2003;111(5):1113–1116. [Policy statement reaffirmed May 2009.]
36. Caplan LS, Erwin K, Lense E, Hicks J. The potential role of breast-feeding and other factors in helping to reduce early childhood caries. *J Public Health Dent.* 2008;68(4):238–241.
37. Centers for Disease Control and Prevention. Iron deficiency: United States, 1999–2000. *MMWR.* 2002;51(40):897–899.
38. Lozoff B, Beard J, Connor J, et al. Long-lasting neural and behavioral effects of iron deficiency in infants. *Nutr Rev.* 2006;64(5):S34–S43.
39. Lozoff B, Corapci F, Burden MJ, et al. Preschool-aged children with iron deficiency anemia show altered affect and behavior. *J Nutr.* 2007;137:683–689.

40. Monsen ER, Hallberg L, Layrisse M, et al. Estimation of available dietary iron. *Am J Clin Nutr.* 1978;31:134–141.
41. Powell CA, Walker SP, Chang SM, Grantham-McGregor SM. Nutrition and education: a randomized trial of the effects of breakfast in rural primary school children. *Am J Clin Nutr.* 1998;68:873–879.
42. Alaimo K, Olsom CM, Frongillo EA. Food insufficiency and American school-aged children's cognitive, academic, and psychosocial development. *Pediatrics.* 2001;108(1):44–51.
43. Kaplan BJ, McNicol J, Conte RA, et al. Dietary replacement in preschool-aged hyperactive boys. *Pediatrics.* 1989;83:7–17.
44. Harper PH, Goyette CH, Conners CK. Nutrient intakes of children on the hyperkinesis diet. *J Am Diet Assoc.* 1978;73:515–519.
45. American Academy of Pediatrics Subcommittee on Attention-Deficit/Hyperactivity Disorder. Clinical practice guideline: treatment of the school-aged child with attention-deficit/hyperactivity disorder. *Pediatrics.* 2001;108(4):1033–1044.
46. Craig WJ, Mangels AR, American Dietetic Association. Position of the American Dietetic Association: vegetarian diets. *J Am Diet Assoc.* 2009;109(7):1266–1282.
47. Kleinman RJ. Nutritional aspects of vegetarian nutrition. In: American Academy of Pediatrics, Committee on Nutrition, ed. *Pediatric Nutrition Handbook,* 6th ed. Elk Grove Village, IL: American Academy of Pediatrics; 2009:201–224.
48. Hediger ML, Scholl TO, Schall JI. Implications of the Camden study of adolescent pregnancy: interactions among maternal growth, nutritional status, and body composition. *Ann N Y Acad Sci.* 1997;817:281–291.
49. Rees JM, Lederman SA. Kiely JL. Birth weight associated with lowest neonatal mortality: infants of adolescent and adult mothers. *Pediatrics.* 1996;98:1161–1166.
50. Substance Abuse and Mental Health Services Administration, Office of Applied Studies. *The NSDUH Report: Trends in Substance Use, Dependence or Abuse, and Treatment Among Adolescents: 2002 to 2007.* Rockville, MD. Substance Abuse and Mental Health Services Administration; 2008.
51. Farrow JA, Rees JM, Worthington-Roberts B. Health, developmental and nutritional status of adolescent alcohol and marijuana abusers. *Pediatrics.* 1987;79:218–223.
52. Centers for Disease Control and Prevention. Tobacco use among middle and high school students—United States, 2002. *MMWR.* 2003;52(45):1096–1098.
53. Primack BA, Walsh M, Bruce C, Eissenberg T. Water-pipe tobacco smoking among middle and high school students in Arizona. *Pediatrics.* 2009;123(2):e282–e288.
54. U.S. Department of Health and Human Services. Physical activity and fitness health indicators. *Healthy People 2010: Understanding and Improving Health,* 2nd ed. Washington, DC: U.S. Government Printing Office; 2000. Available at: http://www.healthypeople.gov/pdf/Volume2/22Physical.pdf. Accessed August 10, 2010.
55. U.S. Department of Health and Human Services. *Physical Activity Guidelines for Americans.* 2008. Available at: http://www.health.gov/paguidelines/guidelines/default.aspx. Accessed July 31, 2011.
56. President's Council on Physical Fitness and Sports. The president's challenge. Available at: http://www.presidentschallenge.org. Accessed July 31, 2011.
57. Goldberg B, Saraniti A, Witman P, et al. Pre-participation sports assessment: an objective evaluation. *Pediatrics.* 1980;66:736–745.
58. Luckstead SR. Cardiac risk factors and participation guidelines for youth sports. *Ped Clin North Am.* 2002;49:4.
59. National Academy of Sciences. Institute of Medicine. Food and Nutrition Board. Dietary reference intakes: recommended intakes for individuals. Available at: http://iom.edu/en/Global/News%20Announcements/~/media/Files/Activity%20Files/Nutrition/DRIs/DRISummaryListing2.ashx. Accessed March 28, 2010.
60. U.S. Department of Agriculture. MyPlate.gov. Available at: http://www.choosemyplate.gov. Accessed July 31, 2011.
61. Story M, Holt K, Sofka D, eds. *Bright Futures in Practice: Nutrition,* 2nd ed. Arlington, VA: National Center for Education in Maternal and Child Health; 2002:203–211.
62. American Academy of Pediatrics Committee on Sports Medicine and Fitness. Medical concerns in the female athlete. *Pediatrics.* 2000;106(3):610–613.
63. Rogoi A. Effects of endurance training on maturation. *Consultant.* 1985;25:68–83.
64. Bar-Or O, Barr S, Bergeron M, et al. Youth in sport: nutritional needs. Gatorade Sports Science Institute. 1997;RT30(8):4. Available at: http://www.gssiweb.com. Accessed July 31, 2011.
65. American Academy of Pediatrics. Use of performance-enhancing substances. *Pediatrics.* 2005;115(4):1103–1106. [Policy statement reaffirmed August 2008.]
66. Daniels SR, Greer FR, Committee on Nutrition. Lipid screening and cardiovascular health in childhood. *Pediatrics.* 2008;122:198–208.
67. National Heart, Lung and Blood Institute, National Cholesterol Education Program. *Report of the Expert Panel on Blood Cholesterol Levels in Children and Adolescents.* Bethesda, MD: National Heart, Lung, and Blood Institute; 1991.
68. Lichtenstein AH, Appel LJ, Brands M, et al. Diet and lifestyle recommendations revision 2006: a scientific statement from the American Heart Association Nutrition Committee. *Circulation.* 2006;114(1):82–96. [Published corrections appear in *Circulation.* 2006;114(23):e629 and *Circulation.* 2006;114(1):e27.]
69. Gidding SS, Dennison BA, Birch LL, et al. Dietary recommendations for children and adolescents: a guide for practitioners: consensus statement from the American Heart Association. *Circulation.* 2005;112(13):2061–2075.
70. Olson RE. The folly of restricting fat in the diet of children. *Nutr Today.* 1995;30(6):234–235.
71. Pugliese MT, Weyman-Daum M, Moses N, et al. Parental health beliefs as a cause of nonorganic failure to thrive. *Pediatrics.* 1987;80:175–182.
72. Luepker RV, Perry CL, McKinlay SM, et al. Outcomes of a field trial to improve children's dietary patterns and physical activity. The Child and Adolescent Trial for Cardiovascular Health (CATCH). *JAMA.* 1996:275;768–776.
73. Dixon LB, McKenzie J, Shannon BM, et al. The effect of changes in dietary fat on the food group and nutrient intake of 4- to 10-year-old children. *Pediatrics* 1997;100:863–872.
74. Obarzanek E, Kimm SYS, Barton BA, et al. Long-term safety and efficacy of cholesterol-lowering diet in children with elevated low-density lipoprotein cholesterol: seven-year results of the Dietary Intervention Study in Children (DISC). *Pediatrics.* 2001;107(2):256–264.
75. Kronsberg SS, Obarzanek E, Affenito SG, et al. Macronutrient intake of black and white adolescent girls over than 10 years:

the NHLBI Growth and Health Study. *J Am Diet Assoc.* 2003;103(7):852–860.
76. Casey PH, Szeto K, Lansing S, et al. Children in food-insufficient, low-income families: prevalence, health, and nutrition status. *Arch Pediatr Adolesc Med.* 2001;155(4):508–514.
77. Harnack L, Walters SH, Jacobs DR. Dietary intake and food sources of whole grains among US children and adolescents: data from the 1994–1996 Continuing Survey of Food Intakes by Individuals. *J Am Diet Assoc.* 2003;103(8):1015–1019.
78. Lucas B, Feucht S. Nutrition in childhood. In: Mahan LK, King K, eds. *Krause's Food, Nutrition, & Diet Therapy,* 12th ed. Philadelphia, PA: Saunders/Elsevier; 2008:22–245.
79. Huhman M, Bauman A, Bowles HR. Initial outcomes of the VERB campaign: tweens' awareness and understanding of campaign messages. *Am J Prev Med.* 2008;34(6 Suppl):S241–S248.
80. Contento I, Balch GI, Bronner YL, et al. The effectiveness of nutrition education and implications for nutrition education and policy, programs, and research: a review of research. *J Nutr Educ.* 1995;27:298–311.
81. Sigman-Grant M. Strategies for counseling adolescents. *J Am Diet Assoc.* 2002;102(3 Suppl):S32–S39.
82. Story M, Neumark-Sztainer D, French S. Individual and environmental influences on adolescent eating behaviors. *J Am Diet Assoc.* 2002;102(3 Suppl):S40–S51.

CHAPTER 7

Food Hypersensitivities

Lynn Christie

Introduction

An adverse food reaction is a clinically abnormal response to an ingested food or food additive. Adverse food reactions (food sensitivities) are categorized either as hypersensitivities (food allergy) or as intolerances. Food hypersensitivity is caused by an immunologic reaction resulting from the ingestion of a food or food additive. Food intolerance is an abnormal physiological response to an ingested food or a food additive that has not been proven to be immunologic in nature.

Food hypersensitivity involves either immunoglobulin E (IgE)-mediated or non-IgE–mediated immune mechanisms. IgE-mediated reactions occur after ingestion of a specific food, occur usually within 1 hour, and can be followed by a late-phase reaction. Non-IgE–mediated reactions, such as food protein–induced enterocolitis, proctocolitis, allergic eosinophilic diseases, and gluten-sensitive enteropathy, are cell mediated reactions. Food hypersensitivities are further described in **Table 7-1** by their clinical manifestations and whether the disorder is IgE mediated.

Food intolerances that are proven not to be immunologic in nature are secondary to factors such as toxic contaminants, pharmacological properties of foods, and metabolic disorders. **Table 7-2** provides a differential diagnosis for adverse food reactions.

Eggs, milk, peanuts, soybeans, wheat, tree nuts, fish, and shellfish cause approximately 90% of food hypersensitivities in children in the United States.[1] Milk, egg, peanut, soybean, and wheat are the primary foods responsible for hypersensitivity in children 3 years of age and younger.

Contact with an allergen is necessary before an IgE immunological response can occur. The dermis, gastrointestinal tract (GI), and respiratory tract are involved in an allergic reaction. More severe, life-threatening reactions involve the cardiovascular system. IgE-mediated food allergy is responsible for oral allergy syndrome, exercise-induced anaphylaxis, and possibly colic in infants with milk allergy. Non-IgE–mediated food allergies involve the gastrointestinal tract. Elimination of the allergen is the basis of medical management.

The allergic immune response begins with sensitization to a particular antigen, a glycoprotein in a food. Therefore, the susceptible individual must come into contact with a food before becoming allergic. The plasma cells (mature B-cells) begin producing IgE to a particular food antigen. The food-specific IgE becomes bound to mast cells and basophils, and then recurrent antigen exposure leads to a cross-linking of the food-specific IgE molecules, activating the mast cells and basophils. This activation causes the release of histamine, leukotrienes, and other mediators. These mediators produce vasodilation, smooth muscle contraction, and mucous secretion, resulting in the clinical symptoms detected in the skin, respiratory system, and GI system. The immediate allergic reaction can occur within seconds and up to 2 hours after contact with the food allergen. This cross-linking can lead to the synthesis of proinflammatory cytokines and chemokines that are responsible for a late-phase reaction that might occur within 4 to 48 hours after the initial exposure. A chronic inflammatory response seen primarily with the skin and respiratory systems is thought to be due to the repetitive ingestion of a food allergen.[2]

The organ systems generally related to IgE-mediated allergic reactions are the skin, GI tract, and respiratory tract. Once foods are ingested, immediate oral symptoms such as itching mouth and swelling of the lips, palate, tongue, or throat may occur. In the GI tract, nausea, cramping, gas, distention, vomiting, abdominal pain, or diarrhea may occur. Once the antigen spreads through the bloodstream and lymphatics, degranulation of mast cells may occur in the skin, causing urticaria, angioedema, pruritis, or an erythematous macular rash. Respiratory symptoms include coughing, wheezing, profuse nasal rhinorrhea, sneezing, or laryngeal edema. The eyes may experience edema, tearing, excess mucus, itching, or burning. The relationship of food hypersensitivities to migraine headaches, epilepsy, rheumatoid arthritis, enuresis, and attention deficit hyperactivity

TABLE 7-1 Food Hypersensitivity Disorders

	IgE Mediated	Mixed (May Involve Both IgE-Mediated and Cell-Mediated Mechanisms)	Non-IgE Mediated
Gastrointestinal	Oral allergy syndrome (oral and perioral pruritis and angioedema, throat tightness) Gastrointestinal anaphylaxis (nausea, cramping, emesis, diarrhea) Infantile colic (~15% of infants with colic)	Allergic eosinophilic esophagitis (subset) Allergic eosinophilic gastroenteritis (postprandial nausea, emesis, weight loss)	Food-induced enterocolitis (1 to 3 hours postingestion: emesis, diarrhea, failure to thrive, and rarely, hypotension) Food-induced proctocolitis (2 to 12 hours postingestion; blood in stools) Food-induced malabsorption syndrome ("celiac-like"; nausea, steatorrhea, weight loss) Celiac disease
Cutaneous	Acute (common) and chronic (rare) urticaria Generalized flushing	Atopic dermatitis (pruritic morbilliform rash leading to eczematous lesion)	Dermatitis herpetiformis Contact hypersensitivity Contact irritation (especially with acid fruits and vegetables)
Respiratory	Rhinoconjunctivitis Laryngeal edema	Asthma (both acute wheezing and increased bronchial hyper-reactivity)	Heiner's syndrome (rare form of pulmonary hemosiderosis)
Other: Mechanism Unknown	Migraine (rare)		

Source: Adapted with permission from Sampson HA. Diagnosing food allergies in children. In: Lichtenstein LM, Busse WW, Raif SG (eds). *Current Therapy in Allergy, Immunology, and Rheumatology*, 6th ed. St. Louis, MO: Mosby; 2004:147–153.

remains controversial.[3] Physical findings associated with gluten sensitivity can be found in Chapter 12.

Systemic anaphylaxis is an acute and potentially fatal reaction. Anaphylaxis can begin with any of the symptoms just mentioned plus cardiovascular symptoms, including chest tightness, tachycardia, hypotension, and shock. A fatal reaction may begin with mild symptoms and progress to cardiorespiratory arrest and shock rapidly within 1 to 3 hours. Risk factors include: (1) children with asthma; (2) allergies to peanuts, tree nuts, fish, and/or shellfish; (3) individuals who do not receive epinephrine immediately after the reaction begins; and (4) patients who have had a previous allergic reaction to a food.[4] Milk, egg, and soy are less likely than the previously listed items to produce fatal reactions in children.[5]

Exercise-induced anaphylaxis is associated with the ingestion of a specific food prior to exercise. Then, during or shortly after exercise, the individual experiences allergic symptoms that may progress to anaphylaxis.[6] The individual can usually exercise without any reaction as long as the specific food has not been ingested within the past 8 to 12 hours. Individuals with exercise-induced anaphylaxis typically have a positive skin prick test to foods that provoke symptoms. Management requires identifying the food through a food challenge that includes strenuous exercise after food ingestion and avoiding the food at least 8 to 12 hours prior to any expected exercise.

Oral allergy syndrome (OAS), also referred to as pollen–food allergy syndrome, is another form of IgE-mediated food allergy.[7] OAS occurs mainly in patients allergic to pollens. The proteins in the pollens that cause allergic rhinitis immunologically cross-react to the allergens in related raw fruits and vegetables.[8] The reaction is limited to the lips, tongue, palate, and throat, followed by a rapid resolution of symptoms. Systemic anaphylaxis is rare. People allergic to birch tree pollen may have OAS symptoms when they eat raw carrots, celery, apples, pears, cherries, apricots, and kiwis. Those allergic to ragweed may react when they eat watermelon, cantaloupe, honeydew, and bananas. Generally, cooking fruits and vegetables denatures the relevant proteins, allowing symptom-free consumption.

Infants with cow's milk allergy have a high rate of colic that improves with the use of extensively hydrolyzed formulas.[9] All causes of colic need to be considered, but if there are additional symptoms of cow's milk allergy or a poor response to other measures (e.g., medicines) a trial elimination diet may be reasonable. Infantile colic may represent an early manifestation of food allergy.[10,11]

TABLE 7-2 Differential Diagnosis for Adverse Food Reactions

I. Food additives
  A. Food colors: Azo dye F, D, and C, yellow no. 5 (tartrazine)
  B. Preservatives
    1. Sulfiting agents
    2. Nitrate/nitrite
    3. BHA/BHT
  C. Flavor enhancers: l-monosodium glutamate (MSG)
  D. Sweeteners: aspartame, sorbitol, sucrose
  E. Miscellaneous: antibiotics (penicillin)

II. Unintentional food contaminants
  A. Plant toxins
    1. Cyanogenic compounds: glycosides in fruit pits and cassava
    2. Oxalates: spinach
    3. Solanine alkaloids: potatoes
  B. Microbial toxins
    1. Bacterial
      a. *Staphylococcus aureus, Clostridium botulinum*, etc.
      b. Scromboid poisoning: tuna, mackerel
    2. Fungal (mycotoxins): aflatoxins, ergot
    3. Algal (dinoflagellates)
      a. Ciguatera poisoning: grouper, snapper, barracuda
      b. Saxitoxin: shellfish
  C. Foodborne infectious agents
    1. Bacterial: salmonellosis, *Campylobacter jejuni, Clostridium perfringens*, etc.
    2. Parasitic: *Giardia lamblia, Trichinella spiralis*, flukes, etc.
    3. Viral: hepatitis

III. Naturally occurring pharmacologic agents
  A. Methylxanthines: caffeine, theobromine
  B. Biologically active amines: tyramine, phenylethylamine, serotonin, histamine

IV. Gastrointestinal diseases
  A. Structural abnormalities
    1. Gastroesophageal reflux
    2. Hiatal hernia
    3. Pyloric stenosis
    4. Intestinal obstruction
  B. Carbohydrate intolerance
    1. Congenital carbohydrate deficiency: lactase, sucrase, isomaltase, galactose-4-epimerase
    2. Acquired carbohydrate intolerance: lactase, sucrase, isomaltase
  C. Malignancy
  D. Other conditions
    1. Gastroenteritis
    2. Gastric/duodenal ulcer disease
    3. Cholelithiasis
    4. Pancreatic insufficiency
    5. Irritable bowel syndrome
    6. Inflammatory bowel disease
    7. Mucosal damage secondary to drug therapy

V. Other conditions
  A. Malnutrition
  B. Endocrine disorders: hypothyroidism, hyperthyroidism
  C. Eating disorders

Source: Adapted with permission from Olejer V. Food hypersensitivities. In: Queen PM, Lang CE (eds). *Handbook of Pediatric Nutrition*. Gaithersburg, MD: Aspen Publishers; 1993:206–231.

Food protein–induced enterocolitis syndrome, food protein–induced enteropathy, allergic proctocolitis, and celiac disease (gluten-sensitive enteropathy) are not IgE mediated.[9] Food protein–induced enterocolitis, enteropathy, and protocolitis tend to be outgrown by 12 to 36 months of age. Diagnosis is usually made through clinical history and response to an elimination diet. Management is dietary elimination of the offending foods. Up to half of all cases of cow's milk allergy in childhood may manifest with symptoms limited to the GI tract.

Food protein–induced enterocolitis syndrome (FPIES) presents with projectile emesis and excessive diarrhea that can lead to dehydration, hypotension, and lethargy within 2 to 3 hours after exposure. FPIES usually occurs in formula-fed infants. Most infants present with this classic history of severe reactions and become asymptomatic when the suspected food is eliminated. Oral food challenges of the suspected food are required prior to reintroducing the food back into the diet. Cow's milk, soybeans, grains, vegetables, and/or poultry are often the offending foods.[12]

Dietary protein enteropathy presents within the first 1 to 2 months of life and can be seen as late as 9 months of age in infants fed cow's milk–based formula. The onset of symptoms mimics acute enteritis with transient emesis, anorexia, and protracted diarrhea that leads to failure to thrive. Diagnosis through an intestinal biopsy reveals patchy, subtotal villus injury. The foods commonly associated with food-sensitive enteropathy are cow's milk, soy, egg, rice, chicken, and/or fish.

Allergic proctocolitis presents with rectal bleeding within the first few weeks to months of life in well-nourished infants. These children do not have growth delay or poor weight gain. Biopsy of the large intestine reveals eosinophils in the lamina propria. Cow's milk and soy proteins are the usual offending foods.

Allergic eosinophilic gastroenteropathy is inflammation in the GI tissues caused by eosinophilic inflammation. When eosinophils are found in the esophagus, the disease is labeled allergic eosinophilic esophagitis (AEE). If eosinophils are located in the stomach and intestines, the diagnosis is allergic eosinophilic gastroenteritis (AEG). Symptoms are pain, nausea, poor appetite, vomiting, and diarrhea. Strictures and dysmotility also occur. Endoscopic biopsies are required to establish the diagnosis. Fifty percent are atopic and benefit from removal of identified foods, reducing the need for corticosteroids or repeated esophageal dilations.[13] Medical management is controversial.

Diagnosis

The evaluation of a suspected adverse food reaction requires a thorough process. If food hypersensitivity is suspected, an elimination diet is indicated and food challenges may need to be performed. The medical history is useful in diagnosing food allergy in acute events (e.g., systemic anaphylaxis following the ingestion of peanuts). The history may be helpful in distinguishing IgE-mediated food reactions from other forms of adverse food reactions. The history should include:

- Food suspected to have provoked the reaction
- Quantity of the food ingested
- Length of time between ingestion and development of symptoms
- Description of the symptoms provoked
- What similar symptoms developed on other occasions when the food was eaten
- If other factors (e.g., exercise) are necessary for the reaction to occur
- Length of time since the last reaction

If reactions occur within minutes to 1 to 2 hours of ingesting a specific food and the symptoms are consistent with those previously mentioned, one should suspect a food hypersensitivity. Adverse food reactions or intolerances and disorders that mimic food allergic reactions are listed in Table 7-2.

The physical exam can identify other atopic diseases that increase the chance that the symptoms are related to food hypersensitivity. Atopic diseases are food and environmental allergy, asthma, allergic rhinitis, and atopic dermatitis; they share allergic mechanisms. Many young children with atopic dermatitis have food allergies as a trigger for the condition.[14] Anthropometrics, assessment of growth and development, and nutritional status should be performed (refer to Chapters 2 and 3). Abnormal physical findings and a patient's behavior may suggest a diagnosis other than adverse reactions to foods.

If IgE-mediated food sensitivity is suspected, skin prick testing (SPT) with food extracts will help screen for the responsible food allergens. SPT is the first test used because of its ease of use, low cost, and immediate results. Glycerated food extracts and positive (histamine) and negative (saline) controls are applied by a prick technique.[15,16] After 15 to 20 minutes, the diameter of the wheal is measured. If the wheal, defined as a localized area of edema not including erythema, is at least 3 mm greater than the negative control, it is considered positive; anything else is considered negative. A positive SPT indicates the presence of food-specific IgE, not necessarily that the child will have a clinical reaction to the food. Individuals may or may not be hypersensitive to a specific food, because the positive predictive accuracy of a SPT is less than 50%. A good history is critical when evaluating SPT results. If the SPT is negative, no food-specific IgE has been detected. With a negative history, it is highly unlikely that an IgE allergic reaction would occur to the tested food. The negative predictive value is greater than 95%, but severe reactions may occur in patients with negative test results.[17]

To diagnose OAS, a skin prick test is recommended with the prick-to-prick technique. This involves pricking the fresh food first and then the patient's skin with the same lancet.[18] This induces a minor reaction that does not require a challenge to confirm. It is important to distinguish the OAS from oropharyngeal symptoms that may precede systemic symptoms, including urticaria, GI symptoms, rhinitis, and anaphylactic shock.

A few exceptions to the clinical findings should be considered when interpreting the SPT results. A child younger than 1 year of age may have an IgE-mediated food allergy without a positive SPT because of the lower concentration of IgE present in the skin; a child younger than 2 years of age may have smaller wheals when tested by the SPT method.[19] Therefore, histories of strongly suspected foods for which the SPT is negative should not be discounted. Patients may have a positive SPT long after they have outgrown the food allergy. Another exception is when a SPT is positive to a food; if that food had been ingested in isolation causing a serious systemic anaphylactic reaction, this scenario is considered diagnostic.

In vitro assays are available to detect and quantify food-specific serum IgE antibodies. The Phadia ImmunoCAP (Pharmacia-Upjohn Diagnostics, Uppland, Sweden) system has been validated to show that there are food-specific serum levels of IgE that indicate a ≥95% probability of a reaction if that individual undergoes a food challenge to the specific food.[20] The ImmunoCAP positive values for milk and egg are lower for younger children because of their less developed immune system.[21,22] The ImmunoCAP is helpful in quantifying the amount of food-specific serum IgE for other foods. Like SPT, the ImmunoCAP test for other foods has a false positive rate of less than 50%.

Monitoring food-specific serum IgE levels is clinically important in the follow-up of patients with food hypersensitivity. Pediatric food allergy is a dynamic process, with the majority of children developing oral tolerance. Patients destined to "outgrow" their allergies to milk or egg protein will demonstrate lowering levels of IgE antibodies to the food.[23] Food-specific serum IgE test results indicate an approximately 50% or better chance of tolerance with egg, milk, and peanut IgE.[24] A diagnostic food challenge is indicated when food-specific serum IgE values drop below these levels and if there is no known reaction to that food over the past 6 months. Again, these tests are guidelines rather than set diagnostic points. The food-specific serum IgE levels give no indication of the dose the patient may react to or predict the severity of the reaction.

Cross-reactivity occurs when an individual is allergic to more than one food in a food family. Clinical reactivity to more than one member of an animal species or botanical family is more common with fish, shellfish, tree nuts, and OAS, as previously mentioned.[25,26] A significant amount of cross-reactivity is demonstrated through the food-specific positive SPTs and food-specific serum IgE because of the shared homologous proteins. SPT and food-specific serum IgE cannot determine the clinical relevance of cross-reactivity between foods because of the high rate of false-positive results.

A diet diary may be helpful in identifying a relationship between the foods ingested and the symptoms experienced. Families are asked to keep a timed, chronological record of the amount of formula and/or food (including condiments) ingested for each meal or snack over a specified period of time. It is important to record brand names (with ingredient labels), methods of preparation, and recipes. The families and other caregivers should record any prescription or over-the-counter medications, including vitamin and mineral supplements or herbal preparations, along with the duration and severity of any symptoms experienced during this time. The registered dietitian can evaluate the diet for nutritional adequacy. If a food intolerance is responsible for the symptoms, minor dietary changes may be adequate as opposed to elimination diets.

Food Elimination Diets

Food elimination followed by selected food challenges is important to determine whether a food is responsible for the reported symptoms. The food(s) to be eliminated and tested by oral food challenge are based on patient history, food diary, skin prick test, and/or food-specific serum IgE results. The elimination diet used in diagnosing a food allergy may be the same as one needed in treatment of the diagnosed food hypersensitivity. If used as part of the diagnostic process, it should be for a specified trial period to avoid iatrogenic malnutrition. There are several types of elimination diets.

A single-food elimination diet is used when a child has a history of a sudden acute reaction and positive test for IgE to the food (e.g., egg). If an infant is breastfed, the mother will need to eliminate the food(s) in question from her diet.[27,28]

A multiple-food elimination diet removes a number of foods from the diet based on history and positive tests. Children with chronic disease (e.g., asthma, atopic dermatitis) may not have noticeable reactions to a specific food but will have a positive test. A trial elimination diet for 2 to 6 weeks of the identified foods will determine whether the foods play a role in the child's chronic disease when accompanied by medical management for asthma and/or atopic dermatitis. The purpose of the multiple-food elimination diet is to provide a clean baseline. Food challenges begin with the patient's favorite nutrient-dense foods, if appropriate.

A few-foods diet, also called an "eat-only" or "oligoantigenic" diet, eliminates a large number of food allergens suspected of playing a role in severe chronic diseases such as atopic dermatitis and eosinophilic gastroenteropathies. This diet includes foods that cannot be related to symptoms or that were negative on testing. To begin, select one meat, one grain, three cooked vegetables, three fruits, and all condiments from the following list:

- *Meats:* Chicken, turkey, or lamb
- *Grain:* Rice or corn
- *Vegetables (cooked):* Carrots, broccoli, cauliflower, sweet potato, squash, spinach, or cucumber
- *Fruits:* Apple, pear, peach, plum, canned pineapple, or grapes
- *Condiments:* Salt, pepper, canola and/or olive oil, white vinegar, or sugar

An extensively hydrolyzed or amino acid formula may be needed to provide adequate nutrients for growth and development. Once symptoms resolve on the few-foods diet, slowly expand the diet using additional fruits and vegetables, then meats and grains based on testing and history. Individual condiments may be expanded to help increase palatability of the safe foods. The time frame used to introduce new foods, including condiments to flavor foods, is based on the disease (e.g., every 5 to 7 days with severe atopic dermatitis). Several foods are slowly introduced with eosinophilic gastroenteropathies followed by endoscopic biopsies. Biopsies used with eosinophilic gastroenteropathies occur every 3 to 6 months to determine tolerance of new foods.

An elemental diet requires the use of amino acid–based formulas as the sole source of nutrition. This eliminates all foods to help establish whether food consumption plays a role in the symptoms. Once the patient is symptom-free, foods cited in the previous list may be added slowly to the diet.

Resolution of symptoms during the elimination phase suggests that the symptoms were triggered by one or more of the eliminated foods. An oral food challenge is recommended to reintroduce foods that are not responsible for the clinical reactions. In order to diagnose the allergy or intolerance appropriately, the symptoms must be documented after oral ingestion of the suspected food. If improvement of symptoms is not detected within 2 weeks on the elimination diet, consider the following:

- A food sensitivity is not responsible for the symptoms.
- There is poor dietary compliance.
- The unrecognized offending food continues to be present in the diet.
- Other chronic conditions are causing the flair of symptoms (e.g., asthma, atopic dermatitis).

Food Challenges

Oral food challenges (OFCs) determine whether an individual is, in fact, reactive to a food. The three types of OFCs are (1) open; (2) single-blind; and (3) double-blind, placebo-controlled. The double-blind, placebo-controlled food challenge (DBPCFC) is considered the "gold standard" for accurately diagnosing food allergies and for examining a wide variety of food-related complaints.[20,29,30] Open or single-blind food challenges are useful in the medical practice setting to determine whether symptoms can be reproduced when a food is ingested. Any challenge should be supervised by personnel appropriately trained to recognize and manage any severe food reaction.[31]

During an open food challenge, the patient eats a serving of the food in its traditional form (e.g., a cup of milk, a scrambled egg). Open challenges can be performed following a single-blind or double-blind OFC. A negative open challenge—no reaction within 2 hours after ingestion—will convince the individual that the food does not cause any symptoms. A single-blind OFC is where the patient and parent do not know what food is being challenged. It is easily performed in an office setting to confirm objective symptoms.

The DBPCFC has the patient, parent, and medical personnel performing the challenge "blinded" to what substance is being administered. The DBPCFC uses two servings of a food (vehicle); one contains the food allergen (active arm) and the other contains a safe, similar food (placebo arm). The active and placebo vehicles are randomized and fed to the patient in that order. The DBPCFC may be performed on 1 or 2 days. The DBPCFC is the most objective of the three tests and provides the most accurate information.

For an OFC to be accurate, suspected foods should be totally eliminated for at least 10 to 14 days, or up to 12 weeks in some GI disorders, prior to the challenge. The subject should be symptom-free during the elimination diet. It might be assumed that once symptoms resolve and the skin tests are positive, a diagnosis could be made; however, less than 50% of positive histories will be confirmed by DBPCFC.[32] Children with atopic dermatitis may require aggressive skin care prior to food challenges. If there is a clear history of severe anaphylaxis following an isolated ingestion of a specific food and there is a positive skin test, this patient should *not* be challenged.

Foods to be used in OFCs can be found locally. Powdered milk, individually packed flours, powdered egg, and baby foods are found in grocery and health food stores. The challenge substance and placebo material should be well mixed in a carrier food (vehicle). The vehicle should mask the smell, flavor, and texture of the food to be tested. Vehicles to use in food challenges include baby food fruits, hot cereals, applesauce, ice cream, mashed potatoes, fruit smoothies, and ground chicken or beef patties. Placebos can be safe foods not under suspicion, such as dextrose, cornstarch, another grain, or baby food meat.

The OFC is administered in a fasting state, starting with a dose unlikely to cause symptoms (10 to 100 mg of dry powder food, 0.1–1% of the total amount to be consumed). The dose is doubled every 10 to 60 minutes, depending on the type of reaction that might occur based on the history. Clinical reactivity is generally ruled out once the patient has tolerated 10 grams of a dried food, 100 mL of a wet food, or 30–60 g of meat/fish without symptoms. Following completion of the challenge, the individual should be observed for 2 hours for food allergic reactions and 4 to 8 hours for food intolerances, based on the child's history. If the immediate onset of symptoms is suspected, the DBPCFC can be performed in a day. Refer to the Food Allergy and Anaphylaxis Network (FAAN) for its book titled *A Health Professional's Guide to Food Challenges* for more details.[33]

Education and Management

Once a diagnosis has been made, management of food hypersensitivities is strict avoidance of the offending allergen(s) supported by pharmacological treatment during an allergic reaction, such as injection of epinephrine in the event of anaphylaxis. Education is the cornerstone for good compliance and a nutritionally adequate diet. This requires extensive education for the patient and family regarding all forms of the food to be avoided, how to read food labels, where the food may be hidden, and alternative food sources for the nutrients that may be affected. Follow-up for newly diagnosed individuals is best 1 to 2 months after diagnosis to reinforce education and address issues that have come up with the family. If a child is allergic to a single food, such as peanuts or fish, the nutritional adequacy of the diet may not be compromised; however, the elimination of milk, eggs, soybeans, or wheat can have a major impact on the quality of a diet. These foods are found in the food supply in many forms, making complete elimination difficult. Milk, soy, wheat, and egg food hypersensitivities traditionally can be outgrown. Therefore, long-term follow-up involves repeated testing to determine if a child is still reactive to a food and to prevent unnecessary food avoidance.

Choose MyPlate can be used to quickly assess one's diet for nutrient deficiencies by comparing the diet to a personalized MyPlate and other tools in the preschooler and kids section available on http://www.choosemyplate.gov/specificaudiences.html. This includes a list of foods in each food group that helps to explain what the child can eat. Alternative foods based on the allergens to avoid can be worked into MyPlate to demonstrate a balanced diet.

Label reading is critical to successfully avoiding a food allergen. The patient and family should read all product labels every time they shop because ingredients change without warning. The Food Allergen Labeling and Consumer Protection Act of 2004 (http://www.fda.gov/food/labeling nutrition) requires that major allergens—milk, egg, wheat, soy, peanuts, tree nuts, fish, and seafood—be identified in plain English on packaged foods. Specific tree nut, fish species, and crustacean shellfish must be identified. Mollusks are not considered major allergens and will not be fully disclosed on the food label like crustacean shellfish. The allergen can be listed on the label in the following ways:

- Included in the ingredient list (e.g., milk, wheat)
- Parenthetically following a scientific term (e.g., whey, milk)
- Below the ingredient list in a "contains" statement (e.g., *Contains: egg*)

If a child is allergic to other foods (e.g., chicken), the family must contact manufacturers to determine if the food is allergen-free, especially if terms like *flavors* or *spices* are listed. Only intentional ingredients, not contaminants, are listed on the food product label. Other household products, including pet food, cosmetics, bath products, lotions, sunscreens, and so forth, are known to contain food allergens and may use creative terms for the ingredients on the label. It is advantageous for families to know specific terms for the allergens, such as casein or whey for milk. See the website http://www.foodallergy.org for more on how to read a label for the major allergens.

Advisory labeling declares potential cross-contact. This is completely voluntary and unregulated. Advisory labeling uses phrases such as "may contain (*allergen*)" or "produced in a facility that also produces (*allergen*)." A *D* (dairy) or *DE* (dairy equipment) next to Rabbinical agency symbols (such as a *U* in a circle) is a form of advisory labeling indicating the possible presence of milk protein, which may or may not be found in the ingredient statement. Avoidance of products with advisory labeling is suggested, and contacting the company for more information is recommended.

Cross-contact occurs when an allergen-containing food comes into contact with a "safe" food. As a result, each food now contains a small and usually hidden amount of the other food. Cross-contact happens during the manufacturing, preparation, and serving of a food throughout the food industry and at home.

Packaged and processed foods are at risk for cross-contact because equipment for related products is shared. Failure to clean the equipment satisfactorily between processing different products can leave allergenic food residues. Guidelines for the cleaning and care of equipment for manufactured foods ("good manufacturing practice") do not eliminate all the sources of cross-contact. Formulation errors and packaging or labeling mistakes may also occur.

At the grocery store, cross-contact occurs in the deli, where meats and cheeses are sliced on the same equipment; in the bakery, where pastries with and without nuts are side by side; and in bins, where bulk foods are accidentally mixed. Families should purchase sealed packages with ingredient labels whenever possible.

Food service industry practices can lead to cross-contact. Cooking utensils, serving utensils, and containers may be shared on buffets, salad bars, cafeteria lines, and in ice cream stores. The same frying oil may be used for all of the foods (e.g., potatoes dipped in egg or milk and battered in wheat). Seafood, eggs, and bacon may be prepared on the same grill.

At home, cooking utensils may be used to stir an allergen-containing food and then a safe food, contaminating the safe food. An allergen-containing food may spill or splatter into safe foods. All cooking equipment must be cleaned with soap and water prior to preparing allergen-free foods.

Elimination Diets

All forms of a food to be eliminated must be completely removed from an individual's diet once diagnosed with food hypersensitivity. If in doubt, check online websites for lists of foods containing the allergy ingredient. If cow's milk protein hypersensitivity is suspected in infancy, an extensively hydrolyzed protein-based formula (Alimentum, Nutramigen, or Pregestimil) rather than a soy-based formula is recommended until the child is 1 year of age or has had a negative test to soy.[34]

The breastfed infant with any food allergy benefits from maternal avoidance of the identified allergen from the diet. Partially hydrolyzed milk-based formulas (e.g., Good Start, Enfamil, Gentlease, Lipil) contain whole cow's milk allergens and will continue to cause allergic reactions in the milk-allergic child. In some cases an amino acid–based formula (e.g., Neocate, Elecare, Nutramigen AA) would be required.[35,36] Goat's milk is not an alternative to cow's milk because of the potential cross-reactivity with the beta-lactoglobulins in cow's milk.[37] Parents should be encouraged to continue using milk-free formulas as long as the milk-hypersensitive child will consume them.

Alternative enriched beverages can be considered if the child begins to refuse formula and is able to consume at least two-thirds of the total daily nutrient requirement from a wide variety of solid foods. Some of these products include enriched soy milk, rice milk, hemp, and oat-enriched products. The appropriate amounts of high biological protein must be consumed for normal growth.

The Daily Value of calcium on food labels is a helpful tool that can help families make sure their child is consuming adequate amounts of calcium. A calcium and vitamin D supplement may still be needed, because not all calcium-fortified foods (such as breakfast cereals) are fortified with vitamin D. Vitamin D deficiency has been the culprit for rickets in children with milk allergy.[38,39] If a low intake is suspected, it may be appropriate to check serum levels of 25(OH) vitamin D in infants and children with milk allergy.[40,41]

When cooking from scratch at home, fruit juice, water, rice milk, or soy milk may be appropriate substitutes for milk in recipes depending on the allergy. Whole grains, legumes, meats, and nuts can provide alternative sources of other nutrients, such as phosphorus, riboflavin, and pantothenic acid, that are found in milk.

Nutrients in eggs are easily replaced by other high-protein foods and whole grains. However, eggs are incorporated into many prepared foods, such as breads, pasta, salad dressings, sauces, and candies. The elimination of all these foods containing egg causes problems in providing a nutritionally balanced diet.

Families can be taught how to modify recipes at home to provide substitutes for the binding and leavening properties of eggs. Try one of the following for each egg:

- 1 tsp. of baking powder, 1 Tbsp. of water, 1 Tbsp. of vinegar (add vinegar separately at end)
- 1 tsp. of baking soda, 1 Tbsp. of oil, 2 Tbsp. of baking powder, 1 Tbsp. of vinegar (add vinegar separately at end)
- 1 tsp. of yeast dissolved in ¼ cup of warm water
- 1½ Tbsp. of water, 1½ Tbsp. of oil, 1 tsp. of baking powder
- 1 Tbsp. of apricot (or other fruit) puree (binder)
- 1 packet of plain gelatin mixed with 1 cup of boiling water (binder). Substitute 3 Tbsp. of this liquid for each egg. Refrigerate remainder for 1 week; microwave to liquefy.

Soybean flour and soybean protein are major ingredients used by food manufacturers. Soy can be found in processed grains (e.g., cereals, baked goods) and in many other foods, such as processed meats, salad dressings, sauces, and Asian foods. A balanced diet may be a challenge in this population, and cooking from scratch with basic ingredients may be a necessity. Soybean oil and soy lecithin are considered safe for most soy-allergic individuals because the processing of the oil removes the protein portion.[42,43] The highly refined soybean oil is exempt from allergen labeling, but not soy lecithin. Products that contain soy lecithin may have a "contains soy" statement. To ensure that a product is safe, the manufacturer should be contacted to determine if any soy protein ingredients are included in the product.

Wheat and wheat products are found in many foods and are difficult to eliminate from the diet. Wheat is found in various types of foods, including pastas, cereals, crackers, snacks, and processed meats. Wheat flours are fortified with niacin, riboflavin, thiamine, and iron. A child's diet composed of very few whole-grain products may be deficient in these and other nutrients. The use of fortified or 100% whole grains should be encouraged. Products made with the flours of amaranth, arrowroot, barley, buckwheat, corn, oats, potato, quinoa, rice, rye, soybean, and tapioca are suitable wheat alternatives. Gluten-free products may be good alternatives, but some contain milk or egg products.

Peanuts are legumes, but an allergy to peanuts does not automatically make one allergic to other legumes (soybeans, peas, beans, green beans, and lentils). However, there is a strong possibility of cross-reaction between peanuts and lupine, a legume used predominantly in Europe but that may be found in high-protein and baked products manufactured in the United States.[44] Individuals allergic to peanuts are advised to avoid tree nuts (such as pecans, almonds, and walnuts) for several reasons. Many people who are allergic to peanuts also are allergic to one type of tree nut.[45,46] Peanuts are often substituted for tree nuts in recipes or flavored as tree nuts. Tree nuts are commonly processed on equipment shared with peanuts. Peanuts, especially peanut flour, are found in pastries; candies; fruit nut breads; and ethnic foods, particularly those of Africa, China, and Thailand; as well as in many other products. Peanut oil is considered safe for most individuals with peanut allergies,[43,47] but not crude peanut oil that has been cold pressed, expressed, extruded, or expelled. Nutrients such as vitamin E, niacin, magnesium, manganese, and chromium found in peanuts can also be found in legumes, whole grains, meats, and vegetable oils.

Tree nut hypersensitivity is more common in adults than children and may cause anaphylactic reactions. Almond, Brazil nut, cashew, chestnut, filbert/hazelnut, macadamia, pecan, pine nut, pistachio, and walnut are considered tree nuts. Tree nuts are used in cereals, crackers, ice cream, and many other commercially produced foods, making avoidance more difficult. Nut paste and nut butters are often made on shared equipment. Pure tree nut extracts, such as almond and walnut, may contain allergens.

Individuals hypersensitive to any tree nut are advised to avoid all tree nuts because of potential cross-reactivity.[45,46] Nuts are frequently processed on the same equipment and substituted for each other in recipes. But, if a specific tree nut has previously been eaten and tolerated, that nut is OK to include in the diet if it is shelled at home (e.g., pecans).

An individual may be hypersensitive to one fish and tolerate others,[25] but, in the marketplace, substituting one fish for another is a common occurrence and is dangerous for the fish-allergic individual. In addition, there is a 50% rate of cross-reactivity with fish allergies.[26] Cross-contamination occurs in restaurants because of shared equipment (e.g., frying oil, grill, spatula). Those allergic to fish but not shellfish need to be aware of Surimi, an imitation shellfish made with fish. Nutrients in fish, such as vitamin B_6, vitamin B_{12}, vitamin E, niacin, phosphorus, and selenium, are also found in meats, grains, and oils.

If one is allergic to shellfish, all shellfish need to be avoided due to the risk of cross-reactivity. Crustacean shellfish (crab, crawfish, shrimp, and lobster) are considered major allergens and are listed on product labels. Mollusks (clams, mussels, oysters, scallops, and squid) are not considered major allergens under the food-labeling laws. Therefore, the food company will need to be called to determine whether clams, for example, are used in a seafood flavoring. Shellfish are traditionally not hidden in foods, but beware of cross-contamination in restaurants and in cafeterias serving seafood. Asian dishes use a number of fish and shellfish and should also be avoided. Imitation seafood may not be safe because the flavoring used may be made from shellfish.

Other Management Concerns

The registered dietitian can play a critical role in working with children who have food hypersensitivities and their families. The key is avoiding all of the necessary foods, suggesting alternatives to the avoided foods, providing recipes and meal plans where necessary, evaluating compliance, and ensuring adequacy and enjoyment of the diet. Families need education on all aspects of cooking and eating out.

Ideally, everyone in the family follows the allergen-free diet at home so the home can be a safe place for the child. Families may need to be educated on basics of cooking, how to adapt recipes, and how to make appropriate safe substitutions. Various cookbooks and websites on eating allergy free can be valuable resources at home.

If the allergen is brought into the home, extra care should be taken. Hands, cutting boards, mixing bowls/utensils, and cooking pots and pans must be thoroughly washed. The allergen-free meal should be prepared first and protected from cross-contact before mealtime. In a household with an allergy, it is helpful for everyone to always eat at a table and not in other rooms throughout the home; hands are washed after eating to avoid the spread of the allergen throughout the home. It may be helpful to have designated areas in the pantry and refrigerator for allergen-free "safe" foods.

Parents of infants must be warned that they may cause developmental and behavioral feeding issues by continuing to feed jarred baby foods and not preparing allergen-free food or by not feeding the family meal to the older infant. Parents also may rely on "safe" fast foods to avoid allergen-free food preparation that may lead to potentially nutritionally deficient diets.

Eating out creates a high-risk situation for the food-allergic individual. Factors that put one at risk include not telling the staff about a child's food allergy, cross-contact between foods (caused by shared cooking surfaces or utensils), and restaurant errors. Creative or ethnic recipes lead to allergens found in unexpected places. The food-allergic individual or parent may want to contact the manager or chef to decide if the restaurant would be able to provide safe foods. It is best to avoid buffet service, sauces, combination foods, fried foods, and desserts. Select simple, single food items. For clearer communication, written information about one's food allergy can be shared with the manager or food server. Make sure the restaurant staff is informed of a food allergy and make sure they understand what food must be avoided. Safe foods should be available in case there are problems.

Social events can be stressful because there is food everywhere and the parent has no idea how most of the foods were prepared. Other individuals may try to feed the allergic child without knowing of the child's food hypersensitivity. Children need to be taught not to accept any food or candy from anyone without their guardian's approval. Eating before events may help curb the child's hunger.

Schools and day cares need aggressive education for those caring for children with food allergies. Accidental ingestions do occur in spite of the best avoidance efforts, and the family or teachers will need to be educated on how to manage an allergic reaction. Most accidental ingestions that lead to severe systemic anaphylaxis occur when foods are eaten away from home and are disguised. If the allergic reaction is mild (only urticaria or rhinitis), the treatment may be a quick-acting antihistamine. Antihistamines or albuterol (for those with asthma), however, are never a substitute for epinephrine when an allergic reaction becomes more severe. Individuals with food hypersensitivities must be taught how to self-inject epinephrine once an allergic reaction is recognized. Epinephrine is available by prescription for emergency use in premeasured doses. These include EpiPen Jr. and EpiPen; Twinject and Twinject Jr; or generic epinephrine (Adrenaclick). Because accidental ingestions commonly occur away from the home, emergency medicine should be carried at all times. Epinephrine provides valuable time for transport to the hospital emergency room for observation. Once epinephrine is used, the individual must go to a hospital emergency room. The medically supervised observation period is critical for immediate treatment of an unexpected late phase reaction.

A family's quality of life is impacted when a child is diagnosed with a food allergy.[48] Parents may be fearful of a life-threatening allergic reaction, giving rise to anxiety on their part. The more informed the family is about living with a food allergy, the more control they have, and the less stress they will experience.[49] At this time, the only proven treatment is strict elimination of the offending allergen and pharmacological and/or medical intervention if there is an allergic reaction.

Prevention and Changes in Hypersensitivity Status

The general understanding is that most children "outgrow" food hypersensitivities by school age. The allergens responsible for the sensitivities will affect whether one will outgrow the allergic response. Children with peanut, tree nut, fish, or shellfish hypersensitivity rarely lose their allergic reactivity. The exception is that roughly 20% of children with peanut hypersensitivity do lose their clinical reactivity.[50–52] If the child has not had a clinical reaction to peanut for 1 to 2 years and the peanut ImmunoCAP is low (under 2 kU/L), the child may have lost clinical reactivity.

There is no universal guide for the general population for preventing food allergies through dietary intervention. For the at-risk infant, the current evidence suggests:[53]

- Maternal dietary restrictions during pregnancy or lactation do not play a significant role in preventing atopic disease in infants.
- Exclusively breastfeeding the high-risk infant for at least 4 months compared to feeding intact cow's milk protein formula (CMF) decreases the incidence of atopic dermatitis and milk allergy during the first 2 years of life.
- Extensively hydrolyzed formulas and, less effectively, partially hydrolyzed formulas may prevent atopic disease compared to CMF.
- Soy-based formula plays no role in allergy prevention.
- Delaying the introduction of solids until after 4 to 6 months of age does not provide a protective effect, whether the infant is breastfed or CMF fed; this includes potentially allergenic foods such as eggs, peanuts, and fish.
- If a child develops a food allergy or other atopic disease triggered by foods, the food allergen must be identified and restricted.

If an infant is diagnosed with food hypersensitivity and is breastfed, the mother will need to completely remove the allergen from her diet.[28,54] Counseling may be needed on alternative sources of the nutrients that are lost through the avoidance diet, which may be difficult for many reasons.[54] If the mother cannot follow a strict avoidance diet, an extensively hydrolyzed formula may be appropriate.

For the food-allergic infant/child, milk or soy inclusion in the diet should be delayed until after 1 year of age; eggs until 2 years of age; and peanuts, tree nuts, fish, and shellfish until after 3 years of age.[35] Postponing the introduction of food allergens often delays the development of food hypersensitivity and other atopic diseases in high-risk infants.[55,56]

Case Study

Nutrition Assessment of Child with Potential Food Allergy

Patient history: 16-month-old female was a term newborn with no perinatal complications. At 2 months of age she developed atopic dermatitis that keeps getting worse, not better, with medically directed skin care.

Family history: There is a family history of seasonal allergies in the child's mother.

Food/nutrition-related history: Infant was breastfed and had mild reflux that worsened when supplemented with a milk-based formula around 5 months of age. The child's physician placed the child on an extensively hydrolyzed formula at 6 months; reflux improved. Mom took child off formula at 12 months and tried whole milk; 15 minutes later the child vomited and broke out in hives. The physician told mom to avoid milk, measured food-specific serum IgE, and referred the child to an allergy and immunology clinic. Mom has been avoiding milk and cheese in the child's diet. The child is eating table food; eats a wide variety of fruits, vegetables, grains, and meats; and drinks juice, no milk alternative. She has not been offered peanuts or tree nuts, but eats salmon and catfish and has had shrimp without any problems. She takes no vitamin or mineral supplement.

Anthropometric Measurements

Weight: 9.8 kg (25th percentile)

Height: 78 cm (50th percentile)

Weight for length: (25th–50th percentile)

Estimated energy needs: 792 kcal [(89 × wt (kg) − 100) + 20]

Estimated protein needs: 11 grams [1.1 × wt (kg)]

Medical test: ImmunoCAP (kU/L): milk—13, egg—0.9, soy—0.35, wheat—0.35, peanut—1.1, walnut—0.35, cod—0.35 (*Note:* 0.35 is considered negative.)

Diet order: Avoidance diet for milk, egg, peanuts, and tree nuts

Nutrition Diagnoses

1. Food and nutrition-related knowledge deficit related to newly diagnosed food allergy as evidenced by allergy test
2. Inadequate mineral (calcium) intake and inadequate vitamin intake (vitamin D) related to food allergy as evidenced by current diet restrictions requiring the avoidance of dairy foods

Intervention Goals

1. Remove all forms of milk, egg, peanut, and tree nuts from diet.
2. Increase consumption of calcium and vitamin D to meet AI.

Nutrition Interventions

1. Comprehensive nutrition education:
   - Instructed on strict avoidance of milk, egg, peanut, and tree nuts
   - Reviewed how to read labels
   - Discussed sources of cross-contact
   - Explained how to eat out
   - Instructed how to prepare safe foods at home
   - Provided sources of information on food allergies and day cares for the future
2. Vitamin/mineral supplement:
   - Offer a fortified soy beverage instead of juice at meals (minimum of 16 ounces/day to provide > 500 mg of calcium/day to meet AI).
   - Begin a multiple vitamin for vitamin D (to provide a minimum of 200 IU of vitamin D/day to meet AI).

Monitoring and Evaluation

- Evaluate for accidental ingestions associated with allergens at follow-up clinic visits.
- Assess intake of calcium and vitamin D (goal of 16 oz of fortified soy beverage and a multiple vitamin) at follow-up clinic visits.
- Monitor atopic dermatitis improvement with elimination of food allergy triggers.
- Educate parents regarding possible food challenge to egg in future.

Questions for the Reader

What will you do during the follow-up visit 2 months later:

1. If the child only has the fortified soy beverage on their cereal in the morning, and refuses to drink it?
2. If the child's atopic dermatitis has not improved?
3. If the child has not gained any weight since her last visit?

REFERENCES

1. Sicherer SH, Sampson HA. Food allergy. *J Allergy Clin Immunol.* 2006;117:S470–S475.
2. Sellge G, Bischoff SC. The immunological basis of IgE-mediated reactions. In: Metcalfe DD, Sampson HA, Simon RA, eds. *Food Allergy: Adverse Reactions to Foods and Food Additives,* 4th ed. Malden, MA: Blackwell Science; 2008:15–28.
3. Metcalfe DD, Sampson HA, Simon RA. *Food Allergy: Adverse Reactions to Foods and Food Additives,* 4th ed. Malden, MA: Blackwell Science; 2008.
4. Sampson HA. Anaphylaxis and food allergy. In: Metcalfe DD, Sampson HA, Simon RA, eds. *Food Allergy: Adverse Reactions to Foods and Food Additives,* 4th ed. Malden, MA: Blackwell Science; 2008;157–170.
5. Munoz-Furlong A, Weiss CC. Characteristics of food-allergic patients placing them at risk for a fatal anaphylactic episode. *Curr Allergy Asthma Rep.* 2009;9:57–63.
6. Castells MC, Horan RF, Sheffer AL. Exercise-induced anaphylaxis. *Curr Allergy Asthma Rep.* 2003;3:15–21.
7. Tatachar P, Kumar S. Food-induced anaphylaxis and oral allergy syndrome. *Pediatr Rev.* 2008;29:23–27
8. Ortolani C, Ispano M, Pastorello EA, et al. Comparison of results of skin prick test (with fresh foods and commercial food extracts) and RAST in 100 patients with oral allergy syndrome. *J Allergy Clin Immunol.* 1989;83:683–690.
9. Sicherer SH. Clinical aspects of gastrointestinal food allergy in childhood. *Pediatrics.* 2003;111:1609–1616.
10. Iacono G, Carroccio A, Montalto G, et al. Severe infantile colic and food intolerance: a long-term prospective study. *J Pediatr Gastroenterol Nutr.* 1991;12:332–335.
11. Lothe L, Lindberg T, Jakobsson I. Cow's milk formula as a cause of infantile colic: a double-blind study. *Pediatrics.* 1982;70:7–10.
12. Norwak-Wegrzyn A, Sampson HA, Wood RA, et al. Food protein-induced entercolitis syndrome caused by solid food proteins. *Pediatrics.* 2003;111:829–835.
13. Liaciuras CA, Spergel JM, Ruchelli E, et al. Eosinophilic esophagitis: a 10-year experience in 381 children. *Clin Gastroenterol Hepatol.* 2005;95:336–343.
14. Burks AW, James JM, Hiegel A, et al. Atopic dermatitis and food hypersensitivity reactions. *J Pediatr.* 1998;132:132–136.
15. Bock SA, Buckley J, Houst A, May CD. Proper use of skin test with food extracts in diagnosis of food hypersensitivity. *Clin Allergy.* 1978;8:559–564.
16. American Academy of Allergy, Asthma and Immunology. The use of standardized allergen extracts. *J Allergy Clin Immunol.* 1997;99:583–586.
17. Sampson HA. Utility of food specific IgE concentration in predicting symptomatic food allergy. *J Allergy Clin Immunol.* 2001;107:891–896.
18. Ortoloni C, Ispano M, Partorella EA, et al. Comparison of results of skin prick test (with fresh foods and commercial food extracts) and RAST in 100 patients with oral allergy syndrome. *J Allergy Clin Immunol.* 1989;83:683–689.

19. Menurdo JL, Bousquet J, Rodiere M, et al. Skin test reactivity in infancy. *J Allergy Clin Immunol.* 1985;74:646–651.
20. Nowak-Wegrzyn A, Assa'ad AH, Bahna SL, et al. Work Group report: Oral food challenge testing. *J Allergy Clin Immunol* 2009;123:S365–S383.
21. Garcia-Ara C, Boyano-Martinez T, Diaz-Pena JM, et al. Specific IgE levels in the diagnosis of immediate hypersensitivity of cows' milk protein in the infant. *J Allergy Clin Immunol.* 2001;107:185–190.
22. Boyano-Martinez T, Garcia-Ara C, Diaz-Pena JM, et al. Validity of specific IgE antibodies in children with egg allergy. *Clin Exp Allergy.* 2001;31:1464–1469.
23. Shek LP, Soderstrom L, Ahlstedt S, et al. Determination of food specific IgE levels over time can predict the development of tolerance in cow's milk and hen's egg allergy. *J Allergy Clin Immunol.* 2004;114:385–391.
24. Perry TT, Matsui EC, Conover-Walker MK, et al. The relationship of allergen-specific IgE levels and oral food challenge outcome. *J Allergy Clin Immunol.* 2004;114:144–149.
25. Bernhisel-Broadbent J, Scanlon SM, Sampson HA. Fish hypersensitivity: in vitro and oral challenge results in fish allergic patients. *J Allergy Clin Immunol.* 1992;89:730–737.
26. Sicherer SH. Clinical implications of cross-reactive food allergens. *J Allergy Clin Immunol.* 2001;108:881–890.
27. Jarvinen KM, Makinen-Kiljunen S, Suomalainen H. Cow's milk challenge through human milk evokes immune responses in infants with cow's milk allergy. *J Pediatr.* 1999;135:506–512.
28. Vadas P, Wai Y, Burks AW, et al. Detection of peanut allergens in breast milk of lactating women. *JAMA.* 2001;106:346–349.
29. Sicherer SH. Food allergy: when and how to perform oral food challenges. *Pediatr Allergy Immunol.* 1999;10:226–234.
30. Reibel S, Rohr C, Zeigert M, et al. What safety measures need to be taken in oral food challenges in children? *Allergy.* 2000;55:940–944.
31. Executive Committee of the Academy of Allergy and Immunology: Reactions caused by immunotherapy with allergic extracts (position statement). *J Allergy Clin Immunol.* 1986;77:271–273.
32. Sampson HA, Albergo R. Comparison of results of skin test. RAST and double-blind, placebo-controlled food challenge in children with atopic dermatitis. *J Allergy Clin Immunol.* 1984;74:26–33.
33. Mofidi S, Bock SA. *A Health Professional's Guide to Food Challenges.* Fairfax, VA: Food Allergy and Anaphylaxis Network; 2004.
34. American Academy of Pediatrics, Committee on Nutrition. Hypoallergenic infant formulas. *Pediatrics.* 2000;106:346–349.
35. Niggerman B, Christaine B, Dupont C, et al. Prospective, controlled, multi-center study on the effect of an amino acid based formula in infants with cow's milk allergy/intolerance and atopic dermatitis. *Pediatr Allergy Immunol.* 2001;12:78–82.
36. Sicherer SH, Noone SA, Koerner CB, et al. Hypoallergenicity and efficacy of an amino acid–based formula in children with cow's milk and multiple food hypersensitivities. *J Pediatr.* 2001;138:688–693.
37. Bellioni-Businco B, Paganelli R, Lucenti P, et al. Allergenicity of goat's milk in children with cow's milk allergy. *J Allergy Clin Immunol.* 1999;103:1191–1194
38. Fox AT, Du Toit G, Lang A, Lack G. Food allergy as a risk factor for nutritional rickets. *Pediatr Allergy Immunol.* 2004;15:566–569.
39. Yu JW, Pekeles G, Legault L, McCusker CT. Milk allergy and vitamin D deficiency rickets: a common disorder associated with an uncommon disease. *Ann Allergy Asthma Immunol.* 2006;96: 615–619.
40. Holick MF. Vitamin D deficiency. *N Engl J Med.* 2007;357:266–281.
41. Holick MF, Chen TC. Vitamin D deficiency: a worldwide problem with health consequences. *Am J Clin Nutr.* 2008;87:1080S–1086S.
42. Bush RK, Taylor CL, Nordlee JA, Busse WW. Soybean oil in not allergenic to soybean-sensitive individuals. *J Allergy Clin Immunol.* 1985;76:242–245.
43. Crevel RWR, Kerhoff MAT, Konig MMG. Allergenicity of refined vegetable oils. *Food Chem Toxicol.* 2000;109:385–293.
44. Moneret-Vuatrin DA, Guerin L, Kanny G, et al. Cross-allergenicity of peanut and lupine: the risk of lupine allergy in patients allergic to peanuts. *J Allergy Clin Immunol.* 1999;104:883–888.
45. Sicherer S, Burks AW, Sampson H. Clinical features of acute allergic reactions to peanut and tree nuts in children. *Pediatrics.* 1998;102:6.
46. Sampson HA. Update on food allergy. *J Allergy Clin Immunol.* 2004;113:805–819.
47. Taylor SL, Busse WW, Sachs MI, et al. Peanut oil is not allergenic to peanut-sensitive individuals. *J Allergy Clin Immunol.* 1981;68:372–375.
48. Sicherer SH, Noone SA, Munoz-Furlong A. The impact of childhood food allergy on quality of life. *Ann Allergy Asthma Immunol.* 2001;87:461–464.
49. Munoz-Furlong A. Daily coping strategies for patients and their families. *Pediatrics.* 2003;111:S1654–S1661.
50. Hourihane JO, Roberts SA, Warner JO. Resolution of peanut allergy: case-control study. *BMJ.* 1998;316:1271–1275.
51. Skolnick HS, Conover-Walter MK, Barnes-Koerner C, et al. The natural history of peanut allergy. *J Allergy Clin Immunol.* 2001;107:265–274.
52. Fleischer DM, Conover-Walker MK, Christie L, et al. The natural progression of peanut allergy: resolution and the possibility of recurrence. *J Allergy Clin Immunol.* 2003;112:183–189.
53. Greer FR, Sicherer SH, Burks AW, Committee on Nutrition and Section on Allergy and Immunology. Effects of early nutritional interventions on the development of atopic disease in infants and children: the role of maternal dietary restriction, breastfeeding, timing of introduction of complementary foods, and hydrolyzed formulas. *Pediatrics.* 2008;121:183–191.
54. Isolauri E, Tahvanainen A, Peltola T, et al. Breast-feeding of allergic infants. *J Pediatr.* 1999;134:27–32.
55. Kjellman MIM. Atopic disease in seven-year-old children. Incidence in relation to family history. *Acta Paediatr Scand.* 1977;66:465–471.
56. Zeiger RS, Heller S. The development and prediction of atopy in high-risk children: follow-up at age 7 years in a prospective randomized study of combined maternal and infant food allergen avoidance. *J Allergy Clin Immunol.* 1995;95:1179–1190.

CHAPTER 8

Weight Management

Laura V. Hudspeth, Bonnie A. Spear, and Haley W. Lacey

The growing epidemic of childhood overweight and obesity is one of the most significant public health concerns facing the United States today. Excessive weight gain is a result of several factors, including genetic predisposition and biological issues related to weight regulation; environmental and behavioral influences, such as dietary and exercise habits; and sociocultural influences.

In a culture that glorifies being thin, many youth become overly preoccupied with their physical appearance and, in an effort to achieve or maintain a thin body, begin to diet obsessively. A minority of these youth eventually develops an eating disorder such as anorexia nervosa, bulimia nervosa, or eating disorders not otherwise specified. Symptoms of eating disorders usually first become evident early in adolescence.

Adults and health professionals should take it seriously when children or adolescents express concerns about their body weight. Health professionals can help children and their parents understand the importance of physical activity and appropriate nutrition for maintaining health.

Overweight/Obesity

Childhood obesity is the most prevalent pediatric nutritional problem, and children are becoming obese at younger ages. This increased prevalence is problematic because obesity that occurs early in life and persists throughout childhood is more difficult to reverse.

Many infants and toddlers are at or above the 95th percentile of the weight for recumbent length growth charts. About 20% of children 6 to 11 years of age and 18.1% of children 12 to 19 years of age are at or above the 95th percentile of body mass index (BMI)-for-age.[1,2] The increases are occurring in both boys and girls, across all states and socioeconomic lines, and among all racial and ethnic groups. African American and Hispanic children and adolescents are disproportionately affected.[1] The probability that obese school-age children will become obese adults is estimated at 50%, and the likelihood that obese adolescents will become obese adults is at least 70%.[3]

Risk Factors of Obesity

Obesity is associated with significant health problems in children and adolescents and is an important early risk factor for much of adult morbidity and mortality. Medical problems are common and can affect cardiovascular health, the pulmonary system, the musculoskeletal system, the endocrine system, the gastrointestinal system, and mental health.[4]

The cardiovascular complications associated with obesity include the following:

- Hypertension
- Dyslipidemia
- Left ventricular hypertrophy
- Pulmonary hypertension

Obese children have increased risks for elevated cholesterol, elevated triglycerides, and low high-density lipoprotein cholesterol. Blood pressure tends to track with BMI; as BMI increases, so does blood pressure. The risk for elevated blood pressure in children is three times greater in obese children compared to nonobese children. The correlation of BMI and hypertension is independent of race, gender, or age.

Childhood obesity results in pulmonary complications, such as sleep apnea, exercise intolerance, and asthma. More obese children have asthma than do non obese, although the severity of asthma is not related to obesity. In many children, asthma is triggered by exercise (exercise-induced asthma); if left untreated, it limits the child's ability to be active, which may increase the risk for obesity. However, weight loss improves lung function in individuals who have asthma and obesity.

Obstructive sleep apnea (OSA) is a common condition in children characterized by episodes of stopped breathing during sleep. Loud snoring, mouth breathing, daytime sleepiness, depression, and hyperactive behavior in children are all indicators of possible OSA. Consequences of untreated OSA include the following:

- Delayed growth
- Bedwetting
- Behavior problems
- Poor academic performance
- Cardiopulmonary disease

Although obesity is not the only cause of obstructive sleep apnea, children who have high BMIs have obstructive sleep apnea more frequently than their peers.[5] Daytime sleepiness and fatigue secondary to obstructive sleep apnea may impair the ability of a child to get adequate physical activity. The diagnosis of obstructive sleep apnea should be confirmed by polysomnography (sleep study).

Overweight also is associated with increased incidence of slipped capital femoral epiphysis, the most common hip disorder among young teenagers. Slipped capital femoral epiphysis happens when the cartilage plate (epiphysis) at the top of the thighbone (femur) slips out of place. Symptoms include a limp and hip or knee pain. This can only happen during growth, before the epiphysis plates fuse.

Blount disease, also known as tibia vera, presents as a bowing of the tibia and femur, affecting one or both knees. Patients usually present with a limp with or without pain. Obesity has been reported in two-thirds of the patients with Blount disease.

Metabolic syndrome is defined as a link between insulin resistance and hypertension, dyslipidemia, type 2 diabetes, and other metabolic abnormities and is associated with an increased risk of atherosclerotic cardiovascular disease. Obesity is the most common cause of insulin resistance in children and is associated with dyslipidemia, type 2 diabetes, and long-term vascular complications. Children and adolescents have metabolic syndrome if they meet three or more of the following criteria:

- BMI for age and gender above the 97th percentile
- A triglyceride level above the 95th percentile
- An HDL cholesterol level below the 5th percentile
- Systolic or diastolic blood pressure above the 95th percentile (for age, gender, and height)
- Impaired glucose tolerance

Many of the children diagnosed with metabolic syndrome develop type 2 diabetes in a very short period of time.[6] Type 2 diabetes now accounts for up to 45–50% of newly diagnosed cases of diabetes in children and adolescents, especially minority youth.[7] This increase in adolescent diabetes is almost completely attributable to childhood obesity. Family history is strongly associated with type 2 diabetes in children. Acanthosis nigricans is often associated with insulin resistance and type 2 diabetes. It is seen in 85–90% of individuals with insulin resistance. This condition is characterized by hyperpigmentation and a velvety thickening that occurs in the skin of the neck, axillae, and groin. Skin tags are seen in more severe cases. Many patients present with complaints of a dirty neck that they cannot get clean with soap and water.

Polycystic ovarian syndrome is one of the most common endocrine problems in females.[8] Patients usually present with menstrual irregularities. It is characterized by insulin resistance in the presence of elevated androgens. Patients present with irregular menstrual periods or amenorrhea, hirsutism, acne, polycystic ovaries, and obesity. Hair usually forms mid-line with hair on the face, chest, abdomen, and back. Weight loss will improve symptoms, but treatment with hormones will often help in the short term. A new diagnosis, teen polycystic ovarian syndrome, has the following symptoms: normal or high BMI, hyperinsulinemia, abnormal lipid profile, anovulatory/polycystic ovaries, and early development of auxiliary (underarm) hair.

Obesity is a major risk factor for the development of cholelithiasis (gallstones) and cholecystitis. Symptoms include right upper quadrant abdominal pain and tenderness. It is mostly seen in females, and 50% of adolescents presenting with cholelithiasis are obese. Gallstones are three times more common in obese individuals than nonobese subjects.

Nonalcoholic fatty liver disease (NAFLD) has increased with the increased rate of childhood obesity. NAFLD is the early stages of hepatic steatosis and is associated with the degree of obesity, elevated triglycerides, and insulin resistance. Patients with NAFLD usually have no symptoms, although some may present with right upper quadrant abdominal pain or tenderness. Serum alanine aminotransferase (ALT) and aspartate aminotransferase (AST) levels are usually elevated and can be used as good screening tests for NAFLD. ALT or AST levels two times normal levels should prompt a consult with a hepatologist.[9]

Obesity occurs in 30–80% of children diagnosed with pseudotumor cerebri. This is often diagnosed due to an elevated intracranial pressure, but no tumor or other abnormalities are seen. Pseudotumor cerebri presents with headache, dizziness, diplopia, and mild unsteadiness, and generally has a gradual onset. Neck, shoulder, and back pain also have been reported. Weight loss is recognized as the best treatment.[9]

Children and adolescents are at risk of developing psychosocial problems related to being obese in a society that values thinness. Overweight children and youth with decreased levels of self-esteem report increased rates of loneliness, sadness, and nervousness.[10] Overweight adolescents also are more likely to be socially isolated than normal weight adolescents. Additionally, obese children and adolescents are more likely than healthy children to report impaired school function. Psychological effects may also contribute to worsening obesity.[10]

Nutrition Screening and Assessment

The assessment of an obese child or adolescent is critical in the treatment of childhood obesity. The assessment should include factors such as age, sex, family history, developmental stage, ethnicity, and social environment. Each of these factors will influence the treatment goal, the selection of type of treatment, and the course of therapy. Obesity is a complex disease, and even with excellent adherence to treatment recommendations progress may be slow.

BMI is the preferred measure for evaluating obesity in children and adolescents 2 to 19 years of age. Weight-for-length is still recommended to assess children younger than 2 years of age. BMI expresses the weight-for-height relationship as a ratio: weight (kg)/height (m^2). BMI is recommended because it is easily obtained, is highly correlated with body fat percentage, and can correctly identify the fattest individuals (BMI > 95th percentile) with acceptable accuracy (e.g., greater than 95th percentile).[8] For children and teens, age- and sex-specific percentiles are used to interpret the BMI because the amount of body fat changes with age and differs between girls and boys. The CDC growth charts take into account these differences and allow the BMI number to be translated into a percentile for a child's sex and age. A BMI in the 85th to 94th percentile defines overweight. Children and adolescents with BMI in this range often have excess body fat and health risks, although for some, the BMI category will reflect high lean body mass rather than fat. A BMI ≥ 95th percentile defines obesity. Almost all children and adolescents with BMI in this range are likely to have excess body fat and associated health risks.[4]

Children and adolescents with BMI at or above the 99th percentile have a higher health risk, and therefore intervention is more urgent. The 97th percentile may be used to determine the highest risk children and adolescents and can be used to implement a higher degree of assessment and treatment.[9]

BMI changes substantially with age. After about 1 year of age, BMI-for-age begins to decline, and it continues falling during the preschool years until it reaches a minimum around 4 to 6 years of age. After 4 to 6 years of age, BMI-for-age begins a gradual increase through adolescence and most of adulthood. The rebound or increase in BMI that occurs after it reaches its lowest point is referred to as *BMI rebound*. This is a normal pattern of growth that occurs in all children. The age when the BMI rebound occurs may be a critical period in childhood for the development of obesity as an adolescent or adult.

Although skinfold measurements are predictive of total body fat in children and adolescents, they are not done routinely because they are difficult to measure and require expertise in assessment techniques.

Screening for obesity risk is an ongoing process. It starts with a BMI evaluation and then incorporates evaluation of medical conditions and risks, current behaviors, family attitudes, and psychosocial situations. In general, children with BMI below the 85th percentile will benefit from prevention counseling, which will guide them toward healthier behaviors or reinforce current healthy behaviors. This counseling should be framed as growing healthy bodies rather than achieving a specific weight.

Children whose BMI is in the overweight category (85th–95th percentile) are unlikely to have excess body fat; however, they should receive standard obesity prevention counseling without necessarily a goal of a lower BMI percentile. These children and adolescents should be seen more frequently to ensure that the BMI is remaining stable and not increasing. If BMI begins to increase, these children would need more in-depth intervention.

Steps in nutrition screening/assessment include:

1. *BMI assessment:* BMI calculation and plotting at least once a year to identify current category.
2. *Screening*: Screening includes:
   - *Parental obesity:* Parental obesity is one of the strongest risk factors in childhood obesity that persists into adulthood—similar genetics as well as eating and fitness habits.
   - *Family medical history:* A positive family history includes history of early cardiovascular disease, parental hypercholesterolemia, parental hypertension, or a first- or second-generation relative with type 2 diabetes (e.g., parents and grandparents). Providers should regularly review and update family history, especially for at-risk children.
   - *Blood pressure:* Elevated systolic blood pressure is seen in 13% of obese children. Blood pressure should be checked at all health supervision visits. Children's and adolescents' blood pressure evaluation should be based on age, gender, and height. Blood pressures greater than the 90th percentile for age/gender/height is considered at risk; blood pressure greater than the 95th percentile for age/gender/height is considered high if elevated on three or more occasions.[8]
3. *Assessment of weight-related problems:* A review of systems through a detailed family and patient history as well as a physical examination for current obesity-related conditions should be performed. Even with a thorough history, some of the comorbidities have no symptoms or signs.[9] Laboratory assessment may be necessary to complete the assessment.
4. *Laboratory assessment/testing:* History and physical examination cannot effectively screen for abnormal cholesterol, NAFLD, and type 2 diabetes mellitus; therefore, these conditions must be identified by laboratory tests. Children with BMI between the 85th and 94th percentiles should have a lipid panel performed. If risk factors are present,

then a fasting glucose and ALT and AST should also be measured every 2 years for individuals age 10 years or older. When the BMI is ≥ 95th percentile, a fasting glucose and ALT and AST should be done every 2 years starting at age 10 years, regardless of other risk factors. Elevation of ALT or AST on two occasions may indicate the need for further evaluation, probably with guidance from a pediatric gastroenterology/hepatology expert.[9]

5. *Behavior assessment:* Providers often find it helpful for parents and/or the child (depending on age) to complete a quick screening form in the waiting room prior to being seen for their first visit. This allows the provider to target the assessment and counseling to potential problem areas. Behavior assessment includes:
    - *Dietary:* A brief assessment of foods and beverages typically consumed and the pattern of consumption can uncover modifiable behaviors associated with excess caloric intake. Not all areas can be assessed or addressed at one visit. Questions assessed during subsequent visits include:
        1. Frequency of eating food prepared outside the home, including restaurants, school and work cafeterias, fast-food establishments, and food purchased for take-out
        2. Amount of sugar-sweetened beverages consumed each day
        3. Amount of 100% juice consumed each day
        4. Frequency and quality of breakfast
        5. Energy density in the diet, such as high-fat foods
        6. Number of fruit and vegetable servings each day
        7. Number of meals and snacks each day, including frequency and quality of snacks
        8. Number of meals eaten together as a family
        9. Portion sizes
        10. Number of calcium sources
        11. Number of fiber sources
        12. History of breast-feeding
    - *Physical activity:* It is important to assess age-appropriate vigorous activity, and routine activity. Areas to be addressed include:
        1. Time spent in moderate to vigorous physical activity each day, to estimate whether the goal of 60 minutes of activity daily is met. One hour or more should be vigorous intensity at least 3 days a week.[11]
        2. Frequency of participating in muscle- and bone-strengthening activities (such as running). This should be occurring at least 3 days per week.
        3. Barriers to physical activity.
    - *Physical inactivity:* Asking about hours of television viewing and other "screen time" will uncover a very important opportunity to modify behavior for improved energy balance. Hours of television, video/DVD, and video game viewing, and nonhomework computer use should be limited to less than 2 hours per day, with no television for children younger than 2 years of age.[12]
    - *Sleep and obesity:* Assessment of sleeping habits and sleep time need to be part of an initial nutritional assessment. Acute sleep deprivation leads to increased food intake, increased norepinephrine levels, and decreased body temperatures. An increase in BMI may be associated with shorter sleep duration.
6. *Attitude assessment:* Prior to providing counseling about new behaviors, clinicians should assess the attitude, capacity, and motivation for change of the parents and child.

Obesity Prevention and Treatment

Fruits and vegetables have been promoted for the prevention of childhood obesity due to their low energy density, high fiber content, and satiety value. When children have higher intakes of fruits and vegetables, they have lower risk of obesity and a lower BMI. Unfortunately, these are the foods that are less likely to be consumed by children. Nationwide, only 21.4% of high school students eat at least five servings of fruits and vegetables per day.[13]

Soft drinks represent the number one source of calorie intake in the diets of U.S. adolescents.[14] Soft drinks are often substitutes for healthier options, such as low-fat milk, water, or 100% fruit juices. Consuming excessive quantities of low-nutrient, energy-dense foods such as sugar-sweetened beverages are a risk factor for obesity.

The intake of dairy products does not increase obesity, whereas lower intakes of dairy products and/or calcium may be associated with obesity in children.[15] An increased intake of calcium and dairy foods also may play a role in the prevention of weight gain in youth.

All children should be encouraged to eat high-fiber foods. High-fiber foods induce greater satiation. The recommendation for children's fiber intake is an "age + 5" rule; for example, a 5-year-old should consume at least 10 grams of fiber per day. Unfortunately, dietary fiber intake throughout childhood and adolescence averages approximately 12 grams per day.[16] Fiber-rich diets containing nonstarchy vegetables, fruits, whole grains, legumes, and nuts may be effective in the prevention and treatment of obesity in children.

Breakfast is an important meal and one that obese children are more likely to skip. Skipping breakfast may be a risk factor for increased obesity, particularly among older children or adolescents. Many of these children, particularly adolescents, end up consuming more food later in the day.

Eating out can negatively impact the diets of children, and consumption of foods away from home is common. This increase may be associated with obesity, especially among adolescents.[15] The frequency of eating foods away from home is associated with greater intakes of total energy, sugar-sweetened beverages, and trans fats, as well as lower consumption of low-fat dairy foods and fruits and vegetables.[17] Portion sizes can significantly influence energy intake. Additionally, children and adolescents who consume fast food more frequently have higher energy intakes, poorer diet quality, and higher BMIs.[8] Frequent eating at fast-food restaurants may be a risk factor for obesity in children, and fast-food ingestion year after year may accumulate to larger weight gains that can be clinically significant.[9]

Portion size may contribute to the increasing prevalence of overweight among children by promoting excessive energy intake.[18] Reducing food portion sizes may be an effective strategy for decreasing energy intake[8] when eating out or in the home.

Snacking frequency or snack food intake is not likely to be a major risk factor associated with obesity in children.[15] Growing children need snacks, and snacking is not a problem unless the frequency of snacking increases (greater than two or three per day) among children of all age groups. Typically, between one-fourth and one-third of the energy intake of adolescents is derived from snacks.[12] Snack foods tend to have higher energy density and fat content than meals, and frequent snacking has been associated with high intakes of fat, sugar, and calories. The primary snacks selected by teens include foods such as potato chips, ice cream, candy, popcorn, and carbonated beverages. It is important not to eliminate snacks but to help children choose healthy snacks and watch portion sizes.

Exercise

Physical activity is a key factor in energy balance. In addition to helping to control weight, physical activity provides numerous mental and physical benefits to health, including reduction in the risk of cardiovascular disease, hypertension, diabetes, depression, and cancer. Children and adolescents should participate in 60 minutes or more of physical activity every day.[11] Physically active children are more likely to remain physically active throughout adolescence and possibly into adulthood.

Particular individuals are at increased risk of having low levels of physical activity, including the following:

- Children from ethnic minorities
- Those living in poverty
- Children with disabilities
- Those residing in apartments or public housing
- Children living in neighborhoods where outdoor physical activity is restricted by climate or safety concerns

Many barriers exist that may prevent children and youth from getting the recommended 60 minutes of daily physical activity, such as the lack of community recreation facilities.

Interventions

In order to successfully treat obesity, providers must address diet, exercise, and behavior change. Understanding of behavioral interviewing and counseling is critical to successfully working with overweight and obese children and adolescents.

Motivational interviewing (MI) is a directive, client-centered counseling style for eliciting behavioral change by helping clients explore and resolve ambivalence.[19] The resolution of ambivalence is one of the central purposes of MI and is particularly effective for individuals who are initially not ready to make changes. The tone of MI is non-judgmental, empathetic, and encouraging. It provides a supportive environment where clients feel comfortable expressing both positive and negative aspects of their current behaviors.[19] The MI approach has the patient do much of the psychological work; that is, the client is responsible for making the change. MI operates under the premise that behavior change is affected more by motivation than by information. Specific techniques and strategies, when used effectively, help to ensure that the spirit of MI is evoked. Clients are motivated to change what they value as important. Other core MI techniques include setting an agenda, rolling with resistance, building discrepancy, and eliciting self-motivation statements.

Intervention programs are few, and program cost may prevent many from being able to participate in or integrate into school curriculums. Prevention is the responsibility of the provider, the family, the child, the school, and the community as well as the insurer and government agencies.[20] The following provides an overview of prevention activities for each segment:

Primary Care Provider

- Early recognition of overweight/obesity. Plot BMI routinely, and if the BMI percentile increases, address this prior to reaching more than 95%.
- Identify those at risk. Risk factors can include
  - Parents are overweight.
  - Sibling is overweight.
  - Lower socioeconomic status.
  - Children with less cognitive stimulation.
- Provide anticipatory guidance in nutrition and physical activity. Anticipatory guidance is information and counseling that helps patients and families understand what to expect during a child or adolescent's current and/or approaching stage of development (e.g., growth spurts, ways to prevent obesity through exercise and nutrition).

- Promote water and milk consumption over juice and soda.
- Eat as a family.
- Encourage nonsedentary family activities.
- Do not use food as a reward.
- Limit television/computer/video games to 1 to 2 hours per day.
- Do not eat in front of the television.
- Do not put a television in the child's room.
- Family
  - Parents act as a role model for nutrition and physical activity.
  - Limit eating out.
  - Eat family meals.
  - "Special times" do not have to involve food or sedentary activities.

School
- Promote physical activity.
- Provide nutritious meals.
- Have recess prior to lunch when possible.
- Control vending machines/healthy vending.
- Have nutrition and activity education integrated into school curriculum.
- Encourage children to walk or bike to school when safe.

Community
- Have safe playgrounds.
- Provide safe places for bike riding and walking.
- Promote physical activity outside of school.

Insurance and Government
- Acknowledge obesity as a medical condition for which one can be reimbursed.
- Provide reimbursement for anticipatory guidance on nutrition and physical activity.

Treatment of childhood obesity is often time consuming, frustrating, difficult, and expensive. Choosing the most effective methods is complex, especially for healthcare providers who have limited resources to offer interventions. It also is complicated by the lack of third-party reimbursement for healthcare services related to obesity.[12] Comprehensive interventions that include behavioral therapy along with changes in nutrition and physical activity appear to be the most successful approaches to improving long-term weight and health status.[15]

Nutrition/Diet Component

The following dietary interventions are components of most obesity treatment programs:

- *Fruits and vegetables:* Five or more a day.
- *Fruit juice:* 100% fruit juice consumption should be limited to 4 oz. per day for children 1 to 6 years of age and 8 to 12 oz. per day for children 7 to 18 years of age.[21] Parents and caregivers should be educated about the difference between fruit drinks and 100% fruit juice and ways to limit 100% juice in children who drink excessive amounts.
- *Sweetened beverages:* Reducing the intake of these type of beverages may be one of the easiest and most effective ways to reduce energy intake and thereby decease weight.[12]
- *Dairy foods and calcium:* Increasing fat-free or low-fat dairy products to three to four servings a day while consuming a lower calorie diet may assist with weight loss.
- *Dietary fiber:* Increasing fiber increases satiety, causing the child to eat less. Additionally, high-fiber foods tend to be lower calorie foods and high in nutrients (high-nutrient density), which also contributes to weight loss.[12]
- *Breakfast:* Incorporating breakfast as one of the key elements in an intervention program may assist with weight reduction.
- *Snacking:* Choosing healthy snacks should be encouraged in any intervention program.
- *Eating out:* Interventions should target education in eating out and increases in family meals.

Increasing Exercise

In general, children and adolescents 6 to 17 years of age should have 60 or more minutes of physical activity each day. This should include moderate- or vigorous-intensity activities, such as walking briskly or running, and muscle- and bone-strengthening activities, such as jumping rope.[11]

Behavioral Modification

Behavior intervention for pediatric obesity uses a number of techniques that modify and control children's food and activity environment to bring about weight loss. These interventions include removing unhealthy foods from the home, monitoring behavior by asking children or parents to keep logs of behavioral components (e.g., food consumed, television time, physical activity amounts), setting goals for nutrient intake and physical activity, and rewarding children's and sometimes parents' successful changes in diet and physical activity.

Staged Treatment Approach for Childhood Obesity

A staged approach to intervention that is tailored to the individual child and family is recommended.[9,12] Stages 1 and 2 occur in the primary care setting, stage 3 in the community, and stage 4 in tertiary care centers.

Stage 1

All children should receive prevention counseling in the form of healthy lifestyle eating and activity habits. For children ages 2 to 18 years who are above the 85th percentile, stage 1 (Prevention Plus) should be implemented. This differs from basic prevention counseling by recommending that providers spend more time and intensity while providing closer follow-up every 3 to 6 months. All intervention in this stage should be based on the family's and/or child's readiness to change. Intervention should focus on basic prevention behavior strategies. The outcome goal for this stage is based on the age of the child and improving the BMI status of the child or adolescent. Specific behavioral components to address in this stage include:

Eating Behaviors

- Minimize or eliminate sugar-sweetened beverages.
- Consume at least five servings of fruits and vegetables daily. Families may subsequently increase to nine servings a day.
- Limit eating out and purchasing restaurant food.
- Eat at the table as a family (family meals).
- Consume a healthy breakfast daily.
- Involve the whole family in lifestyle changes.

Physical Activity Behaviors

- Decrease television viewing as well as other forms of nonhomework screen time to 2 or fewer hours a day and remove the television from a child's bedroom. Children younger than 2 years of age should not watch any television.
- Engage in 1 hour or more of physical activity per day. It is important to gradually increase physical activity for sedentary children. Unstructured play is appropriate for young children; older children may enjoy sports, dancing, bike riding, and walking.

Follow-up visit frequency should be tailored to the individual family, and MI techniques may be useful to set the frequency. After 3 to 6 months, if the child has not made appropriate improvement, the provider can offer the next level of obesity care, Structured Weight Management.

Stage 2: Structured Weight Management

This stage targets the same behaviors as stage 1 (food consumption, activity, and screen time) and offers additional support and structure to help the child and family achieve healthy behaviors in eating and physical activity. This stage requires the primary provider to have additional training in behavioral counseling. The eating plan requires a dietitian or a clinician who has received additional training in creating this kind of eating plan for children. Additionally, this stage requires monitoring. Patients who monitor behavior change through such things as behavior logs, food diaries, or exercise logs have greater success in weight changes. This stage is characterized by closer follow-up, more structure, and monitoring of activities. The outcome goal for this stage is based on the age of the child and improving the BMI status. Positive outcomes can be maintaining weight until BMI is less than the 85th percentile or gradual weight loss until BMI is less than the 85th percentile. Specific behavioral components to address in this stage include:

Eating Behaviors

- Planned and structured daily meals and snacks (breakfast, lunch, dinner, with one or two snacks) with the following characteristics:
  - Balanced macronutrients based on the U.S. Dietary Guidelines
  - Emphasis on foods low in energy density, such as those with high fiber or water content
  - Mild energy (caloric) deficit
- Behavioral monitoring, such as the use of food, activity, and screen time logs
- Planned reinforcement for achieving targeted behavior goals

Physical Activity Behaviors

- Planned and supervised physical activity or playing for 60 minutes daily
- Reduction of screen time for leisure to 60 minutes or less each day
- Keeping a record of the amount of time spent watching television and a 3-day recording of foods and beverages consumed

Ideally, monthly office visits are most effective at this level. After 3 to 6 months, if the child has not made significant improvement based on age and BMI level, the provider can offer the next level of obesity care, Comprehensive Multidisciplinary Intervention.

Stage 3: Comprehensive Multidisciplinary Intervention

The eating and activity goals associated with the Comprehensive Multidisciplinary Intervention stage are generally the same as those of the other treatment stages. The distinguishing characteristics of this stage are an increased intensity of behavioral change strategies, greater frequency of patient–provider contact, and more disciplines/specialists involved. Specific behavioral components to address in this stage include:

Eating Behaviors

- Negative energy balance achieved through structured diet and physical activity (e.g., lower calorie diets that will help with weight reduction, decreasing high intake of sugar-sweetened beverages in children who have excessive consumption, decreased television viewing)
- Planned and structured daily meals and snacks (breakfast, lunch, dinner, and one or two snacks) with the following characteristics:

    - Balanced macronutrients based on the U.S. Dietary Guidelines
    - Emphasis on foods low in energy density, such as those with high fiber or water content
- Behavioral monitoring, such as the use of food, activity, and screen time logs
- Planned reinforcement for achieving targeted behavior goals
- Education for parents to improve home environment

Physical Activity Behaviors

- Planned and supervised physical activity or active play for at least 60 minutes daily
- Planned and supervised muscle-strengthening and bone-strengthening activity at least 3 days per week[11]
- Reduction in nonhomework screen time for leisure to 60 minutes or less each day

Frequent office visits, weekly for a minimum of 8 to 12 weeks, appears most efficacious. Subsequently, monthly visits will help maintain new behaviors. Patients, ages 6 to 18 years old, who do not show improvement in weight after participating in stage 3 for 3 to 6 months may benefit from a referral to a tertiary care center. However, when these centers are not available or if families are motivated they may achieve success with longer implementation of components in Stage 3 with closer follow-up by healthcare providers.

Stage 4: Tertiary Care Intervention

The intensive interventions in this category may be an option for some severely obese youth who have significant comorbidities. These interventions are more intensive and need more supervision than recommendations in the other stages. Candidates being considered for this stage should have attempted weight loss at the level of stage 3, Comprehensive Multidisciplinary Intervention; have the maturity to understand possible risks associated with stage 4 interventions; and be willing to maintain physical activity, follow a prescribed diet, and participate in behavior monitoring. However, lack of success with stage 3 is not by itself a qualification for stage 4 treatment. It is recommended that programs that provide these intensive treatments operate under established protocols to evaluate patients, implement the program, and monitor patients.

Although the interventions included in this stage have been used in adolescents, careful consideration should be made in implementing the components of this stage. The appropriateness of each of these interventions depends on the patient, family resources, age, and the geographic area's resources. Interventions to consider include the following:

- *Very-low-calorie diet/meal replacement:* A restrictive diet may be employed as the first step in a childhood weight management program, followed by a mildly restrictive diet.[22]
- *Pharmacotherapy/medication:* Only two medications have been approved for use in adolescents: sibutramine (for those over 16 years of age) and orlistat (for those older than 12 years of age). Both have significant side effects and require close monitoring. This approach may be beneficial if the medication is used in conjunction with nutrition, physical activity, and behavioral counseling.
- *Weight control surgery:* A few centers offer bariatric surgery. The adolescent must understand that lifelong behavioral changes and nutritional intervention will be expected after surgical interventions.

Weight Goals

The general goal is for the BMI to deflect downwards until it is less than the 85th percentile. This may be done by maintaining weight while height increases, or gradual weight loss may be needed to reach a BMI less than the 85th percentile. Although monitoring BMI over the long term is ideal, in the short term (< 3 months), weight changes may be an easier parameter to measure.

Bariatric Surgery

Often, severe obesity is persistent even when treated through diet and lifestyle change and weight management medications. For some very obese adolescents, bariatric surgery may be a justifiable treatment option. There are stringent guidelines for the use of bariatric surgery in adolescents.[23] Only experienced surgeons in a pediatric center with a multidisciplinary team capable of long-term follow-up should perform adolescent bariatric surgery. **Table 8-1** shows criteria for bariatric surgery in adolescents.

Ongoing assessments of skeletal health should be performed in patients who have had bariatric surgery. Bariatric surgery results in consistent initial weight loss in most patients. Patients are expected to lose about 20–30 pounds in the first month following surgery and an additional 10 pounds per month until weight loss plateaus after about 12 to 18 months. Persistent and long-lasting weight loss occurs in many adolescents following surgery, although it is possible to regain excess body weight.[24]

Success in maintaining weight loss long term depends on the patient's ability to adhere to behavior changes and a reduced calorie diet. Meticulous, lifelong medical supervision of patients who undergo bariatric procedures during adolescence is essential. This is needed to ensure optimal postoperative weight loss and eventual weight maintenance while maintaining optimal nutritional status and overall health.[23,25] Postoperative vitamin and mineral supplementation is critical in a reduced-calorie diet and usually consists of a chewable adult multivitamin, calcium supplement, B-complex vitamins, and folic acid in females.[24]

TABLE 8-1 Criteria for Adolescents Receiving Bariatric Surgery

To be eligible for bariatric surgery, the patient must:

- Have reached physical maturity. (Adolescents who have achieved 95% of adult stature on skeletal exam and Tanner stage 4 can be cleared for surgery.)
- Have a BMI ≥ 50 or a BMI ≥ 40 with significant co-morbidities.
- Have failed a formal 6-month weight loss program.
- Be capable of adhering to the long-term lifestyle changes that are required postoperatively.
- Understand that the surgery is not a cure for obesity, but instead is an effective weight loss tool when used in conjunction with recommended dietary and physical activity regimens.
- Be aware of the known risks and possible side effects of the surgery.
- Undergo preoperative testing focusing on identifying co-morbidities associated with obesity and routine lab screenings including:
  - Fasting insulin and glucose
  - Oral glucose tolerance test
  - Lipid profile
  - Liver profile
  - Complete blood count
  - Vitamin B_1, B_{12}, and folate levels

Sources: Adapted from Inge TH, Krebs NF, Garcia VF, et al. Bariatric surgery for severely overweight adolescents: concerns and recommendations. *Pediatrics.* 2004;114:217–223; and Helmrath MA, Brandt ML, Inge TH. Adolescent obesity and bariatric surgery. *Surg Clin North Am.* 2006;86(2):441–454.

Weight regain and nutritional complications can be avoided by the patient's adherence to five basic rules:

1. Eat low-fat, high-protein foods first at mealtimes.
2. Drink at least 64 ounces of low-calorie liquids per day.
3. Do not snack between meals.
4. Get at least 30 minutes of exercise daily.
5. Take vitamin and mineral supplements as instructed.[24]

Resources

A variety of weight-loss programs are available for individuals, families, schools, and communities. Unfortunately, many do not have long-term outcomes. Many programs that are nationally available provide nutrition and physical activity programming/resources or obesity prevention/treatment in a variety of settings.

Clinical weight loss interventions delivered in the healthcare setting have many advantages. Disadvantages include a higher costs and dropout rates. Programs that utilize behavior modification (as opposed to education alone) result in a greater change in weight status.

Eating Disorders

Eating disorders are the third most common chronic illness in adolescents behind obesity and asthma. They remain a serious cause of morbidity in children, adolescents, and young adults.[26] Eating disorders are considered medical illnesses with diagnostic criteria based on psychological, behavioral, and physiologic characteristics.[27] As a general rule, these illnesses are characterized by abnormal eating patterns and cognitive distortions related to food and weight, which, in turn, result in adverse effects on nutrition status, medical complications, and impaired health status and mental function.[28–31] The major characteristics of eating disorders are a disturbed body image in which the person perceives his or her body as being fat (even at normal or low weight), an intense fear of weight gain or becoming fat, and a relentless obsession to become thinner. Primary prevention combined with early recognition and treatment help decrease the rate of morbidity and mortality in adolescents suffering from these illnesses.[32]

Diagnostic Criteria

Diagnostic criteria for anorexia nervosa, bulimia nervosa, and eating disorders not otherwise specified (EDNOS) are identified in the fourth edition of the *Diagnostic and Statistical Manual of Mental Disorders* (DSM-IV) and shown in **Table 8-2**.[33] These clinical diagnoses are based on psychological, behavioral, and physiologic characteristics. It is important to note that patients cannot be diagnosed with both anorexia nervosa (AN) and bulimia nervosa (BN) at the same time. AN can develop from about 8 years of age, reaching a peak around 15 to 18 years old, whereas bulimia nervosa is rare younger than age of 13 but becomes more common than anorexia by young adulthood. Atypical forms occur at higher rates than full syndrome disorders.[34] Patients with EDNOS do not fall into the diagnostic criteria for either AN or BN but account for about 50% of the population with eating disorders and up to 70% of children and adolescents with eating disorders. Binge eating disorder is currently classified within the EDNOS grouping.

In a medical setting, the psychiatric diagnoses of AN and BN often are not used because medical providers often are not covered for psychiatric diagnoses. Because they are treating medical problems, their diagnoses are related to medical problems/symptoms such as severe malnutrition, bradycardia, hypotension, amenorrhea, vomiting, and esophageal pain.

Because of the complex biopsychosocial aspects of eating disorders, the optimal assessment and ongoing management of these conditions are under the direction of an interdisciplinary team consisting of professionals from medical, nursing, nutrition, and mental health disciplines.[30,31] Medical nutrition therapy (MNT) provided by a registered dietitian

TABLE 8-2 Diagnostic Criteria for Eating Disorders

Anorexia Nervosa (Diagnostic Code 307.10)

A. Refusal to maintain body weight at or above a minimally normal weight for age and height, e.g., weight loss leading to maintenance of body weight less than 85% of that expected; or failure to make expected weight gain during period of growth, leading to body weight less than 85% of that expected.
B. Intense fear of gaining weight or becoming fat, even though underweight.
C. Disturbance in the way in which one's body weight, size, or shape is experienced, undue influence of body weight or shape on self-evaluation, or denial of the seriousness of the current low body weight.
D. In postmenarcheal females, amenorrhea, i.e., the absence of at least three consecutive menstrual cycles. (A woman is considered to have amenorrhea if her periods occur only following hormone, e.g., estrogen, administration.)

Specific type:

Restricting Type: during the current episode of Anorexia Nervosa, the person has not regularly engaged in binge-eating or purging behavior (i.e., self-induced vomiting or the misuse of laxatives, diuretics, or enemas)

Binge-Eating/Purging Type: during the current episode of Anorexia Nervosa, the person has regularly engaged in binge-eating or purging behavior (i.e., self-induced vomiting or the misuse of laxatives, diuretics, or enemas)

Bulimia Nervosa (Diagnostic Code 307.51)

A. Recurrent episodes of binge eating. An episode of binge eating is characterized by both of the following:
   1. eating, in a discrete period of time (e.g., within any 2-hour period), an amount of food that is definitely larger than most people would eat in a similar period of time under similar circumstances
   2. a sense of lack of control over eating during the episode (e.g., a feeling that one cannot stop eating or control what or how much one is eating)
B. Recurrent inappropriate compensatory behavior in order to prevent weight gain, such as self-induced vomiting; misuse of laxatives, diuretics, enemas, or other medications; fasting or excessive exercise.
C. The binge eating and inappropriate compensatory behaviors both occur, on average, at least twice a week for three months.
D. Self-evaluation is unduly influenced by body shape and weight
E. The disturbance does not occur exclusively during episodes of Anorexia Nervosa.

Specific Type:

Purging Type: during the current episode of Bulimia Nervosa, the person has regularly engaged in self-induced vomiting or the misuse of laxatives, diuretics or enemas

Nonpurging Type: during the current episode of Bulimia Nervosa, the person has used other inappropriate compensatory behaviors, such as fasting or excessive exercise, but has not regularly engaged in self-induced vomiting or the misuse of laxatives, diuretics or enemas.

Eating Disorder Not Otherwise Specified (EDNOS) (Diagnostic Code 307.5)

The Eating Disorder Not Otherwise Specified category is for disorders of eating that do not meet the criteria for any specific Eating Disorders. Examples include:

1. For females, all of the criteria for Anorexia Nervosa are met except that the individual has regular menses.
2. All of the criteria for Anorexia Nervosa are met except that despite significant weight loss, the individual's current weight is in the normal range.
3. All of the criteria for Bulimia Nervosa are met except that the binge eating and inappropriate compensatory mechanism occurs at a frequency of less than twice a week or for a duration of less than 3 months.
4. The regular use of inappropriate compensatory behavior by an individual of normal body weight after eating small amounts of food (e.g., self-induced vomiting after the consumption of two cookies).
5. Repeatedly chewing and spitting out, but not swallowing large amounts of food.
6. Binge-eating disorder: recurrent episodes of binge eating in the absence of the regular use of inappropriate compensatory behaviors characteristic of Bulimia Nervosa.

Binge Eating Disorder (Research Criteria of Eating Disorders Not Otherwise Specified EDNOS)

A. Recurrent episodes of binge eating. An episode of binge eating is characterized by both of the following:
   1. eating, in a discrete period of time (e.g., within any 2-hour period), an amount of food that is definitely larger than most people would eat in a similar period of time under similar circumstances
   2. a sense of lack of control over eating during the episode (e.g., a feeling that one cannot stop eating or control what or how much one is eating)
B. The binge-eating episodes are associated with three (or more) of the following:
   1. eating much more rapidly than normal
   2. eating until feeling uncomfortably full
   3. eating large amounts of food when not feeling physically hungry
   4. eating alone because of being embarrassed by how much one is eating
   5. feeling disgusted with oneself, depressed, or very guilty after overeating
C. Marked distress regarding binge eating is present.
D. The binge eating occurs, on average, at least 2 days a week for 6 months.
E. The binge eating is not associated with the regular use of inappropriate compensatory behaviors (e.g., purging, fasting, excessive exercise) and does not occur exclusively during the course of Anorexia Nervosa or Bulimia Nervosa.

Source: Reprinted with permission from the *Diagnostic and Statistical Manual of Mental Disorders*, Fourth Edition, Text Revision, (Copyright©2000). American Psychiatric Association.

(RD) trained in the area of eating disorders and pediatrics is an integral component of treatment of children and adolescents with eating disorders. The main objective of MNT is to normalize the eating patterns and nutritional status of the patient.[27]

The incidence of eating disorders in children and adolescents, especially in females, is about 5%. Atypical eating disorders are estimated to occur in 3–6% of middle-school-age females and 2–13% of high-school-age females.[32,35-37] Large numbers of adolescents who have disordered eating do not meet the strict DSM-IV criteria for either AN or BN but can be classified as EDNOS.

Medical complications in adolescents that are potentially irreversible include growth retardation if the disorder occurs before closure of the epiphyses, pubertal delay or arrest, impaired acquisition of peak bone mass during the second decade of life, increased risk of osteoporosis in adulthood, and structural brain changes.[38,39]

Healthcare Team

Adolescents with eating disorders require evaluation and treatment focused on biological, psychological, family, and social features of these complex, chronic health conditions. The expertise and dedication of the members of a treatment team who work specifically with adolescents and their families are more important than the particular treatment setting. Smooth transition from inpatient to outpatient care can be facilitated by an interdisciplinary team that provides continuity of care in a comprehensive, coordinated, developmentally oriented manner. The healthcare team needs to be familiar with working with the patient, the family, school, coaches, and others who are important influences on healthy adolescent development.[37,40] Many patients with eating disorders have a fear of eating in front of others. Often it can be difficult for the patient to achieve adequate intake from meals at school. Because school is a major element in the life of adolescents, treatment team members need to be able to help adolescents and their families work within the system to achieve a healthy and varied nutrition intake. In working with the family of an adolescent, it is important to remember that the adolescent is the patient and that all nutritional therapy should be planned on an individual basis. It often is helpful to have the dietitian meet with adolescent patients and their parents separately to provide nutrition education and to clarify and answer questions.

Prognosis

Limited prognostic indicators are available to predict outcome.[30-32,41] Generally, poor prognosis has been reported when adolescent patients have been treated almost exclusively by mental health professionals.[35,42] Data from treatment programs based in adolescent medicine show more favorable outcomes.

Adolescents who recover medically and are able to maintain a healthy weight usually have no long-term medical side effects of the malnutrition. The only exception may be that total peak bone mass density may not reach the genetic potential. This is especially critical to individuals who suffer from malnutrition during peak growth phases. Bone density may be in the normal range, but may not be as high as it would have been without the eating disorder. This may be linked to high cortisol levels and growth hormone resistance in adolescents with AN, which can contribute to decreased bone turnover and bone mass density, leading to suppressed bone formation.[43,44]

Nutrition Assessment

The initial interview/visit provides the dietitian with the first opportunity to develop a therapeutic alliance with the patient while gathering information critical to the assessment. Developing an alliance with the patient is important in building a trusting relationship. **Table 8-3** lists the topics to cover during the initial interview. In addition to the information gathered from the initial interview, a nutrition assessment should include the data listed in **Table 8-4**.

Nutritional factors and dieting behaviors may influence the development and course of eating disorders.[31,38,40,45] Higher prevalence rates among specific groups, such as athletes and patients with diabetes mellitus,[46] support the concept that increased risk occurs with conditions in which dietary restraint or control of body weight assumes great importance. In many cases, psychological and cultural pressures must exist along with physical, emotional, and societal pressures for an individual to develop an eating disorder.

Anorexia Nervosa

Essential to the diagnosis of anorexia nervosa (AN) is that patients weigh less than 85% of that expected (see Table 8-2). Whether a patient is less than the 85th percentile can be determined in a number of ways. For postmenarchal adolescents and young adults, the Hamwi method can be used to determine expected weight for height.[47] This method allows 100 pounds for 5 feet of height plus 5 pounds for each inch over 5 feet tall, ± 10%, to determine 90–110% expected weight for height, which is a normal healthy range. The 85th percentile of expected weight for height can be diagnostic of AN.[30,48-49] Additionally, for children and younger adolescents the percentage of expected weight for height can be calculated by using CDC growth charts or the CDC BMI charts. (See Appendix B.) Individuals with BMIs less than the 10th percentile are considered at risk for underweight, and BMIs less than the 5th percentile are at risk for AN.[31,50] In all cases, the patient's body build, weight history, and stage of sexual development should be considered.

Physical characteristics of anorexia include lanugo hair on face and trunk; brittle, listless hair; cyanosis of the hands

TABLE 8-3 Important Topics for Initial Interviews

1. Background information
   - Diagnosis
   - Current age and age of onset
   - Treatment history: previous treatment plans, time in treatment
   - Weight: premorbid and current
   - Height
   - Menstruation history: last menstrual period, typical cycle
2. Food/dieting
   - "Usual" intake prior to diagnosis
   - Typical day's intake or food frequency or 24-hour recall
   - Safe and forbidden foods
   - Food likes and dislikes
   - Weight loss techniques employed
3. Exercise history
   - Exercise and activity level: current and premorbid, including
     - Type of exercise (e.g., running, weight training, riding bike)
     - Intensity (e.g., how long to run 1 mile, how many miles)
     - Setting (e.g., alone in room, at gym)
4. Weight history
   - History of weight conflicts
   - Weight high/low
   - Patient's goal/desired weight
   - Total weight loss
5. Binge/purge activity
   - Frequency of binges
   - Method of purging
   - Frequency of purging
   - Subjective report on severity of bingeing/purging
6. Family history
   - Family members at home
   - Food/dieting/exercise/weight conflicts among other members
   - History of psychiatric illness, especially affective illness
   - Mother or sibling with eating disorder
7. Social history
   - School and grade
   - Overall school performance: current and premorbid
   - Peer interactions: current and premorbid
8. Physical status
   - General observations: hair loss; dry, flaking skin; swollen parotid glands; calluses on knuckles (Russell sign)
   - Reported clinical effects of starvation: decreased tolerance to cold, poor sleep habits, lightheadedness, dizziness, symptoms of hypoglycemia, increased moodiness
9. Medication and substance use
   - Prescription medication
   - Over-the-counter medication, including laxatives, diuretics, and vomiting agents, such as ipecac
   - Alcohol use
   - Other substance use

TABLE 8-4 Data Needed for the Initial Nutritional Assessment

1. Growth data
   - Height
   - Weight
   - BMI percentile
   - Expected weight range for height (using Hamwi method)
   - Percent of expected weight for height
2. Energy
   - Basal energy expenditure (BEE) for ideal body weight for height
   - Requirement for weight gain (BEE × 1.5)
3. Body composition data (if appropriate)
   - Skinfolds: tricep, bicep, subscapular, suprailiac
   - Calculate percent body fat
4. Physical assessment
   - Subjective muscle wasting (e.g., glutial wasting)
   - Symptoms of gastroesophageal reflux (GER) or *H. pylori*
   - Symptoms of hypoglycemia (lightheadedness, dizziness)
   - Calluses on knuckles
   - Dental erosions
5. Biochemical data (labs are based on symptoms; not all will be needed)
   - CBC
   - Electrolytes
   - Glucose
   - Bone density (only recommended if > 6 months amenorrheic)
   - Lipid status (cholesterol level)
   - Phosphorus status
   - Urine specific gravity
   - Amylase
   - Stool antigen for *H. pylori*
   - T4, TSH

and feet; and dry skin. Cardiovascular changes include bradycardia (HR < 60 beats/min), hypotension (systolic < 90 mm Hg), and orthostatic changes in pulse and blood pressure.[28,31,38] A reduced heart mass is also associated with reduced blood pressure and pulse rate.[48,49,51] Cardiovascular complications have been associated with death in AN patients.

AN also can significantly affect the gastrointestinal tract and brain mass of these individuals. Self-induced starvation can lead to delayed gastric emptying, decreased gut motility, and severe constipation. Long-term rehabilitation, as opposed to short-term refeeding, has been shown to improve these symptoms.[52] There is also evidence of structural brain abnormalities (tissue loss) with prolonged starvation, which appears early in the disease process and may be of substantial magnitude. To minimize the potential long-term physical complications of AN, early recognition and aggressive treatment are essential for young people who develop this illness.[39,53,54]

Amenorrhea is a primary characteristic of AN. Amenorrhea is associated with a combination of hypothalamic dysfunction, weight loss, decreased body fat, stress, and excessive exercise. The amenorrhea appears to be caused by an alteration in the regulation of gonadotropin-releasing hormone. In AN, gonadotropins revert to prepubertal levels and patterns of secretion.[38] Complications of amenorrhea, often seen in athletes, include impaired endothelium-dependent arterial vasodilation, which reduces the perfusion of the working muscle; impaired skeletal muscle oxidative metabolism; and elevated low-density lipoprotein cholesterol levels.[55]

Low bone mineral density (BMD) is an established risk in AN. Fifty percent of anorexics develop osteopenia within 20 months of experiencing amenorrhea. Thirty-eight percent subsequently develop osteoporosis after having amenorrhea for less than 24 months. BMD declines as the number of missed menstrual cycles increases. Osteopenia and osteoporosis, like brain changes, are serious and possibly irreversible medical complications of AN. This may be serious enough to result in vertebrae compression and stress fractures. Stress fracture occurrence is more common in physically active women with amenorrhea and/or low BMD.[49,56,57] Optimal intervention is to promote weight restoration early, before bone mineral loss has occurred.[58] In younger adolescents, more bone recovery may be possible. Calcium supplementation alone (1500 mg/day) or in combination with estrogen has not been observed to promote increased bone density;[28] however, adequate calcium intake may help to lessen bone loss.[38] Only weight restoration to > 90% expected weight for height has been shown to increase bone density.

In patients with AN, laboratory values usually remain in normal ranges until the illness is far advanced; however, true laboratory values may be masked by chronic dehydration. Some of the earliest lab abnormalities include bone marrow hypoplasia, including varying degrees of leukopenia and thrombocytopenia.[59] Despite low-fat and low-cholesterol diets, patients with AN often have elevated cholesterol and abnormal lipid profiles. Reasons for this include mild hepatic dysfunction, decreased bile acid secretion, abnormal eating patterns, and increased cholesterol metabolism.[60] Additionally, serum glucose tends to be low, secondary to a deficit of precursors for gluconeogenesis and glucose production.[61] Patients with AN may have repeated episodes of hypoglycemia.

Despite dietary inadequacies, vitamin and mineral deficiencies are rarely seen in AN. This has been attributed to a decreased metabolic need for micronutrients in a catabolic state. Additionally, many patients take vitamin and mineral supplements, which may mask true deficiencies. Despite low iron intakes, iron deficiency anemia is rare. This may be due to decreased needs due to amenorrhea, decreased needs in a catabolic state, and altered states of hydration.[62] Prolonged malnutrition, however, may lead to low levels of zinc, vitamin B_{12}, and folate. Any low nutrient levels should be treated appropriately with food and supplements, as needed.

Treatment for AN may be inpatient- or outpatient-based, depending on the severity and chronicity of the medical and behavioral components of the disorder. An interdisciplinary team approach is necessary for the individual undergoing inpatient or outpatient treatment. In AN, the goals of outpatient treatment are to focus on nutritional rehabilitation, weight restoration, cessation of weight reduction behaviors, improvement in eating behaviors, and improvement in psychological and emotional state. Individualized guidance and a meal plan that provides a framework for meals and snacks and food choices (but not a rigid diet) is helpful for most patients.

The registered dietitian determines the individual caloric needs and with the patient develops a nutrition plan that allows the patient to meet these nutrition needs. In the early treatment of AN, this may be done by gradually increasing the caloric prescription in increments to reach the necessary caloric intake. The dietitian helps the patient to select foods that the patient feels he or she can accept, thereby starting the process of relearning how to eat normally. A critical balance exists between allowing gradual, small changes in a patient with very restricted eating patterns and ensuring adequate nutrition and weight gain. Guidelines for nutritional intervention for AN are shown in **Table 8-5**.

MNT should be targeted at helping the patient understand nutritional needs and helping the patient begin to make wise food choices by increasing variety in diet and practicing appropriate food behaviors.[28] Cognitive behavioral therapy is an effective counseling technique which involves challenging erroneous beliefs and thought patterns with more accurate perceptions and interpretations regarding dieting, nutrition, and the relationship between starvation and physical symptoms.[62,63]

Monitoring skinfold measurements can be helpful in determining composition of weight gain and as an educational tool to show the patient the composition of any weight gain (lean body mass vs. fat mass). The percentage of body fat can be estimated from the sum of four skinfold measurements (triceps, biceps, subscapular, and suprailiac crest) using the calculations of Durnin.[64] The results of skinfold measurements correlated well with dual energy x-ray absorptiometry (DEXA) measurements of body fat percentage.[61,65]

Dietary supplements may be needed to meet nutritional needs. Physical activity recommendations need to be based on medical status, psychological status, and nutritional intake. Physical activity may need to be limited or initially eliminated with the compulsive exerciser who has AN so weight restoration can be achieved. Supervised strength

TABLE 8-5 Nutrition Intervention with Anorexia Nervosa

A. General guidelines
   1. Provide a nutritionally balanced diet with some individual preferences included (e.g., vegetarian).
   2. Provide multivitamin/mineral supplements at recommended dietary allowance (RDA) levels.
   3. Provide dietary fiber from grain sources to enhance elimination.
   4. Whenever possible, permit small, frequent feedings to reduce sensation of bloating.
   5. Use liquid supplements only when the patient cannot achieve goal intake via foods.
   6. Provide cold or room-temperature food to reduce satiety sensations.
   7. Reduce caffeine intake, if appropriate.
   8. Provide parenteral nutrition only in severe cases.
   9. Provide interactive nutritional counseling on an ongoing basis.

B. Energy recommendations
   1. Initial nutrition counseling (outpatient)
      a. Determine average kcal intake.
      b. Develop nutrition plan with patient that:
         i. Contains three meals and one or two snacks a day.
         ii. Provides increasing energy levels (50–75% of DRI for energy or approximately 1000–1500 kcal/day). This depends on the current intake. It may take several visits to reach this level of kcal intake because of fears of food and weight gain.
      c. Continue to assess for refeeding syndrome.
   2. Follow-up counseling
      a. Increase diet prescription in small, progressive increments to provide for:
         i. 0.5–1 lb gain/week—outpatient
         ii. 2–4 lb gain/week—inpatient
      b. Maintain kcal level as long as appropriate weight gain continues.
      c. Increase kcal level if weight gain stops or weight loss occurs.
      d. Because of increased energy demands for repair and growth, patients may require higher than expected energy intake (½ to 2 times DRI for energy).
      e. If patient continues to lose or fails to gain on adequate kcal level evaluate for vomiting, discarding food, increased exercise, or increased activity.

C. Micronutrients
   1. Protein
      a. RDA in g/kg ideal body weight
      b. 15–20% of calories
      c. High biological value
   2. Carbohydrates
      a. 50–60% of calories
      b. High fiber for treatment of constipation
   3. Fat
      a. 20–25% of calories
      b. Encourage small increases in fat intake until goal attained

D. Micronutrients
   1. 100% of RDA for micronutrients with supplements as needed.
   2. 1300–1500 mg of calcium from food and supplements may help to prevent rapid bone loss.
   3. Iron supplement may aggravate constipation.

E. Physical activity
   1. Monitor physical activity levels; increases in physical activity will affect kcal recommendations.
   2. Increase physical activity levels as weight restoration occurs.
      a. Begin with flexibility exercises (~80% expected weight for height).
      b. Next add strength exercises (e.g., free weights, pushups, crunches) (~85% expected weight for height).
      c. Last add aerobic activities. Begin with 10 minutes and increase time as long as weight restoration continues (~88–90% expected weight for height).

training using a low level of weights is less likely to impede weight gain than other forms of activity and may be psychologically helpful for patients.[42] Nutrition therapy must be ongoing to allow the patient to understand his or her nutritional needs as well as to adjust and adapt the nutrition plan to meet the patient's medical and nutritional requirements.

Some patients may not respond to outpatient therapy. Weight should never be used as the only criterion for hospital admission. Most patients with AN are knowledgeable enough to falsify weights through such strategies as excessive water/fluid intake. If body weight alone is used for hospital admission criteria, these behaviors (e.g., excessive water intake) may result in acute hyponutremia or dangerous degrees of unrecognized weight loss. All criteria for admission such as weight < 75% expected weight for height, hypokalemia, and cardiac dysrhythmia should be considered.[38]

The goals of inpatient therapy are the same as for outpatient management except more intense. If admitted for medical instability, medical and nutrition stabilization is the first and most important goal of inpatient treatment. This is often necessary before psychological therapy can be optimally effective. A medical malnutrition protocol is used to stabilize a patient with AN. The goals are to establish adequate energy intake, maintain hydration status, maintain medical stability, and prevent purging activity through supervision.[50] The dietitian team member guides the nutrition plan which should help the patient, as quickly as possible, to consume a nutritionally well-balanced diet. Energy intake and body composition should be monitored to ensure that appropriate weight gain is achieved. In very rare instances, enteral or parenteral feeding may be necessary; however, risks associated with aggressive nutrition support include hypophosphatemia, edema, cardiac failure, seizures, aspiration of enteral formula, and death.[28] Reliance on foods (rather than enteral or parenteral nutrition support) as the primary method of weight restoration contributes significantly to successful long-term recovery. The overall goal is to help the patient normalize eating patterns and learn that behavior must involve planning and practicing with real food.

During the refeeding phase (especially early in the refeeding process), the patient needs to be monitored closely for signs of refeeding syndrome. Refeeding syndrome is characterized by sudden and sometimes severe hypophosphatemia, sudden drops in potassium and magnesium, glucose intolerance, hypokalemia, gastrointestinal dysfunction, and cardiac arrhythmias.[48] Refeeding syndrome can follow sudden increases in nutritional intake after a period of starvation.[34] Water retention during refeeding should be anticipated and discussed with the patient. Guidance with food choices to promote normal bowel function should be provided as well. A weight gain goal of 1–2 pounds per week for outpatients and 2–3 pounds for inpatients is recommended. In the beginning of therapy, the dietitian will need to see the patient on a frequent basis. If the patient responds to medical, nutritional, and psychiatric therapy, nutrition visits may be less frequent. After a normal, safe weight is achieved, caloric intake should be adjusted for weight maintenance.[34] Refeeding syndrome can be seen in both the outpatient and inpatient setting. However, refeeding syndrome is more common in the inpatient setting, especially when being fed parenterally.[34]

Bulimia Nervosa

Most patients with bulimia nervosa (BN) tend to be of normal weight or moderately overweight and therefore are often undetectable by appearance alone. They place a strong emphasis on physical appearance and are often frustrated because they cannot maintain underweight status. The average onset of BN occurs between mid-adolescence and the late 20s, with a great diversity of socioeconomic status.[50] The individual at risk for the disorder may also have a risk for depression that may be exacerbated by a chaotic or conflicting family as well as the stress of social expectations.[66,67] Some patients with BN began bingeing before dieting and tend to have a higher body weight.[67]

The patient with BN has an eating pattern that is typically chaotic, with self-imposed rules of what should be eaten, how much, and what constitutes good and bad foods. These thoughts occupy the thought process for the majority of the patient's day. Although the amount of food consumed that is labeled a binge episode is subjective, the criteria for BN requires other measures, such as the feeling of being out of control during the binge (see Table 8-2).

The diagnostic criteria for this disorder focus on the binge/purge behavior; however, much of the time the person with BN is restricting her or his diet. The dietary restriction can be the physiological or psychological trigger to subsequent binge eating. Any sensation of stomach fullness may trigger the person to purge. Common purging methods consist of self-induced vomiting (with or without the use of syrup of ipecac) and other compensatory behaviors, including laxative use, diuretic use, and excessive exercise.[68] After purging, the patient may feel some initial relief, which is often followed by feelings of guilt and shame. However, resuming normal eating commonly leads to gastrointestinal complaints, such as bloating, constipation, and flatulence.

In the initial assessment, it is important to assess and evaluate medical conditions that may play a role in the purging behavior. Conditions such as gastroesophageal reflux (GER) and *Helicobacter pylori* may increase the pain and the need for the patient to vomit. Medical interventions for these conditions may help in reducing the vomiting and allow the treatment for BN to be more focused. Nutritional abnormalities for patients with BN depend on the amount of restriction during the nonbinge episodes. Purging behaviors do not completely prevent the utilization of calories from the binge; an average retention of calories occurs from binges, depending on their size and content.[27]

Muscle weakness, fatigue, cardiac arrhythmias, dehydration, and electrolyte imbalance can be caused by purging, especially self-induced vomiting and laxative abuse. Hypokalemia and hypochloremic alkalosis as well as gastrointestinal problems involving the stomach and esophagus are common. Some patients may have calluses on one or both hands around the knuckles (Russell signs) caused by the teeth hitting the hand when patients use their fingers to induce vomiting. Dental erosion from self-induced vomiting can be quite serious. Laxative use is ineffective in purging calories. Chronic ipecac use has been shown to cause skeletal myopathy, electrocardiographic changes, and cardiomyopathy with consequent congestive heart failure, arrhythmia, and sudden death.[28,40]

Multidisciplinary team management is essential to care for BN. The majority of patients with BN are treated in an outpatient setting. Indications for inpatient hospitalization include severe disabling symptoms that are unresponsive to outpatient treatment or additional medical problems such as uncontrolled vomiting, metabolic abnormalities, or suicidal ideations.[50]

The primary goal of nutrition therapy intervention is to normalize eating patterns and eliminate chaotic eating habits by recommending three meals a day with snacks as needed. Any weight loss that is achieved would occur as a result of a normalized eating plan and the elimination of bingeing. Helping patients combat food myths often requires specialized nutrition knowledge.[27] Bulimic patients often present with a history of attempts to control weight through severe caloric restriction. Foods become categorized as "good" and "bad" or "safe" and "forbidden." Low-fat foods (e.g., fruits, vegetables, rice cakes, nonfat yogurt) become the staples at meals, leading to decreased satiety at meals and an increased vulnerability to bingeing. Food intake patterns are usually quite rigid, and bulimic patients feel that this is the only way to eat to lose or maintain weight. These unrealistic diet restrictions need to be met with clear guidelines that promote satiety, thereby reducing the risk of bingeing. Specific recommendations for nutrition intervention in BN are shown in **Table 8-6**.

Cognitive-behavioral therapy (CBT), in conjunction with nutrition education and dietary guidance, is a well-established treatment modality for BN. Meal planning, assistance with a regular pattern of eating, and discouraging dieting are all included in CBT. Nutrition education consists of teaching about body weight regulation, energy balance, effects of starvation, misconceptions about dieting and weight control, and the physical consequences of purging behavior. Meal planning consists of three meals a day with one to three snacks per day prescribed in a structured fashion to help break the chaotic eating pattern that continues the cycle of bingeing and purging. Caloric intake should initially be based on the maintenance of weight to help prevent hunger, because hunger has been shown to substantially increase the susceptibility to bingeing. Normalizing the eating pattern of a person with BN includes expanding the diet to include the patient's self-imposed "forbidden" or "feared" foods. CBT provides a structure to expose patients to these foods from least feared to most feared while in a safe, structured, supportive environment.

TABLE 8-6 Nutrition Intervention with Bulimia Nervosa

A. General guidelines
   1. Eat regularly planned, nutritionally balanced meals and snacks.
   2. Adequate but not excessive energy intake.
   3. Include warm foods rather than cold or room-temperature foods to increase meal satiety.
   4. Avoid dieting behavior.
   5. Minimize food avoidance.
   6. Increase the variety of foods consumed.
   7. Increase dietary fiber for meal satiety and to aid elimination.
   8. Develop control strategies for high risk situations.
B. Energy intake
   1. 75–100% DRI for age/height/weight at physical activity level (PAL) 1 (sedentary).
   2. Monitor anthropometric status and adjust caloric intake to ensure weight maintenance.
   3. Depending on beginning entry weight, adjust kcal to help patient achieve healthy weight.
   4. Initial plans are around 1500 kcal/day.
C. Macronutrients
   1. Protein
      a. RDA in g/kg/ideal body weight
      b. 15–20% of total kcal
   2. Carbohydrate
      a. 50–55% of total kcal
      b. Fiber to help with constipation
   3. Fat
      a. 20–30% of total kcal
D. Micronutrients
   1. 100% of RDA through food or supplements.

Discontinuing purging and normalizing eating patterns are a key focus of treatment. A common symptom of stopping purging is fluid retention. Education should include information about the length of time to expect the fluid retention. The patient must also be taught that continual purging or other methods of dehydration, such as restricting sodium or using diuretics or laxatives, will prolong the fluid retention. If the patient is laxative dependent, a protocol for laxative withdrawal should be implemented. The patient should be instructed on a high-fiber diet with adequate fluids while the physician monitors the slow withdrawal of laxatives.

Self-monitoring tools can be helpful in revealing to the patient his or her food beliefs and eating patterns. Records or journals should include facts, state of mind, and some reflection about his or her emotional world, for example:

- Type and amount of food eaten
- Time of day
- Degree of hunger (low, medium, high) and fullness (low, medium, high)
- Binge/purge activity

Medication management is more effective in treating BN than AN, especially with patients who present with comorbid conditions.[47,69] Combined medication management and CBT is the most effective method in treating BN.[70]

Eating Disorders Not Otherwise Specified

The majority of adolescents seeking treatment for an eating disorder do not classify as having AN or BN and, therefore, are considered to have eating disorders not otherwise specified (EDNOS).[71] The nature and intensity of the medical and nutritional problems and the most effective treatment modality will depend on the severity of impairment and the symptoms. These patients may have met all criteria for anorexia except that they have not missed three consecutive menstrual periods. Or, they may be of normal weight and purge without bingeing. Although the patient may not present with medical complications, they do often present with medical concerns.

EDNOS also includes binge eating disorder (BED) (see Table 8-2), in which the patient has bingeing behavior without the compensatory purging seen in BN. Binge episodes must occur at least twice a week and have occurred for at least 6 months. Most patients diagnosed with BED are overweight and suffer the same medical problems faced by the nonbinging obese population, such as diabetes, high blood pressure, heart disease, and other conditions. The patient with BED often presents with weight management concerns rather than eating disorder concerns. Treatment using the CBT model used for BN is also used for patients with BED.[72–74]

High Risk Groups

Specific population groups who focus on food or thinness, such as athletes, models, and young people who may be required to limit their food intake because of a disease state, are at risk for developing an eating disorder. Additionally, risks for developing an eating disorder may stem from predisposing factors such as a family history of mood, anxiety, or other disorders. A family history of an eating disorder or obesity and factors such as the dynamic interactions among family members and societal pressures to be thin are additional risk factors.[75] Eating disorders are becoming increasingly common in athletes in particular due to increased physiologic demands imposed by high-intensity and high-volume sports training.

The female athlete triad can impact all physically active females, not just elite competitors.[76] Common signs and symptoms of the female athlete triad include abnormal menses, chronic fatigue, difficulty sleeping, cold hands and feet, restricted food intake, and stress fractures or injuries. A food-restricted diet with vomiting, diuretic use, and other purging methods as a form of weight control may be practiced during the particular sport's season or year round.[55,77,80] The three components of the triad are the following:

1. Energy availability
2. Menstrual function
3. BMD

Clinical manifestations of the triad can be eating disorders, amenorrhea, and/or osteoporosis. It is important for athletes to maintain a positive energy balance and to practice good eating habits.

Early intervention by education on a well-balanced diet is the key to preventing female athletes from developing the triad. Proper screening for eating disorders should be done annually during preperformance physicals.[79,80] A multidisciplinary approach focused on education is generally the most effective form of treatment. An eating disorder can impair athletic performance, increase injury risk, and lead to other serious medical complications.[55,81–83]

Young men who develop AN are usually members of subgroups that emphasize weight loss. Sport-specific eating behaviors are more common in men. The male anorexic is more likely to have been obese before the onset of symptoms. Both a dietary and activity history should be taken and screening done for androgenic steroid use. The DSM-IV diagnostic criterion for AN of < 85th percentile of ideal body weight is less useful in males. A focus on the BMI, nonlean body mass (body fat percentage), and the height:weight ratio are far more useful in assessing a male with an eating disorder. Adolescent males below the 25th percentile for BMI, upper arm circumference, and subscapular and triceps skinfold thicknesses should be considered to be in an unhealthy, malnourished state.[84–87]

Case Study

Nutrition Assessment of an Obese 12-Year-Old Male

Patient and family history: Adam is a 12-year-old white male who presents in clinic today with complaints of stomach pain for > 6 months. Family history reveals that his parents have been divorced for approximately 1 year and he is not able to see his father as often as he would like. Because of the divorce, mom and Adam have moved to a new neighborhood. Mom often works late and is unable to prepare home-cooked meals on a regular basis. Adam is not allowed to cook when mom is not at home. Mother has just recently been diagnosed with diabetes, and his father is overweight and has hypertension. His mother is concerned about Adam's rapid weight gain but feels the new neighborhood is not safe and does not allow Adam to be outdoors unsupervised. He watches television or plays video games after school. Adam's main concern is stomach pain, although he does identify concerns about his weight gain.

Food/nutrition-related history: Diet history shows an average intake of 3100 kcal (range 2900–3400). Average protein intake is 90 g/day (range 60–120 g/day). Fat intake is approximately 37% of total kcal. Fiber intake is approximately 14 g/day. Average intake of calcium is approximately 1000 mg/day, iron 14 mg/day, and sodium 3800 mg/day from food. Estimated beverage intake is ~ 40 oz/day of sweetened beverages. Physical activity history reveals television viewing/computer games 3 to 4 hours/day.

Anthropometric Measurements

Height: 64.5 inches (156 cm)

Weight: 130 lbs (59 kg)

BMI: 21.9 (85th–90th percentile)

One year ago, Adam was 62 inches (157.5 cm) and 100 lbs (45.45 kg). His BMI was 18.2 (50th–75th percentile). Patient has had a 30-pound weight gain over the past year. Sexual Maturity Rating or Tanner State 2. Blood pressure and heart rate are normal for age and height. Bowel history shows two bowel movements per week.

Nutrition Diagnoses

Nutrition diagnoses may include lack of physical activity, high level of physical inactivity, unhealthy snacking, and high intake of sugar sweetened beverages.

Intervention Goals

The overall goal of treatment is to decrease overall caloric intake and increase activity to maintain current weight until appropriate height for weight is achieved. Increasing fluid and fiber intake will address the patient's concern of constipation.

Monitoring and Evaluation

The expert committee recommends monthly follow-up for children in stage 2 treatment. The patient and his mother should be encouraged to monitor suggestions and return for weight checks and nutrition counseling to ensure BMI maintenance or BMI trending downward during growth spurt. Weight loss is not necessarily recommended.

Questions for the Reader

1. What does Adam's BMI percentile mean? Where was he one year ago?
2. What are Adam's energy and protein needs?
3. What factors are affecting Adam's nutrient and physical activity requirements?
4. Write at least one PES statement for this patient.
5. Identify interventions in at least two domains of nutrition intervention to use in counseling Adam and his mother.

REFERENCES

1. Ogden CL, Carroll MD, Curtin LR, et al. Prevalence of high body mass index in US children and adolescents, 2007–2008. *JAMA.* 2010;303(3):242–249.
2. Centers for Disease Control and Prevention. NCHS Health E-Stat. Available at: http://www.cdc.gov/nchs/data/hestat/obesity_child_07_08/obesity_child_07_08.html. Accessed August 9, 2011.
3. Whitaker RC, Wright JA, Pepe MS, et al. Predicting obesity in young adulthood from childhood and prenatal obesity. *New Engl J Med.* 1997;337:869–873.
4. American Academy of Pediatrics. Policy statement: prevention of pediatric overweight and obesity. *Pediatrics.* 2003;112(2):424–430.
5. Rosen C, Storfer-Isser A, Taylor HG, et al. Increased behavioral morbidity in school aged children with sleep-disordered breathing. *Pediatrics.* 2004;114:1640–1648.
6. Weiss R, Dziura J, Burget TS, et al. Obesity and the metabolic syndrome in children and adolescents. *N Engl J Med.* 2004;350:2362–2374.
7. American Diabetes Association. Type 2 diabetes in children and adolescents. *Diabetes Care.* 2000;286:1427–1430.
8. Krebs NF, Himes JH, Jacobson D, et al. Assessment of child and adolescent overweight and obesity. *Pediatrics.* 2007;120:S193–S288.
9. Barlow SE. Expert committee recommendations regarding the prevention, assessment and treatment of child and adolescent overweight and obesity: summary report. *Pediatrics.* 2007;120:S164–S192.
10. Feld LG, Hyams JS. Childhood obesity. *Consensus Pediatr.* 2007;1(4):1–36.
11. U.S. Department of Health and Human Services. Physical activity guidelines for Americans. Office of Disease Prevention and Health Promotion. 2008. Available at: http://hhs.gov/new/press/2008press/10/20081007a.html. Accessed August 9, 2011.
12. Spear BA, Barlow SE, Ervin C, et al. Recommendations for treatment of child and adolescent overweight and obesity. *Pediatrics.* 2007;120:S254–S288.
13. Centers for Disease Control and Prevention. Youth risk behavior surveillance (YRBS), United States, 2007. *MMWR.* 2008;57:SS-4.
14. Murphy M, Douglass J, Latulippe M, et al. Beverages as a source of energy and nutrients in diets of children and adolescents. *FASEBJ.* 2005;19 (3) 434:275.
15. American Dietetic Association. What we know about childhood overweight. Evidence Analysis Library. 2009. Available at: http://www.adaevidencelibrary.com. Accessed August 9, 2011.
16. Pereira MA, Ludwig DS. Dietary fiber and body weight regulation: observations and mechanisms. *Pediatr Clin North Am.* 2001;48:969–980.
17. Guthrie JF, Lin BH, Frazao E. Role of food prepared away from home in the American diet, 1977–78 versus 1994–96: changes and consequences. *J Nutr Educ Behav.* 2002;34(3):140–150.
18. McConahy KL, Smiciklas-Wright H, Mitchell DC, Picciano MF. Portion size of common foods predicts energy intake among preschool-aged children. *J Am Diet Assoc.* 2004;104(6):975–979.
19. Rollnick S, Miller WR. What is motivational interviewing? *Behav Cogn Psychother.* 1995;23:325–334.
20. Society for Nutrition Education, Weight Realities Division. Guidelines for childhood obesity prevention programs: promoting healthy weight in children. *J Nutr Educ Behav.* 2003;35:1–5.
21. American Academy of Pediatrics. Policy statement. Identifying and treating eating disorders. *Pediatrics.* 2003;111:204–211.
22. Sothern MS, Gordon ST, von Almen TK. *Handbook of Pediatric Obesity.* Boca Raton, FL: Taylor and Francis; 2006:38.
23. Inge TH, Krebs NF, Garcia VF, et al. Bariatric surgery for severely overweight adolescents: concerns and recommendations. *Pediatrics.* 2004;114:217–223
24. Helmrath MA, Brandt ML, Inge TH. Adolescent obesity and bariatric surgery. *Surg Clin North Am.* 2006;86(2):441–454.
25. Apovian CM, Baker C, Ludwig DS, et al. Best practice guidelines in pediatric/adolescent weight loss surgery. *Obes Res.* 2005;13:274–282.

26. Gonzalez A, Kohn MR, Clarke SD. Eating disorders in adolescents. *Aust Fam Physician.* 2007;36(8):614–619.
27. American Dietetic Association. Position of the American Dietetic Association: nutrition intervention in the treatment of anorexia nervosa, bulimia nervosa, and other eating disorders. *J Am Diet Assoc.* 2006;106(12):2073.
28. Rock CL. Nutritional and medical assessment and management of eating disorders. *Nutr Clin Care.* 1999;2:332–343.
29. Kreipe RE, Durkarm CP. Outcome of anorexia nervosa related to treatment utilizing an adolescent medicine approach. *J Youth Adolesc.* 1996;25:483–497.
30. Gralen SJ, Levin MP, Smolak L. Dieting and disordered eating during early and middle adolescence: do the influences remain the same? *Int J Eating Disord.* 1990;9:501–512.
31. Kreipe RE, Birndorf DO. Eating disorders in adolescents and young adults. *Medical Clin North Am.* 2000;84(4):1027–1049.
32. Rome ES. Children and adolescents with eating disorders: the state of the art. *Pediatrics.* 2003;111(1):e98.
33. American Psychiatric Association. Practice guidelines for the treatment of patients with eating disorders. *Am J Psychol.* 2000;157(Suppl):1–39.
34. Gowers SG. Management of eating disorders in children and adolescents. *Arch Dis Child.* 2008;93(4):331.
35. Bryant-Waugh R, Markham L, Kreipe RE, Walsh BT. Feeding and eating disorders in childhood. *Int J Eat Disord.* 2010;43(2):98–111.
36. Patrick LL. Eating disorders: a review of the literature with emphasis on medical complications and clinical nutrition. *Alt Med Rev.* 2002;7(3):184.
37. Fisher M, Golden NH, Datzman KD, et al. Eating disorders in adolescents: a background paper. *J Adolesc Health Care.* 1995;16:420–437.
38. Becker AE, Grinspoon SK, Klibanski A, Herzog DB. Current concepts: eating disorders. *N Engl J Med.* 1999;340(14):1092–1098.
39. Katzman DK, Zipursky RB. Adolescents with anorexia nervosa: the impact of the disorder on bones and brains. *Ann N Y Acad Sci.* 1997;817:127–137.
40. Harris JP, Kriepe RE, Rossback CN. QT prolongation by isoproterenol in anorexia nervosa. *J Adolesc Health.* 1993;14:390–393.
41. Ebbeling CB, Feldman HA, Osganian SK, et al. Effects of decreasing sugar-sweetened beverage consumption on body weight in adolescents: a randomized controlled pilot study. *Pediatrics.* 2006;117:673–680.
42. Szabo CP. Hospitalized anorexics and resistance training: impact on body composition and psychological well-being. A preliminary study. *Eating Weight Disord.* 2002;7(4):293.
43. Misra MM. Alterations in growth hormone secretory dynamics in adolescent girls with anorexia nervosa and effects on bone metabolism. *J Clin Endocrinol Metab.* 2003;88(12):5615.
44. Misra MM. Alterations in cortisol secretory dynamics in adolescent girls with anorexia nervosa and effects on bone metabolism. *J Clin Endocrinol Metab.* 2004;89(10):4972.
45. Ressler A. A body to die for: eating disorders and body-image distortion in women. *Int J Fertil Womens Med.* 1998;43(3):133–138.
46. Rodin GG. Eating disorders in young women with type 1 diabetes mellitus. *J Psychosom Res.* 2002;53(4):943.
47. Hammond KA. Dietary and clinical assessment. In: Mahan K, Escott-Stump S (eds). *Krause's Food, Nutrition and Diet Therapy,* 11th ed. Philadelphia: Saunders; 2004: 407–435.
48. Swenne I. Heart risk associated with weight loss in anorexia nervosa and eating disorders: electrocardiographic changes during the early phase of refeeding. *Acta Paediatr.* 2000;89:447–452.
49. Jayasinghe Y. Current concepts in bone and reproductive health in adolescents with anorexia nervosa. *Br J Obstet Gynaecol.* 2008;115(3):304.
50. Sturdevant MS, Spear BA. Eating disorders and obesity. In: Burg F, Infelfinger J, Polin R, Gershon A (eds). *A Current Pediatric Therapy.* Philadelphia, PA: Saunders; 2006:334–336.
51. Schebendach J, Reichert-Anderson P. Nutrition in eating disorders. In: Mahan K, Escott-Stump S (eds). *Kraus's Nutrition and Diet Therapy.* New York: McGraw-Hill; 2000:594–615.
52. Benini LL. Gastric emptying in patients with restricting and binge/purging subtypes of anorexia nervosa. *Am J Gastroenterol.* 2004;99(8):1448.
53. Cooke RA, Chambers JB. Anorexia nervosa and the heart. *Br J Hosp Med.* 1995;54:313–317.
54. Lantzouni E, Frank GR, Golden NH, Shenker RI. Reversibility of growth stunting in early onset anorexia nervosa: a prospective study. *J Adolesc Health.* 2002;31:162–165.
55. American College of Sports Medicine. American College of Sports Medicine position stand. The female athlete triad. *Med Sci Sports Exerc.* 2007;39(10):1867.
56. Bachrach LK, Guido D, Datzman C. Decreased bone density in adolescent girls with anorexia nervosa. *Pediatrics.* 1990;86:440–447.
57. Biller BMK, Saxe V, Herzog DB. Mechanisms of osteoporosis in adult and adolescent women with anorexia nervosa. *J Clin Endocrinol Metab.* 1989;68:548–554.
58. Mehler PS. Treatment of osteopenia and osteoporosis in anorexia nervosa: a systematic review of the literature. *Int J Eating Disord.* 2009;42(3):195.
59. Hütter G. The hematology of anorexia nervosa. *Int J Eating Disord.* 2009;42(4):293.
60. Ohwada R, Hotta M, Oikawa S, Takano K. Etiology of hypercholesterolemia in patients with anorexia nervosa. *Int J Eat Disord.* 2006;39(7):598–601.
61. Probst M. Body composition in female anorexia nervosa patients. *Br J Nutr.* 1996;76:639–644.
62. Kennedy A. Iron status and haematological changes in adolescent female inpatients with anorexia nervosa. *J Paediatr Child Health.* 2004;40(8):430.
63. Wilson GT. Cognitive behavior therapy for eating disorder: progress and problems. *Behavior Research Ther.* 1999;37(Suppl 1):S79–S95.
64. Durnin JVGA, Rahaman MM. The assessment of the amount of body fat in the human body from measurements of skinfold thickness. *Br J Nutr.* 1967;21:681–685.
65. Kerruish KP. Body composition in adolescents with anorexia nervosa. *Am J Clin Nutr.* 2002;75(1):31.
66. Kirkley BG. Bulimia: clinical characteristics, development and etiology. *J Am Diet Assoc.* 1986;86:468–475.
67. Haiman C, Devlin MJ. Binge eating before the onset of dieting: a distinct subgroup of bulimia nervosa. *Int J Eating Disord.* 1999;25:151–157.
68. Shapiro JR. Bulimia nervosa treatment: a systematic review of randomized controlled trials. *Int J Eating Disord.2007* 40(4):321.
69. Boardley D. The treatment of eating disorders: role of the dietitian. *Academy for Eating Disorders Newsletter.* Winter 2000;1–4.

70. Sysko R, Hildebrandt T. Cognitive-behavioural therapy for individuals with bulimia nervosa and a co-occurring substance use disorder. *Eur Eat Disord Rev.* 2009;17(2):89–100.
71. Eddy J, Kamryn TK. Eating disorder not otherwise specified in adolescents. *J Am Acad Child Adolesc Psychiatry.* 2008;47(2):156.
72. Grilo CM. The assessment and treatment of binge eating disorder. *J Practical Psychiatry Behav Health.* 1998;4:191–201.
73. Williamson DA, Martin CK. Binge eating disorder: a review of the literature after publication of the DSM-IV. *Eating Weight Disord Stud Anorexia Bulimia Obes.* 1999;4(3):103–114.
74. Goldfein JA, Devlin JH, Spitzer RL. Cognitive behavioral therapy for the treatment of binge eating disorder: what constitutes success? *Int J Eating Disord* 2000;157(7):1051–1056.
75. Woodside DB, Field LL, Garfinkel PE, Heinman M. Specificity of eating disorder diagnoses in families of probands with anorexia nervosa and bulimia nervosa. *Compr Psychiatry.* 1998;39(5):261–264.
76. Hobart JA, Smucker DR. The female athlete triad. American Academy of Family Physicians. Available at: http://www.aafp.org/afp/20000601/3357.html. Accessed October 11, 2007.
77. Sanborn CF, Horea M, Simers BJ, Dieringer KL. Disordered eating and the female athlete triad. *Clin Sports Med Athletic Woman.* 2000;19:199–213.
78. Otis C. *The Athletic Women's Survival Guide.* Indianapolis, IN: Human Kinetics; 2000.
79. American Academy of Pediatrics Committee on Sports Medicine and Fitness. Promotion of healthy weight-control practices in young athletes. *Pediatrics.* 2005;116:1557–1564.
80. Gable KA. Special nutritional concerns for the female athlete. *Curr Sports Med Reports.* 2006;5:187–191.
81. International Olympic Committee Medical Commission. Working group on women in sport: position stand on the female athlete triad. Available at: http://multimedia.olympic.org/pdf/en_report_917.pdf. Accessed January 4, 2010
82. Cabera D. *Eating Disorders Across the Lifespan.* Remuda Ranch Program for Eating Disorders; Wickenburg, AZ, 2007.
83. Hoch AZ. Prevalence of the female athlete triad in high school athletes and sedentary students. *Clin J Sport Med.* 2009;19(5):421.
84. Farrow JA. The adolescent male with an eating disorder. *Pedia Ann.* 1992;21:769–773.
85. Carlat DJ, Camargo CA, Herzog DB. Eating disorders in males: a report on 135 patients. *Am J Psychiatry.* 1997;154(8):1127–1132.
86. Braun D, Sunday SR, Huang A, Halmi KA. More males seek treatment for eating disorders. *Int J Eating Disord.* 1999;25(4):415–424.
87. Ogden CL, Carroll MD, Flegal KM. High body mass index for age among U.S. children and adolescents, 2003–2006. *JAMA.* 2008;299(20):2401–2405.

CHAPTER 9

Inborn Errors of Metabolism

Phyllis B. Acosta

Nutrition support of infants and children with inborn errors of metabolism (IEMs) requires in-depth knowledge of metabolic processes; the science and application of nutrition, growth, and development; and food science. The specific nutrient needs of each patient, based on individual genetic and biochemical constitution, must be considered. Nutrient requirements established for normal populations[1] may not apply to individuals with IEMs.[2] Some chemical compounds may not be synthesized in patients with a metabolic defect. Consequently, based on the inborn error, the subsequent organ damage that accrues, and the rate of loss of specific chemicals from the body, several compounds become conditionally essential. Among these are the amino acids arginine,[3] carnitine,[4] cystine,[5] and tyrosine[6] and the "vitamin" tetrahydrobiopterin (BH_4).[7] Failure to adapt nutrient intakes to the needs of each patient can result in mental retardation, metabolic crises, neurological crises, growth failure, and, with some inborn errors, death. Quality care is best achieved by an experienced team in a genetic/metabolic center.[8]

This chapter addresses newborn screening for IEMs and principles and practical considerations in nutrition support of IEMs first suspected by newborn screening[9,10] and later diagnosed by appropriate methods. For a detailed guide to nutrition support, see *Nutrition Management of Patients with Inherited Metabolic Disorders*.[11]

Newborn Screening

The American College of Medical Genetics recommends the core panel for screening newborns that includes tests for 24 inherited metabolic disorders in which nutrition management is important (see **Table 9-1**). Twenty-four metabolic disorders that are secondary targets include some for which it is as yet unknown whether diet therapy will be beneficial. Disorders in the core panel were chosen based on:

1. Availability and sensitivity of a specific screening test that can be carried out within 24 to 48 hours after birth
2. Efficacious therapy
3. Adequate knowledge of the natural history of the disease[9,10]

Diseases in the secondary target are conditions essential in the differential diagnosis of a disorder in the core panel. Differential diagnosis by other analytes, enzymes, or mutation analysis is necessary for appropriate therapy. Marker analytes for disorders recommended for newborn screening by mass spectrometry (MS/MS) are noted in Table 9-1.[10]

Many other IEMs are known for which newborn screening does not occur. These may be diagnosed at a later age by clinical symptoms, and diet therapy may be used to ameliorate or prevent worsening of symptoms.[11] However, early identification, diagnosis, and treatment are essential to prevent the disastrous effects of IEMs.

Principles and Practical Considerations in Nutrition Support

The appropriate approach to the nutrition support of IEMs is dependent on the biochemistry and pathophysiology of disease expression. Several therapeutic strategies may be used simultaneously:[2]

- *Enhancing anabolism and depressing catabolism:* This involves the use of high-energy feedings with appropriate amounts of amino acid mixtures, carbohydrates, and fats and administration of insulin, if needed. Fasting should be prevented. This therapeutic maneuver is important to the management of all inborn errors involving catabolic pathways.
- *Correcting the primary imbalance in metabolic relationships:* This correction reduces accumulated toxic substrate(s) through diet restriction. Examples for which this is used are phenylketonuria (PKU),[12] maple syrup urine disease (MSUD),[13] galactosemia,[14] and mitochondrial medium-chain, long-chain, and very-long-chain fatty acid oxidation[15] defects where phenylalanine;

TABLE 9-1 Core and Secondary Targets of Inborn Errors of Metabolism Recommended for Newborn Screening and Marker Analytes Used with MS/MS Screening

Inborn Error	Marker Analyte
Core Targets	
Amino Acid Disorders	
Argininosuccinic acidemia (ASA)	Citrulline (CIT)
Citrullinemia (CIT)	CIT
Homocystinuria (HCY)	Methionine (MET)
Maple syrup urine disease (MSUD)	Leucine (LEU) ± Valine (VAL)
Phenylketonuria (PKU)	Phenylalanine (PHE), PHE/Tyrosine (TYR)
Tyrosinemia type I (TYR I)	TYR
Fatty Acid Oxidation Disorders	
Carnitine uptake deficiency (CUD)	C[a]O[b]
Long-chain-hydroxy-acyl-CoA dehydrogenase deficiency (LCHAD)	C16-OH[c]; C[a]18:1[d]-OH
Medium-chain acyl-CoA dehydrogenase deficiency (MCAD)	C[a]8/C[a]10 ± C[a]6, C[a]10:1, C8[a]
Trifunctional protein deficiency (TFP)	C[a]16-OH, C[a]18:1-OH
Very-long-chain acyl-CoA dehydrogenase deficiency (VLCAD)	C14:1, C14:1/C12:1 (± C14, C16, C18:1)
Organic Acid Disorders	
β-ketothiolase deficiency (BKT)[e]	C[a]5:1, ± C[a]5OH[c]
β-methylcrotonyl-CoA carboxylase deficiency (3MCC)[e]	C[a]5-OH[c], ± [a]C5:1
Cobalamin A and B defects (Cbl A, B)[e]	C[a]3, C[a]3/C[a]2
Glutaric acidemia type I (GA I)[e]	C[a]5-DC[f]
HMG-CoA lyase deficiency (HMG)[e]	C[a]5-OH, ± C[a]6-DC[f]
Isovaleric acidemia (IVA)[e]	C[a]5
Methylmalonic acidemia (MUT)[e]	C[a]3, C[a]3/C[a]2
Multiple carboxylase deficiency (MCT)[e]	C[a]5-OH, ± C[a]3
Propionic acidemia (PROP)[e]	C[a]3, C[a]3/C[a]2
Other Disorders	
Biotinidase deficiency (BIOT)[e]	± C[c]5-OH[c], C[a]5:1
Cystic fibrosis (CF)	
Galactose-1-phosphate uridyltransferase deficiency (GALT)[g]	
Secondary Targets	
Amino Acid Disorders	
Argininemia (ARG)	ARG
Biopterin regeneration deficiency (Biopt REG)	PHE, PHE/TYR
Biopterin synthesis defect (BS)	PHE, PHE/TYR
Citrin deficiency (CIT II)	CIT
Hypermethioninemia (MET)	MET
Hyperphenylalaninemia (Hyper-PHE)	PHE
Tyrosinemia type II (TYR II)	TYR
Tyrosinemia type III (TYR III)	TYR
Fatty Acid Oxidation Disorders	
Carnitine acylcarnitine transporter defect (CACT)	C[a]16:1; C[a]18:1
Carnitine palmitoyltransferase I defect (CPT IA)	Carnitine
Carnitine palmitoyltransferase II defect (CPT II)	C[a]16:1, C[a]18:1
Dienoyl-CoA reductase deficiency (DE RED)	
Glutaric acidemia type II (GA2)[e]	C[a]4, C[a]5, C[a]5-DC[d], C[a]6, 8, 12, 14, 16
Medium-chain ketoacyl-CoA thiolase deficiency (MCKAT)	C[a]8, C[a]8/C[a]10, ± C[a]6, C[a]10:1
Medium-/short-chain hydroxy-acyl-CoA dehydrogenase deficiency (M/SCHAD)	C[a]4-OH[c]
Short-chain acyl-CoA dehydrogenase deficiency (SCAD)	C[a]4

TABLE 9-1 *(Continued)*

Inborn Error	Marker Analyte
Organic Acid Disorders	
α-methyl-β-hydroxy-butyric acidemia (2M3HBA)[e]	C[a]5, C[a]5:1, C[a]5-OH[c]
α-methylbutyryl-CoA dehydrogenase deficiency[e] (2MBG)	C[a]5
β-methylglutaconyl hydratase deficiency (3MGA)[e]	C[a]5-OH[c]
Cobalamin C and D defects (Cbl C, D)[e]	C[a]3/C[a]2
Isobutyryl-CoA dehydrogenase deficiency (IBG)[e]	C[a]4
Malonic acidemia (MAL)	C[a]3
Other Disorders	
Galactokinase deficiency (GALK)[g]	
Galactose epimerase deficiency (GALE)[g]	

[a] C = acyl group or carbon chain.
[b] O = number of carbons: 0 to 18.
[c] OH = hydroxy.
[d] Colon (:) followed by number represents double bonds.
[e] One or more amino acids involved in disorder.
[f] DC = dicarboxyl.
[g] Screened for by measuring blood galactose.

Sources: American College of Medical Genetics. Newborn screening: toward a uniform screening panel and system. *Genet Med.* 2006;8(Suppl 1):1S–252S; Chace DH, Lim T, Hansen CR, et al. Quantification of malonylcarnitine in dried blood spots by use of MS/MS varies by stable isotope internal standard composition. *Clin Chim Acta.* 2009;402(1–2):14–18; Frazier DM. Newborn screening by mass spectrometry. In: Acosta PB (ed). *Nutrition Management of Patients with Inherited Metabolic Disorders.* Burlington, MA: Jones & Bartlett Learning; 2010:21–67; Gillingham MB. Nutrition management of patients with inherited disorders of mitochondrial fatty acid oxidation. In: Acosta PB (ed). *Nutrition Management of Patients with Inherited Metabolic Disorders.* Burlington, MA: Jones & Bartlett Learning; 2010:369–403; Korman SH. Inborn errors of isoleucine degradation. *Mol Genet Metab.* 2006;89:289–299; Matalon KM. Introduction to genetics and genetics of inherited metabolic disorders. In: Acosta PB (ed). *Nutrition Management of Patients with Inherited Metabolic Disorders.* Burlington, MA: Jones & Bartlett Learning; 2010:1–19; Miinalainen IJ, Schmitz W, Huotari A, et al. Mitochondrial 2, 4-dienoyl-CoA reductase deficiency in mice results in severe hypoglycemia with stress intolerance and unimpaired ketogenesis. *PLoS Genet.* 2009;5:e1000543; Molven A, Matre GE, Duran M, et al. Familial hyperinsulinemia and hypoglycemia caused by a defect in the SCHAD enzyme of mitochondrial fatty acid oxidation. *Diabetes.* 2004;53:221–227; and Sim KG, Wiley V, Carpenter K, et al. Carnitine palmitoyltransferase I deficiency in neonate identified by dried blood spot free carnitine and acylcarnitine profile. *J Inherit Metab Dis.* 2001;24:51–59.

leucine, isoleucine, and valine; galactose; and long-chain fatty acids are limited, respectively.

- *Providing alternate metabolic pathways to decrease accumulated toxic precursors in blocked reaction sequences:* For example, isovalerylglycine is formed from accumulating isovaleric acid if supplemental glycine is provided to drive glycine-N-transacylase.[13]
- *Supplying products of blocked primary pathways:* Some examples are arginine in most disorders of the urea cycle,[3] cystine in homocystinuria,[5,16] tyrosine in PKU,[6,12] and BH_4[7] in biopterin synthesis defects.
- *Supplementing conditionally essential nutrients:* Examples are carnitine,[4] cystine,[5,16] and tyrosine[6] in secondary liver disease or with excess excretion of carnitine in organic acidemias.[17]
- *Stabilizing altered enzyme proteins:* The rate of biologic synthesis and degradation of holoenzymes is dependent on their structural conformation. In some holoenzymes, saturation by a coenzyme increases their biologic half-life and, thus, overall enzyme activity at the new equilibrium. This therapeutic mechanism is illustrated in homocystinuria and MSUD. Pharmacologic intake of pyridoxine in homocystinuria[16] and of thiamine in MSUD[2,13] increases intracellular pyridoxal phosphate and thiamine pyrophosphate, respectively, and increases the specific activity of any functional cystathionine β-synthase and branched-chain α-ketoacid dehydrogenase complex, respectively.
- *Replacing deficient coenzymes:* Many vitamin-dependent disorders are due to blocks in coenzyme production and are "cured" by pharmacologic intake of a specific vitamin precursor. This mechanism presumably involves overcoming a partially impaired enzyme reaction by mass action. Impaired reactions required to produce methylcobalamin and adenosylcobalamin result in homocystinuria and methylmalonic aciduria/acidemia. Daily intakes of appropriate forms of milligram quantities of vitamin B_{12} may cure the disease.[18]

- *Inducing enzyme production:* If the structural gene or enzyme is intact but suppressor, enhancer, or promoter elements are not functional, abnormal amounts of enzyme may be produced. The structural gene may be "turned on or off" to enable normal enzymatic production to occur. In the acute porphyria of type I tyrosinemia, excessive δ-aminolevulinic acid (ALA) production may be reduced by suppressing transcription of the δ-ALA synthase gene with excess glucose.[2,19]
- *Supplementing nutrients that are inadequately absorbed or not released from their apoenzyme:* An example is biotin in biotinidase deficiency.[20]
- *Preventing absorption of a nutrient that may be toxic in excess:* Large neutral amino acids (LNAA) other than PHE are available for preventing absorption of PHE from the intestinal tract and passage across the blood–brain barrier (BBB).[21]

The primary approach to therapy of patients with an IEM is via nutrition management. Each infant or child with an IEM requires individualized medical and nutrition care. Diet restrictions required to correct imbalances in some metabolic relationships usually require the use of elemental medical foods. These medical foods are normally supplemented with small amounts of intact protein that supply the restricted nutrient(s). These foods may supply up to 90%, but sometimes less, of the protein requirement of patients with disorders of amino acid or nitrogen metabolism. Other nitrogen-free foods that provide energy are limited in their range of nutrients. Fat, linoleic acid, α-linolenic acid, minerals, and vitamins must be supplied in adequate amounts. To ensure normal nutrition status indices, most mineral intakes must be greater than the RDAs (see Appendix F) due to poor absorption by patients ingesting elemental diets; they also should be ingested in at least three meals per day for best absorption.[22]

Elemental medical foods used in amino acid disorders may result in an osmotic load causing abdominal cramping, diarrhea, distention, nausea, or vomiting. More serious consequences can occur in infants, such as hypertonic dehydration, hypovolemia, hypernatremia, and death. Thus, neonates should not be fed an elemental formula that contains greater than 450 mOsm/kg water.

Medical foods for IEM of amino acid or nitrogen metabolism are formulated from free amino acids, carbohydrates, and often fat, minerals, and vitamins. The Maillard reaction is a complex group of chemical reactions in foods in which reacting amino acids, peptides, and proteins condense with sugars, forming bonds for which no digestive enzymes are available. The Maillard reaction is accelerated by heat and is characterized by a caramel-like color and roasted aromas. Medical foods should not be heated beyond 100°F (37.8°C) because the Maillard reaction causes loss of some sugars and amino acids.[3,23,24]

Puréed foods (beikost baby foods) should be introduced into the diet at about 4 months of age if the infant shows developmental readiness by a decrease in tongue thrust. Beikost is important in the diet to provide unidentified nutrients and fiber and, when table foods are eaten, to develop jaw muscles important for speech.[24]

Management Factors

As soon as nutrition support is well established in an infant or child, the prescription should be adjusted frequently. The frequency depends on the age of the child; infants require at least weekly changes whereas older children who are growing more slowly may only require a diet change monthly or every 2 to 3 months. Small, frequent changes in prescription prevent "bouncing" of plasma amino acid, glucose, organic acid, or ammonia concentrations and allow the intake to grow with the child, thus precluding the child's "growing out of the prescription."[24] This is especially important in the preteen and teenage years to prevent inadequate intake of nutrients that result in poor linear growth. Frequent diet changes are often needed during pregnancy based on biochemical indices.

Successful management of IEMs requires frequent monitoring to verify the adequacy of the nutrition support prescription. Premature and full-term infants to at least 6 months of age require twice weekly monitoring. Thereafter, weekly monitoring may be adequate if the child is compliant with the diet prescription.

Inborn Errors of Amino Acid Metabolism

Most of the organic acid disorders require restriction of a branched-chain amino acid as part of nutrition management (see **Table 9-2** and **Table 9-3**). The nutrition management of cystic fibrosis is addressed in Chapter 11.

When specific amino acids require restriction, total deletion for 1 to 3 days or until the plasma concentration reaches the upper limit of the reference range is the best approach to initiating therapy. Longer term deletion or overrestriction may precipitate deficiency of the amino acid(s). The most limiting nutrient determines growth rate in all disorders, and overrestriction of an amino acid, nitrogen (N), or energy will result in further intolerance of the toxic nutrient. Results of amino acid and N deficiencies are described in **Table 9-4**.

Restricted amino acid requirements are based on genotype, age, gender, health status, and amount of total protein fed (intact and protein equivalent = N, g × 6.25 = g protein equivalent from elemental medical food containing free amino acids). For example, patients with PKU may fall into one of the following three classifications, depending on genotype:[25]

- *Classical PKU:* Blood/plasma PHE concentration greater than 1200 µmol/L if untreated
- *Mild PKU:* Blood/plasma PHE concentration 600–1199 µmol/L if untreated
- *Non-PKU hyperphenylalaninemia (HPA):* Blood/plasma PHE concentration 120–599 µmol/L if untreated

TABLE 9-2 Nutrition Support of Inborn Errors of Metabolism

Inborn Error and Defect	Nutrient(s) to Modify	Vitamin Responsive?
Inborn Errors of Amino Acid Metabolism		
Aromatic Amino Acids[2,12]		
Phenylketonuria, classical (phenylalanine hydroxylase)	Restrict PHE, increase TYR, provide protein, mineral, and vitamin intakes greater than RDA.	No
Phenylketonuria, mild (phenylalanine hydroxylase)	Same as for PKU, classical.	±, Yes, BH_4 10–20 mg/day
Non-PKU hyperphenylalaninemia (phenylalanine hydroxylase)	Same as for PKU, if needed.	Yes, BH_4 10–20 mg/day
Hyperphenylalaninemia (dihydropteridine reductase)	Same as for PKU, if needed.	Yes, 1–10 mg/kg/day
GTP cyclohydrolase I, (6-pyruvoyltetrahydropterin synthase, sepiapterin reductase)	Seldom necessary to provide diet.	Yes, 1–10 mg/kg/day
Tyrosinemia type I (fumarylacetoacetate hydrolyase)	Restrict PHE and TYR. Provide greater than RDA for protein, energy, mineral, and vitamin intakes.	No
	Drug: 2-(2-nitro-4-trifluromethylbenzyl)-1-3-cyclohexanedione.	—
Tyrosinemia type II (tyrosine aminotransferase)	Restrict PHE and TYR. Provide protein, mineral, and vitamin intakes greater than RDA.	No
Tyrosinemia type III (phenylpyruvic acid dioxygenase)	Same as for tyrosinemia type II.	No
Branched-Chain Amino Acids[2,13]		
Maple syrup urine disease (branched-chain ketoacid dehydrogenase complex)	Restrict ILE, LEU, and VAL. Provide protein energy, mineral, and vitamin intakes above RDA.	Yes, thiamine-responsive if any residual enzyme activity. Response to thiamine inadequate to alleviate need for restriction of BCAAs.
Isovaleric acidemia (isovaleryl-CoA dehydrogenase); β-methylcrotonylglycinuria (β-methylcrotonyl-CoA carboxylase)	Restrict LEU; supplement with L-carnitine and GLY. Provide protein, energy, mineral, and vitamin intakes above RDA.	No
β-methylglutaconic aciduria type I (β-methylglutaconyl-CoA hydratase)	Same as for isovaleric acidemia except no GLY supplement. Unknown if beneficial if started neonatally.	No
β-ketothiolase deficiency (mitochondrial acetoacetyl-CoA thiolase deficiency)	Restrict ILE, supplement L-carnitine. Provide protein, energy, vitamin, and mineral intakes above RDA. Supplement L-LEU and L-VAL.	No
HMG-CoA lyase deficiency (β-hydroxy-β-methylglutaryl-CoA lyase deficiency)	Restrict LEU and fat; avoid fasting, supplement L-carnitine, provide protein, energy, minerals, and vitamins greater than RDA.	No
Isobutyryl-CoA dehydrogenase deficiency	As yet unknown whether VAL should be restricted, L-carnitine supplemented, or protein, energy, minerals, and vitamins should be increased. If yes, supplement L-LEU and L-ILE.	No
Sulfur Amino Acids[2,16]		
Homocystinuria, pyridoxine-nonresponsive (cystathionine-β-synthase)	Restrict MET, increase CYS, supplement folate, and betaine. Provide protein, energy, mineral, and vitamin intakes above RDA.	No
Homocystinuria, pyridoxine-responsive (cystathionine-β-synthase)	None unless plasma homocystine remains elevated. If so, treat as B_6 nonresponsive.	Yes, vitamin B_6
Hypermethioninemia I/III (methionine-s-adenosyltransferase deficiency)	Not treated by diet but with oral adenosylmethionine.	No

(continues)

TABLE 9-2 *(Continued)*

Inborn Error and Defect	Nutrient(s) to Modify	Vitamin Responsive?
Other Inborn Errors of Amino Acid Metabolism[2,17]		
Glutaric acidemia type I (glutaryl-CoA dehydrogenase)	Restrict LYS and TRP. Supplement L-carnitine. Provide protein, energy, mineral, and vitamin intakes above RDA.	Yes. Some patients have a partial response to oral riboflavin 100–300 mg daily. Administer 15–25 mg, with food, several times daily.
Methylmalonic acidemia (methylmalonyl-CoA mutase^0 or mutase-)	Restrict ILE, MET, THR, VAL, odd chain fatty acids, and long-chain unsaturated fatty acids. Supplement L-carnitine. Provide greater than RDA for protein, energy, mineral, and vitamin intakes.	No
Methylmalonic acidemia (cobalamin reductase; adenosyltransferase)	Minimum restriction of ILE, MET, THR, and VAL. Supplement L-carnitine.	Yes, 1–2 mg hydroxycobalamin daily
Propionic acidemia (propionyl-CoA carboxylase)	Restrict ILE, MET, THR, VAL, and long-chain fatty acids. Provide greater than RDA for protein, energy, mineral, and vitamin intakes. Supplement with L-carnitine daily.	Questionable. Some clinicians supplement D-biotin daily
Cobalamin A and B	Vitamin B_{12}.	Yes, 1–2 mg hydroxycobalamin IM
Cobalamin C and D	Supplement vitamin B_{12}, folate, betaine, and L-carnitine IM. Restrict ILE, MET, THR, VAL, if necessary.	Yes, hydroxycobalamin up to 20 mg as needed, and folate daily
Inborn Errors of Nitrogen Metabolism[2,38,39,40,64]		
Carbamylphosphate synthetase deficiency; Ornithine transcarbamylase deficiency	Restrict protein. Add EAAs, L-carnitine, L-ARG, and L-CIT. Provide greater than RDA for energy, mineral, and vitamin intakes.	No
Citrullinemia (argininosuccinate synthetase deficiency)	Restrict protein. Add EAAs, L-carnitine, and L-ARG. Provide greater than RDA for energy, mineral, and vitamin intakes.	No
Argininosuccinic aciduria (arginonosuccinate lyase)	Restrict protein. Add EAAs and L-ARG. Provide greater than RDA for energy, mineral, and vitamin intakes.	No
Citrin deficiency (aspartate-glutamate carrier)	High protein, low carbohydrate, L-ARG; increase water-miscible lipid-soluble vitamins until liver enzymes normal. MCT.	No
Inborn Errors of Carbohydrate Metabolism[2,14,65,66]		
Galactosemias		
Epimerase deficiency	Delete galactose. Add specific known amount of galactose. Provide RDA for protein, energy, minerals, and vitamins.	No
Galactokinase deficiency	Delete galactose. Provide RDA for protein, energy, mineral, and vitamin intakes.	No
Galactose-1-phosphate uridyl transferase deficiency	Delete galactose. Provide RDA for protein, energy, mineral, and vitamin intakes. Administer daily 750 mg calcium, 10 μg vitamin D, and 1 mg vitamin K_1 in addition to RDA. Unknown how strict diet should be in adults.	No
Inborn Errors of Fatty Acid Oxidation (Mitochondrial)[15,50]		
Carnitine acylcarnitine translocase defect; Carnitine palmitoyltransferase I defect	Avoid fasting; use low-fat, MCT-supplemented diet. Administer linoleic and α-linolenic acids. Uncooked cornstarch for hypoglycemia. Water-miscible, fat-soluble vitamins.	L-carnitine therapy if plasma carnitine low

TABLE 9-2 *(Continued)*

Inborn Error and Defect	Nutrient(s) to Modify	Vitamin Responsive?
Very-long-chain acyl-CoA dehydrogenase deficiency; Long-chain acyl-CoA dehydrogenase deficiency; Long-chain hydroxyacyl-CoA dehydrogenase deficiency; Trifunctional protein deficiency	Restrict long-chain fats, administer MCT, linoleic and α-linolenic acids. Uncooked cornstarch for hypoglycemia. Avoid fasting. Water-miscible fat-soluble vitamins. High-protein, moderate carbohydrates. Administer DHA for TFP.	No
Medium-chain acyl-CoA dehydrogenase deficiency	Restrict long-chain and avoid medium-chain fats; administer linoleic and α-linolenic acids. Uncooked cornstarch for hypoglycemia. Avoid fasting.	Yes?
Short-chain acyl-CoA dehydrogenase deficiency; Short-chain 3Hydroxyacyl CoA dehydrogenase deficiency	Restrict fat; administer linoleic and α-linolenic acids. Uncooked cornstarch for hypoglycemia. Avoid fasting, moderate protein.	No

Abbreviations: ALA, alanine; BCAAs, branched-chain amino acids; CYS, cystine; EAAs, essential amino acids (includes conditionally essential cystine and tyrosine); GLY, glycine; ILE, isoleucine; IM, intramuscular; LEU, leucine; LYS, lysine; MCT, medium-chain triglycerides; MET, methionine; MSUD, maple syrup urine disease; PHE, phenylalanine; THR, threonine; TRP, tryptophan; TYR, tyrosine; VAL, valine.

Sources: Anderson HC, Marble M, Shapiro E. Long-term outcome in treated combined methylmalonic acidemia and homcystinuria. *Genet Med.* 1999;1:146–150; Carrillo-Carrasco J, Sloan J, Valle D, et al. Hydroxocobalimin dose escalation improves metabolic control in cblC. *J Inherit Metab Dis.* 2009;52:728–731; Huemer M, Simma B, Fowler B, et al. Prenatal and postnatal treatment in cobalamin C defect. *J Pediatr.* 2005;147:469–472; Urbon Artero A, Aldona Gomez J, Reig Del Moral C, et al. Neonatal onset methylmalonic aciduria and clinical improvement with betaine therapy. *An Esp Pediatr.* 2002;56:337–341; Singh RH. Nutrition management of patients with inherited disorders of urea cycle enzymes. In: Acosta PB (ed). *Nutrition Management of Patients with Inherited Metabolic Disorders.* Burlington, MA: Jones & Bartlett Learning; 2010:405–429; and Smith DL, Bodamer OA. Practical management of combined methylmalonic aciduria and homocystinuria. *J Child Neurol.* 2002;17:353–356.

Patients with classical PKU and some with mild PKU excrete phenylpyruvic acid (PPA) in the urine if the blood/plasma PHE concentration is elevated. Because of the urinary loss of PPA and mental retardation found in patients with PKU, the disease was initially called imbecillitis phenylpyruvica or phenylpyruvic oligophrenia (little brains because of phenylpyruvic acid).[26]

Other patients with IEMs have variable nutrient requirements. Thus, each patient's nutrition prescription must be individualized to her or his specific needs. Tetrahydrobiopterin (BH_4) has been found to lower blood PHE concentration when administered to many patients with non-PKU HPA and some with mild PKU, but very few with classical PKU have been tested.[27,28]

Following the establishment of a firm diagnosis of classical PKU, a prescription must be given for the nutrition management of the patient. For the neonate who weighs 3.4 kg and has an initial blood PHE concentration of 1600 μmol/L with a blood tyrosine (TYR) concentration of 50 μmol/L, the initial prescription may be as follows for the first 3 days:

PHE, mg: 0×3.4 kg = 0 mg/day
TYR, mg: 348×3.4 kg = 1183 mg/day
Protein, g: 3.5×3.4 kg = 11.9 g/day
Energy, kcal: 120×3.4 kg = 408 kcal/day

Plan the diet by first determining which medical food (exempt infant formula) will be used.

Food	Amount	PHE (mg)	TYR (mg)	Protein (g)	Energy (kcal)
Phenex-1 powder	79 g	0	1185	11.9	379
Polycose powder[a]	6 g	0	0	0	30
Total		0	1185	11.9	409
Per kg body weight		0	348	3.5	120

Add water to make 621 mL (21 fl oz).
[a]380 kcal/100 g powder.

PHE must be added to the diet to prevent its deficiency as blood/plasma PHE concentration declines.

PHE, mg: 35×3.4 kg = 119 mg/day
TYR, mg: 304×3.4 kg = 1034 mg/day
Protein, g: 3.5×3.4 kg = 11.9 g/day
Energy, kcal: 120×3.4 kg = 408 kcal/day

First add proprietary infant formula to supply the required PHE. For example, Similac Advance with Iron powder contains 465 mg PHE, 10.8 g protein, and 521 kcal per 100 g powder. To determine the amount of Similac Advance powder to add, divide 119 g by the 465 mg PHE and multiply by 100; this yields 26 g. To determine the remaining protein to give as medical food, subtract the 2.8 g protein in 26 g Similac Advance powder from 11.9 g to get 9.1 g. Phenex-1 contains 1500 mg TYR, 15 g protein, and 480 kcal per 100 g powder.

TABLE 9-3 Recommended Nutrient Intakes (with Ranges) for Beginning Therapy

Nutrients to Modify	Age (years)					
	0.0 < 0.5	0.5 < 1.0	1 < 4	4 < 7	7 < 11	11 < 19
Inborn Errors of Amino Acid Metabolism						
Aromatic Amino Acids						
Phenylketonuria and hyperphenylalaninemia[2,11,12,34]						
PHE (mg)	55 (70–20)/kg	30 (50–15)/kg	325 (200–450)/d	425 (225–625)/d	450 (250–650)/d	500 (300–750)/d
TYR (mg)	195 (210–180)/kg	185 (200–170)/kg	2800 (1400–4200)/d	3150 (1750–4550)/d	3500 (2100–4900)/d	3850 (2100–5600)/d
Protein (g)	3.5–3.0/kg	3.0–2.5/kg	≥ 30/d	≥ 35/d	≥ 40/d	≥ 50–65/d
Energy (kcal)	120/kg	110/kg	900–1800/d	1300–2300/d	1650–3300/d	1500–3300/d
Tyrosinemia type I[2,11,12,24]						
PHE (mg)	100 (125–65)/kg	80 (105–45)/kg	600 (500–700)/d	650 (550–750)/d	700 (600–800)/d	800 (700–900)/d
TYR (mg)	75 (95–45)/kg	55 (75–30)/kg	400 (300–500)/d	450 (350–550)/d	500 (400–600)/d	550 (450–650)/d
Protein (g)	3.5–3.0/kg	3.0–2.5/kg	≥ 30/d	≥ 35/d	≥ 40/d	≥ 50–65/d
Energy (kcal)	← 100–120% of RDA →					
Tyrosinemia type II, III[2,11,12,24]						
PHE (mg)	100 (125–65)/kg	80 (105–45)/kg	450 (400–500)/d	500 (450–550)/d	550 (500–600)/d	600 (550–700)/d
TYR (gm)	75 (100–40)/kg	55 (80–20)/kg	400 (350–450)/d	450 (400–500)/d	500 (450–550)/d	475 (400–550)/d
Protein (g)	3.5–3.0/kg	3.0–2.5/kg	≥ 30/d	≥ 35/d	≥ 40/d	≥ 50–65/d
Energy (kcal)	120/kg	110/kg	900–1800/d	1300–2300/d	1650–3300/d	1500–3300/d
Branched–Chain Amino Acids						
Maple syrup urine disease[2,13,24]						
ILE (mg)	60 (90–30)/kg	50(70–30)/kg	50 (70–20)/kg	25 (30–20)/kg	25 (30–20)/kg	25 (30–10)/kg
LEU (mg)	80 (100–40)/kg	55 (75–40)/kg	55 (70–40)/kg	50 (65–35)/kg	45 (60–30)/kg	40 (50–15)/kg
VAL (mg)	70 (95–40)/kg	55 (80–30)/kg	50 (70–30)/kg	40 (50–30)/kg	28 (30–25)/kg	22 (30–15)/kg
Protein (g)	3.5–3.0/kg	3.0–2.5/kg	≥ 30/d	≥ 35/d	≥ 40/d	≥ 50–65/d
Energy (kcal)	← 100–125% of RDA →					
Isovaleric acidemia, β-methylglutaconyl hydratase deficiency type I[2,11,13,24]						
LEU (mg)	95 (110–65)/kg	75 (90–50)/kg	975 (800–1150)/d	1275 (1050–1500)/d	1445 (1190–1700)/d	1955 (1610–2300)/d
L-carnitine (mg)	300–100/kg	300–100/kg	300–100/kg	300–100/kg	300–100/kg	300–100/kg
GLY (mg)	← 125 (150–100)/kg →					
Protein (g)	3.5–3.0/kg	3.0–2.5/kg	≥ 30/d	≥ 35/d	≥ 40/d	≥ 50–65/d
Energy (kcal)	← 100–125% of RDA →					

HMG-CoA lyase deficiency[2,11,12,24]						
LEU (mg)	120 (140–100)/kg	110 (130–90)/kg	90 (100–80)/kg	80 (90–70)/kg	60 (80–40)/kg	50 (60–40)/kg
L-carnitine (mg)	← 50–100/kg →					
Protein (g)	3.5–3.0/kg	3.0–2.5/kg	≥ 30/d	≥ 35/d	≥ 40/d	≥ 50–65/d
Fat (g)	← 25–30% of energy →					
Energy (kcal)	← 100–125% of RDA →					
Avoid fasting	← →					
β-ketothiolase deficiency[2,11,13,24]						
ILE (mg)	70 (80–60)/kg	65 (75–55)/kg	60 (70–50)/kg	55 (65–45)/kg	55 (65–45)/kg	45 (55–35)/kg
L-carnitine (mg)	← 100–200 mg/kg →					
Protein (g)	3.5–3.0/kg	3.0–2.5/kg	≥ 30/d	≥ 35/d	≥ 40/d	≥ 50–65/d
Fat (g)	← 25–30% of energy →					
Energy (kcal)	← 100–125% of RDA →					
Avoid fasting	← →					
Supplemental L-LEU and L-VAL	← To maintain normal plasma concentrations →					
Isobutyryl-CoA dehydrogenase deficiency[13]						
ILE (mg)	70 (80–60)/kg	60 (70–50)/kg	55 (65–45)/kg	55 (65–45)/kg	50 (60–40)/kg	45 (55–35)/kg
GLY (mg)	100 (150–100)/kg	← 125 (150–100)/kg →				
L-carnitine (mg)	← 100–300/kg →					
Protein (g)	3.5–3.0/kg	3.0–2.5/kg	≥ 30/d	≥ 35/d	≥ 40/d	≥ 50–65/d
Energy (kcal)	← 100–125% of RDA →					
Sulfur Amino Acids						
Homocystinuria, cystathionine-β-synthase deficiency (pyridoxine nonresponsive)[2,11,16,24]						
MET (mg)	35 (50–20)/kg	28 (40–15)/kg	20 (30–10)/kg	15 (20–10)/kg	15 (20–10)/kg	15 (20–10)/kg
CYS (mg)	300–250/kg	250–200/kg	150 (200–100)/kg	150 (200–100)/kg	150 (200–100)/kg	75 (60–50)/kg
Betaine (g)	← 1–3/d →		← 3–6/d →			
Folate (mg)	← 0.5–1.0/d →		← 1–3/d →			
Protein (g)	3.5–3.0/kg	3.0–2.5/kg	≥ 30/d	≥ 35/d	≥ 40/d	≥ 50–65/d
Energy (kcal)	120/kg	115/kg	900–1800/d	1300–2300/d	1650–3300/d	1500–3300/d
Other Amino Acids						
Glutaric acidemia type I[2,11,17,24]						
LYS (mg)	85 (100–70)/kg	65 (90–40)/kg	55 (80–30)/kg	50 (75–25)/kg	45 (65–25)/kg	40 (60–20)/kg
TRP (mg)	25 (40–10)/kg	15 (30–10)/kg	12 (16–8)/kg	12 (16–8)/kg	8 (10–5)/kg	6 (8–4)/kg

(continues)

TABLE 9-3 *(Continued)*

Nutrients to Modify	Age (years) 0.0 < 0.5	0.5 < 1.0	1 < 4	4 < 7	7 < 11	11 < 19
L-carnitine (mg)	← 300–100/kg →					
Riboflavin (mg)	← 300–100 d, administer in 25-mg doses orally with food →					
Protein (g)	3.5–3.0/kg	3.0–2.5/kg	≥ 30/d	≥ 35/d	≥ 40/d	≥ 50–65/d
Energy (kcal)	120/kg	115/kg	900–1800/d	1300–2300/d	1650–3300/d	1500–3300/d
Do not overrestrict TRP	← →					
Propionic acidemia; methylmalonic acidemia[2,11,17,34]						
ILE (mg)	95 (120–60)/kg	70 (90–40)/kg	610 (485–735)/d	795 (630–960)/d	900 (715–1090)/d	1215 (956–1470)/d
MET (mg)	35 (50–15)/kg	25 (40–10)/kg	330 (275–390)/d	435 (360–510)/d	495 (410–580)/d	665 (550–780)/d
THR (mg)	90 (135–50)/kg	55 (75–20)/kg	505 (415–600)/d	660 (540–780)/d	745 (610–885)/d	1010 (830–1195)/d
VAL (mg)	85 (105–60)/kg	66 (75–30)/kg	690 (550–830)/d	900 (720–1080)/d	1020 (815–1225)/d	1380 (1105–1655)/d
D-biotin (mg)	← 5–10/d for propionic acidemia →					
Hydroxy-cobalamin (mg)	← 1–2/d for cobalamin-responsive methylmalonic acidemia →					
L-carnitine (mg)	← 300–100/kg →					
Protein (g)	3.5–3.0/kg	3.0–2.5/kg	≥ 30/d	≥ 35/d	≥ 40/d	≥ 50–65/d
Energy (kcal)	← 100–125% of RDA →					
Multiple carboxylase deficiency; Biotinidase deficiency[17]						
Biotin (mg)	← 10–20/d →					
Inborn Errors of Nitrogen Metabolism						
Citrullinemia; Argininosuccinic aciduria[2,11,24,38,64]						
L-ARG (mg)	700–350/kg	700–350/kg	500–250/kg	500–250/kg	500–250/kg	400–200/kg
Protein (g)	2.5–1.10/kg	1.9–1.0/kg	1.8–0.7/kg	1.3–0.7/kg	1.7–0.9/kg	1.4–0.8/kg
Energy (kcal)	← 125–150% of RDA →					
Carbamylphosphate synthetase deficiency; Ornithine transcarbamylase deficiency[2,11,34,63,66]						
L-CIT (mg)	700–350/kg	700–350/kg	500–250/kg	500–250/kg	500–250/kg	400–200/kg
Protein (g)	2.5–1.7/kg	1.9–1.0/kg	1.8–0.7/kg	1.3–0.7/kg	1.7–0.9/kg	1.4–0.8/kg
Energy (kcal)	← 125–150% of RDA →					
Argininemia[2,11,24,38,64]						
Protein (g)	2.5–1.0/kg	1.9–1.0/kg	1.8–0.7/kg	1.3–0.7/kg	1.7–0.9/kg	1.4–0.8/kg
Energy (kcal)	← 125–150% of RDA →					

Citrin deficiency[40]						
Protein (g)	4.5–4.0/kg	4.0–3.5/kg	3.5–3.0/kg	3.0–2.5/kg	3.0–2.5/kg	2.5–2.0/kg
L-ARG (mg)	← 600–100/kg →					
Carbohydrate (g)	← Low →					
Energy (kcal)	← 100–125% RDA for age →					
Inborn Errors of Carbohydrate Metabolism						
Galactosemias[2,11,14,65,66]						
Epimerase deficiency						
Galactose (mg)	← 1000–1500/d →		← 500–1000/d →			
Protein (g)	>2.2/kg	>2.0/kg	>23/d	>30/d	>35/d	>45–65/d
Energy (kcal)	120/kg	115/kg	900–1800/d	1300–2300/d	1650–3300/d	1500–3300/d
Galactokinase deficiency						
Protein (g)	>2.2/kg	>2.0/kg	>23/d	>30/d	>35/d	>45–65/d
Energy (kcal)	120/kg	115/kg	900–1800/d	1300–2300/d	1650–3300/d	>1500–3300/d
Galactose-1-phosphate uridyltransferase deficiency						
Calcium (mg)[a]	360	540	800	800	800	1200
Vitamin D (μg)[b]	10	10	10	10	10	10
Vitamin K (μg)[c]	30	4	5	6	7	8
Protein (g)	>2.2/kg	>2.0/kg	>30/d	>35/d	>40/d	>45–65/d
Energy (kcal)	120/kg	115/kg	900–1800/d	1300–2300/d	1650–3300/d	1500–3300/d
Inborn Errors of Fatty Acid Oxidation[11,15,24,67]						
Carnitine acylcarnitine translocase defect; Carnitine palmitoyltransferase defect						
Avoid fasting	← →					
Uncooked cornstarch	← To avoid hypoglycemia, 1 g/kg at bedtime →					
Protein (g)	← 15–20% of energy →					
Fat, long chain	← 10% of energy →					
Linoleic acid	← 3–4% of energy →					
α-linolenic acid	← 0.6–1% of energy →					
MCT oil	← 20% of energy →					
Energy	← RDA for age. Avoid obesity. →					
Glucose	← As needed for hypoglycemia →					
Water-miscible fat-soluble vitamins	← RDA for age →					

(continues)

TABLE 9-3 *(Continued)*

Nutrients to Modify	Age (years)					
	0.0 < 0.5	0.5 < 1.0	1 < 4	4 < 7	7 < 11	11 < 19
Very-long-chain acyl-CoA dehydrogenase deficiency; Long-chain acyl-CoA dehydrogenase deficiency; Long-chain hydroxy-acyl-CoA dehydrogenase deficiency; Trifunctional protein defect						
As above except protein	← 30% of energy →					
Add docosahexaenoic acid (DHA)	←→					
Medium-chain acyl-CoA dehydrogenase deficiency; Short-chain acyl-CoA dehydrogenase deficiency; Short-chain β-hydroxyacyl-CoA dehydrogenase deficiency						
Avoid fasting	←→					
Protein (g)	← 15–20% of energy →					
Fat	← 20–30% of energy →					
Linoleic acid	← 3–4% of energy →					
α-linolenic acid	← 0.6–1% of energy →					
Uncooked cornstarch	← To prevent hypoglycemia, 1 g/kg at bedtime →					
Energy (kcal)	← RDA, avoid obesity →					

a. In addition to 750 mg/day after 1 year of age, should be given in addition to recommendations for at least 2 years.

b. 10 μg vitamin D should be given for at least 2 years after 1 year of age in addition to recommendations.

c. 1 mg vitamin K should be given for 2 years after 1 year of age in addition to recommendations.

Abbreviations: ARG, arginine; CIT, citrulline; CYS, cystine; GLY, glycine; ILE, isoleucine; LEU, leucine; LYS, lysine; MET, methionine; PHE, phenylalanine; THR, threonine; TRP, tryptophan; TYR, tyrosine; VAL, valine.

TABLE 9-4 Results of Amino Acid and Nitrogen Deficiencies

Amino Acid	Manifestations of Deficiency
Arginine	Elevated blood ammonia Elevated urinary orotic acid Generalized skin lesions Poor wound healing Retarded growth
Carnitine	Fatty myopathy Cardiomyopathy Depressed liver function Neurologic dysfunction Defective fatty acid oxidation Hypoglycemia Hypertriacylglycerolemia
Citrulline	Elevated blood ammonia
Cysteine	Impaired nitrogen balance Impaired sulfur balance Decreased tissue glutathione Hypotaurinemia
Isoleucine	Weight loss or no weight gain Redness of buccal mucosa Fissures at corners of mouth Tremors of extremities Decreased plasma cholesterol Decreased plasma isoleucine Elevations in plasma lysine, phenylalanine, serine, tyrosine, and valine Skin desquamation, if prolonged
Leucine	Loss of appetite Weight loss or poor weight gain Decreased plasma leucine Increased plasma isoleucine, methionine, serine, threonine, and valine
Lysine	Weight loss or poor weight gain Impaired nitrogen balance
Methionine	Decreased plasma methionine Increased plasma phenylalanine, proline, serine, threonine, and tyrosine Decreased plasma cholesterol Poor weight gain Loss of appetite
Phenylalanine	Weight loss or poor weight gain Impaired nitrogen balance Aminoaciduria Decreased serum globulins Decreased plasma phenylalanine Mental retardation Anemia
Taurine	Impaired visual function Impaired biliary secretion
Threonine	Arrested weight gain Glossitis and reddening of the buccal mucosa Decreased plasma globulin Decreased plasma threonine
Tryptophan	Weight loss or no weight gain Impaired nitrogen retention Decreased plasma cholesterol
Tyrosine	Impaired nitrogen retention Catecholamine deficiency Thyroxine deficiency
Valine	Poor appetite, drowsiness Excess irritability and crying Weight loss or decrease in weight gain Decreased plasma albumin
Nitrogen	No or decreased weight gain Impaired nitrogen retention

Divide 9.1 g protein by 15.0 to get 60.6 g powder. Round to 61 g. Multiply 480 kcal per 100 g by 0.61 g to obtain 293 kcal. Remaining energy, if any is required, is determined by adding 135 kcal of Similac Advance with 293 kcal of Phenex-1. This yields 428 kcal. No further energy is required.

Food	Amount	PHE (mg)	TYR (mg)	Protein (g)	Energy (kcal)
Similac Advance with Iron powder	26 g	121	117	2.8	135
Phenex-1 powder	61 g	0	915	9.1	293
Total		121	1032	11.9	422
Per kg body weight		36	304	3.5	124

Add water to yield 628 mL (21 fluid ounces).

Several clinical phenotypes of branched-chain ketoaciduria (MSUD) exist, and the amount of each branched-chain amino acid required will differ by genotype, age, gender, state of health, and protein intake.[13] Patients with intermediate or intermittent MSUD will require less strict diet management than patients with classical MSUD. However, introduction of BCAA-free medical food to these patients with consistent daily use, especially during febrile illness, will help prevent acidosis. Nutrition therapy of the patient with classical MSUD should be introduced with the first suspicion of disease to prevent severe illness. The 3.4-kg child should be offered a BCAA-free medical food for the first 3 days of therapy. A prescription that includes protein and at least 140 kcal/kg should be written:

Protein, g: 3.5×3.4 kg $= 11.9$ g

Energy, kcal: 140×3.4 kg $= 476$ kcal

Food	Amount	Protein (g)	Energy (kcal)
Ketonex-1 powder	79 g	11.9	379
Polycose powder[a]	26 g	—	99
Total		11.9	478
Per kg body weight		3.5	140

Add water to yield 710 mL (24 oz).

[a]380 kcal/100 g powder

The three BCAAs must be added to the diet to prevent deficiency, and ILE must be added on or before day 4 to prevent skin desquamation. The amount of LEU added at this time may be less than when the plasma concentration has reached the treatment range. The amount of VAL added may be the full prescription depending on the plasma concentration.

ILE, mg: 60×3.4 kg $= 204$ mg

LEU, mg: 75×3.4 kg $= 255$ mg

VAL, mg: 70×3.4 kg $= 238$ mg

Protein, g: 3.5×3.4 kg $= 11.9$ g

Energy, kcal: 140×3.4 kg $= 476$ kcal

Fill the LEU prescription with Similac Advance with Iron powder, which contains 575 mg ILE, 1080 mg LEU, and 640 mg VAL per 100 g powder.

Food	Amount	ILE (mg)	LEU (mg)	VAL (mg)	Protein (g)	Energy (kcal)
Similac Advance with Iron powder	24 g	138	259	154	2.6	125
Ketonex-1 powder	62 g	0	0	0	9.3	298
ILE solution[a]	6.6 mL	66	0	0	0	0
VAL solution[a]	8.4 mL	0	0	84	0	0
Polycose powder[b]	14 g	0	0	0	0	53
Total		204	259	238	11.9	476
Per kg body weight		60	76	70	3.5	140

[a]10 mg/mL.

[b]380 kcal/100 g powder.

Add water to make 650 mL (22 fl oz). As plasma LEU concentration decreases a greater amount of Similac Advance may be added to help maintain plasma ILE, LEU, and VAL in the treatment range and to support normal growth.

All patients with IEMs have nutrient requirements that may differ widely. Thus, the diet prescription must be individualized to support normal growth of each patient. Protein requirements of infants and children with IEMs are normal if liver or renal function is not compromised. Because nitrogen retention from free amino acid formulations differs from that of amino acids derived from intact protein, the recommended protein intakes of infants and children with inborn errors of amino acid metabolism are 125–150% greater than the RDAs.[1,29] Other factors may also contribute to the need by patients with inherited amino acid disorders for greater protein intakes than recommended for normal persons.[30] Fat intakes and the essential fatty acids, linoleic and α-linolenic, should meet RDAs,[1] except in mitochondrial fatty acid oxidation defects.

Energy intakes of infants and children with inborn errors of metabolism must be adequate to help support normal rates of growth. Provision of apparently adequate amino acids and N without sufficient energy will lead to growth failure. Energy requirements are greater than normal when L-amino acids supply the protein equivalent. Maintenance of adequate energy intake is essential for normal growth and development and to prevent catabolism. If the RDA[1] for energy cannot be achieved through oral feeds, nasogastric, gastrostomy, or parenteral feeds must be employed. Care must be taken to prevent overweight or obesity because weight loss results in elevated plasma amino acid concentrations. Fluid intake should be 1.5 mL/kcal for infants and 1.0 mL/kcal for children.

Major, trace, and ultratrace mineral and vitamin intakes should exceed RDA for age.[1,31–34] If the medical food mixture fails to supply ≥ 100% of requirements for infants and children, appropriate supplements should be given. In patients with PKU, plasma phenylalanine concentrations > 480 μmol/L may lead to loss of bone matrix in spite of adequate calcium, phosphorous, and vitamin D intakes.[32–36] All organic acidemias, unless well controlled, will result in bone mineral loss.[37]

Inborn Errors of Nitrogen Metabolism

Eight enzyme defects have been reported in the urea cycle resulting in elevated concentrations of blood ammonia.[38,39] Four of the defects are suspected by elevated concentrations of blood arginine (ARG) or citrulline (CIT) on newborn screening (see Table 9-1). Consequently, differential diagnosis is essential for appropriate therapy.

The urea cycle normally contributes large amounts of ARG to the body ARG pool. When the urea cycle is nonfunctional, ARG becomes an essential amino acid.[2,28] Consequently, L-ARG must be administered in all disorders of the urea cycle except arginase deficiency (see Table 9-2). In carbamyl phosphate synthetase (CPS) or ornithine transcarbamylase (OTC) deficiency, L-CIT may be given in place of or with L-ARG. When administered in adequate amounts, these amino acids also enhance waste N excretion.[39] L-ARG, when given orally, should be in the base form, because the hydrochloride form will cause acidosis.

Protein restriction resulting in N restriction is the primary approach to prevention of elevated blood ammonia (see Table 9-2 and Table 9-3) in all except citrin deficiency (CIT II), which requires a high-protein, low-carbohydrate diet.[40] Citrin is an aspartate-glutamate carrier. Ornithine translocase transports ornithine into the mitochondria; a deficiency results in hyperornithinemia, hyperammonemia, and homocitrullinuria (HHH syndrome). Protein synthesis and N utilization are more efficient when all amino acids are present in appropriate amounts at the same time. Severe restriction of intact protein leads to inadequate intake of several essential and conditionally essential amino acids, as well as minerals and vitamins. Because of this, medical foods consisting of essential and conditionally essential amino acids, minerals, and vitamins have been devised (see Table 9-5 in *Pediatric Nutrition, Fourth Edition*). Carnitine, cystine, taurine, and tyrosine may not be synthesized in adequate amounts when liver parenchymal cells are damaged. Thus, any medical food used for therapy of urea cycle disorders should contain carnitine, cystine, taurine, and tyrosine. Overrestriction of an essential amino acid or N leads to decreased protein synthesis or body protein catabolism and increased blood ammonia concentration. To provide adequate amounts of essential amino acids in the protein-restricted diet, one-half to two-thirds of the protein prescription should be supplied by medical food,[24] as long as growth is proceeding. During the prepubertal growth spurt, greater amounts of protein may be required than previously needed. Maintenance of anabolism is essential to prevent hyperammonemia.

The protein quality of medical foods must be evaluated based on their amino acid, mineral, and vitamin content, because intact protein sources (dairy products, meat, fish and other seafood, poultry) normally supply large amounts of minerals and vitamins. Medical foods devised for patients with urea cycle disorders must supply all minerals and vitamins not contributed by the small quantities of low-protein breads/cereals, fruits, fats, and vegetables the patient may ingest. Because protein intake is severely restricted in urea cycle enzyme defects in all except CIT II, energy (kcal) intake should be increased to prevent use of muscle protein for energy purposes, thereby preventing catabolism of body protein. The best energy-to-protein ratio is unknown in these disorders; however, obesity should be avoided. Energy is the first requirement of the body, and inadequate energy intake for protein synthesis and other needs will lead to elevated blood ammonia concentration.[2]

Waste N excretion is enhanced through treatment with sodium benzoate, sodium phenylacetate, or sodium phenylbutyrate. Sodium benzoate is conjugated with glycine primarily in hepatic and renal cell mitochondria to form hippurate, which is cleared by the kidney.[41] Sodium phenylacetate conjugates with glutamine in kidney and liver cells to form phenylacetylglutamine, which is excreted by the kidney.[42,43] Phenylacetic acid conjugates with taurine in the kidney.[42] Glycine is readily made from serine. Tetrahydrofolate is required for this reaction to occur. Glycine also can be synthesized from glutamate. Pyridoxal phosphate (PLP) and an aldolase are required for this set of reactions. Because several coenzymes are required to maintain serine, nicotinamide-adenine dinucleotide (NAD), PLP, and glycine pools and the use of CoA in synthesis of hippurate, folate, pantothenate, pyridoxine, and niacin should be administered at greater than RDAs[1] for age when sodium benzoate is given therapeutically. Because dietary intake of potassium is often low and use of drugs to enhance waste N loss can lead to its urinary excretion, frequent monitoring of plasma potassium (K^+) concentration is essential to maintain it within the normal range.[38] Daily supplements of KCl may be required because very low plasma K^+ concentration can lead to death.

Inborn Errors of Carbohydrate Metabolism: Galactosemias

Three forms of galactosemia have been reported: galactokinase deficiency, galactose-4-epimerase deficiency, and galactose-1-phosphate uridyl transferase (GALT)[14] deficiency. Deletion of galactose in all forms of galactosemia must be accompanied by adequate intakes of protein, energy, minerals, and vitamins (see Table 9-2 and Table 9-3). Galactose binds with phosphate in patients with GALT deficiencies. This intracellular sequestering of phosphorus in combination with excess urinary phosphate loss (Fanconi syndrome) suggests the need for phosphorus intake greater than RDA.[1] Inadequate calcium intake coupled with hypogonadism results in depressed bone mineral density in patients with galactosemia.[44,45]

Therapy of galactosemia due to GALT deficiency, although lifesaving in the infant, has resulted in less than optimum outcomes. Poor outcomes may be the result of small but significant intakes of naturally occurring galactose in fruits, vegetables, grains, legumes (dried beans and peas), and other foods. Infant formula powders made from soy protein isolate without added lactose contain significantly less galactose than do liquid soy protein isolate formulas, formulas for lactase deficiency, or formulas made from hydrolyzed casein, due to the added carrageenan.[14] Milk products, including all soft cheeses and some hard cheeses, and organ meats must be eliminated. Careful label reading for the presence of lactose, casein, or whey and examination of all drug ingredients should be practiced before suggesting the use of any food or drug.[14] Lactobionic acid, found in Neocalglucon, should not be used in patients with galactosemia due to the presence of galactose.[46]

Rates of decline in erythrocyte galactose-1-phosphate differ in infants with differing genotypes. Infants with a genotype of Q188R/Q188R, all receiving the same diet management, had an erythrocyte galactose-1-phosphate of 4.9 mg/dL at 5 to 8 months of age, and patients with a genotype of Q188R/other had a concentration of 3.3 mg/dL at the same age. Patients with a genotype of other/other had an erythrocyte galactose-1-phosphate of 2.5 mg/dL when in the same age range.[47] Use of the breath test to measure galactose oxidation also indicates differences in utilization of galactose in patients by genotype.[48]

Inborn Errors of Fatty Acid Oxidation (Mitochondrial)

Fatty acids are a primary fuel for the body when fasting is prolonged and are a direct source of fuel for heart and skeletal muscle. Ketones such as acetoacetate and β-hydroxybutyric acid, obtained during hepatic fat metabolism, are an important energy source for the brain and other tissues.[49] Consequently, all fat must not be removed from the diet and care must be taken to supply required energy, linoleic acid, and α-linolenic acid. Fat restriction in long-chain and very-long-chain fatty acid oxidation defects; replacement of most fat with MCT; addition of the docosahexaenoic acid precursor, α-linolenic acid, with the use of canola, soy, walnut, or flaxseed oils;[15] avoidance of fasting; glucose therapy as needed; and uncooked cornstarch have improved outcomes. Patients with a defect in medium- or short-chain fatty acid oxidation require avoidance of fasting and of MCT oil, addition of glucose for hypoglycemia, and uncooked cornstarch as needed. The recommendation for fat is 30–35% of energy for children and adults.

Patients with VLCAD, LCHAD, TFP, or CPT 2 deficiency require about 10% of energy as long-chain fats and about 20% of energy as MCT. With this restriction of long-chain fats, supplementation with a water-miscible form of vitamin E should be considered if plasma α-tocopherol concentrations are below reference range. Ingested vitamins A and D should remain in normal ranges. Nutrition guidelines to manage patients with VLCAD or MCAD deficiency are available at http://www.gmdi.org/Resources/NutritionGuidelines/VLCADGuidelines and http://www.gmdi.org/Resources/NutritionGuidelines/MCADGuidelines.

Protein intake at much greater than RDA may be beneficial in helping to control hypoglycemia and in preventing the obesity that occurs in patients fed high-carbohydrate diets. Patients with medium- and short-chain fatty acid oxidation defects may benefit with up to 20% of energy as protein to help control hypoglycemia. Some patients with SCAD deficiency respond to riboflavin supplementation. Because riboflavin is extremely insoluble, 15–25 mg should be given orally with meals up to three times daily.[1]

Malonyl-CoA decarboxylase is present in high amounts in human heart and skeletal muscle and the liver, kidney, and pancreas.[50] Malonyl-CoA decarboxylase plays a key role in peroxysmal systolic and mitochondrial fatty acid oxidation and appears to inhibit CPT I.[51] Malonyl-CoA decarboxylase deficiency results in variable clinical symptoms, including hypoglycemia, hypotonia, cardiomyopathy, developmental delay, acidosis, seizures, and elevated urinary malonic acid.[52,53] Moderate long-chain fat restriction, MCT,

TABLE 9-5 Functions of the Dietitian in Nutrition Support of Patients with Inborn Errors of Metabolism

During Diagnosis	Evaluate nutrient intake. Prepare nutrition support plan. Implement nutrition support plan. Evaluate nutrition support plan. Evaluate nutrition status. Record findings in medical records. Adjust amino acid prescription (e.g., glycine). Adjust selected medications (e.g., sodium benzoate, sodium phenylbutyrate).
During Critical Illness	Recommend composition of feedings. Develop tube feedings when needed. Monitor nutrition support. Record in medical record. Recommend amount to feed per hour. Recommend continuous or intermittent feedings. Recommend route of alimentation. Recommend necessary laboratory tests. Recommend peripheral or central line feeding. Recommend size of feeding tube.
During Long-Term Care	Formulate diet prescription/nutrition care plan. Record in medical record. Monitor for diet compliance. Revise nutrition care plan as needed. Evaluate effectiveness of nutrition care plan. Coordinate with other agencies. Prepare sample menus. Modify diet prescription during illness. Prescribe medical food. Prescribe very-low-protein foods. Recommend methods of feeding. Evaluate research findings and apply to clinical care. Fill diet prescription. Monitor for gastrointestinal complications. Refer to other specialists. Monitor potential nutrient–drug interactions. Help caretaker prepare patient-specific food lists, if needed. Help caretaker prepare shopping lists, if needed.

Source: Acosta PB. *Nutrition Management of Patients with Inherited Metabolic Disorders.* Burlington, MA: Jones & Bartlett Learning; 2010.

and L-carnitine supplementation with frequent feedings appear to be beneficial (see Table 9-2).[53,54] Glutaric aciduria type II (multiple acyl-CoA dehydrogenase deficiency) is caused by defects in electron transport lipoprotein (ETF) or ETF-ubiquinone oxidoreductase (ETF-QO) and results in three main phenotypes: neonatal onset with congenital anomalies, neonatal onset without congenital anomalies, and mild or later onset.[55] Patients with milder or later onset of symptoms treated with oral riboflavin, L-carnitine, and diets low in protein and fat (see Table 9-2) have had little better outcomes than infants who present neonatally.[55-58]

Functions of the Dietitian in Nutrition Support of Patients with IEM

The roles of the dietitian in nutrition support are outlined in **Table 9-5.** The crucial role of the dietitian in long-term management of the patient with an IEM mandates excellent interpersonal skills as well as a knowledge base far in excess of entry-level requirements.

Nutrigenomics

Some nutrients are considered capable of interacting with the genome to change gene expression, structure, and function.[59] Patients with multifactorial diseases usually not seen in medical genetics clinics are the usual persons for whom the dietitian provides diet counseling; these patients' diseases may include conditions such as cancer, diabetes mellitus, and heart disease. Diet alone is seldom the exclusive therapy, and if it must be followed long-term it is seldom adequately adhered to.

The risk for developmental and degenerative diseases increases with increasing DNA damage, which is dependent on nutrition status and optimal concentration of micronutrients for prevention of genome damage.[59] Overfeeding and failure to ingest foods with bioactive compounds, minerals, vitamins, and protein in adequate amounts may lead to DNA methylation and chronic disease, whereas ingestion of a diet rich in minerals and vitamins may help prevent disease.[60-63]

REFERENCES

1. Otten JJ, Hellwig JP, Meyers LD. *Dietary Reference Intakes: The Essential Guide to Nutrient Requirements.* Washington, DC: National Academies Press; 2006.
2. Elsas LJ, Acosta PB. Inherited metabolic disease: amino acids, organic acids, and galactose. In: Shils ME, Shike M, Olson J, Ross AC, Caballero B, Cousins RJ (eds). *Modern Nutrition in Health and Disease,* 10th ed. Philadelphia: Lippincott Williams & Wilkins; 2005:909–959.
3. Goldblum OM, Brusilow SW, Maldonado YA, Farmer ER. Neonatal citrullinemia associated with cutaneous manifestations and arginine deficiency. *J Am Acad Dermatol.* 1986;14:321–326.
4. Borum PR, Bennett SG. Carnitine as an essential nutrient. *J Am Coll Nutr.* 1986;5:177–182.
5. Sansaricq C, Garg S, Norton PM, et al. Cystine deficiency during dietotherapy of homocystinemia. *Acta Paediatr Scand.* 1975;64:215–218.
6. Laidlaw SA, Kopple JD. Newer concepts of the indispensable amino acids. *Am J Clin Nutr.* 1987;46:593–605.
7. Blau N, Thony B, Cotton RGH, Hyland K. Disorders of tetrahydrobiopterin and related biogenic amines. In: Scriver CR, Beaudet AL, Sly WS, Valle D (eds). *The Metabolic and Molecular Bases of Inherited Disease,* 8th ed. New York: McGraw-Hill; 2001:1725–1776.
8. Acosta PB. Nutrition support for inborn errors. In: Samour PQ, King K (eds). *Handbook of Pediatric Nutrition,* 3rd ed. Burlington, MA: Jones & Bartlett Learning; 2005:239–286.
9. Frazier DM. Newborn screening by mass spectrometry. In: Acosta PB (ed). *Nutrition Management of Patients with Inherited Metabolic Disorders.* Burlington, MA: Jones & Bartlett Learning; 2010:21–65.
10. American College of Medical Genetics. Newborn screening: toward a uniform screening panel and system. *Genet Med.* 2006;8(Suppl 1):1S–252S.
11. Acosta PB. *Nutrition Management of Patients with Inherited Metabolic Disorders.* Burlington, MA: Jones & Bartlett Learning; 2010.
12. Acosta PB, Matalon KM. Nutrition management of patients with inherited disorders of aromatic amino acids. In: Acosta PB (ed). *Nutrition Management of Patients with Inherited Metabolic Disorders.* Burlington, MA: Jones & Bartlett Learning; 2010:119–174.
13. Marriage B. Nutrition management of patients with inherited disorders of branched-chain amino acid metabolism. In: Acosta PB (ed). *Nutrition Management of Patients with Inherited Metabolic Disorders.* Burlington, MA: Jones & Bartlett Learning; 2010:175–236.
14. Acosta PB. Nutrition management of patients with inherited disorders of galactose metabolism. In: Acosta PB (ed). *Nutrition Management of Patients with Inherited Metabolic Disorders.* Burlington, MA: Jones & Bartlett Learning; 2010:343–367.
15. Gillingham MB. Nutrition management of patients with inherited disorders of mitochondrial fatty acid oxidation. In: Acosta PB (ed). *Nutrition Management of Patients with Inherited Metabolic Disorders.* Burlington, MA: Jones & Bartlett Learning; 2010:369–403.
16. van Calcar S. Nutrition management of patients with inherited disorders of sulfur amino acid metabolism. In: Acosta PB (ed). *Nutrition Management of Patients with Inherited Metabolic Disorders.* Burlington, MA: Jones & Bartlett Learning; 2010:237–281.
17. Yannicelli S. Nutrition management of patients with inherited disorders of organic acid metabolism. In: Acosta PB (ed). *Nutrition Management of Patients with Inherited Metabolic Disorders.* Burlington, MA: Jones & Bartlett Learning; 2010:283–341.
18. Rosenblatt DS, Fenton W. Inherited disorders of folate and cobalamin transport and metabolism. In: Scriver CR, Beaudet AL, Sly WS, Valle D (eds). *The Metabolic and Molecular Bases of Inherited Disease,* 8th ed. New York: McGraw-Hill; 2001:3897–3934.
19. Bonkowsky HL, Magnussen CR, Collins AR, et al. Comparative effects of glycerol and dextrose on porphyrin precursor excretion in acute intermittent porphyria. *Metabolism.* 1976;25:405–414.

20. Wolf B. Disorders of biotin metabolism. In: Scriver CR, Beaudet AL, Sly WS, Valle D (eds). *The Metabolic and Molecular Bases of Inherited Disease,* 8th ed. New York: McGraw-Hill; 2001: 3935–3962.
21. Matalon R, Michals-Matalon K, Bhatia G, et al. Double blind placebo control trial of large neutral amino acids in treatment of PKU: effect on blood phenylalanine. *J Inherit Metab Dis.* 2007;30:153–158.
22. Alexander JW, Clayton BE, Delves HT. Mineral and trace-metal balances in children receiving normal and synthetic diets. *Q J Med.* 1974;169:80–111.
23. Erbersdobler HF, Somoza V. Forty years of furosine—forty years of using Maillard reaction products as indicators of the nutritional quality of foods. *Mol Nutr Food Res.* 2007;51:423–430.
24. Acosta PB, Yannicelli S. *Nutrition Support Protocols,* 4th ed. Columbus, OH: Ross Products Division, Abbott Laboratories; 2001.
25. Scriver CR, Waters PJ, Sarkissian C, et al. PAHdb: a locus-specific knowledgebase. *Hum Mutat.* 2000;15:99–104.
26. Folling A. The original detection of phenylketonuria. In: Bickel H, Hudson FP, Woolf LI (eds). *Phenylketonuria and Some Other Inborn Errors of Amino Acid Metabolism.* Stuttgart: Georg Thieme Verlag; 1971:1–3.
27. Kure S, Hou DC, Ohura T, et al. Tetrahydrobiopterin-responsive phenylalanine hydroxylase deficiency. *J Pediatr.* 1999;135:375–378.
28. Hennermann JB, Buhrer C, Blau N, et al. Long-term treatment with tetrahydrobiopterin increases phenylalanine tolerance in children with severe phenotype of phenylketonuria. *Mol Genet Metab.* 2005;86(Suppl 1):S86–S90.
29. Acosta PB. Evaluation of nutrition status. In: Acosta PB (ed). *Nutrition Management of Patients with Inherited Metabolic Disorders.* Burlington, MA: Jones & Bartlett Learning; 2010:67–98.
30. Loots DT, Mienie LJ, Erasmus E. Amino-acid depletion induced by abnormal amino-acid conjugation and protein restriction in isovaleric acidemia. *Eur J Clin Nutr.* 2007;61:1323–1327.
31. Acosta PB, Yannicelli S, Singh RH, et al. Iron status of children with phenylketonuria undergoing nutrition therapy assessed by transferrin receptors. *Genet Med.* 2004;6:96–101.
32. Yannicelli S, Medeiros DM. Elevated plasma phenylalanine concentrations may adversely affect bone status of phenylketonuric mice. *J Inherit Metab Dis.* 2002;25:347–361.
33. Acosta PB, Yannicelli S. Plasma micronutrient concentrations in infants undergoing therapy for phenylketonuria. *Biol Trace Elem Res.* 1999;67:75–84.
34. Pasquali M, Singh R, Kennedy MJ, et al. Pyridinium cross-links: a parameter of bone matrix turnover in phenylketonuria. *Book of Abstracts,* 5th Meeting of the International Society for Neonatal Screening, June 26–29, 2002. Genoa, Italy.
35. Acosta PB, Yannicelli S. Nutrient intake and biochemical status of children with phenylketonuria undergoing nutrition management. Unpublished data. Columbus, Ohio: Ross Products Division, Abbott Laboratories; 2003.
36. Yannicelli S, Acosta PB, Velazquez A, et al. Improved growth and nutrition status in children with methylmalonic or propionic acidemia fed an elemental medical food. *Mol Genet Metab.* 2003;80:181–188.
37. Bushinsky DA. Acid-base imbalance and the skeleton. *Eur J Nutr.* 2001;40:238–244.
38. Singh RH. Nutritional management of patients with urea cycle disorders. *J Inherit Metab Dis.* 2007;30:880–887.
39. Brusilow S, Horwich A. Urea cycle enzymes. In: Scriver CR, Beaudet AL, Sly WS, Valle D (eds). *The Metabolic and Molecular Bases of Inherited Disease,* 8th ed. New York: McGraw-Hill; 2001:1909–1963.
40. Dimmock D, Kobayashi K, Iijima M, et al. Citrin deficiency: a novel cause of failure to thrive that responds to a high-protein, low-carbohydrate diet. *Pediatrics.* 2007;119:e773–e777.
41. Moldave K, Meister A. Synthesis of phenylacetylglutamine by human tissue. *J Biol Chem.* 1957;229:463–476.
42. Ambrose AM, Powder FW, Sherwin CP. Further studies on the detoxification of phenylacetic acid. *J Biol Chem.* 1933;101: 669–675.
43. James MO, Smith RL, Williams RT, Reidenberg M. The conjugation of phenylacetic acid in man, sub-human primates and some non-primate species. *Proc R Soc Lond B Biol Sci.* 1972;182:25–35.
44. Kaufman FR, Loro ML, Azen C, et al. Effect of hypogonadism and deficient calcium intake on bone density in patients with galactosemia. *J Pediatr.* 1993;123:365–370.
45. Rubio-Gozalbo ME, Hamming S, van Kroonenburgh MJ, et al. Bone mineral density in patients with classic galactosaemia. *Arch Dis Child.* 2002;87:57–60.
46. Harju M. Lactobionic acid as a substrate of ß-galactosidases. *Milchwissenschaft.* 1990;45:411–415.
47. Singh RH, Kennedy MJ, Jonas CR, et al. Whole body oxidation and galactosemia genotype: prognosis for galactose tolerance in the first year of life. *J Inherit Metab Dis.* 2003;26:123A.
48. Berry GT, Singh RH, Mazur AT, et al. Galactose breath testing distinguishes variant and severe galactose-1-phosphate uridyltransferase genotypes. *Pediatr Res.* 2000;48:323–328.
49. Roe CR, Ding J. Mitochondrial fatty acid oxidation disorders. In: Scriver CR, Beaudet AL, Sly WS, Valle D (eds). *The Metabolic and Molecular Bases of Inherited Disease,* 8th ed. New York: McGraw-Hill; 2001:2297–2326.
50. Sacksteder KA, Morrell JC, Wanders RJ, et al. MCD encodes peroxisomal and cytoplasmic forms of malonyl-CoA decarboxylase and is mutated in malonyl-CoA decarboxylase deficiency. *J Biol Chem.* 1999;274:24461–24468.
51. Saggerson D. Malonyl-CoA, a key signaling molecule in mammalian cells. *Annu Rev Nutr.* 2008;28:253–272.
52. Ficicioglu C, Chrisant MR, Payan I, Chace DH. Cardiomyopathy and hypotonia in a 5-month-old infant with malonyl-CoA decarboxylase deficiency: potential for preclinical diagnosis with expanded newborn screening. *Pediatr Cardiol.* 2005;26:881–883.
53. Salomons GS, Jakobs C, Pope LL, et al. Clinical, enzymatic and molecular characterization of nine new patients with malonyl-coenzyme A decarboxylase deficiency. *J Inherit Metab Dis.* 2007;30:23–28.
54. Yano S, Sweetman L, Thorburn DR, et al. A new case of malonyl coenzyme A decarboxylase deficiency presenting with cardiomyopathy. *Eur J Pediatr.* 1997;156:382–383.
55. Frerman FE. Defects of electron transfer lipoprotein and electron transfer lipoprotein oxidoreductase: glutaric acidemia type II. In: Scriver CR, Beaudet AL, Sly WS, Valle D (eds). *The Metabolic and Molecular Bases of Inherited Disease,* 8th ed. New York: McGraw-Hill; 2001:2357–2365.

56. Angle B, Burton BK. Risk of sudden death and acute life-threatening events in patients with glutaric acidemia type II. *Mol Genet Metab.* 2008;93:36–39.
57. Maillart E, Acquaviva-Bourdain C, Rigal O, et al. Multiple acyl-CoA dehydrogenase deficiency (MADD): a curable cause of genetic muscular lipidosis. *Rev Neurol (Paris).* 2010:166:289–294.
58. Vockley J. Glutaric aciduria type 2 and newborn screening: commentary. *Mol Genet Metab.* 2008;93:5–6.
59. Bull C, Fenech M. Genome-health nutrigenomics and nutrigenetics: nutritional requirements or 'nutriomes' for chromosomal stability and telomere maintenance at the individual level. *Proc Nutr Soc.* 2008;67:146–156.
60. Ferguson LR. Nutrigenomics approaches to functional foods. *J Am Diet Assoc.* 2009;109:452–458.
61. Plagemann A, Harder T, Brunn M, et al. Hypothalamic proopiomelanocortin promoter methylation becomes altered by early overfeeding: an epigenetic model of obesity and the metabolic syndrome. *J Physiol.* 2009;587:4963–4976.
62. Jang SH, Lim JW, Kim H. Mechanism of beta-carotene-induced apoptosis of gastric cancer cells: involvement of ataxia-telangiectasia-mutated. *Ann N Y Acad Sci.* 2009;1171:156–162.
63. Kim KC, Friso S, Choi SW. DNA methylation, an epigenetic mechanism connecting folate to healthy embryonic development and aging. *J Nutr Biochem.* 2009; 20:917–926.
64. Acosta PB, Yannicelli S, Ryan AS, et al. Nutritional therapy improves growth and protein status of children with a urea cycle enzyme defect. *Mol Genet Metab.* 2005;86:448–455.
65. Panis B, Vermeer C, van Kroonenburgh MJ, et al. Effect of calcium, vitamins K1 and D3 on bone in galactosemia. *Bone.* 2006;39:1123–1129.
66. Acosta PB, Gross KC. Hidden sources of galactose in the environment. *Eur J Pediatr.* 1995;154:S87–S92.
67. Spiekerkoetter U, Lindner M, Santer R, et al. Treatment recommendations in long-chain fatty acid oxidation defects: consensus from a workshop. *J Inherit Metab Dis.* 2009;32:498–505.

CHAPTER 10

Developmental Disabilities

Harriet H. Cloud

The nutritional needs of children with developmental disabilities vary and primarily involve energy, growth, regulation of the biochemical processes, and repair of cells and body tissue. Nutritional risk factors often include growth deficiency, obesity, gastrointestinal disorders, metabolic problems, feeding problems, and drug–nutrient interactions.[1]

A developmental disability is defined as a severe chronic disability of a person that is attributable to a mental or physical impairment or combination of mental and physical impairments with the following characteristics:

- Manifests before the person attains age 22
- Likely to continue indefinitely
- Results in substantial functional limitations in three or more areas of life activity (e.g., self-care, learning, mobility, self-sufficiency)
- Reflects the person's need for a combination of special interdisciplinary or generic care, treatments, or other services that are lifelong or of extended duration and are individually planned and coordinated[2]

Children with special healthcare needs are those who have or are at increased risk for a chronic physical, developmental, behavioral, or emotional condition and who require health and related services of a type or amount beyond that required by children generally.[3] The etiology of developmental disabilities includes chromosomal aberrations such as Down syndrome (trisomy 21) and Prader-Willi syndrome; neurologic insults in the prenatal period; prematurity; infectious diseases; trauma; congenital defects, such as cleft lip and palate; neural tube defects, such as spina bifida; and other syndromes.[4]

Nutrition considerations that involve the child with developmental disabilities include assessment of growth and the problems surrounding energy balance, such as failure to thrive, obesity, or slow growth rate in height. Another major consideration includes feeding from the standpoint of oral motor problems, developmental delays of feeding skills, inability to self-feed, behavioral problems, and tube feedings. Other areas of nutritional concern include drug–nutrient interaction, constipation, dental caries, urinary tract infections, and use of alternative therapies. **Table 10-1** includes a list of developmental disorders and their nutrition considerations.[5]

Nutritional Considerations

Energy needs for children with developmental disabilities vary as they do for normal children. A decreased energy need is most apparent in chromosomal aberrations such as Down syndrome; conditions accompanied by limited gross motor activity, such as in spina bifida; and syndromes characterized by low muscle tone, such as in Prader-Willi syndrome. Energy needs of infants and children with other developmental disabilities, such as cerebral palsy and Rett syndrome, are highly individualized and vary widely. See Appendix F for equations to calculate energy needs.

Children with Down syndrome, Prader-Willi syndrome, or spina bifida have a slower growth rate and lower basal energy needs and muscle tone, leading to diminished motor activity when compared to the normal child.[6] Children with these types of developmental disabilities tend to become overweight and obese when fed according to normal standards. Monitoring the growth of these children is essential to prevent excessive weight gain or becoming overweight. Children with cerebral palsy (CP) often tend to be seriously underweight for height.[7] Growth failure and an abnormal pattern of REE are related to inadequate energy intake.[8,9]

Commonly used methods for determining the energy needs of this population include use of a nomogram for calculating body surface area and standards based on kcal/m^2/hour (see Appendix E).[9] This method can be used for males and females who are 6 years of age and older. The DRIs are generally not appropriate to use in determining the energy levels of children with developmental disabilities. It is important for the dietitian and physician to evaluate the child's nutritional needs individually.

TABLE 10-1 Developmental Disorders and Corresponding Nutrition Considerations

Syndrome or Developmental Disability	Nutrition Diagnostic Terms	Indicators of this Nutrition Diagnosis
Autism spectrum disorders (ASD) Characterized by delayed speech and language development, ritualistic or repetitive behaviors, and impairments in social interactions.	Inadequate energy intake	Limited or restricted food choices
	Excessive energy intake	High intake of food (kcal) due to food obsessions or use of food by behavioral interventions
	Food-medication interactions	Potential interactions between food and a variety of medications used for individuals with ASD
	Underweight	Inadequate energy intake Body mass index (BMI) <5th percentile for children 2–19 y Refusal to eat Restricted or limited food choices that result in low energy intake
	Overweight	BMI >85th percentile for children 2–19 y Excessive energy intake Infrequent, low duration, and/or low intensity physical activity Large amounts of sedentary activities Limited food choices that result in excessive energy intake
	Harmful beliefs/attitudes about food	Eating behavior serves a purpose other than nourishment Pica Food fetish
	Undesirable food choices	Intake that reflects an imbalance of nutrients/food groups Avoidance of foods/food groups Complementary and alternative medicine treatments, often nutrition-based (vitamin B_6 supplements, gluten-free casein-free diet) may place child at risk for nutrient deficiencies Intake inconsistent with Dietary Reference Intakes, US Dietary Guidelines, MyPyramid, or other methods of measuring diet quality Inability, unwillingness, or disinterest in selecting food consistent with the guidelines Condition associated with diagnosis, ASD–food selectivity, rigid eating patterns
Cerebral palsy A disorder of muscle control or coordination resulting from an injury to the brain during early fetal, perinatal, and early childhood development. There may be associated problems with intellectual, visual or other system functions.	Increased energy expenditure	Unintentional weight loss Evidence of need for accelerated or catch-up growth or weight gain; absence of normal growth Condition associated with a diagnosis (eg. cerebral palsy)
	Inadequate energy intake	Failure to gain or maintain appropriate weight Insufficient energy intake from diet compared to needs Inability to independently consume foods/fluids
	Excessive energy intake	Increased body adiposity Weight gain greater than expected Enteral nutrition more than measured/estimated energy expenditure
	Swallowing difficulty	Abnormal swallow study Prolonged feeding time

		Coughing, choking, prolonged chewing, pouching of food, regurgitation, facial expression changes during eating Decreased food intake Avoidance of food Mealtime resistance
	Altered gastrointestinal (GI) function	Constipation Condition associated with diagnoses: internal muscle tone in cerebral palsy can be affected as well as more visible external muscle tone
	Food-medication interactions	Seizure medications: food and medication interactions
	Underweight	Inadequate energy intake BMI <5th percentile for children 2–19 years Decreased muscle mass, muscle wasting Inadequate intake of food compared to estimated or measured needs
	Overweight	History of physical disability or malnutrition BMI >85th percentile for children 2–19 years Excessive energy intake Infrequent, low duration and/or low-intensity physical activity Large amounts of sedentary activities
Cystic fibrosis An inherited disorder of the exocrine glands, primarily the pancreas, pulmonary system, and sweat glands, characterized by abnormally thick luminal secretions.	Increased energy expenditure	Unintentional weight loss Evidence of need for accelerated or catch-up growth or weight gain; absence of normal growth Condition associated with a diagnosis (eg. cystic fibrosis)
	Altered gastrointestinal function	Abnormal digestive enzyme and fecal fat studies Malabsorption Steatorrhea
	Impaired nutrient utilization	Abnormal digestive enzyme and fecal fat studies Growth stunting or failure Evidence of vitamin and/or mineral deficiency Steatorrhea Condition associated with diagnoses: cystic fibrosis
Down syndrome A genetic disorder that results from an extra no. 21 chromosome, causing developmental problems such as congenital heart disease, mental retardation, short stature, and decreased muscle tone	Excessive energy intake	Increased body adiposity Energy intake higher than estimated need Reduced energy needs related to short stature, low muscle tone
	Breastfeeding difficulty	Poor sucking ability as an infant (due to low tone) Poor weight gain
	Altered GI function	Constipation (related to low muscle tone, low activity, and/or low fiber intake) Celiac disease (higher incidence in Down syndrome)

(continues)

TABLE 10-1 *(Continued)*

Syndrome or Developmental Disability	Nutrition Diagnostic Terms	Indicators of this Nutrition Diagnosis
Prader-Willi syndrome (PWS) A genetic disorder marked by poor feeding skills in infancy, hypotonia, short stature, hyperphagia, and cognitive impairment. When not carefully managed, hyperphagia leads to obesity. May be treated with growth hormone.	Excessive energy intake	Increased body adiposity Energy intake higher than estimated need Condition associated with diagnosis (eg. hyperphagia and PWS) Reduced energy needs related to short stature, low muscle tone
	Breastfeeding difficulty	Poor sucking ability as an infant (due to low tone) Poor weight gain
	Harmful beliefs/attitudes about food	Eating behavior serves a purpose other than nourishment Pica Food obsession
	Undesirable food choices	Intake inconsistent with diet quality guidelines Unable to select foods, independently, that are consistent with food quality, kcal controlled guidelines Condition associated with diagnosis, PWS-food hyperphagia, obsession with food
Spina bifida (myeolomeningocele) results from a midline defect of the skin, spinal column and spinal cord. It is characterized by hydrocephalus, lack of muscular control, and mental retardation	Excessive energy intake	Increased body adiposity Energy intake higher than estimated need Reduced energy needs related to altered body composition, short stature
	Swallowing difficulty	Abnormal swallow study Noisy wet upper airway sounds Condition associated with diagnosis of Arnold Chiari malformation of the brain
	Altered gastrointestinal function	Constipation Condition associated with diagnosis: neurogenic bowel

Source: Van Riper C, Wallace L. Position of the American Dietetic Association: providing nutrition services for people with developmental disabilities and special health care needs. *J Am Diet Assoc.* 2010;110:296–307.

Careful monitoring of protein intake is essential in the child with developmental disabilities. It is recommended that 15–20% of total calories come from proteins, which may be difficult for a child with an oral motor feeding problem such as in CP. These children often suffer from serious malnutrition manifested by little or no weight gain and limited growth in height.

At least 50% of calories should come from carbohydrates, with no more than 10% coming from sucrose. Children with developmental disabilities often have a high percentage of their carbohydrate calories coming from foods highly concentrated in sucrose, such as candy, and carbonated beverages. Dietary counseling and education on better food choices is frequently needed.

Fats should provide 30–35% of the total caloric intake, increasing palatability and satiety, as well as providing a supply of essential fatty acids. For the child who tends to be overweight or obese, fat intake should be carefully evaluated and controlled. For the underweight child, fat can provide an important source of supplemental calories. Infant formulas containing a higher percentage of the fatty acids arachidonic acid (ARA) and docosahexanoeic acid (DHA) should be used for the infant with special needs when the infant is not breastfed.[10]

In general, children with developmental disabilities do not have higher than normal vitamin and mineral needs. However, children on anticonvulsant medications (such as phenobarbital, Dilantin, Depakote, and Topamax) may experience poor absorption of both vitamins and minerals.[11–13]

Diminished bone density and a propensity to fracture with minimal trauma are common in children and adolescents with moderate to severe cerebral palsy. Many children with CP have osteopenia correlated with medication, feeding problems, and lower triceps skinfold measures.[14]

All adolescents of childbearing age should consume extra 400 mcg of folate daily.[15] A concern related to children with spina bifida has been their allergic reaction to latex brought about by multiple surgeries.[16] For those children affected, it has been recommended that they avoid certain foods:

- Bananas
- Water chestnuts
- Kiwi
- Avocados

Mild reactions can occur from apples, carrots, celery, tomatoes, papaya, and melons.[16]

A special concern regarding adequacy of vitamin and mineral intake is the effect of certain medications commonly prescribed to developmentally disabled children on utilization of certain vitamins and minerals. Among these medications are antibiotics, anticonvulsants, antihypertensives, cathartics, corticosteroids, stimulants, sulfonamides, and tranquilizers. (See **Table 10-2** for more information on drug–nutrient interactions.) Their nutritional effects can include nausea and vomiting, gastric distress, constipation, and interfere with the absorption of vitamins and minerals. In some cases, vitamin and mineral supplements are recommended.[17]

Nutrition Assessment

Assessment of the child with developmental disabilities includes all components of nutrition assessment for normal children (as addressed in Chapter 3), plus the inclusion of an evaluation of feeding skills and development. Taking anthropometric measurements of children who are unable to stand and who have gross motor handicaps will require some ingenuity. Weights may be difficult to obtain on standing calibrated balance beam scales for the child with spina bifida or CP. Chair and bucket scales are available for use, and bed scales are indicated for the severely affected. Recumbent boards can be constructed or commercially obtained. Alternate measures for height measurements include arm span, knee-to-ankle height, or sitting height.[18]

Standards for comparison of weight, height, and head circumference are found on the CDC growth charts (see Appendix B).[19] Because these standards were developed using a normal population, the child with developmental disabilities may plot as short, especially when length or height for age is considered. This is particularly true for children with chromosomal aberrations such as Down syndrome[20] or those with a neural tube defect such as spina bifida. Growth charts have been developed for children with a number of disabilities (see **Table 10-3**), but for the most part the CDC charts should be used.

Weight-for-age, interpreted for the developmentally disabled, is also an important indicator of nutritional status and requires comparison with height-for-age. Again, it is the child with Down syndrome, spina bifida, CP, Cornelia De Lange syndrome, Prader-Willi, or chromosomal aberrations in general whose height/weight relationship should be carefully monitored. Early identification of inappropriate relationships is critical so nutrition counseling can be given. The CDC BMI charts for age can be very helpful for the child with developmental disabilities. However, it may not always identify overweight in children who are overfat because of decreased muscle mass. Growth velocity is also important because this information assists the dietitian in evaluating changes in rate of growth over a specified period of time. Incremental growth curves are available for plotting growth velocity.[21] Skinfold thickness is a useful measurement for estimating body fat and is recommended along with arm circumference.[22]

Biochemical measures for the child with developmental disabilities should include the following:

- Hemoglobin and hematocrit levels
- Complete blood count
- Urinalysis
- Semi-quantitative amino acid screening

TABLE 10-2 Drug-Nutrient Interaction

Generic Name	Brand Name	Drug-Nutrient Interaction
Cardiovascular Disease		
Digoxin	Lanoxin	Anorexia Nausea
Furosemide	Lasix	Hyponatremia Hypokalemia Hypomagnesemia Calcium loss
Respiratory Disease		
Prednisone	Deltisone Orasone Liquid Prednisone	Weight gain due to drug-induced appetite increase or edema Stunting of growth in children Hyperglycemia
Trimethaprim	Bactrim	Can cause folate depletion Sulfa in the product can cause anemia
Amoxicillin	Amoxil	Absorption provided by increased fluids
Gastrointestinal Disease		
Ranitidine	Zantac	May cause nausea/diarrhea Constipation
Metoclopramide	Reglan	Nausea and diarrhea
Seizure Disorders		
Carbamazepine	Tegretol	Unpleasant taste Anorexia Sore mouth
Phenobarbital	Phenobarbital	Can induce folate deficiency vitamin D deficiency vitamin K deficiency High intake of folic acid (> 5 mg per day) can interfere with seizure control Folate depletion can lead to megaloblastic anemia
Phenytoin	Dilantin	Same as phenobarbital
Primidone	Mysoline	Folate depletion leading to megaloblastic anemia
Valproic Acid	Depakene and Depakote	Carnitine deficiency Coagulating defects may occur with risk of bleeding and anemia
Hyperactivity		
Methylphenidate	Ritalin	Anorexia when given before a meal

Source: Pronsky ZM, Redfern CM, Crowe J, Epstein J, Young V. *Food Medication Interactions*, 13th ed. Birchrunville, PA: Food-Medication Interactions; 2007.

Other tests may be indicated for children on an anticonvulsant medication who may have low serum levels of folic acid, carnitine, ascorbic acid, calcium, vitamin D, alkaline phosphatase, phosphorus, and pyridoxine. A glucose tolerance test is recommended for individuals with Prader-Willi syndrome.[23] For children with Down syndrome, after an initial screening, thyroid levels should be checked annually.

The methods used to obtain dietary information about a child with developmental disabilities are the same as those used with a normal child, such as a 3-day food diary. In addition to dietary information, an assessment of feeding skills and identification of feeding problems that influence the child's food intake is indicated. This part of the evaluation may include members of the healthcare team such as the physical therapist, occupational therapist, dentist, and psychologist. Observation of an actual feeding session is often very helpful. The feeding evaluation should also include assessment of the following:

- Oral mechanism
- Neuromuscular development
- Head and trunk control

TABLE 10-3 List of Some Special Growth Charts

Condition	Reference(s)	Printed Copies Available
Achondroplasia	Horton WA, Rotter JI, Rimoin DL, Scott CI, Hall JG. Standard growth curves for achondroplasia. *J Pediatr.* 1978;93(3):435–438.	Cedars-Sinai Medical Center Birth Defects Center 444 S. San Vincente Blvd., Los Angeles, CA 90048 (213) 855-2211 Camera-ready copies
Brachmann-(Cornelia) de Lange syndrome	Kline AD, Stanley C, Belevich J, Brodsky K, Barr M, Jackson LG. Developmental data on individuals with the Brachmann-de Lange syndrome. *Am J Med Genet.* 1993;47(7):1053–1058.	
Cerebral palsy (quadriplegia)	Krick J, Murphy-Miller P, Zeger S, Wright E. Pattern of growth in children with cerebral palsy. *J Am Diet Assoc.* 1996:96:680–685.	Kennedy Krieger Institute 707 N. Broadway, Baltimore, MD 21205 www.kennedykrieger.org
Down syndrome	Cronk CE. Growth of children with Down's syndrome: birth to age 3 years. *Pediatrics.* 1978;61(4):564–568.	
Marfan syndrome	Pyeritz RE. Marfan Syndrome and Related Disorders. In Emery AH, Rimoirn LD (eds). *Principles and Practice of Medical Genetics.* New York: Churchill Livingstone; 1983:3579–3624. Pyeritz RE, Murphy EA, Lin SJ, Rosell EM. Growth and anthropometrics in the Marfan syndrome. *Prog Clin Biol Res.* 1985;200:355–366.	Camera-ready copies in article
Myelomeningocele	Ekvall S (ed). *Ped Nutrition in Chronic Disease and Developmental Disorders: Prevention, Assessment and Treatment.* New York: Oxford Press; 1993: Appendix 2.	
Noonan syndrome	Witt DR, Keena BA, Hall JG, Allanson JE. Growth curves for height in Noonan syndrome. *Clin Genet.* 1986; 30(3).150–153.	Camera-ready copies in article
Prader-Willi syndrome	Greenswag L, Alexander R. *Management of Prader-Willi Syndrome*, 2nd ed. New York: Springer-Verlag; 1995: Appendix B growth chart.	
Sickle cell disease	Phebus CK, Gloninger MF, Maciak BJ. Growth patterns by age and sex in children with sickle cell disease. *J Pediatr.* 1984;105:28–33. Tanner JM, Davies PS. Clinical longitudinal standards for height and height velocity for North American children. *J Pediatr.* 1985;107:317–329.	

- Eye-hand coordination
- Position for feeding
- Social-behavioral components

Children with developmental disabilities frequently have oral motor feeding and positioning problems and tend to be very easily distracted.[24]

Once the nutritional problems have been identified for the child with developmental disabilities, various types of intervention programs can be implemented. All approaches should be family-centered, community-based, comprehensive, and culturally competent. Intervention should include all aspects of a child's treatment program.[25,26]

Nutritional Problems

Many infants and children with developmental disabilities develop other problems, such as obesity, failure to thrive, constipation, and dental diseases.

Obesity

Weight management of the child with developmental disabilities is indicated for any child who tends to plot higher than the 75th percentile for BMI. Conditions that predispose a child to obesity are low muscle tone, limited physical activity, isolation, lack of knowledge about food, and slow growth in height, all of which are found in children with Down syndrome, Prader-Willi syndrome, spina bifida, Turner's syndrome, myelomeningocele, and CP.

Prevention is the best way to avoid obesity. Counseling in appropriate feeding practices, increasing physical activity, and frequent monitoring of height and weight are essential. Successful programs for the obese individual should be individually planned with a written meal plan. Dietary modification of the school meal can be ordered by the physician or a registered dietitian and may address calories, protein, carbohydrates, and allergy/food intolerances. Childhood weight management must be carefully planned in order to avoid poor growth or nutritional deficiencies. In the school setting, it should become a part of the Individualized Education Plan (IEP). Dietary records maintained by the parent and others caring for the child are useful for monitoring intake. The diet plan for the older developmentally disabled child who is also mentally delayed must be presented in a way the child can understand.

Lack of exercise often is common in the child or adolescent with developmental disabilities. The availability of exercise programs for such children varies with the school system, as does the availability of general community-based programs of exercise. Special Olympics events exist in most states and are associated with school sports in which the child with developmental disabilities can participate and compete.

Behavioral considerations are also an important aspect of weight management programs for the child with developmental disabilities. Important behavioral assessments to make include:

- Speed of eating
- Meal frequency
- Length of time spent eating
- Where meals are eaten

Frequently used behavior strategies include establishing a reward system for compliance with diet, increasing exercise, and targeting eating behaviors to change.

Intervention for obesity for the child with Prader-Willi syndrome requires special involvement of both the family and healthcare providers.[27] Total environmental control of food access plus a low-calorie diet combined with consistent behavior management techniques and physical exercise are necessary. Environmental control may include locking the refrigerator, cupboards, and kitchen. Individuals with Prader-Willi syndrome often hide and hoard food and exhibit emotional outbursts when food is withheld. Physical exercise is challenging due to the hypotonia that is characteristic of the syndrome, a poor sense of balance, and reluctance to exercise. The child tires easily and often has limited gross motor skills.

The energy needs of the child with Prader-Willi syndrome are 37–77% of normal for weight maintenance. Weight loss occurs at 8 to 9 calories per centimeter of height, and maintenance of appropriate weight can be accomplished at 10 to 11 calories per centimeter of height.[27] Several hypocaloric regimens have been used with variable success. The use of a modified diabetic exchange list has been successful along with a balanced low-calorie diet, a ketogenic diet, and a protein-sparing modified fast.[23]

Increasing physical activity and exercise are important strategies with a daily exercise routine. Adaptive physical education programs in the school should be used with the school-age child with Prader-Willi. The use of growth hormone therapy may be used to increase stature.[28] Advances in the early diagnosis of infants with Prader-Willi syndrome is an important factor in beginning an early intervention program that includes working with failure to thrive followed by hyperphagia and weight management concerns.

Failure to Thrive

Failure to thrive, defined as inadequate weight gain for height, is frequently found in the child with developmental disabilities. It may result from the following:

- Impaired oral motor function and resultant feeding problems
- Excessive energy needs, such as occur in CP
- Gastrointestinal problems, such as reflux and diarrhea
- Infections and frequent illnesses
- Medications that may affect appetite
- Pica consumption leading to lead intoxication or parasites such as giardia
- Parental/caretaker inadequacy related to feeding

Nutrition intervention must begin with a careful assessment, including a feeding evaluation with observation of parent/caregiver–child interaction. Some children with developmental disabilities and failure to thrive require medical evaluations to determine the existence of gastroesophageal reflux and aspiration requiring a tube feeding or total parenteral nutrition on a temporary basis following a surgical procedure for a gastrointestinal disorder. Usually this will be followed with a return to oral feeding (see Chapters 19 and 20).

Constipation

Constipation often afflicts children with developmental disabilities due to lack of activity, generalized hypotonia, or limited bowel muscle function. It also can result from insufficient fluid intake, lack of fiber in the diet, frequent vomiting, and medications. Laxatives and enemas should not be used, because they can lead to dependency. Mineral oil decreases the absorption of the fat-soluble vitamins A, D, E, and K.

Nutrition management may include adjusting the diet to increase fiber and fluid content. General recommendations include the following:

- Maintain adequate fluid intake, exceeding the daily requirement for age, including water and diluted fruit juice.
- Increase fiber content of the diet by replacing white bread and canned fruits with whole-grain breads and cereals, fresh fruits and vegetables, and cereals fortified with 1 to 2 tablespoons of unprocessed bran. Fiber supplements, such as Benefiber, can be added to beverages or soft food. These supplements can generally be used from the age of 6 years on.
- Use yogurt containing pre- and probiotics to improve the intestinal function.
- Increase daily exercise.

Feeding Problems

Feeding problems are defined as the inability or refusal to eat certain foods because of neuromotor dysfunction, obstructive lesions, or psychosocial factors. Most of these problems are due to oral motor difficulties (see **Table 10-4**) caused by neuromotor dysfunction, developmental delays, positioning problems, a poor mother–child relationship, or sensory defensiveness.[24] These problems may contribute to such behavioral problems as a refusal to eat and mealtime tantrums.

Intervention for feeding problems lends itself best to a multidisciplinary team approach.[24] Nutritional intervention may involve increasing calories, altering the texture of foods offered, and determining tube-feeding formulas. Additional nutrition education and counseling, oral motor therapy, and behavior management counseling are part of the feeding plan. A modified barium swallow may be useful in children with oral motor feeding problems to detect the possibility of aspiration. This will allow the team to determine the necessity of thickening liquids. Nectar and honey thickened foods and beverages can help improve food intake of infants and children with oral motor problems.

Dental Issues

Dental caries and gum disease are prevalent in children and adolescents who are developmentally disabled. Prevention includes home care, professional treatment, and nutritional intervention. Nutritional intervention involves decreasing dietary sucrose intake, as discussed in Chapter 5 in the section on dental caries. Supplying adequate fluoride in the drinking water is helpful in the prevention of caries, as is the topical application of fluoride.

Gingival disease is often found where dental hygiene is poor. Children taking Dilantin for seizures may suffer

TABLE 10-4 Oral Motor Problems and Affect on Food Intake

Problem	Description	
Tonic bite reflex	Strong jaw closure when teeth and gums are stimulated	Interferes with actual intake of food
Tongue thrust	Forceful and often repetitive protrusion of an often bunched or thick tongue in response to oral stimulation	Parent or care taker may misinterpret as child's dislike of food
Jaw thrust	Forceful opening of the jaw to the maximal extent during eating, drinking, attempts to speak, or general excitement	Interferes with acceptance of food and swallowing
Tongue retraction	Pulling back the tongue within the oral cavity at the presentation of food, spoon, or cup	Makes swallowing and chewing difficult along with cup drinking
Lip retraction	Pulling back the lips in a very tight, smile-like pattern at the approach of the spoon or cup toward the face	Makes food intake difficult and requires facilitation to relax the lips
Sensory defensiveness	A strong adverse reaction to sensory input (touch, sound, light)	Can lead to refusal to accept a variety of foods due to oral sensitivity

Source: Cloud HH. *Feeding Is a Priority for the Dietetic Professional.* Birmingham, AL: Nutrition Matters; 2009. Available at: http://www.nutritionmatters.us. Accessed July 27, 2011.

gingival hyperplasia, a side effect of the drug. Nutrition counseling to increase intake of raw fruits and vegetables and improve snacking practices, coupled with good dental hygiene instructions and regular dental care, are important components of dental intervention. Late weaning from the bottle and extended use of the "sippy" cup filled with juice, tea, or other sweetened beverages as well as permitting a child to drink constantly from this cup can contribute to dental caries.

Seizures

The ketogenic diet is used in the treatment of epileptic seizures nonresponsive to anticonvulsants.[29] Traditionally, the diet is recommended for children younger than age 5 with myoclonic, absence, and atonic seizures that are medically nonresponsive. This diet is high in fat and very low in protein and carbohydrates and is designed to increase the body's reliance on fatty acids rather than glucose for energy. The classic fat-to-carbohydrate ratio is 4:1. It is thought that the ketosis produced by the high fat to low carbohydrate ratio decreases the number and severity of the seizures. Typically, the diet provides 1 gram of protein per kilogram of body weight, although protein can be increased if linear growth slows unacceptably.[29] The diet is usually high in saturated fat; however, corn oil and MCT oil can be used instead.[29]

The child younger than 18 months of age, older than 12 years, or obese may be started on a 3:1 ratio. Other variants of the ketogenic diet include the MCT diet originated in 1970;[30] the modified Atkins diet; and the low glycemic index treatment, which stabilizes blood glucose and allows more carbohydrate than the classic ketogenic diet. Infants and children fed by either bottle or tube can be given the ketogenic diet as a liquid feeding. Products such as Ketocal, KetoVolve, and Ketonia also are available.

Daily carbohydrate-free vitamin and mineral supplements are required because the diet is low in calcium, magnesium, iron, vitamin C, and other water-soluble vitamins and minerals. The expense of the diet, compliance problems, and lack of palatability have made its use controversial. Concerns also have been raised related to growth.

Close monitoring and frequent follow-up visits are needed. Laboratory studies are required at regularly scheduled clinic visits and include urinalysis, electrolytes, transaminates, bilirubin, glucose, serum calcium, lipid profile, and prealbumin. The diet may be discontinued for children who are seizure-free for 2 years.

Autism, Attention Deficit Disorder, and Attention Deficit Hyperactivity Disorder

There is an increased incidence in the frequency of children with these disorders that affects their nutritional status. Autism is one of five disorders under the category pervasive developmental disorders (PDD) and has grown in incidence since 1980. All types of PDD are neurologic disorders that are usually evident by age 3. In general, children who have one of the types of PDD have difficulty in talking, playing with other children, and relating to others, including their family. The five types of PDD are:

- Autistic disorder
- Rett's disorder
- Childhood disintegrative disorder
- Asperger's syndrome
- Pervasive developmental disorder not otherwise specified

PDDs are four times more common in boys, with the exception of Rett's disorder, which is more commonly found in girls.

Autistic disorders or autism spectrum disorders (ASD) affect 3.4 per 1000 children per year.[31] Children with autistic disorder also have mental retardation. The term *Asperger's syndrome* is most often used to describe children with the problems of ASD but who have normal to high cognitive levels.[31]

Nutrition and eating problems may affect up to three-quarters of children with ASD. Some of these problems include routine intake and refusal to try new foods; short attention span; increased sensitivity to food textures, color, taste, or temperature; food obsessions or ritual; eating nonfood items; compulsive eating or drinking; packing the mouth with food; vomiting; and gag reflex. GI problems include constipation, diarrhea, reflux, vomiting, bloating, pain, and feeding problems.

Attention deficit hyperactivity disorder (ADHD) or ADD is a neurobehavioral problem being seen with increasing frequency in children. It has been associated with learning disorders, inappropriate degrees of impulsiveness, hyperactivity, and attention deficit. Causes of ADHD are unclear. The three subtypes of ADHD developed by the American Psychiatric Association are:

1. Combined type of hyperactivity and attention deficit
2. Predominately inattentive type
3. Predominately hyperactive-impulse behavior[32]

Many of these children are on medications that may affect their weight and growth in height. Medications used to treat these disorders often cause anorexia, so the child's nutrition assessment and follow-up should include anthropometric measures. If the child is on medications, the time of administration is important, generally after eating.

Many dietary treatments have been proposed, such as the Feingold diet; eliminating sugar and caffeine; and the addition of large doses of vitamins. The most effective treatment for the child with ADHD or ADD is a diet based on the Dietary Guidelines or the Food Guide Pyramid with mealtime structure, a distraction-free environment, and no "grazing" on food or liquids throughout the day.

Resources

Several federal programs provide financial coverage for nutrition services for children with developmental disabilities and special healthcare needs. Title V of the Social Security Act includes children with special healthcare needs. Title XIX of the Social Security Act funds Medicaid, which may be used to purchase tube feeding formulas, dietary supplements, eating devices, and formulas for inherited disorders of metabolism. Other programs such as Head Start include children with special needs.[33]

Programs such as the Supplemental Program for Women, Infants and Children (WIC) will provide formulas and food for children from low income families. Children with special needs and developmental disabilities of school age are eligible for meal modification under Section 504 of the Rehabilitation Act of 1973 and the Americans with Disabilities Act of 1990.

Other legislation that provides funding for children with developmental disabilities and funding of nutrition services includes the Child Health Act of 2000 and State Children's Health Insurance Programs. All of these programs are possible resources although many vary from state to state.

Case Study

Nutrition Assessment of Child with Down Syndrome and Obesity

Patient history: A 14-year-old girl with Down syndrome was admitted to a mental health services facility for treatment of sleep apnea, prediabetes, and severe behavioral activities. The contributing factor to the medical problems was her severe obesity. Prior to her admission to the facility she had been in public school in their special education programs, but her behavior was so difficult to control that the school transferred her to the mental health facility. She is the only individual in her family with Down syndrome and was born when her mother was 40. There is a history of diabetes in the family, and food has always been used as a reward for this girl.

Food/nutrition-related history: This child's birth weight was 7 lb., 8 oz, birth length was 19″, and the pregnancy was full term. She was breastfed until 3 months of age, when she was transferred to Similac and reportedly had no feeding problems other than consuming over 36 oz. of milk daily and eating baby food in unusual amounts. Her weaning to a cup was late, at 18 months, and her motor skill development was late with an inability to walk until 28 months of age. She also had low muscle tone.

By the time she was 12 months of age her weight was 28 lbs., placing her above the 95th percentile, and each subsequent year she remained between the 75th and 95th percentile for her weight, but at the 10th percentile for her height. During her preschool and school years the child's intake was reported as very limited in variety with a heavy concentration of foods from fast food restaurants and little intake of fruits and vegetables. She drank milk but preferred soft drinks and sweetened tea. She also consumed many sweetened desserts, cookies, and bakery products. Although her mother reported trying to control this behavior, a grandparent was very indulgent. She also developed behavioral problems with a great deal of acting out behavior both at home and at school. It was this behavior that led to her referral to the mental health facility.

Anthropometric Measures

Weight: 247 pounds, >97th percentile

Height: 56″, 50th–75th percentile

H/W relationship: >97th percentile

BMI: >97%

Estimated protein needs: 1716 kcal

Estimated energy intake at home: 3000 kcal (based on maternal report)

Estimated protein needs: 52 g

Biochemical Data

Hgb: 14 mg

Hct: 36 mg

Cholesterol: 210

Glucose: 120 mg

Medications: Topomax, Clonidine for seizures and behavioral problems

Diet order following physical examination: 1500 calories plus exercise

Nutrition-Focused Physical Findings

1. Excessive appetite
2. Dry skin
3. Inactivity with behavioral outbursts related to walking
4. Feeding problems—very rapid eating with possibility of choking
5. Low muscle tone
6. Constipation

Nutrition Diagnoses

Obesity: Excessive intake of carbohydrates: Inadequate fluid intake due to refusal to eat raw fruits, vegetable and whole grains:

Intervention Goals

1. Weight loss and acceptance of difference in food provided.
2. Increase consumption of high-fiber foods.
3. Limit midmeal snacks to fruit and vegetables.
4. Counsel parents related to meal management and poor behavior related to food.
5. Increase physical activity at school and home.

Nutrition Intervention

1. Modify the menus to provide 1500 calories, including snacks.
2. Provide copies of menu to group home staff and parents.
3. Increase availability of fresh fruit and raw vegetables for snacks.
4. Increase water intake.

Monitoring and Evaluation

1. Weigh monthly and plot continuously with report to parents.
2. Counsel parents monthly or as necessary related to food intake and exercise at home.
3. Walking at school with teachers and other students.

Questions for the Reader

1. Teachers report that the child eats only part of the meal provided and refuses the snacks offered. What would be your response?
2. The parents report in their monthly conference that the child is very rebellious and refuses to participate in the family activities unless provided with a trip to a fast food restaurant for hamburgers and French fries. What could you suggest?
3. Monthly weights show a loss of 2–3 pounds each month. Should there be a reward system followed by motivational interviewing?

REFERENCES

1. Centers for Disease Control and Prevention. Developmental disabilities. Available at: http://www.cdc.gov/ncbddd/dd/default.htm. Accessed August 9, 2011.
2. *Developmental Disabilities Assistance and Bill of Rights Act*, Public Law 106-402; 2000.
3. McPherson M, Arango P, Fox H, et al. A new definition of children with special health care needs. *Pediatrics.* 1998;102:137–140.
4. Cloud HH. Update on nutrition for the children with special needs. *Top Clin Nutr.* 1997;13(1):21–32.
5. Van Riper C, Wallace L. Position of the American Dietetic Association: providing nutrition services for people with developmental disabilities and special health care needs. *J Am Diet Assoc.* 2010;110:296–307.
6. Luke A, Roizen NJ, Sutton M, Schoeller DA. Energy expenditure in children with Down syndrome: correcting metabolic rate for movement. *J Pediatr.* 1994;125:829–838.
7. Sullivan PB, Juszczak E, Lambert BR, et al. Impact of feeding problems on nutritional intake and growth: Oxford Feeding Study II. *Dev Med Child Neurol.* 2002;44(7):461–467.
8. Stallings VA, Cronk CE, Zemme BS, Charney EB. Body composition in children with spastic quadriplegic cerebral palsy. *J Pediatr.* 1995;126(5):833–839.
9. Stallings VA, Zemel BS, Davies JC, et al. Energy expenditure of children and adolescents with severe disabilities: a cerebral palsy model. *Am J Clin Nutr.* 1996;64(4):627–634.
10. Holland M, Murray P. Diet and nutrition. In: Lucas BL (ed). *Children with Special Health Care Needs: Nutrition Care Handbook.* Chicago, IL: American Dietetic Association; 2004:5–22.
11. Bennett FC, McClelland S, Kriegsmann E, et al. Vitamin and mineral supplementation in Down's syndrome. *Pediatrics.* 1983;72:707–713.
12. Bidder RT, Gray P, Newcombe RG, et al. The effects of multivitamins and minerals on children with Down syndrome. *Dev Med Child Neurol.* 1989;31:532–537.
13. Pueschel SM. General health care and therapeutic approaches. In: Pueschel SM, Pueschel JK (eds). *Biomedical Concerns in Persons with Down Syndrome.* Baltimore, MD: Brookes Publishing; 1992:273–287.
14. Henderson RC, Kairalla JA, Barrington JW, et al. Longitudinal changes in bone density in children and adolescents with moderate to severe cerebral palsy. *J Pediatr.* 2005;146:769–775.
15. Green NS. Folic acid supplementation and prevention of birth defects. *J Nutr.* 2002;132(8 Suppl):2356S–2360S.
16. Pittman T. Latex allergy in children with spina bifida. *Ped Neurosurg.* 1995;22(2):96–100.
17. Pronsky ZM, Redfern CM, Crowe J, et al. *Food Medication Interactions,* 13th ed. Birchrunville, PA: Food-Medication Interactions; 2007.
18. Chumlea WC, Guo SS, Steinbaugh ML. Prediction of stature from knee height for black and white adults and children with application to mobility-impaired or handicapped persons. *J Am Diet Assoc.* 1994;94(12):1385–1388.
19. National Center for Health Statistics, National Center for Chronic Disease Prevention and Health Promotion. CDC growth charts. 2000. Available at: http://www.cdc.gov/growthcharts. Accessed August 9, 2011.
20. Cronk C, Crocker AC, Pueschel SM, et al. Growth charts for children with Down syndrome: 1 month to 18 years of age. *Pediatrics.* 1988;81:102.
21. Roche AF, Hines JH. Incremental growth charts. *Am J Clin Nutr.* 1980;33:2041–2052.

22. Frisancho AR. New norms of upper limb fat and muscle areas for assessment of nutritional status. *Am J Clin Nutr.* 1981;34:2540–2545.
23. Cassidy SB. Prader-Willi syndrome. *J Med Genetics.* 1997;34(11):917–923.
24. Cloud HH, Ekvall S, Hicks L. Feeding problems of the child with special health care needs. In: Ekvall SW, Ekvall VK (eds). *Pediatric Nutrition in Chronic Diseases and Developmental Disorders,* 2nd ed. New York: Oxford University Press; 2005.
25. American Dietetic Association. Providing nutrition services for infants, children and adults with developmental disabilities and special health care needs. *J Am Diet Assoc.* 2009;104(1):97–106.
26. Terry RD. Needed: a new appreciation of culture and food behavior. *J Am Diet Assoc.* 1994;95(5):501–503.
27. Hoffman CJ, Abeltman D, Pipes P. A nutrition survey of and recommendations for individuals with Prader-Willi who live in group homes. *J Am Diet Assoc.* 1992;92(7):823–830.
28. Hauffa BP. One-year results of growth hormone treatment of short stature in Prader-Willi syndrome. *Acta Paedia.* 1997;423(Suppl):63–65.
29. Kelly MT, Hays TL. Implementing the ketogenic diet. *Top Clin Nutr.* 1997;13(1):53–61.
30. Freeman JM, Vining EP, Pillas DJ, et al. The efficacy of the ketogenic diet—1998: a prospective evaluation of intervention of 150 children. *Pediatrics.* 1998;102:1358–1363.
31. Yeargin-Allsopp M, Rice C, Karapurkar T, et al. Prevalence of autism in a U.S. metropolitan area. *JAMA.* 2003;289:49–55.
32. American Psychiatric Association. *Diagnostic and Statistical Manual of Mental Disorders,* 4th ed. Washington, DC: American Psychiatric Association; 1994.
33. Office of Head Start, Administration for Children and Families, U.S. Department of Health and Human Services. About Head Start. Available at: http://acf.hhs.gov/programs/ohs. Accessed August 9, 2011.

CHAPTER 11

Pulmonary Diseases

Erin Redding and Shannon Despino

Cystic Fibrosis

Cystic fibrosis (CF), a genetic disorder characterized by widespread dysfunction of the exocrine glands, is the most common lethal hereditary disease of the Caucasian race.[1] The disease is characterized by an abnormality in the CF transmembrane conductance regulator (CFTR) protein, causing increased sodium reabsorption and decreased chloride secretion. The result is the production of abnormally thick and viscous mucus, which affects various organs of the body. In the lungs, the thick mucus clogs the airways, causing obstruction, subsequent bacterial infections, and progressive lung disease. In the pancreas, the thick mucus prevents the release of pancreatic enzymes into the small intestine for the digestion of foods. Blockage of ducts eventually causes pancreatic fibrosis and cyst formation. Most CF patients have pancreatic insufficiency (PI),[2] exhibited by gastrointestinal symptoms, including frequent, foul-smelling stools; increased flatus; and abdominal cramping. In some patients, the ducts and tubules of the liver are obstructed by mucus, resulting in liver disease that may progress to cirrhosis.[3] Common complications include CF-related diabetes (CFRD) and bone disease. A unique characteristic of CF is an increased loss of sodium and chloride in the sweat. Sterility in males and decreased fertility in females is also seen.

Pancreatic enzyme therapy, antibiotic therapy, nutrition therapy, and earlier diagnosis all contribute to the improvement in the prognosis for patients with CF. The median age of survival is now about 37 years.[3]

CF is transmitted as an autosomal recessive trait. Both parents are carriers of the defective gene but exhibit no symptoms of the disease themselves. Each offspring of two carriers of the defective gene has a 25% chance of having the disease, a 50% chance of being a carrier of the defective gene, and a 25% chance of neither having the disease nor being a carrier.

The CF gene is on the long arm of chromosome 7.[4] The CF gene product is a protein called the CFTR, which is a cyclic adenosine monophosphate (cAMP)-regulated chloride channel and regulator of secondary chloride and sodium channels normally present in epithelial cells.[5-10] The most common mutation is called DF508, which accounts for the majority of CF alleles among the Caucasian population worldwide.[11] Over 1500 mutations of the CFTR gene have been identified,[12] which accounts for the wide variability of disease symptoms and severity seen in patients with CF. The incidence of CF is 1 in 3500 births each year. CF is most common in Caucasians, but can be diagnosed in all racial and ethnic groups.[3]

Diagnosis

Manifestations of the disease are numerous and vary greatly from patient to patient, due in part to the large numbers of mutations of the defective gene. Pulmonary manifestations of CF include chronic cough and chronic sinusitis. GI manifestations include failure to thrive; steatorrhea; and frequent, foul smelling stools. Any child who repeatedly exhibits any of these symptoms should be tested for CF. In addition, CF should be considered when a child tastes salty when kissed or experiences heat prostration.

The diagnosis of CF should be based on the presence of one or more characteristic features of the disease:[12]

- Evidence of chronic sinopulmonary disease
- Evidence of GI and nutritional abnormalities
- Evidence of salt-loss syndromes
- Evidence of obstructive azoospermia in males
- Family history of the disease
- A positive newborn screening test result plus an elevated sweat chloride test

Sweat chloride is measured by a quantitative pilocarpine iontophoresis sweat test. A sweat chloride concentration greater than 60 mmol/L is indicative of the diagnosis of CF. Patients with an intermediate sweat chloride concentration (30–59 mmol/L for infants younger than 6 months of age and 40–59 mmol/L for individuals older than 6 months of age) should undergo CFTR mutation analysis to rule out CF. The diagnosis can also be made with the identification of CF mutations on both alleles of the CFTR gene, which is sometimes even seen in patients who have a negative sweat test (<39 mmol/L).[12]

Newborn screening for CF is recommended. Earlier diagnosis of CF is linked with improved growth and lung function and increased life expectancy. A positive CF newborn screen does not always mean that the patient has CF, so further medical testing such as a sweat test must be done to confirm the diagnosis. Because all states conduct routine newborn screening for CF, the median age of survival should continue to increase along with an increased quality of life.[12]

CF Management

Rigorous daily management is required to control the symptoms of the disease. Daily chest percussion therapy and postural drainage, along with aerosolized medications, help to clear the airways of mucus, improve existing lung compromise, and retard future deterioration. Antibiotics are used to control pulmonary infections. Pancreatic enzyme replacement therapy is a crucial part of the management of the GI symptoms in patients who exhibit PI. These patients are required to take pancreatic enzymes prior to each meal and snack containing fat, protein, and/or complex carbohydrates. Dosage of pancreatic enzymes is individualized, depending on factors such as the extent of pancreatic involvement, dietary intake, and the weight and age of the patient. Vitamin, mineral, and salt supplementation are also recommended.

Many aspects of CF stress the nutritional status of the patient by affecting the patient's appetite and subsequent intake (see **Table 11-1**). CFRD and liver disease also impact nutritional status. Bile salts and bile acid losses contribute to fat malabsorption. Gastrointestinal losses occur in spite of pancreatic enzyme replacement therapy. Also, the catch-up growth that is often needed after diagnosis requires additional calories. CF patients generally have an increase in resting energy expenditure as compared with non-CF patients.[13–17] Energy requirements for patients with CF range from 110–200% of the calories recommended for healthy individuals of the same age, gender, and size.[18,19] All of these factors can contribute to a chronic energy deficit, which can lead to a marasmic type of malnutrition. The primary goal of nutritional therapy is to overcome this energy deficit and to promote normal growth and development for CF patients in an effort to optimize lung function and increase longevity.

TABLE 11-1 Aspects of Cystic Fibrosis that Affect Nutritional Status

Pulmonary	Gastrointestinal
Increased work of breathing	Malabsorption of fat
Chronic cough	Loss of fat-soluble vitamins
Cough-emesis cycle	Loss of essential fatty acids
Chronic antibiotic therapy	Malabsorption of protein
Fatigue, anxiety	Anorexia
Decreased tolerance for exercise	Gastroesophageal reflux/ esophagitis
Repeated pulmonary infections	Bile salts and bile acid loss Distal intestinal obstructive syndrome (DIOS) Fibrosing colonopathy

Patients with CF often have very poor appetites and early satiety. Table 11-1 delineates some aspects of CF that can contribute to poor appetite and failure to thrive. Psychosocial issues may cause depression, anxiety, fatigue, and anorexia that will also impact appetite and nutritional status. Behavioral issues related to eating and ineffective parenting strategies may play a role in a child's poor appetite and intake as well. Appetite stimulation medications, such as megastrol acetate, as part of therapy for CF may be helpful.[20]

Children with cystic fibrosis should grow and develop like their peers without CF. In addition, adults are expected to maintain a nutrition status similar to healthy individuals of the same age. Age-specific goals for patients with CF are:[18]

- *Infants and toddlers 2 years or younger:* Achieve weight for length at the 50th percentile by 2 years
- *Children and adolescents 2 years old to 20 years old:* Achieve or exceed the 50th percentile for body mass index (BMI) for age and gender
- *Females 20 years or older:* Achieve or exceed a BMI of 22
- *Males 20 years or older:* Achieve or exceed a BMI of 23

Nutritional status is an important prognostic indicator in the outcome of CF.[21] Patients with CF who have weight-for-height less than 90% of predicted may have lower values on pulmonary function tests than those patients with normal weight-for-height.[21] There is an association between growth parameters and lung function. Progressive lung disease is usually what causes the morbidity and mortality of CF, thus nutrition intervention is important to optimize growth and help improve lung function.

Every patient with CF should be assessed by a registered dietitian at least annually. At diagnosis, a nutrition assessment should include the following:

- Head circumference
- Weight
- Length/height
- MAC
- TSH
- Checking of the parents' heights

The CF Foundation has published a consensus report on pediatric nutrition for patients with CF and the *Clinical Practice Guidelines for Cystic Fibrosis,* which includes nutrition management information.[22–24]

Monitoring growth should occur at regular nutrition clinic visits. For infants and children younger than 36 months of age, weight, recumbent length, weight-for-height, and head circumference should be accurately measured and plotted on the CDC growth curves at each clinic visit or hospitalization.[25] For children 2 years of age or older who are measured standing, weight, height, and BMI-for-age should be measured, plotted, and calculated. (See Appendix B for CDC growth charts and Chapter 3 for additional information.) An age-appropriate BMI method should also be used to assess weight and height, instead of the %IBW method of assessment.[26]

Anthropometric measurements, including mid-arm circumference and triceps skinfold thickness, should be obtained according to standard procedures on all patients with CF older than 1 year of age.[22–24,27] From these measurements, mid-arm muscle circumference, mid-arm muscle area (mm^2) and mid-arm fat area (mm^2) should be calculated and compared with gender- and age-specific normative data.[28] They are useful in monitoring the nutrition status of CF patients with liver disease and ascites because weight is not a good indicator of nutrition status.

It is important to determine whether patients with CF are achieving their full genetic height potential. One method is to determine mid-parental height, plot this height on the growth chart at age 20, and then use this percentile as the target for the individual patient. Calculate the target height as follows: Add 13 centimeters to the mother's height if the patient is a boy, or subtract 13 centimeters from the father's height if the patient is a girl. Obtain the average of the two parents' adjusted heights. To calculate the patient's target height range, adjust +/– 10 cm for a boy and +/– 9 cm for a girl.[22,23]

Laboratory monitoring of nutritional status should be done at diagnosis and annually thereafter to include vitamins A, D, E, and K as well as iron and albumin. Other tests, such as EFA, calcium/bone status, zinc, and sodium, may need to be checked.

Undiagnosed infants, particularly those who are breastfed, often present with hypoalbuminemia and subsequent edema. The malabsorption that occurs in undiagnosed CF causes inadequate absorption of protein. The low protein content of breast milk as compared with modified cow's milk formulas may further compromise the infant's protein status. Upon diagnosis of CF and the initiation of pancreatic enzyme therapy, hypoalbuminemia is usually corrected because the infant is no longer malabsorbing protein. A serum albumin level should be measured in newly diagnosed infants. Any time an inadequate protein intake is suspected, it may be beneficial to assess the albumin or prealbumin level. However, it is important to remember that other potential causes of an abnormal albumin value include infection and other factors such as fluid overload.[29] Patients with CF who chronically have inadequate calorie intakes, usually have a marasmic type of malnutrition. Their visceral protein levels are usually normal, whereas somatic protein stores are low.[29]

Hemoglobin and hematocrit should be checked annually. If there is evidence of anemia, further iron studies should be obtained, including serum iron, iron-binding capacity, ferritin, transferrin, and reticulocyte count.[24] A trial of iron therapy will help determine if the anemia is caused by iron deficiency or anemia of chronic disease.

Even patients who are adequately treated with pancreatic enzymes may continue to malabsorb fat, and consequently fat-soluble vitamins, so it is important to check fat-soluble vitamin levels annually.

- Vitamin A levels should not be drawn during an acute illness because vitamin A is a negative acute phase reactant and will be decreased with acute illness and inflammation.[22,23]
- Many CF patients may not be exposed to enough sunlight to meet vitamin D needs. Measuring 25-hydroxyvitamin D and parathyroid hormone (PTH) annually in the late fall is recommended for monitoring bone disease.[22,23]
- Vitamin E levels should be checked annually to avoid a symptomatic deficiency.[22,23]

Long-term antibiotic therapy commonly used in the treatment of CF alters the gut flora. Because an important source of vitamin K is microbiologic synthesis in the gut, vitamin K status is often negatively affected. Thus, serum vitamin K levels should be monitored. Prothrombin time (PT) is an indirect measurement of vitamin K status; PT also may be a useful measure of hepatic synthetic function in patients with nutritional failure or biliary cirrhosis.[22,23]

Patients with CF are also at risk of essential fatty acid (EFA) deficiency. The etiology of EFA deficiency can be multifactorial, including fat malabsorption and abnormal fatty acid oxidation. Some of the clinical manifestations of EFA deficiency include scaly rash, poor growth, and alopecia. EFA deficiency is also correlated with an increased inflammatory response in patients with CF. A minimum of 3–5% of total calories should come from EFAs to prevent an EFA deficiency.[30]

Diabetes Screening

The increased life expectancy of CF patients has lead to an increase in the frequency of glucose intolerance.[31] Many older individuals with CF have some form of glucose intolerance and some have CFRD.[32] CFRD is a distinct clinical entity because it has features of both type 1 and type 2 diabetes.[31,32] Clinical symptoms of CFRD include polydipsia, polyuria, fatigue, unintentional weight loss, and decreased lung function. **Table 11-2** outlines how CFRD is diagnosed.

CFRD can be classified as CFRD with fasting hyperglycemia or CFRD without fasting hyperglycemia. The former is characterized by a fasting blood glucose (FBG) equal to or

TABLE 11-2 Diagnosis of Cystic Fibrosis-Related Diabetes

Test	Time	Blood Glucose Level	Diagnosis	Action
Casual blood glucose	Done at any time regardless of eating	< 100 mg/dL (< 5.6 mmol/L)	CFRD is not likely	Do blood glucose levels every year or earlier if CFRD symptoms occur.
		100–199 mg/dL (5.6–11.0 mmol/L)	Gray zone	Do a fasting blood glucose test or an OGTT.
		≥ 200 mg/dL (≥ 11.1 mmol/L)	CFRD likely	Do a fasting blood glucose test or an OGTT.
Fasting blood glucose	Done in the morning before breakfast	< 100 mg/dL (< 5.6 mmol/L)	Normal	Do blood glucose levels every year or unless CFRD symptoms occur.
		100–125 mg/dL (5.6–6.9 mmol/L)	Impaired fasting glucose	Make sure the level was fasting. If so, an OGTT should be done.
		≥ 126 mg/dL (≥ 7.0 mmol/L)	CFRD with fasting hyperglycemia	Make sure the level was fasting. More testing may be done to confirm CFRD diagnosis unless patient has symptoms. Other tests may be another fasting glucose test or an OGTT. If the patient has CFRD, he or she will learn to manage it with insulin.
OGTT (with normal fasting glucose)	2 hours after glucose load	< 140 mg/dL (< 7.8 mmol/L)	Normal glucose tolerance	Do blood glucose levels every year or earlier if CFRD symptoms occur.
		140–199 mg/dL (7.8–11.0 mmol/L)	Impaired glucose tolerance	Do an OGTT every year or earlier if CFRD symptoms occur.
		≥ 200 mg/dL (≥ 11.1 mmol/L)	CFRD without fasting hyperglycemia	High risk of getting CFRD with fasting hyperglycemia. Patients will learn to use a blood sugar meter and how to count carbohydrates in the food they eat. The doctor may give insulin if the patient has symptoms, is ill, or is taking steroids.

Source: Courtesy of Hardin D, Brunzell C, Schissel K, et al. *Managing Cystic Fibrosis Related Diabetes (CFRD): An Instruction Guide for Patients and Families,* 5th ed. Bethesda, MD: Cystic Fibrosis Foundation; 2011.

greater than 126 mg/dL. The latter is characterized with a normal FBG but an oral glucose tolerance test (OGTT) equal to or greater than 200 mg/dL. The treatment plan may be affected by the type of CFRD.[31]

Pancreatic Function

Stool fecal elastase-I is a highly sensitive and specific way to measure pancreatic function and is generally tested at diagnosis. Patients who are initially pancreatic sufficient can become pancreatic insufficient over time. These patients should have their pancreatic function evaluated annually.[22,23]

When a patient is pancreatic insufficient and on pancreatic enzyme therapy, it is important to evaluate the appropriateness of their enzyme regimen at regular intervals. In some instances, a 72-hour fecal fat test is useful. This test is conducted as follows:[30]

1. Patient's stool is collected for 72 hours and frozen.
2. An accurate food record is kept for a minimum of the 3 days when the stool is being collected. The goal is to consume 2–3 g fat/kg/day. Using the food diary, the average fat intake per day is calculated in grams.
3. The coefficient of fat absorption (COA) is calculated: (grams of fat consumed – grams of fat excreted)/grams of fat consumed × 100% = COA

The normal COA for premature infants is 60–75%, for full-term newborns 80–85%, for age 10 months to 3 years 85–95%, and for age > 3 years 95%.[30] Any patient with CF who demonstrates a percentage less than is deemed normal in correlation with their age may require an increased dosage of pancreatic enzymes or the initiation of pancreatic enzymes if not already prescribed. Although 72-hour fecal fat tests are an accurate way of assessing fat absorption, the steps that must be completed are cumbersome for patients and families. If a 72-hour fecal fat test cannot be done, adjustments can be made to pancreatic enzyme dosages based on reported symptoms of malabsorption or poor weight gain in the setting of adequate caloric intake.

Health Assessment

An assessment of the patient's overall health status should be obtained, including activity and energy levels. Any missed school or work days should be noted. A general review of systems should be performed and a description of the patient's Tanner stage should be noted.[22-24] (See Appendix C.) Comorbid medical conditions such as active pulmonary or sinus disease, gastroesophageal reflux disease (GERD), CFRD, hepatobiliary disease, or history of gut resection should be noted.[22-24] These conditions will also have a direct impact on the patient's nutritional status by affecting appetite, intake, and disease state. Questions about the patient's use of alternative/complementary medicine therapies should be asked in addition to questions about the use of routine medications.

Information about the patient's stool pattern should be monitored carefully at each clinic visit to evaluate the adequacy of the enzyme therapy. Increased frequency or volume of stool output, notable oil in stools, extremely malodorous stools, increased gassiness and abdominal distention, and/or stools that float instead of sinking to the bottom of the toilet are all signs that a patient may be experiencing malabsorption. Patients with persistent malabsorptive symptoms should also be evaluated for nonpancreatic causes of malabsorption such as lactose intolerance or bacterial overgrowth of the small intestine.[22,25] Constipation, a symptom of distal intestinal obstructive syndrome (DIOS), which is also a complication of PI, can be a problem. Enzyme replacement therapy should be checked during every clinic visit and hospitalization to include the type, brand, amount, timing with meals, method of administration, and where they are stored. It also is important to note if the patient is taking any other medications, such as antibiotics, bronchodilators, H_2 blockers, antacids, prokinetic agents, steroids, appetite stimulants, probiotics, vitamins, and minerals.

The pulmonary status of the patient directly influences the patient's nutritional status. The presence of an acute pulmonary exacerbation and chronic disease should be noted. CF patients older than about 6 years of age will be able to perform pulmonary function tests to assess the extent of their pulmonary involvement.

Patients with CF are at risk for developing osteopenia and osteoporosis. The origin of bone disease in CF appears to be multifactorial (see **Figure 11-1**). Important contributing factors include the following:

- Malabsorption of vitamins D and K
- Failure to thrive

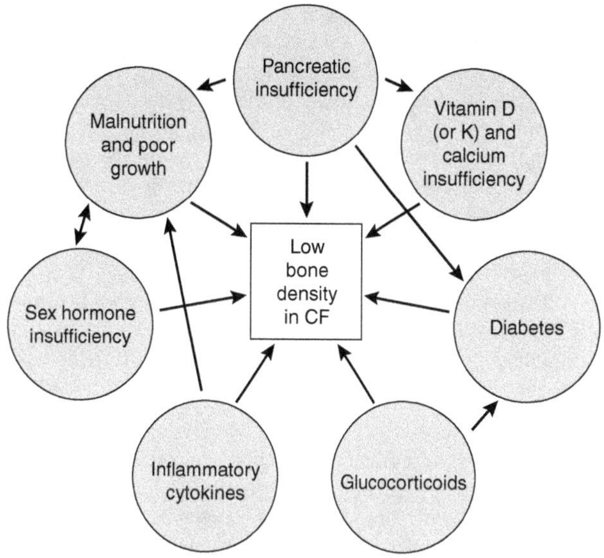

FIGURE 11-1 Pathogenesis of Bone Disease in CF

Source: Courtesy of Aris RM, Merkel PA, Bachrach LK, et al. Consensus statement: guide to bone health and disease in cystic fibrosis. *J Clin Endocrinol Metab.* 2005;90:1888–1896.

- Delayed puberty
- Physical inactivity
- Use of corticosteroid medications

The prevalence of bone disease appears to increase with severity of lung disease and malnutrition.[33] Patients with severe pulmonary disease (FEV_1 < 30%) often have severe bone disease with a high rate of kyphosis and fractures of long bones, vertebrae, and ribs.[34,35]

Patients older than 8 years of age should have a dual energy x-ray absorptiometry (DEXA) scan done as a measure of bone mineral density if < 90% ideal body weight, FEV_1 < 50% predicted, glucocorticoids ≥ 5 mg/day for ≥ 90 days/yr, delayed puberty, or history of fractures.[33] Patients with CF at risk for poor bone health also should have annual tests for serum calcium, phosphorus, intact parathyroid hormone, and 25-hydroxyvitamin D level.[36] All patients should have a DEXA scan done by age 18 years if the scans have not been previously obtained.

Nutrition Assessment

The overall goal of nutrition management is to promote normal growth and development. The main components include the provision of adequate energy, protein, and nutrients; pancreatic enzyme therapy; and vitamin and mineral supplementation. Important information about the CF patient's intake can be obtained from nutrition analysis. A 24-hour dietary recall, 3- to 5-day food record, or food frequency questionnaire can be used to gather data. The diet should be analyzed for energy, protein, and other key nutrients such as calcium and iron. Information about the patient's appetite, eating patterns, consumption of sweetened beverages, and behavioral issues related to feeding should also be noted.[22–24] The Behavioral Pediatrics Feeding Assessment Scale may be administered to identify and evaluate behavioral issues related to eating.[22,23,37]

Drug–nutrient interactions should be assessed because CF patients often consume many different medications and supplements. Factors to consider include the following:

- How these medications may impact the patient's appetite
- If there are dietary restrictions related to any of the patient's medications
- What biochemical data may need to be evaluated with the use of certain medications

As the CF patient's pulmonary disease progresses, issues with fluid status may develop. If diuretics are prescribed, fluid and electrolyte status need to be carefully monitored.

Dietary Intake Composition

Due to improved enzyme replacement therapy, fat restriction is no longer imposed on patients with CF. Higher energy intake results in improved weight gain.[26] Estimated energy recommendations to support age-appropriate growth in children with CF older than age 2 years range from 110–200% of energy needs for the healthy population of similar age, gender, and size.[26] This can be accomplished by increasing both the amount and caloric density of foods consumed. To achieve this energy goal, patients with CF often require a greater amount of dietary fat, 35–40% of total energy.[23] It is appropriate to encourage the use of polyunsaturated fats that are good sources of the EFAs. Vegetable oils are high in calories and a good source of these fats.[22,23] Protein intake is correlated with overall calorie intake and, in general, patients with CF who consume adequate calories also consume adequate protein.[38,39] Formula calculations can be used to determine energy needs, but gain in weight and height, velocity of weight and height gain, and fat stores may provide a more objective measure of energy balance.[40]

Age-specific considerations in the nutritional management of CF are summarized in **Exhibit 11-1.** Infants with CF may be successfully breastfed or fed standard iron-fortified infant formula as long as pancreatic enzymes are administered prior to each feeding. Expensive hydrolyzed formulas are not needed.[41]

To meet the energy needs of the patient with CF, energy-dense foods can be added to the patient's diet. For example, cheese, sour cream, and peanut butter can easily be added to the patient's favorite foods, as tolerated. **Exhibit 11-2** depicts one approach to increasing calories and protein.

Pregnancy

With the increased life expectancy of patients with CF, more women with the disease are becoming pregnant. The increased energy needs of pregnancy must be taken into consideration with an emphasis on proper weight gain. The woman's weight before and during pregnancy has an impact on the outcome for both mother and infant.[42] A pregnant woman with CF must add between 340 to 1000 kcal/day to her usual diet.[42] A diet sufficient in iron and calcium should be emphasized, and salt intake should not be restricted except for medical reasons.[36]

Intake of vitamins and minerals should be monitored and blood levels of fat-soluble vitamins should be obtained before and during pregnancy to determine the correct vitamin dose.[36] Mothers with CF can successfully breastfeed their infants.[43] Breastfeeding further increases the energy demands on the patient with CF.

CF-Related Diabetes

The treatment goal for CFRD is to provide a diet that promotes optimal growth and development in children and adolescents, achievement and maintenance of normal weight in adults, and optimal nutritional status.[31,44] Other treatment goals include controlling hyperglycemia to reduce diabetes complications and avoiding severe hypoglycemia.[31] Carbohydrates have the greatest impact on blood sugar. Simple sugars can be included in the diet plan, but regular sodas and other sweetened beverages should be discouraged. The patient needs to learn how to identify the carbohydrate content of foods, such as carbohydrate counting.[31,44] For those on a fixed insulin regimen, blood sugars can be managed by eating a consistent amount of carbohydrate at each of three meals and three snacks in addition to eating at the same time each day.[32] Fat should continue to contribute about 40% of total calories, and protein intake should provide about 20% of total calories.[31]

Education

Patient and family education on nutrition management and its importance in the patient's overall health care is an integral component of the individual patient's care plan. A qualified, registered dietitian should be available to assist the family and patient with CF in meeting the nutritional needs. The health professional needs to provide anticipatory guidance to the parents/caretakers of these patients to try and avoid battles over eating.[45,46]

Young children with CF or those at risk of growth deficits may benefit from an intensive treatment with behavioral intervention in conjunction with nutrition counseling to promote weight gain.[18] Some strategies include the following:

EXHIBIT 11-1 Nutritional Management of CF Patients

1. Infant
   - Breast milk or standard iron-fortified infant formula should be recommended. Special formulas such as Alimentum (Abbott Laboratories) and Pregestimil (Mead Johnson Nutritionals), protein hydrolysate formulas containing medium-chain triglycerides, can be recommended for infants in special situations, such as gut resection or increased fat malabsorption.
   - Pancreatic enzymes should be given prior to feedings.
   - Vitamin supplements and a source of fluoride should be given.
   - Introduction of solid foods and advancement of diet should proceed as recommended by the American Academy of Pediatrics (AAP). The RD should guide parents toward foods that will enhance weight gain. Meat, a good source of iron and zinc, may be recommended as a first food for infants consuming human milk.
   - Salt should be added to breast milk or infant formula, particularly in hot weather. When solid foods are added to the infant's diet, salt should be added to these foods.
   - Referrals should be made to community programs such as the WIC program.
2. Toddler
   - Toddlers' diets should be based on a normal healthy diet for age with a variety of foods.
   - Parents should be forewarned of the normal decrease in growth and appetite during this age.
   - Regular meal and snack times should be encouraged.
   - Constant snacking or "grazing" should be discouraged.
   - Drinking of sweetened beverages should be discouraged.
   - Pancreatic enzymes and vitamins are continued.
   - Continue communication with community programs such as the WIC program.
3. Preschool and school age
   - A normal healthy diet with a variety of foods should continue to form the basis of the diet.
   - Limit sweetened beverages.
   - Parents lose control of what child eats away from home at preschool, child care, and school.
   - Arrangements need to be made for child to take enzymes during the school day.
   - Vitamin therapy is continued.
   - Diet prescriptions for a high-calorie, high-protein, high-salt diet can be sent to the school.
4. Adolescent
   - Patients are exercising more independence in food choices.
   - Parents can provide appropriate food environment at home.
   - Patients can be taught to include quick-to-prepare high-calorie foods in daily diet.
   - Snack and fast foods can add a significant amount of calories to the diet and should not be discouraged.
   - Limit sweetened beverages.
   - Health professionals should emphasize the importance of high-calorie intake and enzyme and vitamin therapy directly to the patient and not via the parents.
   - Nutrition needs increase prior to and during adolescent growth spurt.

- Complimenting children for appropriate feeding behaviors (e.g., trying a new food)
- Paying minimal attention to behaviors not compatible with eating (e.g., refusing food)
- Limiting mealtimes to 15 minutes, specifically for toddlers[47]

Nutrition Supplements

Milkshakes and other high-calorie drinks can be used to supplement oral intake. Commercial oral beverages (such as Ensure Plus or Boost) can also be used to boost calories. Often in spite of vigorous efforts, it is very difficult to meet the patient's energy needs by the oral route alone. Supplemental tube feedings should be considered when the optimization of feeding behaviors and addition of oral supplements have not achieved adequate weight gain or growth parameters. The patient and family need to be involved in the decision making.[22,23] Various forms of tube feedings, including nasogastric, gastrostomy, and jejunostomy feedings can be used. Tube feedings are often administered on a continuous basis while the patient is asleep. A variety of formulas are available, as discussed in Chapter 19. Some contain MCT

EXHIBIT 11-2 Instructional Handout on Increasing Calories

Calorie-Protein Boosters

—Some ways to hide extra calories and protein—

Powdered milk (33 cal/tbsp, 3 g pro/tbsp)
Add 2–4 tbsp to 1 cup milk. Mix into puddings, potatoes, soups, ground meats, vegetables, and cooked cereal.

Eggs (80 cal/egg, 7 g pro/tbsp)
Add to casseroles, meat loaf, mashed potatoes, cooked cereal, and macaroni & cheese. Add extra to pancake batter and french toast. (Do not use raw eggs in uncooked items.)

Butter or margarine (45 cal/tsp)
Add to puddings, casseroles, sandwiches, vegetables, and cooked cereal.

Cheeses (100 cal/oz, 7 g pro/oz)
Give as snacks or in sandwiches. Add melted to casseroles, potatoes, vegetables, and soup.

Wheat germ (25 cal/tbsp)
Add a tablespoon or two to cereal. Mix into meat dishes, cookie batter, casseroles, etc.

Mayonnaise or salad dressings (45 cal/tsp)
Use liberally on sandwiches, on salads, as a dip for raw vegetables, or as a sauce on cooked vegetables.

Evaporated milk (25 cal/tbsp, 1 g pro/tbsp)
Use in place of whole milk, in desserts, baked goods, meat dishes, and cooked cereals.

Sour cream (26 cal/tbsp)
Add to potatoes, casseroles, dips; use in sauces, baked goods, etc.

Sweetened condensed milk (60 cal/tbsp, 1 g pro/tbsp)
Add to pies, puddings, milkshakes. Mix 1–2 tbsp with peanut butter and spread on toast.

Peanut butter (95 cal/tbsp, 4 g pro/tbsp)
Serve on toast, crackers, bananas, apples, and celery.

Carnation Instant Breakfast (130 cal/pckt, 7 g pro/pckt)
Add to milk and milkshakes.

Gravies (40 cal/tbsp)
Use liberally on mashed potatoes and meats.

High Protein Foods

- MEATS—Beef, Chicken, Fish, Turkey, Lamb
- MILK & CHEESE—Yogurt, Cottage Cheese, Cream Cheese
- EGGS
- PEANUT BUTTER (with Bread or Crackers)
- DRIED BEANS & PEAS (with Bread, Cornbread, Rice)

Source: Courtesy of Pediatric Pulmonary Center, ©1990, University of Alabama at Birmingham, Birmingham, Alabama.

oil, which can help with fat absorption issues. All types of commercially available formulas can be used successfully.[36]

Vitamin A, E, and D supplements are needed for all infants and children with CF.[22,23] CF-specific multivitamin preparations are available on the market that contain high amounts of the fat-soluble vitamins A, D, E, and K in a water-miscible form to meet the needs of patients with CF. **Table 11-3** compares the amounts of fat-soluble vitamins in different CF-specific vitamins to a standard multivitamin. These CF-specific multivitamins simplify patients' vitamin regimen and often improve compliance.[48] Not all of the commercially available products contain the recommended level of vitamin K, so vitamin K status needs to be monitored carefully. Additional vitamin K is often prescribed to patients to prevent vitamin K deficiency, especially due to the frequent usage of antibiotics.[21,49]

Vitamin D deficiency is common in CF.[40] If the 25-OH vitamin D level is less than 30 ng/mL, ergocalciferol should be consumed for 8 weeks according to the following dosing schedule: 12,000 IU weekly for patients younger than 5 years of age and 50,000 IU weekly for patients older than 5 years of age. If 25-OH vitamin D levels remain less than 30 ng/mL 2 to 4 weeks after completion of treatment, then the vitamin D dose is increased to twice per week for 8 weeks.[44] When repleating vitamin D levels, the patient also needs to consume enough calcium. If after this additional treatment, the vitamin D levels are still less than 30 ng/mL, then phototherapy or increased sunlight exposure should be considered or a referral to endocrinology made.[44] Vitamin D treatment recommendations may not correct low vitamin D levels and thus should be closely monitored and supplemented as needed.[50]

Minerals such as zinc, iron, and selenium may need to be supplemented in patients with CF. A trial of zinc supplementation for 6 months may be initiated for patients with CF who have poor growth.[22,23] All patients with CF should be encouraged to consume at least the DRIs for calcium for their age group. Patients with CF who are on steroids, who have decreased dietary intake of calcium, and/or have decreased bone density may benefit from calcium supplementation.

Additional salt should be added to the diet during times of increased sweating, such as during hot weather, with a fever, during strenuous physical activity, or with profuse diarrhea. The additional salt compensates for the increased losses of sodium and chloride through perspiration. In most instances, liberal use of the salt shaker and the inclusion of high-salt foods in the diet will supply the needed sodium and chloride. Salt supplements may be used in cases of very heavy sweating. Both breastfed and formula-fed infants need supplementation with sodium chloride.[22,23] Infants without CF require 2 to 4 mEq/kg/day of sodium.[22,23] It is recommended that infants younger than 6 months of age be given ⅛ teaspoon per day of table salt, and ¼ teaspoon per day

TABLE 11-3 Comparison of CF-Specific Vitamin and Mineral Supplements in the United States to Non–CF-Specific Products[a]

Age	SourceCF[b,c] Drops, Chewables, and Softgels	ADEK Chewables[b,d]	AquADEKs[b,e] Drops and Softgels	Vitamax[b,f] Drops and Chewables	Poly-Vi-Sol Drops[g] and Centrum Chewables and Tablet
Vitamin A (IU): Retinol and Beta Carotene					
0–12 mo	4627 (1 mL) 75% BC[h]	—	5751 (1 mL) 87% BC	3170 (1 mL) 0% BC	1500 (1 mL) 0% BC
1–3 y	9254 (2 mL) 75% BC	—	11502 (2 mL) 87% BC	6340 (2 mL) 0% BC	3000 (2 mL) 0% BC
4–8 y	16,000/chewable 88% BC	9000/chewable 60% BC	Ages 4–10 y: 18,167/1 softgel 92% BC	5000/chewable 50% BC	3500/chewable 29% BC
>9 y	32,000/2 softgels 88% BC	18,000/2 chewables 60% BC	Ages 10 and up: 36,334/2 softgels 92% BC	10,000/2 chewables 50% BC	7000/2 tablets 29% BC
Vitamin E (IU)[i]					
0–12 mo	50 (1 mL)	—	50 (1 mL)[i]	50 (1 mL)	5 (1 mL)
1–3 y	100 (2 mL)	—	100 (2 mL)[i]	100 (2 mL)	10 (2 mL)
4–8 y	200/chewable	150/chewable	Ages 4–10 y: 150/1 softgel[i]	200/chewable	30/chewable
>9 y	400/2 softgels	300/2 chewables	Ages 10 and up: 300/2 softgels[j]	400/2 chewables	60/2 tablets
Vitamin D (IU)					
0–12 mo	500 (1 mL)	—	400 (1 mL)	400 (1 mL)	400 (1 mL)
1–3 y	1000 (2 mL)	—	800 (2 mL)	800 (2 mL)	800 (2 mL)
4–8 y	1000/chewable	400/chewable	Ages 4–10 y: 800/1 softgel	400/chewable	400/chewable
>9 y	2000/2 softgels	800/2 chewables	Ages 10 and up: 1600/2 softgels	800/2 chewables	800/2 tablets
Vitamin K (μg)					
0–12 mo	400 (1 mL)	—	400 (1 mL)	300 (1 mL)	0
1–3 y	800 (2 mL)	—	800 (2 mL)	600 (2 mL)	0
4–8 y	800/chewable	150/chewable	Ages 4–10 y: 700/1 softgel	200/chewable	10/chewable
>9 y	1600/2 softgels	300/2 chewables	Ages 10 and up: 1400/2 softgels	400/2 chewables	50/2 tablets
Zinc (mg)					
0–12 mo	5 (1 mL)	—	5 (1 mL)	7.5 (1 mL)	0
1–3 y	10 (2 mL)	—	10 (2 mL)	15 (2 mL)	0
4–8 y	15/chewable	7.5/chewable	Ages 4–10 y: 10/softgel	7.5/chewable	15/chewable
>9 y	30/2 softgels	15/2 chewables	Ages 10 and up: 20/2 softgels	15/2 chewables	22/2 tablets

[a] The content of this table was confirmed December 2008. Products also contain a full range of water-soluble vitamins; see SourceCF.com for content.

[b] CF-specific products.

[c] SourceCF Liquid, Chewables, and Softgels are registered trademarks of SourceCF Inc., a subsidiary of Eurand Pharmaceuticals, Inc.

[d] ADEK Chewables is a registered trademark of Axcan Pharma, Inc.

[e] AquADEKs Liquid and Softgels are registered trademarks of Yasoo Health Inc.

[f] Vitamax Drops and Chewables are registered trademarks of Shear/Kershman Labs, Inc.

[g] Poly-Vi-Sol Drops is a registered trademark of Mead Johnson and Company. Centrum Chewables and Tablets are registered trademarks of Wyeth Consumer Care.

[h] Beta carotene.

[i] α-Tocopherol.

[j] Contains mixed tocopherols.

Abbreviation: BC, beta carotene.

Source: Reprinted from Pediatric Clinics of North America, Vol. 56, Michel S, Maqbool A, Hanna M, Mascarenhas M. Nutrition management of pediatric patients who have cystic fibrosis. *Pediatric Clin N Am.* 2009;56:1123–1141. Copyright 2009, with permission from Elsevier.

is recommended for infants older than 6 months of age administered in feedings throughout the day.[40]

Table 11-4 lists the three brands of pancreatic enzymes on the market today. They contain varying amounts of lipase, protease, and amylase. The nonproprietary name of these products is pancrelipase. The products are available in capsule form and feature an enteric coating that protects the enzymes from inactivation in the acid environment of the stomach. The enzymes become activated in the alkaline pH of the duodenum.

Dosage/Administration

Standards on the use of pancreatic enzyme supplements are published.[51,52] Extremely high doses can cause fibrosing colonopathy or strictures in the colon in CF patients.[53,54] A recommended starting dose for infants is 2000 to 5000 units of lipase per 4 oz feeding, though this may be less in newborns who take less volume at each feeding.[47] Another dosing schedule starts with 1000 units of lipase/kg body weight/meal for children younger than 4 years of age and 500 units of lipase/kilogram body weight/meal for those older than age 4.[51,52] The usual enzyme dose for snacks is one-half of the mealtime dose. It is recommended not to exceed 2500 units of lipase/kg body weight/meal, with a maximum daily dose of 10,000 units lipase/kg body weight. Careful monitoring of the patient's growth, stool pattern, and the absence or presence of gastrointestinal symptoms will help determine the adequacy of therapy. Monitoring and adjusting the dosage as needed is ongoing. If the patient with CF is still exhibiting symptoms of malabsorption after reaching a maximum enzyme dose, it may be because the stomach contents are too acidic. In this case, the addition of bicarbonate or other drugs that inhibit gastric acidity may be helpful.[51,52] Nonpancreatic reasons for malabsorption also should be considered.

Enzymes should be taken immediately prior to meals and snacks that contain fat, protein, and complex carbohydrate. The enterically coated enzymes should not be chewed or crushed. For infants and small children who are unable to swallow a capsule, the capsule can be opened and the contents mixed with a soft, acidic food, such as applesauce. Enzymes mixed with food should be used within 30 minutes of mixing. When the enterically coated enzymes are mixed with a higher pH food, such as pudding, the enzymes will become activated and begin breaking down the food.

Dosing enzymes for gastrostomy and other types of tube feedings can be difficult. Patients should take their usual meal dose of pancreatic enzymes by mouth prior to the initiation of the feeding.[22,23] If receiving continuous overnight tube feeds, some patients may need to take additional enzymes during the middle of the night or at the end of their feeding.[22,23] Giving enterically coated microspheres or microtablets via the feeding tube may result in clogging of the feeding tube.

Administering enzymes to an extremely young infant can be a frustrating endeavor for the parent. After a few months of age, taking enzymes becomes part of a patient's daily routine. Parents of toddlers should be warned against allowing the child to "graze" throughout the day, because this makes enzyme dosing difficult. In the preadolescent and adolescent age groups, patient compliance with enzyme administration

TABLE 11-4 Examples of Pancreatic Enzymes

Enzyme	Form*	Lipase USP Units	Protease USP Units	Amylase USP Units
Creon 6[1]	Delayed release capsules	6000	19,000	30,000
Creon 12[1]	Delayed release capsules	12,000	38,000	60,000
Creon 24[1]	Delayed release capsules	24,000	76,000	120,000
Pancreaze MT4[2]	Delayed release capsules	4200	10,000	17,500
Pancreaze MT10[2]	Delayed release capsules	10,500	25,000	43,750
Pancreaze MT16[2]	Delayed release capsules	16,800	40,000	70,000
Pancreaze MT20[2]	Delayed release capsules	21,000	37,000	61,000
ZENPEP 5[3]	Delayed release capsules	5000	17,000	27,000
ZENPEP 10[3]	Delayed release capsules	10,000	34,000	55,000
ZENPEP 15[3]	Delayed release capsules	15,000	51,000	82,000
ZENPEP 20[3]	Delayed release capsules	20,000	68,000	109,000

*Form as described by respective company

[1]Solvay Pharmaceuticals: http://www.creon-us.com/default.htm

[2]Ortho-McNeil-Janssen Pharmaceuticals: http://www.pancreaze.net

[3]Eurand: http://www.zenpep.com/site/cfpatient.aspx

can become a big issue. The lack of compliance needs to be discussed with the child and a solution found that is agreeable to the child, parents, and the school. Pancreatic enzyme therapy is very expensive. Enzymes are often covered by third-party payers and some state programs for children with special healthcare needs.

Resources

Referral to food and nutrition resources such as the WIC program and the Food Stamp Program should be made based on the individual's needs. In some states, referrals can be made to the state program for children with special healthcare needs for aid in obtaining supplemental feedings, enzymes, and vitamins. Children who participate in the Child Nutrition Program at their school will need diet prescriptions for high-calorie, high-protein diets provided the school staff. Most CF centers provide an interdisciplinary team approach to the care of these children and their families to better help them meet their many needs.

Complementary Therapies

CF caregivers can advise patients and their families as to the safety and efficacy of various therapies. It is important that CF caregivers ask questions about alternative/complementary medicine practices when interviewing patients with CF and their family members, especially in regard to ingested substances.

Bronchopulmonary Dysplasia

Bronchopulmonary dysplasia (BPD) is a form of chronic lung disease seen in infants with severe hyaline membrane disease who required mechanical ventilation and high concentrations of oxygen for prolonged periods of time. Improved clinical practice has resulted in a decrease in lung injury in larger (greater than 1200 gram birth weight) and more mature infants. At the same time, more and more premature infants are surviving at earlier gestational ages and lower birth weights. The current definition of BPD reflects differing criteria for infants born at less than or greater than 32 weeks gestation.[55] This expanded definition includes different diagnostic criteria for mild, moderate, and severe forms of the disease.[55] For example, the definition of severe BPD for an infant with a gestational age of less than 32 weeks is the need for 30% oxygen or more and/or positive pressure at 36 weeks postmenstrual age or discharge, whichever comes first.[55]

BPD includes infants who have had an acute lung injury with minimal clinical and radiographic findings as well as those with major radiographic abnormalities. BPD represents a continuum of lung disease. The pathogenesis of BPD is multifactorial but includes primarily arrested lung development due to the necessary accelerated maturation of the lungs due to premature birth. Severe, diffuse, acute lung injury and an early inflammatory response exacerbate the abnormal lung development due to primary injury and inadequate immature repair mechanisms. The lungs may be damaged by the barotrauma from the use of intermittent positive pressure ventilation (IPPV) and by oxygen toxicity from the high concentrations of oxygen required by these infants early in life.[56,57] Infection may play a role in the pathogenesis of BPD.[56] Other factors that may contribute to the development of the disease include increased fluids contributing to pulmonary edema[58–60] and inadequate early nutrition impeding lung reparative processes.[56,61]

BPD is one of the most common sequelae of newborn intensive care unit stays. It is rare in premature infants weighing 1500 grams or more with uncomplicated respiratory distress syndrome. This is due to the use of antenatal steroids, surfactant replacement therapy, gentler ventilation that reduces barotrauma, better nutrition, and careful use of supplemental oxygen.[62] However, the incidence of BPD is higher in infants with birth weight under 1000 grams. As BPD patients are followed over time, chronic lung disease remains a major clinical problem into late childhood and early adolescence.[56,61]

Signs of respiratory distress, such as chest retractions, tachypnea, crackles, and wheezing, characterize BPD. Supplemental oxygen therapy may be required. Pulmonary complications may include recurrent atelectasis, pulmonary infections, and respiratory failure requiring mechanical ventilation. Other complications include:

- Pulmonary edema
- Cor pulmonale
- Poor growth
- Neurodevelopmental delays, including delayed feeding skills
- Cardiovascular problems

The primary goal of BPD management is to provide the patient with the necessary pulmonary support during the acute and chronic phases of the disease to minimize lung damage and to maintain optimal oxygen saturation. This may include mechanical ventilation, supplemental oxygen, anti-inflammatory and β-adrenergic aerosols, and diuretic therapy. Of equal importance is the provision of adequate nutrition. Growth of new lung tissue can occur in humans until about 8 years of age. Theoretically, a BPD patient can "outgrow" the disease if adequate pulmonary and nutritional support can be provided.

Nutrient Requirements

Most infants who develop BPD are premature, and these infants have little fat, glycogen, or other nutrients in reserve, particularly iron, calcium, and phosphorus. Several factors increase the energy and nutrient needs of BPD patients, such as increased basal metabolic rate, increased work of breathing, and chronic hypoxia. These infants are also prone to chronic illness/infections and respiratory distress/metabolic complications.

Growth failure is common due to their increased work of breathing and an increased resting oxygen consumption. Their resting energy expenditure is also higher than normal infants.[63-65] Treatment of the BPD patient usually includes a wide array of medications, including diuretics, steroids, and bronchodilators. See **Table 11-5** for more on the impact of these drugs on the patient's nutritional status.

Infants with BPD are extremely fluid sensitive because of their lung disease and the possible complication of cor pulmonale, or right-sided heart failure. Fluid restriction also limits their energy and nutrient intake. As a result, infants with BPD often require a calorically enhanced formula in order to meet their energy needs for adequate growth.

Frequent intubations and mechanical ventilation interfere with the normal feeding sequence and feeding-skill development. Therefore, these infants may be poor oral feeders and develop aversive oral behavior.[66] Also, these infants often get tired out or have decreased oxygen saturation during feeding.[67,68] Gastroesophageal reflux may also be present, causing a further impediment to feeding.[69]

Growth and Nutrition Assessment

It is important to monitor growth and nutritional status of patients with BPD. It is unrealistic to expect true growth to occur when life-threatening events, such as respiratory failure, necrotizing enterocolitis, or other serious problems of prematurity, are taking place. The infant must be fairly stable in order for growth to occur. A poor pattern of growth in patients with BPD is often related to the severity of pulmonary disease.[70] Adequate oxygenation must be maintained in the patient with BPD for growth to occur. Positive growth can occur in infants with BPD who maintain an oxygen saturation of greater than 92% while sleeping.

Daily weights are essential during the early hospitalization(s) and critical stages of the disease. Weight data help to identify fluid overload in a patient, as well as growth. Monitoring weight, length, and head circumference on a regular basis is needed to assess growth. Measurements should be plotted on appropriate growth charts, such as the CDC growth charts and correcting for gestational age or growth charts that allow assessment of infants of varying gestational age, such as those by Babson and Benda.[25,71] When using CDC growth charts for premature infants, weight should be corrected for gestational age until 24 months, length until 36 months, and head circumference until 18 months.[36]

Biochemical monitoring of the BPD patient is individualized. During diuretic therapy, sodium, chloride, and potassium should be monitored. Other helpful measurements include prealbumin or albumin, a complete blood count, alkaline phosphatase, parathyroid hormone, 25-hydroxyvitamin D, and urine specific gravity, especially if the patient is fluid restricted and/or being fed a concentrated formula.

The patient's pulmonary status directly impacts nutritional needs and intake. A patient with BPD who is ventilator dependent has respiratory failure and severe lung disease. These infants with BPD require close follow-up because it may be difficult initially to determine their nutritional needs. Many chronic ventilator-dependent patients with BPD have very low energy needs and yet their other nutrient needs are the same as other infants with BPD. Feedings may need to be adjusted to meet nutrient needs without providing too many calories, which often requires vitamin and mineral supplementation. A patient who has a low arterial partial pressure of oxygen is not properly oxygenating tissue, which may contribute to growth failure. These patients may require supplemental oxygen for tissue oxygenation and growth. An increase in pulmonary symptoms, such as the presence of tachypnea, rales, rhonchi, and bronchiolitis/pneumonia, is indicative of active pulmonary disease. The presence of chronic pulmonary disease and acute pulmonary exacerbations in BPD patients further increases their energy needs and may increase their sensitivity to fluids.

Other medical conditions—such as cor pulmonale; gastroesophageal reflux, with or without aspiration; esophagitis; repeated emesis; and the patient's medication regimen—should also be noted. Table 11-5 lists drug–nutrient interactions of medications commonly prescribed for patients with BPD.

TABLE 11-5 BPD Drug–Nutrient Interactions

Medication	Nutrients Affected (lowers all)	Other Effects
Diuretics (e.g., furosemide)	Na, K, Cl, Mg, Ca, Zn	Volume depletion Metabolic alkalosis Anorexia Diarrhea Hyperuricemia Gastrointestinal irritant
Bronchodilators (e.g., theophylline)		Gastrointestinal distress Nausea Vomiting Diarrhea
Steroids (e.g., dexamethasone)	Ca, P	Growth suppression

Nutrition Intake

The diet intake should be evaluated for calories; protein; fluid; electrolytes; key minerals, such as calcium, phosphorus, and iron; and caloric distribution of fat, protein, and carbohydrate. The type of feeding—oral, tube feeding, or parenteral—should be noted as well as the route and rate of administration. Any vitamin and mineral supplements also should be recorded. This can then be compared to the patient's estimated nutrient and fluid requirements.

Of particular importance is careful monitoring of the patient's ability to suck and swallow and the patient's feeding-skill development. The sucking reflex does not develop until about 34 weeks gestation. Alternate methods of feeding are required until this reflex develops. Neurologic impairment may prevent the patient from being able to coordinate sucking and swallowing. Noxious stimuli to the patient's mouth, such as frequent intubations and suctioning, may seriously affect normal feeding-skill development. Maintaining adequate oxygenation during feedings is essential.[67,68] It is important to note if the patient tires during feedings and whether the infant turns blue around the mouth or fingertips, which indicates a drop in oxygen saturation. These problems must be identified early and appropriate intervention instituted.

The caloric requirement for infants with BPD is higher than normal and ranges from 120–150 kcal/kg/day; those with severe BPD may need more than 150 kcal/kg/day.[69] Meeting these high levels of intake can be a challenge. Nutrition management of an infant with BPD involves three phases:

1. *Acute phase:* The BPD patient during this phase is critically ill and at risk for clinical morbidities, such as PDA and NEC (see also Chapter 4). Efforts should be made to minimize thermal losses. Possible feeding complications include fluid overload and hyperglycemia. Fluid tolerance is decreased because of pulmonary edema and reduced cardiac output. Total energy needs are about 50–70 kcal/kg/day.
2. *Intermediate phase:* This phase is characterized by a period of clinical improvements and a gradual introduction of oral feeding while keeping thermal losses to a minimum. Fluid overload continues to be a concern, but often the patient with BPD is able to tolerate an increase in fluid during this phase. Total energy needs are 95–120 kcal/kg/day.
3. *Convalescent phase:* This is a period of recovery when the patient with BPD is usually feeding orally. Minimizing thermal losses continues to be important, as is monitoring activity, growth, and adequate oxygenation of tissues. Total energy needs are 120–130 kcal/kg/day.

The immature kidney of an infant cannot handle high-protein loads, so protein should constitute about 8–12% of the total calories, with the remainder of the calories evenly divided between carbohydrate and fat.[72]

Vitamin A is essential in the respiratory tract for maintenance of the integrity and differentiation of epithelial cells. Deficiency of vitamin A results in loss of cilia and other changes in the airways, which resemble the changes seen in BPD. Vitamin A adequacy may decrease the incidence of BPD in infants with very low birth weight, and thus plasma serum vitamin A levels should be monitored.[73] Administering 5000 IU vitamin A intramuscularly three times a week to infants at risk for developing BPD may be advantageous.[74,75] Some newborn intensive care units administer vitamin A in an attempt to protect against BPD.[76]

Adequate vitamin E status is also important in premature infants with BPD who are on oxygen therapy because vitamin E is a major antioxidant. Vitamin E acts as an oxygen free-radical scavenger and membrane stabilizer, protecting cell membranes from oxidation. Infants are most likely to receive adequate vitamin E when fed human milk or commercial formulas.

Copper, zinc, selenium, and manganese are especially important in BPD because they are components of an antioxidant enzyme system.[92] Zinc can be decreased with diuretic therapy, and premature infants often are in negative zinc balance.[77] Infants with BPD may be at risk for toxic accumulation of certain trace elements, such as copper and manganese, especially if the patient has cholestasis or other liver disease.[72]

The recommended iron intake is 2–4 mg of elemental iron/kg/day,[78] and the supplementation should begin no later than 2 months of age. Iron can be provided through a supplement or through the use of iron-fortified formulas. Adequate iron status is important in patients with BPD to maximize tissue oxygenation and minimize oxygen consumption.[57]

Infants who are born prematurely do not have the benefit of the calcium and phosphorus accretion during the third trimester of gestation. In addition, the calcium and phosphorus status of premature infants with BPD can be further compromised by diuretics, steroids, long-term use of parenteral nutrition, and feeding delays. Consequently, infants with BPD are at risk for developing rickets of prematurity or osteopenia, which is diagnosed by decreased bone density and an elevated serum alkaline phosphatase. If supplements are needed, preterm human milk can be fortified with a commercial human milk fortifier. Adequate vitamin D (400 IU/d) intake is also needed.[78]

Electrolyte imbalance may result, especially when the infant is receiving diuretic therapy. The infant with BPD can usually tolerate a sodium intake of 1.5–3.5 mEq/kg/d.[57] Potassium (3 mEq/kg/d) and chloride may need to be supplemented, depending on the diuretic therapy.[57,58] The infant should be closely monitored when sodium chloride and/or potassium chloride are being added to the infant's feedings.

The infant with BPD faces many barriers to meet these increased nutrient needs, including:

- Fluid restriction for infants with cor pulmonale, with or without right-sided heart failure, and those who are fluid sensitive
- Gastrointestinal limitations, such as an immature gut
- Immature renal function, making renal solute load of feedings an issue
- Chronic hypoxia, especially during feedings and sleep
- Feeding difficulties, including lack of sucking reflex and feeding aversions
- Significant GERD resulting in vomiting or discomfort with feeding

During the acute phase of BPD, parenteral nutrition (PN) is often employed. See Chapter 4 for further details about PN in premature infants. IV lipids should be started at 0.5–1.0 g/kg/day and slowly increased to a maximum of 2.0–3.0 g/kg/day.[78] Serum triglyceride levels should be monitored and kept below 150 mg/dL.[78]

Glucose should be infused at a rate less than 6 mg/kg/minute and steadily increased to a rate of 11–12 mg/kg/minute.[78] High glucose loads in patients with BPD may result in an increase in resting energy expenditure, basal oxygen consumption, and carbon dioxide production.[63] Infants with borderline respiratory function may not be able to excrete this additional carbon dioxide, and respiratory acidosis can result.

If able to feed enterally, tube feedings should be initiated at a slow rate and gradually advanced. During this transitional phase, PN is often continued to maintain the delivery of adequate energy and protein while tolerance to enteral feedings is being established. This transitional phase can be difficult because an infant must be hungry before an oral feeding will be readily accepted. Continuous infusions of nutrition may suppress natural hunger sensations. Hunger is particularly important when feeding skills are being developed. An appropriate schedule of parenteral feedings, enteral tube feedings, and oral feedings must be determined by members of the interdisciplinary healthcare team and the family.

Fortified breast milk or premature infant formulas, which have higher concentrations of vitamins and minerals, may be used. Breast milk is preferred initially.[69] The infant should continue with breast milk fortified with a human milk fortifier or with premature formula until reaching a weight of 2000–2500 g. At this point, the infant can most likely transition to a premature follow-up formula or a standard infant formula concentrated to 22 or 24 kcal/oz. To meet some infants' very high energy needs, the formula may need to be concentrated to between 26–30 kcal/oz. while maintaining a proper balance of nutrients. Caloric distribution should continue to be approximately 8–12% protein, 40–50% carbohydrate, and 40–50% fat.[76] A high fat intake may be contraindicated in patients who have gastroesophageal reflux.[79] Excessive osmolality and renal solute load should be avoided. Once an infant is on standard formula or breast milk, a supplement of a standard infant multivitamin preparation may be recommended until the infant is taking about 1 L of formula. The usual recommendation is 1 cc of a standard infant multivitamin with breast milk or formula intakes over 16 ounces per day and 0.5 cc for intakes between 16 and 30 ounces per day.[80]

Careful monitoring is needed when high-calorie formulas are used. This is primarily due to a high potential renal solute load if fluid intake is limited. When the infant is growing and nitrogen is being utilized to form new tissue, the infant usually handles the solute load. However, if growth ceases or if there is increased fluid loss, such as with a febrile illness, renal solute load may become a problem for these infants, and azotemia may result. Urine specific gravity should be monitored.[79]

The infant may be unable to consume an adequate amount of formula by mouth. Oral gastric or nasogastric feedings are commonly used for short-term supplementary feedings, whereas gastrostomy feedings are used for long-term tube feeding.

Feeding Problems

The patient's ability to suck and swallow must be assessed. Abnormalities in the developmental patterns of suck-and-swallow rhythms during feeding in preterm infants with BPD can occur.[81] Feeding behavior should be assessed for age appropriateness based on corrected age. Patients with BPD may develop feeding difficulties because of their usual prematurity and because of the nature of the life-sustaining respiratory therapy that they receive. Supplemental oxygen is usually delivered by nasal cannula and does not interfere with oral feedings.

Nonnutritive sucking can be instituted during a tube feeding so that the infant can begin to associate feelings of satiety with sucking. In some instances, feedings thickened with rice cereal may be easier for infants to handle. Overlooking problems in the development of feeding skills can result in serious aversions to eating or decreased and inadequate intake.

When critical steps in feeding skill development have been missed, it may be necessary to design a program that breaks eating down into small steps and to orient the child to each step. Instead of feeding according to chronological age, it is more important to feed the child according to the stage of feeding development. A behavioral program may be necessary to help the patient overcome fears related to eating or when food refusal is used manipulatively.

Problematic feeding interactions between the caregiver and the infant may develop. It is important that the healthcare professional be aware of this potential problem. If the patient's oral intake is not adequate to meet nutritional needs, then tube feedings are necessary. A plan for balancing tube feedings with oral feedings must be designed to establish hunger and appetite for feedings by mouth but providing the balance of nutrition via the tube feeding. Tube feedings can be nasogastric, oral gastric, trans pyloric, or gastrostomy. Drip, bolus, or a combination tube feeding schedule can be developed based on the patient's individual needs.

Education and Follow-Up

The home care of the patient with BPD can be quite complex and may include supplemental oxygen and multiple medications and therapies as well as nutrition management. Family and caretaker education by a registered dietitian is an important component of the nutrition care plan. Written instructions for mixing formulas in common household measures for volumes that will be used in 24 hours or less should be given to families. It is best to have the family member or caretaker demonstrate the proper mixing of formulas, especially formula that is being concentrated or contains additives. Reinforcement of these instructions needs to take place on an ongoing basis in outpatient follow-up. It is important to consistently ask the family how they are mixing the formula at home to ensure they are following the correct recipe and the infant is getting the calories needed for adequate growth. It is important to assess the patient's and family's needs with regard to food and nutrition resources. Appropriate referrals must be made. Often, this can be done in cooperation with the nurse, social worker, or case manager.

After discharge from the hospital, the infant with BPD will require regular medical and nutrition follow-up. Feedings will need to be adjusted as the patient grows and develops. Many patients benefit from being enrolled in early intervention programs, which can provide nutrition, occupational therapy, physical therapy, and speech therapy, as needed by the individual patient.

Asthma

Asthma is the most common chronic disease of childhood, affecting an estimated 7 million children from birth to 18 years of age.[82] The prevalence of childhood asthma has been increasing and is a major public health problem.[83] Disparities exist among racial/ethnic populations, with a higher prevalence seen in non-Hispanic blacks and Puerto Ricans compared to non-Hispanic white children.[83] Non-Hispanic blacks have more emergency department visits, more hospitalizations, and an increase in asthma mortality.[84] There is increased prevalence in childhood among males, children of lower socioeconomic groups, African Americans, and those with a family history of asthma or allergies.[85,86] Underdiagnosis and inappropriate treatment are major contributors to morbidity and mortality.[86]

Asthma is a chronic inflammatory disorder of the airways.[87] Symptoms of this inflammation include recurrent episodes of wheezing, breathlessness, chest tightness, and cough, particularly at night and early in the morning. These asthma episodes are associated with obstruction of airflow, which is often reversible either spontaneously or with treatment. Inflammation of the airways also causes an associated increase in airway responsiveness to a variety of stimuli.[87] Inflammation causes airway narrowing and increased airway secretions. Chronic inflammation can lead to airway remodeling, which can cause progressive loss of pulmonary function.[86] Airway obstruction is caused by bronchoconstriction, airway edema, chronic mucus plug formation, and airway remodeling.[86,87]

The diagnosis of asthma can be made when the clinician determines that episodic symptoms of airflow obstruction are present, that airflow obstruction is at least partially reversible, and when alternative diagnoses have been excluded.[87] Diagnostic tools available to the clinician include:

- Obtaining a thorough history
- Spirometry, which measures pulmonary function but is not feasible to measure in young children younger than 5 to 6 years of age
- Chest radiograph
- Pulse oximetry, a measure of oxygen saturation, to evaluate hypoxemia during an acute episode

Other diagnostic tests available include allergy testing, nasal and sinus evaluation, and gastroesophageal reflux assessment.[87] Differential diagnoses include aspiration, cystic fibrosis, cardiac or anatomical defects, and upper and lower respiratory tract infections.[86]

Asthma can be classified by severity: intermittent, mild persistent, moderate persistent, and severe persistent. These classifications reflect the clinical manifestations of asthma and are based on frequency of daytime and nighttime symptoms, spirometry if available, and severity of asthma flare-ups.[87]

A major goal of asthma treatment is to reduce inflammation. The first step toward this is for the patient to recognize and avoid the triggers of asthma. Triggers may include indoor allergens, such as dust mites, and outdoor allergens, such as trees.[86] Environmental tobacco smoke and air pollutants are major precipitants of asthma symptoms in children.[87] Viral respiratory infections are the primary cause of severe asthma flare-ups. Other factors contributing to asthma severity include rhinitis, sinusitis, gastroesophageal reflux, and sulfite sensitivity.[87] In some children, weather or humidity changes, or exercise—especially in cold and dry air—may produce inflammation of the airways.[90] Food allergies may also cause asthma symptoms.[88]

In addition to reducing factors that increase the patient's asthma symptoms, pharmacologic therapy is an important component of asthma management.[87,89] The goal is to optimize pharmacotherapy while minimizing side effects. Long-term control medicines include inhaled corticosteroids, long-acting beta$_2$ agonists, cromolyn sodium and nedocromil sodium (mast cell stabilizers), methylxanthine, leukotriene modifiers, oral corticosteroids, and inhaled corticosteroids and long-acting $beta_2$ agonists in combination. Quick-relief medications, inhaled short-acting $beta_2$ agonists, anticholinergics, and short-course systemic corticosteroids may be used while short-acting $beta_2$ agonists are used to pretreat exercise-induced asthma.[86,87,89] Patient *and* family education are important. Long-term follow-up is essential to adjust medication as needed and for education reinforcement.

The rates of food allergies and asthma are rising, and they may be correlated. Infants diagnosed with an allergy have an increased risk of asthma.[90,91] An even stronger association exists between the diagnosis of food allergies and asthma in children who have multiple or more severe food allergies.[92]

Patients with asthma are more likely to have a life-threatening reaction if they are exposed to foods they are allergic to because of the potential for respiratory system involvement.[91] It is important that patients receive thorough education on how to safely avoid foods they have been diagnosed as allergic to while still maintaining a balanced diet. (See Chapter 7 on food hypersensitivities.)

It is a common misconception among lay people that drinking milk causes an increased production of mucus and may be a trigger for asthma. However, there is no scientific evidence to support this claim. This belief may persist because milk, particularly whole milk, coats the tongue and mouth, and some people may have the sensation that they have an increase in mucus production or that their mucus is thicker after milk consumption. Indiscriminate elimination of a whole food group such as dairy products from the diet of a child with asthma may be totally unnecessary and may deprive the child of an important source of nutrients such as calcium.

The association of overweight and asthma in pediatrics include the following:

- There is a higher prevalence of overweight in children with asthma.
- Overweight children with asthma have increased asthma symptoms.
- Overweight may influence asthma risk.

Nutrition Concerns

Nutrients that have been studied with regards to asthma include vitamin C, fish oils, selenium, and electrolytes, including sodium and magnesium.[89] Antioxidants protect cell membranes from damage caused by free radicals and chemical oxidants. Of the antioxidant vitamins, vitamin C has received the most attention with regards to airway responsiveness.[89] No conclusive evidence links vitamin C levels to asthma or identifies the role that vitamin C may play in the treatment of asthma.[89] However, encouraging children with asthma to include a daily source of vitamin C in their diets is sound advice.

The ingestion of fish oils, which contain omega-3 fatty acids, causes arachidonic acid (AA) to be replaced by eicosapentaenoic acid (EPA) and docosahexaenoic acid (DHA) in cell membranes. This replacement leads to a decrease in the production of the inflammatory metabolites of AA, including leukotrienes. It is thought that this change in metabolites could have potential effects on airway inflammation.[89,93] Most studies do not show significant clinical improvement in asthma patients with the use of fish oils, despite some changes seen in inflammatory cell functions.[94] Recommending the inclusion of fatty fish in the diets of children with asthma is consistent with current healthy diet recommendations.

The relationship of selenium to asthma has been studied because of selenium's role as an antioxidant. Currently, there is not sufficient evidence to advocate the use of selenium supplementation in the treatment of asthma.[89] The relationship of increased sodium intake and asthma has been investigated by several groups of researchers.[89] Other electrolytes have been studied, but no data support the use of supplements.

Nutritional Status

Most of the effects of asthma treatment on the nutritional status of patients are related to the use of oral steroids and high-dose inhaled steroids. Medium- to high-dose inhaled corticosteroids may be needed daily for long-term control in patients whose disease is classified as moderate-persistent.[87] For patients whose disease is in the severe-persistent classification, long-term control may require high-dose inhaled corticosteroids as well as a long-acting bronchodilator plus oral corticosteroids.[87] The primary goal is to treat the asthma with the smallest doses of medicines that will control the symptoms in order to minimize side effects.

Poorly controlled asthma may delay growth in children.[87] In general, children with asthma tend to have longer periods of reduced growth rates prior to puberty.[87] However, this delay in puberty does not appear to affect final adult height.[95] This delay in puberty is not associated with the use of inhaled corticosteroids.[96] The potential for adverse effects on linear growth from inhaled corticosteroids appears to be dose-dependent.[87,96–99] High doses of inhaled corticosteroids have greater potential for growth suppression than lower doses.[87] Using high doses of inhaled corticosteroids with children having severe persistent asthma has less potential for decreasing linear growth than does using oral systemic corticosteroids.[87] The use of oral corticosteroids on a prolonged basis does stunt linear growth.[95]

Chronic corticosteroid use induces osteoporosis.[100] Corticosteroids decrease calcium absorption from the gastrointestinal tract and decrease renal calcium reabsorption, which leads to a decrease in plasma calcium. At the same time, there is an increase in parathyroid hormone secretion and an increase in bone resorption, all of which lead to osteoporosis. This is why it is important that the smallest possible dose be used to control asthma symptoms. Inhaled corticosteroids may have a negligible effect on bone mineral density.[101]

Maintaining adequate calcium and vitamin D intake in patients on chronic steroid therapy is important.[100] Calcium supplementation may be necessary, especially if dietary intake of calcium is low.[102] Calcium supplementation alone may be insufficient to completely block the progression of corticosteroid-dependent osteoporosis.[103] Other factors that may benefit the patient are weight-bearing exercise and the avoidance of other inhibitors of osteoblast production, such as alcohol excess.[101] This is another reason why indiscriminate elimination of dairy products from the diet of a child with asthma may be harmful.

Excessive Weight Gain

Common side effects of oral corticosteroid therapy include appetite stimulation, central distribution of fat, sodium and fluid retention, and steroid-induced glucose intolerance. For the asthma patient with persistent severe disease who may require chronic oral steroid therapy to control asthma symptoms, anticipatory dietary guidance as to how to combat some of these side effects, such as limiting salt intake or limiting concentrated sweets, will be beneficial.

The growth of children with asthma should be monitored on a regular basis. Any deviation in growth parameters should be investigated. BMI should be calculated, and the BMI-for-age growth charts used to monitor overweight asthma patients and those at risk for overweight.[27] Nutrition counseling and lifestyle changes need to be emphasized by the healthcare practitioner at the first sign that an asthma patient may be at risk for overweight.

A diet that provides a variety of foods, including fruits, vegetables, and dairy products, should be encouraged. Educational tools—such as the USDA ChooseMyPlate[104], MyPyramid Tracker[105] for children, or the USDA/HHS Dietary Guidelines for Americans[106]—can be utilized. Patients and family members should be warned against eliminating whole food groups from the diet indiscriminately. Preadolescent and adolescent patients should receive information about healthy weight control practices, including regular exercise.

Some patients with asthma who have a true food allergy will require an allergen-elimination diet. (See Chapter 7 on food hypersensitivities for further details.) For asthma patients who must take oral corticosteroids on a regular basis, additional factors should be closely monitored. Adequate calcium and vitamin D intake is essential. These patients should be receiving at least the DRIs for calcium and in some instances may require calcium supplementation.[107] The patient may need to modify energy intake to maintain weight control. The registered dietitian can assist the patient in identifying ways to accomplish a healthy diet, especially if the patient develops steroid-induced hyperglycemia. Moderate exercise should be encouraged.

Complementary Medicine

Many asthma patients and their families have turned to alternative/complementary medicine therapies. Relaxation techniques, such as biofeedback training and yoga, are commonly practiced. It is important to ask about the use of specific herbal products when obtaining a diet history. Traditional Chinese medicine (TCM) herbal formulas are safe and can have a positive effect on symptoms and/or lung function in children when used as monotherapy or complementary therapy.[100]

Case Study

Nutrition Assessment of Child with Cystic Fibrosis

Client history: GB is an 11.5-year-old male with cystic fibrosis, mild lung disease, and PI. He presents to the outpatient nutrition clinic for annual nutrition evaluation.

Food/nutrition-related history: Patient reports that he generally has a good appetite. He always eats three meals per day and two to three snacks. Dietary intake from yesterday reported as:

- *Breakfast:* 1 slice of toast with peanut butter, 8 oz. whole milk with chocolate syrup, ½ banana
- *Snack:* 1 cup pretzels, water
- *Lunch:* ½ hamburger, 1 cup French fries, ½ cup peaches, 8 oz apple juice
- *Dinner:* 1 cup spaghetti with beef marinara sauce, ½ cup cooked carrots, 8 oz. whole milk
- *Snack:* apple with peanut butter

Patient and mom both agree that above intake is consistent with a typical day of eating for GB. Caloric intake is estimated approximately 1900 kcal/day. He appears to be eating a variety of foods and choosing some higher fat options for additional calories.

GB is currently swimming three to four times a week outdoors on his local swim team. He also plays basketball and baseball with his friends for fun. Mom reports that he is usually pretty active and likes to be outside with his friends.

Current nutrition-related medications include 1 AquADEK gel tab daily, ZENPEP 20 (3 with meals, 1 with snacks), and Prevacid. GB reports compliance with these meds as they are ordered every day. Mom confirms his compliance and states, "He always takes his enzymes before eating. I don't even have to remind him." He has been taking all of these medications at their current dosage for at least a year.

Nutrition-related physical findings: He complains of increased gassiness and abdominal pain after some of his meals over the past 3 to 4 months. He is stooling two to three times a day. He reports that his stools float about half of the time and recently he's noticed that there is an oil ring in the toilet. He denies weight loss.

Biochemical data, medical tests, and procedures: Chem 10 WNL, CRP WNL, vitamin A slightly low, vitamin E slightly low, vitamin D (WNL), PT WNL

Anthropometric Measurements

35 kg, 144 cm

Comparative Standards

REE: (Schofield) 1289 kcal/day (37 kcal/kg) × 1.5–1.7 = 1950–2190 kcal/day

Estimated energy needs: (RDA) 1 g protein/kg/day

Nutrition Intervention

High-calorie, high-protein diet, compliance with enzymes, and CF-specific vitamin

Nutrition Monitoring and Evaluation

1. Growth pattern indices/percentile rankings
2. Biochemical data (vitamins A and E)
3. Total energy intake
4. Intestinal (signs and symptoms of malabsorption)

Questions for the Reader

1. How many units of lipase/kg/meal is GB's current enzyme regimen providing? What is the maximum recommended unit of lipase/kg/meal?
2. His serum vitamin A and E are slightly low. Is he on the recommended dose of his CF-specific MVI (AquADEK gel tab) for his age?
3. Calculate GB's BMI and plot on the correct NCHS growth chart to determine his BMI percentile for age. What is the CF Foundation's goal BMI percentile for his age? Is he currently meeting this goal?
4. Using this data and taking into account the information presented above, please develop at least one appropriate nutrition diagnosis.
5. Using NCP terminology, identify an appropriate nutrition intervention based on the etiology of your PES statement(s). Define an ideal goal of your intervention based on the signs and symptoms mentioned in your PES statement.

REFERENCES

1. Welsh MJ, Tsui L, Boat TF, Beaudet AL. Cystic fibrosis. In: Scriver CR (ed). *The Metabolic Basis of Inherited Disease.* New York: McGraw-Hill; 1989:3799–3876.
2. Borowitz D, Durie PR, Clarke LL, et al. Gastrointestinal outcomes and confounders in cystic fibrosis. *J Pediatr Gastroenterol Nutr.* 2005;41:273–285.
3. Cystic Fibrosis Foundation. *Cystic Fibrosis Foundation Patient Registry 2008 Annual Data Report.* Bethesda, MD: Cystic Fibrosis Foundation; September 2009.
4. Riordan JR, Rommens JM, Kerem B, et al. Identification of the cystic fibrosis gene: cloning and characterization of complementary DNA. *Science.* 1989;245:1066–1073.
5. Anderson MP, Gregory RJ, Thompson S, et al. Demonstration that CFTR is a chloride channel by alteration of its anion selectivity. *Science.* 1991;253:202–205.
6. Bear CE, Li CH, Kartner N, et al. Purification and functional reconstitution of the cystic fibrosis transmembrane conductance regulator (CFTR). *Cell.* 1992;68:809–818.
7. Cheng SH, Rich DP, Marshall J, et al. Phosphorylation of the R domain by cAMP-dependent protein kinase regulates the CFTR chloride channel. *Cell.* 1991;66:1027–1036.
8. Schwiebert EM, Egan ME, Hwang TH, et al. CFTR regulates outwardly rectifying chloride channels through an autocrine mechanism involving ATP. *Cell.* 1995;81:1063–1073.
9. Stutts MJ, Canessa CM, Olsen JC, et al. CFTR as a cAMP-dependent regulator of sodium channels. *Science.* 1995;269:847–850.
10. Welsh MJ, Smith AE. Molecular mechanisms of CFTR chloride channel dysfunction in cystic fibrosis. *Cell.* 1993;73:1251–1254.
11. Cystic Fibrosis Genetic Analysis Consortium. Population variation of common cystic fibrosis mutations. *Hum Mutat.* 1994;4:167–177.
12. Farrell PM, Rosenstein BJ, White TB, et al. Guidelines for diagnosis of cystic fibrosis in newborns through older adults: Cystic Fibrosis Foundation consensus report. *J Pediatr.* 2008;153(2):4–14.
13. Tomezsko JL, Stallings VA, Kawchak DA, et al. Energy expenditure and genotype of children with cystic fibrosis. *Pediatr Res.* 1994;35:451–460.
14. O'Rawe A, McIntosh I, Dodge JA, et al. Increased energy expenditure in cystic fibrosis is associated with specific mutations. *Clin Sci.* 1992;82:71–76.
15. Murphy M, Ireton-Jones CS, Hilman BC, et al. Resting energy expenditures measured by indirect calorimetry are higher in preadolescent children with cystic fibrosis than expenditures calculated from prediction equations. *J Am Diet Assoc.* 1995;95:30–33.

16. Shepherd RW, Vasques-Velasquez L, Prentice A, et al. Increased energy expenditure in young children with cystic fibrosis. *Lancet.* 1988;135:1300–1303.
17. Vaisman N, Pencharz PB, Corey M, et al. Energy expenditure of patients with cystic fibrosis. *J Pediatr.* 1987;111:137–141.
18. Stallings VA. *New nutrition guidelines.* Presented at North American Cystic Fibrosis Conference, Baltimore, MD; October 22, 2005.
19. Food and Nutrition Board. *Recommended Dietary Allowances,* 10th ed. Washington, DC: National Academies Press; 1989.
20. Eubanks V, Koppersmith N, Wooldridge N, et al. Effects of megestrol acetate on weight gain, body composition, and pulmonary function in patients with cystic fibrosis. *J Pediatr.* 2002;140:393–395.
21. Steinkamp G, Wiedemann B, on behalf of the German CFQA Group. Relationship between nutritional status and lung function in cystic fibrosis: cross sectional and longitudinal analyses from the German CF quality assurance (CFQA) project. *Thorax.* 2002;57:596–601.
22. Cystic Fibrosis Foundation. *Pediatric Nutrition for Patients with Cystic Fibrosis. Consensus Conferences: Concepts in CF Care.* Bethesda, MD: Cystic Fibrosis Foundation; 2001:1–39.
23. Borowitz D, Baker RD, Stallings V. Consensus report on nutrition for pediatric patients with cystic fibrosis. *J Pediatr Gastroenterol Nutr.* 2002;35:246–259.
24. Cystic Fibrosis Foundation. *Clinical Practice Guidelines for Cystic Fibrosis.* Bethesda, MD: Cystic Fibrosis Foundation; 1997.
25. Sproul A, Huang N. Growth patterns in children with cystic fibrosis. *J Pediatr.* 1964;65:664–676.
26. Stallings VA, Stark LJ, Robinson KA, et al. Evidence-based practice recommendations for nutrition-related management of children and adults with cystic fibrosis and pancreatic insufficiency: results of a systematic review. *J Am Diet Assoc.* 2008;108:832–839.
27. Centers for Disease Control and Prevention, National Center for Health Statistics. CDC growth charts: United States. Available at: http://www.cdc.gov/growthcharts/clinical_charts.htm Accessed August 16, 2010.
28. Frisancho AR. New norms of upper limb fat and muscle areas for assessment of nutritional status. *Am J Clin Nutr.* 1981;34:2540–2545.
29. Heimburger DC, Weinsier RL. *Handbook of Clinical Nutrition,* 3rd ed. St. Louis, MO: Mosby; 1997.
30. Hendricks K, Duggan C. *Manual of Pediatric Nutrition,* 4th ed. Hamilton, Ontario: BC Decker; 2005.
31. Hardin DS. The diagnosis and management of cystic fibrosis related diabetes. *The Endocrinologist.* 1998;8:265–272.
32. Brunzell C, Hardin D, Schissel K, et al. Managing cystic fibrosis related diabetes (CFRD). In: *An Instruction Guide for Patients and Families,* 4th ed. Bethesda, MD: Cystic Fibrosis Foundation; 2008.
33. Aris RM, Merkel PA, Bachrach LK, et al. Consensus statement: guide to bone health and disease in cystic fibrosis. *J Clin Endocrinol Metab.* 2005;90:1888–1896.
34. Aris R, Renner JB, Winders AD, et al. Increased rate of fractures and severe kyphosis: sequelae of living to adulthood with cystic fibrosis. *Ann Intern Med.* 1998;128:186–193.
35. Shane E, Silverberg S, Silverberg SJ, et al. Osteoporosis in lung transplantation candidates with end stage pulmonary disease. *Am J Med.* 1996;101:262–269.
36. American Dietetic Association, Pediatric Nutrition Practice Group. *Pediatric Manual of Clinical Dietetics,* 2nd ed. Washington, DC: Author; 2008.
37. Crist W, McDonnell P, Beck M, et al. Behavior at mealtimes in the young child with cystic fibrosis. *J Devel Behav Pediatr.* 1994;15:157–161.
38. Kawchak D, Zhoa H, Scanlin TF, et al. Longitudinal, prospective analysis of dietary intake in children with cystic fibrosis. *J Pediatr.* 1996;129:119–129.
39. White H, Morton A, Peckham DG, et al. Dietary intakes in adult patients with cystic fibrosis—do they achieve guidelines? *J Cystic Fibrosis.* 2003;3:1–7.
40. Michel SH, Maqbool A, Hanna MD, et al. Nutrition management of pediatric patients who have cystic fibrosis. *Pediatr Clin N Am.* 2009;56:1123–1141.
41. Ellis L, Kalnins D, Corey M, et al. Do infants with cystic fibrosis need a protein hydrolysate formula? A prospective, randomized, comparative study. *J Pediatr.* 1998;132:2 70–276.
42. Winick M. *Nutrition and Pregnancy and Early Infancy.* Baltimore, MD: Williams and Wilkins; 1989.
43. Michel SH, Mueller DH. Impact of lactation on women with cystic fibrosis and their infants: a review of five cases. *J Am Diet Assoc.* 1994; 94:159–165.
44. Cystic Fibrosis Foundation. *Consensus Document: Diagnosis, Screening, and Management of Cystic Fibrosis Related Diabetes Mellitus. Consensus Conferences: Concepts in CF Care.* Bethesda, MD: Cystic Fibrosis Foundation; 1999;1–26.
45. Stark LJ, Jelalian E, Mulvihill MM, et al. Eating in preschool children with cystic fibrosis and healthy peers: behavioral analysis. *Pediatrics.* 1995;95:210–215.
46. Stark LJ, Mulvihill MM, Jelalian E, et al. Descriptive analysis of eating behavior in school-age children with cystic fibrosis and healthy control children. *Pediatrics.* 1997;99:665–671.
47. Borowitz D, Robinson KA, Rosenfield M, et al. Cystic Fibrosis Foundation evidence-based guidelines for management of infants with cystic fibrosis. *J Pediatr.* 2009;155:S73–S93.
48. Fomon SJ. *Nutrition of Normal Infants.* Philadelphia, PA: Mosby; 1993.
49. Peterson ML, Jacobs DR, Milla CE. Longitudinal changes in growth parameters are correlated with changes in pulmonary function in children with cystic fibrosis. *Pediatrics.* 2003;112:588–592.
50. Green D, Carson K, Leonard A, et al. Current treatment recommendations for correcting vitamin D deficiency in pediatric patients with cystic fibrosis are inadequate. *J Pediatr.* 2008;153:554–559.
51. Cystic Fibrosis Foundation. *Use of Pancreatic Enzyme Supplements for Patients with Cystic Fibrosis in the Context of Fibrosing Colonopathy. Consensus Conferences: Concepts in Care.* Bethesda, MD: Cystic Fibrosis Foundation; 1995:1–11.
52. Borowitz DS, Grand RJ, Durie PR, Consensus Committee. Use of pancreatic enzyme supplements for patients with cystic fibrosis in the context of fibrosing colonopathy. *J Pediatr.* 1995;127:681–684.

53. FitzSimmons SC, Burkhart GA, Borowitz D, et al. High-dose pancreatic enzyme supplements and fibrosing colonopathy in children with cystic fibrosis. *N Eng J Med.* 1997;336:1283–1289.
54. Schwarzenberg SJ, Wielinski CL, Shamieh I, et al. Cystic fibrosis-associated colitis and fibrosing colonopathy. *J Pediatr.* 1995;127:565–570.
55. Jobe AH, Bancalari E. Bronchopulmonary dysplasia. *Am J Respir Crit Care Med.* 2001;163:1723–1729.
56. Abman SH, Groothius JR. Pathophysiology and treatment of bronchopulmonary dysplasia. Current issues. *Pediatr Clinics.* 1994;41:277–315.
57. Cox JH. Bronchopulmonary dysplasia. In: Groh-Wargo S, Thompson M, Cox J (eds). *Nutritional Care for High-Risk Newborns,* 3rd ed. Chicago: Precept Press; 2000:369–390.
58. Tammela OKT, Lanning FP, Koivisto ME. The relationship of fluid restriction during the 1st month of life to the occurrence and severity of bronchopulmonary dysplasia in low birth weight infants: a 1-year radiological follow up. *Eur J Pediatr.* 1992;151:367–371.
59. Wilson DC, McClure G, Halliday HL, et al. Nutrition and bronchopulmonary dysplasia. *Arch Dis Child.* 1991;66:37–38.
60. Frank L, Sosenko IR. Undernutrition as a major contributing factor in the pathogenesis of bronchopulmonary dysplasia. *Am Rev Respir Dis.* 1988;138:725–729.
61. Giacoia GP, Venkataraman PS, West-Wilson KI, Faulkner MJ. Follow-up of school-age children with bronchopulmonary dysplasia. *J Pediatr.* 1997;130:400–408.
62. Northway WH. Bronchopulmonary dysplasia: thirty-three years later. *Pediatr Pulmonol.* 2001; Suppl 23:5–7.
63. Yunis KA, Oh W. Effects of intravenous glucose loading on oxygen consumption, carbon dioxide production, and resting energy expenditure in infants with bronchopulmonary dysplasia. *J Pediatr.* 1989;115:127–132.
64. Yeh TF, McClenan DA, Ajayi OA, Pildes RS. Metabolic rate and energy balance in infants with bronchopulmonary dysplasia. *J Pediatr.* 1989;114:448–451.
65. deGamarra E. Energy expenditure in premature newborns with bronchopulmonary dysplasia. *Biol Neonate.* 1992;61:337–344.
66. Farrell PA, Fiascone JM. Bronchopulmonary dysplasia in the 1990s: a review for the pediatrician. *Curr Probl Pediatr.* 1997;27:129–163.
67. Singer L, Martin RJ, Hawkins SW, et al. Oxygen desaturation complicates feeding in infants with bronchopulmonary dysplasia after discharge. *Pediatrics.* 1992;90:380–384.
68. Garg M, Kurzner SI, Bautista DB, Keens TG. Clinically unsuspected hypoxia during sleep and feeding in infants with bronchopulmonary dysplasia. *Pediatrics.* 1988;81:635–642.
69. Biniwale MA, Ehrenkranz RA. The role of nutrition in the prevention and management of bronchopulmonary dysplasia. *Semin Perinatol.* 2006;30:200–208.
70. Shankaran S, Szego E, Eizert D, Siegel P. Severe bronchopulmonary dysplasia: predictors of survival and outcome. *Chest.* 1984;86:607.
71. Babson SG, Benda GI. Growth graphs for the clinical assessment of infants of varying gestational age. *J Pediatr.* 1976;89:814–820.
72. Niermeyer S. Nutritional and metabolic problems in infants with bronchopulmonary dysplasia. In: Bancalari E, Stocker JT (eds). *Bronchopulmonary Dysplasia.* Washington, DC: Hemisphere Publishing; 1988;313–336.
73. Robbins ST, Fletcher AB. Early vs. delayed vitamin A supplementation in very-low-birth-weight infants. *J Parenter Enteral Nutr.* 1993;17:220–225.
74. Kennedy KA, Stoll BJ, Ehrenkranz RA, et al. Vitamin A to prevent bronchopulmonary dysplasia in very-low-birth-weight infants: has the dose been too low? *Early Human Dev.* 1997;49:19–31.
75. Tyson JE, Wright LL, Oh W, et al. Vitamin A supplementation for extremely-low-birth-weight infants. *New Eng J Med.* 1999;340:1962–1968.
76. Shenai JP. Vitamin A supplementation in very low birth weight neonates: rationale and evidence. *Pediatrics.* 1999;104:1369–1374.
77. Higashi A, Ikeda T, Iribe K, Matsuda I. Zinc balance in premature infants given the minimal dietary zinc requirement. *J Pediatr.* 1988;112:262–266.
78. American Academy of Pediatrics, Committee on Nutrition. Kleinman RE (ed). *Pediatric Nutrition Handbook,* 5th ed. Elk Grove Village, IL: American Academy of Pediatrics; 2004.
79. Reimers KJ, Carlson SJ, Lombard KA. Nutritional management of infants with bronchopulmonary dysplasia. *Nutr Clin Prac.* 1992;7:127–132.
80. Johnson D. Gaining and growing: assuring nutritional care of preterm infants. University of Washington. Available at: http://depts.washington.edu/growing. Accessed August 16, 2010.
81. Gewolb IH, Bosma JF, Taciak VL, Vice FL. Abnormal developmental patterns of suck and swallow rhythms during feeding in preterm infants with bronchopulmonary dysplasia. *Dev Med Child Neur.* 2001;43:454–459.
82. Centers for Disease Control and Prevention, National Center for Health Statistics. Summary health statistics for U.S. children: National Health Interview Survey, 2008. Available at: http://www.cdc.gov/nchs/data/series/sr_10/sr10_244.pdf. Accessed January 14, 2010.
83. Centers for Disease Control and Prevention, National Center for Health Statistics. The state of childhood asthma: United States, 1980–2005. Available at: http://www.cdc.gov/nchs/data/ad/ad381.pdf. Accessed January 27, 2010.
84. Centers for Disease Control and Prevention. Asthma prevalence and control characteristics by race/ethnicity: United States, 2002. *MMWR.* 2004;53:145–148.
85. Rodriguez MA, Winkleby MA, Ahn D, et al. Identification of population subgroups of children and adolescents with high asthma prevalence. *Arch Pediatr Adolesc Med.* 2002;156:269–275.
86. Johnston J. Lower respiratory disorders. In: Millonig VL, Mobley C (eds). *Pediatric Nurse Practitioner Certification Review Guide,* 4th ed. Potomac, MD: Health Leadership Associates, Inc. 2004;135–151.
87. National Heart, Lung and Blood Institute. Expert panel report 3: guidelines for the diagnosis and management of asthma. August 2007. Available at: http://www.nhlbi.nih.gov/guidelines/asthma/asthgdln.htm. Accessed January 27, 2010.
88. Sampson HA. IgE-mediated food intolerance. *J Allergy Clin Immunol.* 1988;81:495–504.
89. National Asthma Education and Prevention Program, National Heart, Lung and Blood Institute. *Expert Panel Report: Guidelines for the Diagnosis and Management of Asthma—Update of Selected Topics 2002.* Bethesda, MD: National Institutes of Health; 2002. Pub no. 02-5075.

90. Ozol D, Mete E. Asthma and food allergy. *Curr Opin Pulm Med.* 2008;14(1):9–12.
91. Beausoleil J, Fiedler J, Spergel J. Food intolerance and childhood asthma: what is the link? *Paediatr Drugs.* 2007;9(3):157–163.
92. Schroeder A, Kumar R. Food allergy is associated with an increased risk of asthma. *Clin Exp Allergy.* 2009;39(2):261–270.
93. Spector SL, Surette ME. Diet and asthma: has the role of dietary lipids been overlooked in the management of asthma? *Ann Allergy Asthma Immunol.* 2003;90:371–377.
94. Morris A, Noakes M, Clifton PM. The role of Ω-6 polyunsaturated fat in stable asthmatics. *J Asthma.* 2001;38:311–319.
95. Price JF. Asthma, growth and inhaled corticosteroids. *Resp Med.* 1993;87:23–26.
96. Merkus PJFM, van Essen-Zandvliet EEM, Duiverman EJ, et al. Long-term effect of inhaled corticosteroids on growth rate in adolescents with asthma. *Pediatrics.* 1993;91:1121–1126.
97. Agertoft L, Pedersen S. Effects of long-term treatment with an inhaled corticosteroid on growth and pulmonary function in asthmatic children. *Resp Med.* 1994;88:373–381.
98. Allen DB, Bronshky EA, LaForce CF, et al. Growth in asthmatic children treated with fluticasone propionate. *J Pediatr.* 1998;132:472–477.
99. Sharek PJ, Bergman DA. The effect of inhaled steroids on the linear growth of children with asthma: a meta-analysis. *Pediatr.* 2000;106. Available at: http://www.pediatrics.org/cgi/content/full/106/1/e8. Accessed February 1, 2002.
100. Hosking DJ. Effects of corticosteroids on bone turnover. *Resp Med.* 1993;87:15–21.
101. Allen DB. Inhaled corticosteroid therapy for asthma in preschool children: growth issues. *Pediatrics.* 2002;109:373–380.
102. Boner AL, Piacentini GL. Inhaled corticosteroids in children. Is there a "safe" dosage? *Drug Safety.* 1993;9:9–20.
103. Picado C, Luengo M. Corticosteroid-induced bone loss. *Drug Safety.* 1996;15:347–359.
104. U.S. Department of Agriculture. MyPlate. Available at: http://www.choosemyplate.gov. Accessed July 15, 2011.
105. U.S. Department of Agriculture. Center for Nutrition Policy and Promotion. Available at: http://www.mypyramidtracker.gov. Accessed August 9, 2011.
106. U.S. Department of Agriculture, U.S. Department of Health and Human Services. Dietary Guidelines for Americans, 2010. Available at: http://www.health.gov/dietaryguidelines/dga2010/DietaryGuidelines2010.pdf. Accessed August 9, 2011.
107. Institute of Medicine, Food and Nutrition Board. *Dietary Reference Intakes for Calcium, Phosphorus, Magnesium, Vitamin D, and Fluoride.* Washington, DC: National Academies Press; 1997.
108. Xiu-Min L. Complementary and alternative medicine in pediatric allergic disorders. *Curr Opin Allergy Clin Immunol.* 2009;9:161–167.

CHAPTER 12

Gastrointestinal Disorders

Amanda Croll, Sarah Weston, Jennifer Autodore, and Jenni Beary

The gastrointestinal (GI) tract can be thought of as a tube that processes and absorbs nutrients. The function of the GI tract can be disrupted by disease, injury, chemotherapy drugs, antibiotics, parasites, environmental toxins, or bacterial overgrowth, resulting in alteration of nutritional requirements. Many nutrients are absorbed throughout the intestinal tract, whereas others are absorbed only at specific sites. Absorption of the latter class of nutrients is particularly vulnerable to disease or surgical resection. **Figure 12-1** graphically portrays the principal sites of absorption of macro- and micronutrients, vitamins, and minerals.

Symptoms of GI disease can arise from disorders located in a specific region of the bowel, the entire bowel, or distant sites (e.g., vomiting can occur due to pyloric stenosis or a brain tumor). Common pediatric GI disorders are listed in **Table 12-1**; common diagnostic tests are provided in **Table 12-2**. Many tests are available to evaluate GI function as well as the presence or absence of disease.

Acute Diarrhea

Diarrhea is defined as the passage of three or more loose, watery stools per day or as 10 mL/kg liquid stool per day.[1,2] A child having diarrhea for 3 to 7 days is among the most common reasons for seeking a pediatrician.[3,4] Practice parameters and guidelines delineate treatment depending on the presence of dehydration.[3,5,6] General principles of diarrhea management include replacement of fluid and electrolyte losses and nutritional therapy with age-appropriate feeding.[1] The composition of commonly used oral maintenance and rehydration solutions is presented in **Table 12-3**.

Nutrition Management

Nutrition management varies with the degree of dehydration. The different stages of dehydration are based on the following physical signs:

- *Mild:* Slightly dry mucous membranes, increased thirst
- *Moderate:* Sunken eyes, sunken fontanelle, loss of skin turgor, dry mucous membranes
- *Severe:* Signs of moderate dehydration plus one or more of the following: rapid thready (scarcely perceptible) pulse, cyanosis, rapid breathing, delayed capillary refill time, lethargy, coma[3]

A normal diet should be continued throughout periods of mild diarrhea with no dehydration, including breastfeeding or full-strength infant formula and a regular diet. Beverages high in sugar, such as juices and sodas, should be excluded. Increased fluid intake is necessary to compensate for losses. Infants and children who are not dehydrated can be kept hydrated using frequent breastfeeding, infant formula, or milk. The use of lactose-free formula is not recommended in managing acute diarrhea.[3,7] Using a regular diet as treatment for mild diarrhea does not change the volume of diarrhea and requires education of parents concerning treatment goals of maintaining a regular diet and hydration.[3] Most infants and children demonstrate hunger and thirst during mild, acute diarrheal illness, and parents can respond to these cues. The BRAT diet (bananas, rice, applesauce, tea, and toast) should be avoided because it is low in calories and is not a balanced source of nutrition. However, foods that are high in carbohydrates, such as rice, wheat, peas, and potatoes, may slow diarrheal output.

Increased fluid intake is necessary to compensate for losses during periods of mild to moderate diarrhea.[3] The use of oral rehydration solutions (ORS) helps to replace fluid and electrolyte losses from diarrhea. Dehydration can be treated at home by giving an ORS solution by syringe at the rate of 1 teaspoon (5 mL) per minute over 4 hours for a child less than 15 kg or 2 teaspoons (5–10 mL) for children 15–20 kg. This method of fluid administration is adequate to replace the fluid deficit within a 4-hour period. After 1 to 2 hours of this treatment, the infant or child may begin voluntarily accepting the rehydration liquid. If the child or infant is not cooperative, a nasogastric (NG) tube may be used at home or in the hospital. After correction of dehydration, age-appropriate feeding should be initiated as described above.

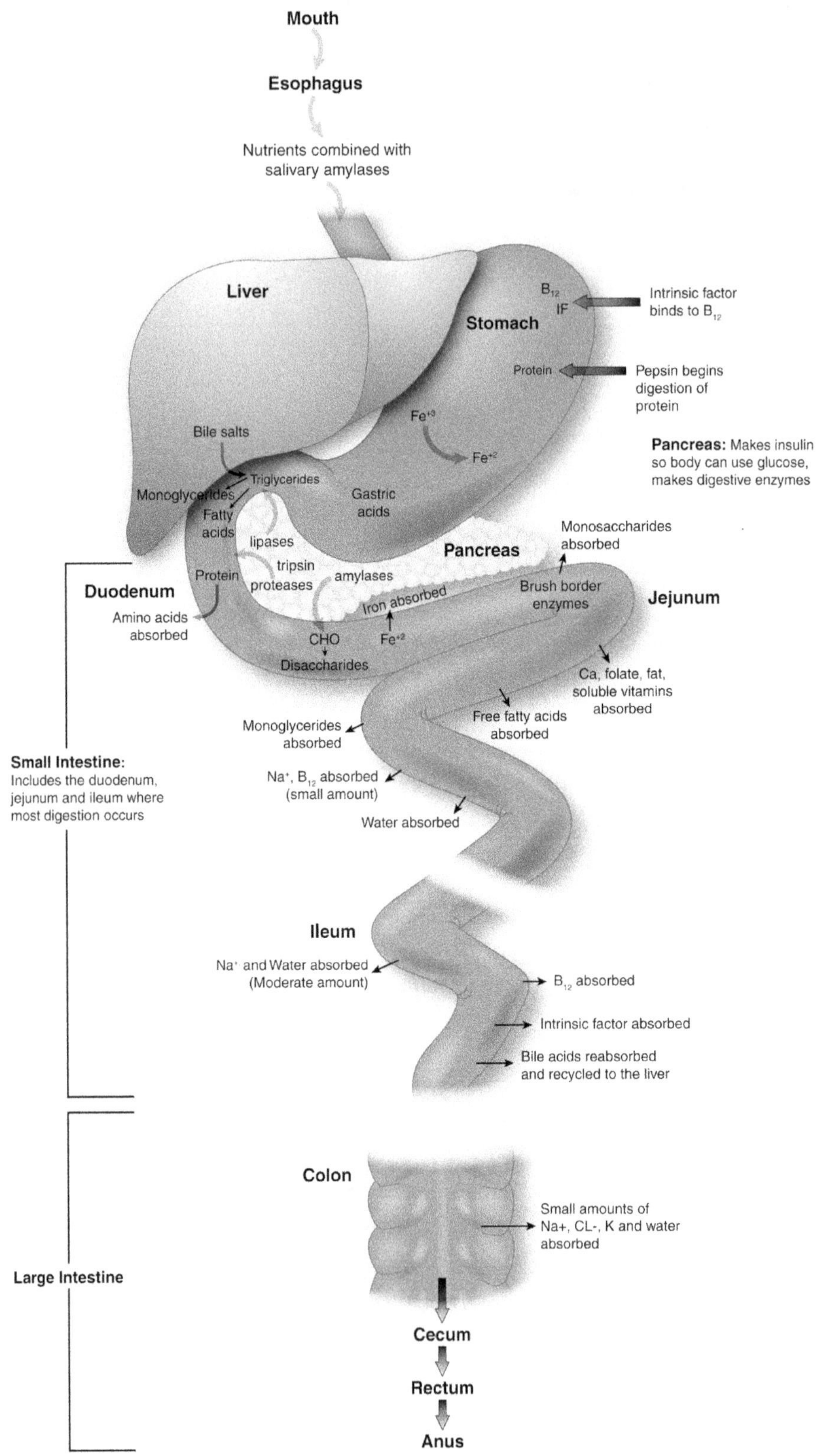

FIGURE 12-1 Principle Sites of Absorption

TABLE 12-1 Common Pediatric Gastrointestinal Disorders

Presenting Symptom	Differential Diagnosis	Treatment
Stomach and Esophagus		
Vomiting/regurgitation	Congenital anomaly of the gastrointestinal tract	Surgery
	Gastroesophageal reflux	Infants: positioning, medications such as antacids, H2 blockers, and proton pump inhibitors (PPI). If preceding fails, consider surgical treatment.
		All ages: medications, antacids, H2 blockers, PPI, avoid caffeine-containing foods and other personal triggers
	Eosinophilic esophagitis	Elimination diet, swallowed steroids
	Eosinophilic gastritis	Steroids, immunosuppressive medication
	Peptic disease	Medications such as antacids, H2 blockers, and PPI; avoid caffeine-containing foods and other personal triggers
	H. pylori	Antibiotics, PPI
	Gastroparesis	Prokinetics, diet changes such as multiple small low-fat meals per day, or postpyloric feeds
Dysphagia (choking after eating), odynophagia (pain with swallowing)	Congenital anomalies, strictures, webs	Surgery
	Eosinophilic esophagitis	Elimination diet, swallowed steroids
	Esophageal spasms/dysmotility	Calcium channel blockers and nitrates; avoid extreme temperatures in foods
	Peptic strictures	Medications such as antacids, H2 blockers, and PPI; dilation
Liver and Pancreas		
Jaundice	Extrahepatic biliary tract obstruction, such as biliary atresia	Surgical correction; diet/formula with medium chain triglycerides (MCT), fat-soluble vitamin supplementation, choleretic agents such as ursodeoxycholate
	Autoimmune hepatitis	Steroids, evaluation for fat malabsorption, fat-soluble vitamin supplementation, protein restriction only if encephalopathic
Jaundice with recurrent abdominal pain	Gallstones	Surgery
	Choledochal cyst	Surgery
Nausea, vomiting, abdominal pain	Pancreatitis	NPO; if severe or prolonged course expected then postplyoric tube feeds or parenteral nutrition; pain control, H2 blockers; when clinically able, resume low-fat oral diet
	Pancreatic pseudocyst	Monitor cyst size; if cyst increases with enteral nutrition, may require parenteral nutrition
Chronic diarrhea, failure to thrive	Pancreatic insufficiency, such as cystic fibrosis	Enzyme replacement therapy, fat-soluble vitamin supplementation, high calorie balanced diet
	Cholestatic disease	Diet/formula with MCT, fat-soluble vitamin supplementation
Small Bowel and Colon		
Anemia, gastrointestinal bleeding	Congenital malformations, such as Meckel's diverticulum, duplication cysts	Surgery
Vomiting	Food allergies	Hydrolysate formula, elimination diet
	Infectious enteropathies	Oral rehydration solutions, followed by lactose and/or sucrose restrictions
Diarrhea in neonatal period	Congenital disorders of carbohydrate absorption and transport	Restriction of the problematic carbohydrate, balanced nutrition, vitamin/mineral supplementation, enzyme replacement
Diarrhea, perioral and perianal rash	Zinc deficiency	Zinc supplementation

(continues)

TABLE 12-1 *(Continued)*

Presenting Symptom	Differential Diagnosis	Treatment
Diarrhea	Food allergies	Elemental formula and/or elimination diet
	Infectious enteropathies	Intravenous fluids, oral rehydration solutions, followed by lactose and/or sucrose restrictions if clinically indicated
	Crohn's disease	Enteral feeds for therapy and/or malnutrition, replete iron, fat-soluble vitamins, and zinc as necessary; monitor vitamin B_{12} if severe ileal disease or resection
	Ulcerative colitis	Enteral feeds for weight gain, replete iron as necessary, low-residue diet if strictures
	Celiac disease	Gluten-free diet
	Short bowel syndrome	Parenteral nutrition progressing to enteral nutrition to oral feeds; vitamin and mineral supplements specific to patient's condition
	Fructose intolerance	Dietary restrictions of fructose-containing foods
	Lactose intolerance	Dietary restrictions of lactose-containing foods
Diarrhea, normal growth pattern	Irritable bowel syndrome, chronic nonspecific diarrhea, toddler's diarrhea	Normal diet for age, increased soluble fiber intake, decreased intake of sorbitol-containing beverages (apple and pear juice) and other personal triggers
Abdominal distention/ pain	Celiac disease	Gluten-free diet
	Short bowel syndrome	Total parenteral nutrition progressing to MCT-predominate hydrolysate formula; vitamin and mineral supplements
	Functional constipation	Complete bowel clean-out using saline enemas, mineral oil, Miralax; high-fiber diet and adequate fluids; bowel habit training
	Congenital disorders of carbohydrate absorption and transport	Restriction of the problematic carbohydrate, balanced nutrition, vitamin/mineral supplementation, enzyme replacement
	Fructose intolerance	Dietary restrictions of fructose-containing foods
	Lactose intolerance	Dietary restrictions of lactose-containing foods
Constipation	Hirschsprung's disease; post-NEC strictures	Surgery
	Functional constipation	Complete bowel clean-out using saline enemas, mineral oil, Miralax; high-fiber diet and adequate fluids; bowel habit training

TABLE 12-2 Common Diagnostic Tests for Pediatric Gastrointestinal Disorders

Test	Description	Useful to Help Diagnose
Barium enema	Barium sulfate administered by enema; colonic lumen and mucosa visualized by fluoroscopy.	Colonic strictures and obstructions Hirschsprung's disease Polyps
Barium swallow	Barium sulfate administered orally; upper gastrointestinal tract is visualized by fluoroscopy.	Aspiration Dysmotility disorders Hiatal hernias Strictures Varices
Breath hydrogen test	Oral administration of sugar and expiratory collection of hydrogen as an indirect measure of bacterial fermentation of unabsorbed carbohydrate.	Fructose malabsorption Lactose malabsorption Bacterial overgrowth
DXA (dual energy X-ray absorptiometry)	Measures bone density in the spine, hip, or forearm.	Osteomalacia Osteopenia Osteoporosis

TABLE 12-2 *(Continued)*

Test	Description	Useful to Help Diagnose
Colonoscopy	Insertion of flexible fiber optic tube via anus into large bowel; visual examination of colonic lining, biopsies obtained.	Colitis Polyps
CT (computed tomography scan) of abdomen	Multiple radiographs of abdomen with or without intraluminal and/or intravenous contrast; computer reconstructs multiple images to generate "slices" through the abdomen.	Areas of inflammation (e.g., abscess) Blood vessel anatomy and obstructions Organ size and consistency Tumors
EGD (esophagogastroduodenoscopy)	Fiber optic tube is inserted into upper gastrointestinal tract allowing mucosal lining of upper GI tract to be visualized and biopsies to be taken.	Celiac disease Duodenitis Esophagitis, including esosinophilic esopahgitis (EE) Gastritis Peptic ulcer disease
Fecal fat test	Concurrent 3-day diet record of fat intake and stool collection; comparison as percentage of total fat in 24 hours excreted in stool. Malabsorption indicated in children if greater than 7% of fat is excreted; for infants less than 6 months of age if greater than 15% of fat is excreted.	Fat malabsorption Pancreatic insufficiency
pH probe	Tube with pH sensor is inserted into esophagus for 24 hours with feeding at regulated intervals.	Gold standard for gastroesophageal reflux
Scintigraphy ("milk scan")	Barium ingested with X-rays capturing movement through upper GI tract	Delayed gastric emptying Pulmonary aspiration
Ultrasound	Can be of all abdominal organs or individual organs such as the stomach, intestines, gallbladder, liver, spleen, pancreas, kidney, and bladder	Anatomical abnormalities Cysts Obstructions Stones Tumors
Upper GI/upper GI with small bowel follow-through.	Barium ingested with X-ray monitoring of path in GI tract to duodenum or to ileum if small bowel follow through.	Anatomical abnormalities Inflammation Tumors
X-ray of abdomen		Bowel dilatation or obstruction Calcified gall bladder stones Gas patterns and free air Presence of stool in GI tract Pnuematosis Toxic megacolon

Sources: Corkins MR, Scolapino J. Diarrhea. In: Merritt R (ed). *The ASPEN Nutrition Support Practice Manual,* 2nd ed. Silver Spring, MD: ASPEN; 2005:207–210; Graham-Maar RC, French HM, Piccoli DA. Gastroenterology. In: Frank G, Shah SS, Catallozzi M, Zaoutis LB (eds). *The Philadelphia Guide: Inpatient Pediatrics.* Philadelphia, PA: Lippincott, Williams, and Wilkins; 2003:100–115; and Leonberg BL. *ADA Pocket Guide to Pediatric Nutrition Assessment.* Chicago: American Dietetic Association; 2008:106.

Severe dehydration in infants and children with diarrhea is a medical emergency and requires immediate hospitalization. Once rehydration is complete, age-appropriate feeding can be resumed.

Nutrients and GI Effects

Lactose-containing products, especially when given with complex carbohydrates, do not increase diarrheal output or prolong the illness unless stool output clearly increases on a lactose-containing diet.[8]

For infants, the use of soy formula with added fiber is not a standard of care because continuation of breast feeding or usual formula works to correct dehydration in most cases. The key is to return to age-appropriate feedings as soon as rehydration is accomplished.

TABLE 12-3 Oral Rehydrating Solutions (ORS)

Solution	Glucose/ CHO (g/L)	Sodium (mEq/L)	Potassium (mEq/L)	Osmolality (mmol/L)	CHO/Sodium
Pedialyte (Abbott, Columbus, Ohio)	25	45	20	250	3.1
Pediatric Electrolyte (PendoPharm, Montreal, Quebec)	25	45	30	250	3.1
Kaolectrolyte (Pfizer, New York, New York)	20	48	20	240	2.4
Rehydralyte (Abbott, Columbus, Ohio)	25	75	20	310	1.9
WHO, ORS, 2002 (reduced osmolarity)	75	75	30	224	1
WHO, ORS, 1975 (original formulation)	111	90	20	311	1.2
Cola*	126	2	0.1	750	1944
Apple juice*	125	3	32	730	1278
Gatorade* (Gatorade, Chicago, Illinois)	45	20	3	330	62.5
Whole cow's milk	12 (lactose)	40	1226	285	Not available

*Cola, juice, and Gatorade are shown for comparison only; they are not recommended for use.

Abbreviations: CHO, carbohydrate; WHO, World Health Organization.

Sources: Adapted from Oral therapy for acute diarrhea. In: Kleinman RE (ed). *Pediatric Nutrition Handbook*, 6th ed. Elk Grove Village, IL: American Academy of Pediatrics; 2009:651–659; and Roberts J, Shilkofski N. *The Harriet Lane Handbook*, 17th ed. Elsevier Mosby; 2005:559,Table 20–14a.

Use of probiotics and prebiotics in infant and enteral formulas and in foods may be beneficial in the treatment of acute and chronic diarrhea of infancy and childhood. *Probiotics* are live microorganisms, historically available in fermented foods such as yogurt, that promote health by improving the balance of healthy organisms in the intestinal tract.[5] *Prebiotics* are complex carbohydrates, not microorganisms, that promote the growth of healthy microorganisms in the intestinal tract.[5] Human milk contains oligosaccharides (a type of prebiotic) that promote the growth of *Lactobacilli* and *Bifidobacteria* in the colon of breastfed infants.[5,9] Higher intake of breast milk is associated with a lowered incidence of acute diarrhea.[10]

Questions about consuming live probiotic bacteria and prebiotics include whether long-term consumption is safe and whether it has positive health effects. There is still no consensus concerning the types and amounts of probiotics that are beneficial. Infant formulas with prebiotics and probiotics include Nutramigen with Enflora LGG (probiotic, *Lactobacillus rhamnosus* GG) by Mead Johnson, Similac Advance EarlyShield (galactooligosaccharide) by Abbott, and Enfamil PREMIUM with Triple Health Guard (galactooligosaccharide) by Mead Johnson.

An example of an enteral formula for children older than 1 year of age supplemented with probiotics is Boost Kids Essentials 1.0 and 1.5 (*L. reuteri* inserted in optional straw to use for drinking) by Nestle. Examples of products using prebiotics include Pediasure enteral formula with fiber (NutraFlora and scFOS) by Abbott; Vital Jr (NutraFlora and scFOS), also from Abbott; and Peptamen Jr with fiber (contains insoluble fiber and Prebio, a blend of FOS and inulin) and Peptamen Jr with Prebio (no insoluble fiber) by Nestle.

Chronic Diarrhea

Diarrheal illnesses in children follow a continuum from acute to chronic or persistent diarrhea. Persistent or chronic diarrhea is defined as "diarrhea episodes of presumed infectious etiology that begin acutely but last at least 14 days."[11] Persistent diarrhea has also been defined as "the passage of ≥ 3 watery stools per day for > 2 weeks in a child who either fails to gain or loses weight."[12] Persistent diarrhea has many triggers, including acute diarrhea caused by an enteric infection, HIV infection, and AIDS.[12]

The four kinds of chronic diarrheal disease include osmotic, secretory, dysmotility, and inflammatory:

- *Osmotic diarrhea* may result from congenital or acquired disease and is often associated with failure to absorb a specific carbohydrate, such as lactose, or with excessive carbohydrate intake, such as excessive juice intake in toddlers, or dietary fructose intolerance.[13] Diarrhea stops when the dietary cause is removed.
- *Secretory diarrhea* does not respond to cessation of oral intake. Disorders include congenital choridorrhea and neural crest tumors.[13]
- *Diarrhea from dysmotility* may be associated with rapid transit or irritable bowel syndrome.
- *Inflammatory diarrhea* may result from enteric infection, inflammation secondary to celiac disease, or inflammatory bowel disease. Chronic or persistent diarrhea (also called intractable diarrhea of infancy) has been thought of as a nutritional disorder, and certainly requires nutritional treatment for recovery.[14–18]

Malnutrition is considered the most important risk factor for persistent diarrhea when no specific congenital, inherited, or acquired disorders are identified. Other associated risk factors are:

- Younger than 6 months of age
- Acute diarrheal episode within the past 2 months
- Zinc deficiency
- Lack of breastfeeding
- Male sex
- Infection with enteropathogenic or enteroaggregative *Escherichia coli* or *Cryptosporidium*
- A history of intrauterine growth retardation[12]

If infection as a cause is excluded, other etiologies must be considered. These include food allergy, dietary protein intolerances, celiac disease, lactose or other disaccharide intolerances, cystic fibrosis and other causes of pancreatic insufficiency, and inflammatory bowel disease.[19] (See Chapters 7 and Chapter 11 for information on food allergies and cystic fibrosis, respectively.) Chronic diarrhea is dangerous if not treated promptly and appropriately, because it can result in dehydration and severe malnutrition.[16]

Nutrition Management

The first step is appropriate fluid resuscitation. Next, cautious refeeding through a combination of enteral feedings and/or parenteral nutrition is started slowly due to the possibility of metabolic alterations from refeeding syndrome.[20] Key nutrients such as potassium, phosphorus, magnesium, calcium, and trace elements should be monitored closely. Continued use of breast milk is recommended during infancy.[12] Continuously infused breast milk loses calories through adherence of protein and lipids on the tube walls; this factor should be considered when making calorie determinations.[21,22] Alterations in the continuous infusion-feeding method can be made to maximize nutrient delivery by using the shortest amount of tubing available and slanting the feeding syringe.[23] Another option is to use a formula for the continuous infusion for greater lipid delivery, saving the expressed breast milk for oral feedings.[24] Oral zinc supplementation may be needed, especially in infants and children with malnutrition or history of multiple episodes of acute or persistent diarrhea.[25–27] Carbohydrate intolerance may or may not exist, and tolerance should be monitored. Adequate normal amounts of foods containing energy, protein, fat, and vitamins can be given.[28]

Absorption of many nutrients may be improved by continuous enteral feedings. Small bolus oral feedings may be retained for oral motor stimulation. The calories needed for catch-up growth may be in the range of 140–200 kcal/kg.[29] Nutritional support may start at 75 kcal/kg/day and increase over 5 to 7 days to 130–150 kcal/kg/day. Protein is started at 1–2 g/kg/day, increasing to 3–4 g/kg/day as caloric intake increases.[11] Mild zinc deficiency may play a role in both acute and chronic diarrhea. Zinc supplementation may result in a decrease in number of stools per day and decreased number of days with watery diarrhea.[30] In children with acute and persistent diarrhea, zinc supplementation is recommended:

- 10 mg/day for 10 to 14 days for infants younger than 6 months of age
- 20 mg/day for 10 to 14 days for infants and children older than 6 months of age[25]

Cereal and other infant foods should be continued as tolerated; however, juices and sodas should be avoided due to their high osmolality. For infants with malnutrition or who are severely dehydrated, use of a lactose-free formula may lead to quicker recovery.[8] Semi-elemental protein hydrolysate formulas such as Alimentum (Abbott) or Pregestimil (Mead Johnson) may be also used. A semi-elemental formula may be superior to an elemental amino acid–based formula such as Neocate (SHNA), Elecare (Abbott), or Nutramigen AA (Mead Johnson).

As the infant improves, parenteral nutrition or IV hydration can be weaned, and enteral nutrition gradually increased in the form of continuous feedings. Gradually larger bolus oral feedings can be added as tolerated. If this period of progressing from parenteral to enteral nutrition is prolonged, the transition from continuous feeding to oral bolus feedings can be done in the home setting.

Constipation

Constipation is common in childhood and is defined as "a delay or difficulty in defecation, present for two or more weeks and sufficient to cause significant stress to the patient."[31] Treatment in infants may include juices that contain natural sorbitol, such as apple, pear, or prune (0.5 g/100 g, 2.1 g/100 g, and 12.7 g/100 g, respectively); increasing fluids; and verifying that infant formula is mixed correctly.[31] Rice cereal, a common first food for infants, may also cause constipation that resolves when infant oatmeal is used instead. Inadequate fluid intake also can be a cause of constipation.[32] High fiber diets with adequate fluids are recommended as the first line of therapy in children. Recommended fiber intake for children by age is listed in Appendix G-1. "Age plus 5" is an easy way to estimate fiber intake.[33] This estimation never exceeds, but may underestimate, fiber requirements. Fiber supplements may be used when dietary intake is inadequate. When fiber alone fails, lubricants and laxatives may be required. The fiber content of common foods is presented in **Table 12-4.**

Medications such as phenytoin may slow peristalsis, and diuretics that alter fluid balance may cause constipation as well.[32] Mothers may believe the iron contained in formula causes constipation, but iron in formula is not associated with adverse side effects, including constipation.[32,34–37] Iron-fortified infant formula is recommended for the first year of life to prevent anemia.[37]

TABLE 12-4 Good Sources of Dietary Fiber

	Grams of Fiber	Serving Size
Fruit		
Apple	2.2	1 med. w/skin
Apple	2	1 med. w/o skin
Apricot, dried	7.8	3 oz
Blueberries	4.4	1 cup raw
Dates, dried	4.2	10
Kiwi	3.4	3 oz
Pear	4.1	1 med. raw
Prunes, dried	7.2	3 oz
Prunes, stewed	6.6	3 oz
Raisins	5.3	3 oz
Raspberries	5.8	1 cup
Strawberries, raw	2.8	1 cup
Vegetables and Legumes		
Avocado, California, raw	3	1 med.
Beans, black, boiled	7.2	1 cup
Beans, great northern, boiled	6	1 cup
Beans, kidney, boiled	6.4	1 cup
Beans, lima, boiled	6.2	1 cup
Beans, baby lima, boiled	7.8	1 cup
Beans, navy, boiled	6.6	1 cup
Beans, green, canned	6.8	½ cup
Broccoli, boiled	2.2	½ cup
Chickpeas (garbanzo beans)	5.7	1 cup
Cowpeas (black-eyed peas)	4.4	1 cup
Lentils, boiled	7.9	1 cup

	Grams of Fiber	Serving Size
Ready-to-Eat Cereal		
FiberOne (General Mills)	14	½ cup
All-Bran (Kellogg's)	10	½ cup
100% Bran (Post)	9	⅓ cup
Shredded Wheat and Bran (Post)	8	1¼ cup
Raisin Bran (Post)	8	1 cup
Grape-Nuts (Post)	7	½ cup
Multi Bran Chex (General Mills)	6	¾ cup
Cracklin' Oat Bran (Kellogg's)	6	¾ cup
Mini Wheats (Kellogg's)	6	1 cup (30 biscuits)
Frosted Mini Wheats with raisins (Kellogg's)	6	¾ cup (24 biscuits)
Shredded Wheat (Post)	6	1 cup
Mini Wheats with strawberries (Kellogg's)	5	¾ cup (24 biscuits)
Wheat Chex (General Mills)	5	¾ cup
Bran Flakes (Post)	5	¾ cup
Banana Nut Crunch (Post)	4	1 cup
Raisin Bran Pecan Date Crunch (Post)	4	½ cup
Cranberry Almond Crunch	3	¾ cup
Low Fat Granola (Kellogg's)	3	½ cup
Grape-Nut Flakes (Post)	3	¾ cup

Source: Data for sections on fruits and vegetables/legumes from Pennington JAT. *Bowes and Church's Food Values of Portions Commonly Used*, 15th ed. Philadelphia: JB Lippincott; 1989; and U.S. Department of Agriculture. *USDA Provisional Table on the Dietary Fiber Content of Selected Foods*; 1988. HNIS/PT-106; data for section on ready-to-eat cereals from a survey of manufacturer's Websites as of November 2009.

When stooling is chronically difficult or painful, children may withhold stool, aggravating the existing problem. Encopresis may result due to the stretched rectal wall, allowing softer stool to leak out involuntarily.[32] A bowel program after a thorough clean-out often includes a high-fiber diet, adequate fluid, and increased physical activity.

Gastroesophageal Reflux

Gastroesophageal reflux (GER) is the passage of gastric contents into the esophagus and is a normal physiologic process that occurs throughout the day.[38] GER may include regurgitation and vomiting. Recurrent vomiting usually peaks at 4 months of age and resolves by 10 to 12 months when the infant achieves a more upright posture. When GER causes multiple vomiting episodes or interferes with growth, it is called gastroesophageal reflux disease (GERD).[38]

The "happy spitter" is an infant who has frequent episodes of regurgitation but continues to grow well. Parental education concerning the expected improvement as the infant develops is all that is necessary. If the infant is not growing well or has increased irritability, changes in feeding are recommended. If GER is a symptom of an allergy to cow's milk protein, symptoms may resolve with a change to an extensively hydrolyzed or amino acid formula. If the infant is breastfed, elimination of cow's milk and egg from the mother's diet may also improve symptoms. Discontinuation of breastfeeding is rarely recommended. Decreasing volume of each feeding and offering more frequent feedings may also improve GER symptoms; however, total intake may decrease with this change.[39] Thickened formula may decrease the number of vomiting episodes but does not reduce the number of reflux episodes.[39,40] Use of infant rice or oatmeal cereal to thicken formula may result in too rapid weight gain and decrease the percentage of calories provided by protein and fat. Use of antiregurgitant formulas such as Enfamil AR (Mead Johnson) may similarly reduce the number of vomiting episodes but not decrease the number of reflux episodes. If the infant is diagnosed with failure to thrive, increasing the caloric density of formula is recommended, especially if extensively hydrolyzed or amino acid formulas have improved symptoms. Although GER symptoms do improve in the flat prone position, prone positioning is not recommended with infants because of its association with sudden infant death syndrome (SIDS). The semi-supine position, such as in a car seat, worsens symptoms. Simple GER usually resolves around 18 months of age. GERD usually requires medical management.[39]

In older children and adolescents, there is no evidence that changes in diet improve symptoms. Children and adolescents should eliminate caffeine, chocolate, spicy foods, and alcohol.[39] Left-sided sleeping in adolescents also may improve symptoms.

Lactose

Lactose intolerance is the inability to metabolize and digest lactose, which is the sugar most commonly found in milk and milk products. It is caused by a shortage of the enzyme lactase, which is produced by the cells that line the small intestine.[41] People who lack this enzyme are unable to metabolize and completely digest lactose into its simpler forms—glucose and galactose. This results in digestive discomfort such as abdominal cramping, bloating, flatulence, and diarrhea.

Lactose intolerance is commonly diagnosed noninvasively via a breath hydrogen test. Following the ingestion of a lactose-containing beverage, the patient blows into a balloon-like bag at intervals for a specified amount of time. Intermittent samples are taken and analyzed. Carbohydrate that is malabsorbed in the small intestine is fermented by colonic bacteria and releases hydrogen gas.[42] A raised hydrogen breath level signifies the inability to digest lactose. For details on a lactose-controlled diet, please refer to the *Pediatric Manual of Clinical Dietetics*.[43]

Primary lactase deficiency is common.[41,44,45] Prevalence and age of onset vary secondary to ethnicity and overall use of dairy products in the diet.[45] It is estimated that 20% of Hispanic, Asian, and black children younger than age of 5 "have evidence of lactase deficiency and lactose malabsorption" as opposed to Caucasian children, who typically do not develop symptoms of lactose intolerance until after the age of 4 or 5.[41,46] Children who present with symptoms of lactose intolerance before the age of 2 to 3 years should receive a more complete evaluation, because secondary lactase deficiency may have developed from an unknown etiology.[41]

Secondary lactase deficiency may occur if the lining of the small intestine that houses lactase-containing epithelial cells is destroyed as a direct result of the following:

- Underlying disease (e.g., celiac disease)
- Small intestinal resection
- Gastrectomy
- Chemotherapy treatments
- Parasitic infections (e.g., giardiasis)
- Acute diarrheal disease

Elimination of lactose from the diet is generally not required for the treatment of secondary lactase deficiency and lactose malabsorption.[41] Treatment of the underlying condition is key. Once the primary issue is resolved, lactose-containing products can be reintroduced according to individual tolerance.[41]

In utero, lactase is the last of the major intestinal disaccharidases to develop.[47] Lactase activity is low prior to 24 weeks gestation.[48] It then begins to increase but remains deficient until 34 weeks gestation.[41,48] As a direct result, premature infants have lower levels of lactase activity and may be unable to digest and absorb lactose as well as normal term infants.[47,49] The use of lactase to hydrolyze lactose in preterm formulas and maternal breast milk may aid in decreasing "lactose malabsorption in preterm infants" and further lead to enhanced weight gain and improved feeding tolerance.[47]

Congenital lactase deficiency is an extremely rare autosomal recessive disorder that primarily affects those of Finnish decent.[50] It is caused by "mutations in the gene coding for the lactase enzyme (LC)."[51] Affected newborns present with severe diarrheal disease that occurs immediately following introduction of maternal breast milk or lactose-containing formula.[41,50] If left untreated, congenital lactase deficiency can be life threatening as a result of dehydration and loss of electrolytes.[41] Treatment includes complete removal of lactose from the diet and consumption of a lactose-free formula during infancy and lactose-free diet after infancy.[41]

Celiac Disease

Celiac disease (CD) is a multisystem, T-cell-mediated chronic autoimmune intestinal disorder that occurs in genetically predisposed individuals.[52–54] At-risk populations include first-degree relatives of people with celiac disease, along with those previously diagnosed with type 1 diabetes mellitus, autoimmune thyroid disease, selective IgA deficiency, trisomy 21, Turner syndrome, or Williams syndrome.[52,53,55] The prevalence in children between the ages of 2.5 and 15 years is about 3 to 13 per 1000 children, or approximately 1:300 to 1:80.[52,55]

Classic GI-related symptoms of celiac disease include diarrhea, constipation, chronic abdominal pain, abdominal distention, and vomiting with associated failure to thrive.[52,55] Non-GI or extraintestinal symptoms include short stature, inadequate weight gain, weight loss, delayed puberty, dental enamel defects, dermatitis herpetaformis, and reduced bone mineral density. Iron deficient anemia that is resistant to oral iron supplementation, fatigue, migraines, and joint pain may also present as symptoms.[52–55]

Those who present with symptoms suspicious of celiac disease must first receive serology testing, which includes immunoglobulin A (IgA) antibody and tissue transglutaminase (TTG), along with tissue transglutaminase immunoglobulin G (TTG IgG) if IgA deficiency is present. It is important that gluten remain in the diet to ensure reliable serology testing. Formal diagnosis must be further confirmed via intestinal biopsy. In some cases, diagnosis may be uncertain. If this is the case, human leukocyte antigen (HLA) typing and repeat biopsy can be performed. Trialing the gluten-free diet may also be considered. After trialing the gluten-free diet, repeat serology testing and intestinal biopsy are recommended. If once positive serology tests become negative following the trial of the gluten-free diet, this is tangible and supportive evidence for the diagnosis of celiac disease.[52,55]

Once formal diagnosis has been made, individuals with celiac disease have a permanent intolerance to gluten and must adhere to a gluten-free diet. Nutritive sources of gluten (such as wheat, rye, barley, and its derivatives) and non-nutritive sources of gluten (such as toothpaste) should be completely eliminated from the diet. As a result, GI and often extraintestinal symptoms, serologic test results, histology, and growth and development should normalize as celiac symptoms improve and move into a state of remission.[52,56]

Celiac disease remains underdiagnosed.[57] The only known treatment for celiac disease is the gluten-free diet. Strict dietary adherence proves beneficial. If left untreated, celiac disease can result in nutritional deficiencies, decreased bone mineral density, and neurological disorders. Additionally, if left untreated, affected individuals are at increased risk for developing intestinal lymphoma, infertility, spontaneous abortion, and the delivery of low-birth-weight infants.[52,58,59] A gluten-free diet will allow for normal growth and development as well as relief from symptoms.

Gluten is composed of two proteins, gliadin and glutenin. Gluten is the name for storage proteins, or prolamins, that are found in wheat, rye, and barley. Gliadin is the specific prolamin found in wheat, secalin in rye, and hordein in barley.[53,58,59] When ingested, it is these specific prolamins that cause villous atrophy, which may further result in nutrient malabsorption and/or deficiency.

Iron, calcium, and folate are key nutrients often affected in those with celiac disease, because these nutrients are absorbed in the proximal small bowel.[53,58,60] If the disease progresses further down the small intestinal tract, malabsorption of carbohydrates, fat, fat-soluble vitamins, and protein may occur. The most common causes of anemia in those with celiac disease are iron, folate, or vitamin B_{12} deficiency. Calcium, phosphorus, and vitamin D deficiencies may also occur secondary to malabsorption or decreased intake of dairy products if lactose intolerance is present.[53] Secondary lactose intolerance is commonly observed.[53,58,61] Those diagnosed with celiac disease are considered at higher risk for developing bone disease and should receive dual energy x-ray absorpiometry (DXA scan), quantitative CT scan, or computerized bone age estimation at the time of diagnosis.[52,53,62] Strict adherence to the gluten-free diet during childhood will result in improved bone mineral density in adulthood.[52,62]

Whether an individual with celiac disease can safely consume oats remains controversial, because oats may become contaminated by gluten during the harvesting and milling process.[52,53,58] Most children with celiac disease can safely consume 20–25 grams per day (¼ cup dry rolled gluten-free oats).[59] The patient should discuss the inclusion of gluten-free oats with his or her gastroenterologist and/or registered dietitian prior to ingestion because individual tolerance varies and monitoring of antibody levels is required.

Immediately following diagnosis, affected individuals should be referred to a registered dietitian with expertise in celiac disease for comprehensive nutrition education on the gluten-free diet and the gluten-free lifestyle.[52,53,58,60] Nutrition counseling should focus on nutritive and non-nutritive sources of gluten, gluten-free alternatives, hidden sources of gluten, various aspects of cross-contamination, where one can purchase gluten-free products; credible resources and support groups, and eating outside of the home.[52,53,58,60] Periodic assessment and reassessment should occur paying close attention to anthropometric measurements, growth trends, nutritional intake, and the need for multivitamin and mineral supplementation to aid in preventing and/or correcting nutrient deficiency.[52,53,58,60] Assessment also includes determining the comprehension level of the patient and family, addressing individual questions/concerns, and providing continued support in an effort to achieve optimal quality of life.[52,53,58,60]

Evidence-based nutrition practice guidelines have been published by the American Dietetic Association (ADA) for the dietary treatment of celiac disease. These formal guidelines can be viewed online at http://www.eatright.org within the Evidence Analysis Library (EAL).[60]

Inflammatory Bowel Disease

The two major types of inflammatory bowel disease (IBD) are Crohn's disease and ulcerative colitis (UC). Crohn's disease may occur in any portion of the GI tract. Ulcerative colitis is by definition confined to the colon with minimal involvement of the terminal ileum.[63] Patients who develop nonspecific IBD-like symptoms are often temporarily termed as having indeterminate colitis. The two diseases have many features in common:

- Diarrhea
- GI blood and protein loss
- Abdominal pain
- Weight loss
- Anemia
- Growth failure

Children with IBD may experience growth failure due to inadequate intake, malabsorption, excessive nutrient losses, drug–nutrient interaction, and increased nutrient needs. Inadequate intake may be due to abdominal pain, gastritis, personal effort to decrease the incidence of diarrhea, and taste changes with zinc deficiency. Nutrient deficits are common in adolescents and children with IBD.[64] At the time of diagnosis, the majority of pediatric patients with Crohn's disease or ulcerative colitis present with weight loss.[65]

Patients who present in a flare, or active disease state, often have multiple macro- and micronutrient losses. Inflammation of the mucosa and bowel resections can lead to general malabsorption. Depending on the location and length of the bowel resection, specific nutrients may no longer be absorbed and will need to be supplemented. Bacterial overgrowth due to altered motility or strictures can also lead to malabsorption.

There is a lack of consensus for estimated caloric needs in pediatric patients with IBD. The REE (resting energy expenditure) of Crohn's patients appears to be similar to that of normal people per kg of lean body mass. The REE per kg of body mass is not down-regulated as it is in the starvation state.[66] In adults with IBD, total energy expenditure is not significantly elevated in active disease compared to remission or inactive disease.[67]

Protein requirements are likely elevated due to protein losses as well as increased needs for healing, especially in patients after surgery. In patients with IBD who present with protein-losing enteropathy, the body cannot synthesize new proteins as fast as they are lost through the GI tract.[68] The resulting hypoalbuminemia cannot be corrected by the addition of protein to the diet.

Bile malabsorption leads to decreased absorption of long-chain fatty acids but not medium-chain fatty acids, because bile is not required for the transport of medium-chain fatty acids through the mucosa. Fat malabsorption contributes to the malabsorption of fat-soluble vitamins.

All patients should be assessed for micronutrient deficiencies and repleted as necessary. Blood losses via the stool can lead to iron deficiency. Folate deficiency can result from drug–nutrient interactions as well as decreased intake of folate-rich food sources. The fat-soluble vitamins as well as zinc, magnesium, and calcium are lost when steatorrhea is present. Zinc deficiency may be related to diarrheal, high-output fistula losses and inadequate dietary intake. Magnesium and potassium also are lost via diarrhea. Patients with resections of the stomach or ileum or severe disease of the terminal ileum may not be able to absorb sufficient vitamin B_{12}.[69,70] Patients should be on a daily multivitamin unless they are receiving enteral formula, which provides the equivalent of a multivitamin.[71]

Although bone disease in IBD is multifactorial, vitamin D and calcium are important nutrients to monitor and are supplemented as needed. Steroids are known to affect bone mineral density,[72] and inflammatory cytokines lead to lower bone mineral density.[73] Fat malabsorption can lead to low vitamin D levels, and vitamin D plays many roles beyond bone health in the body. A general recommendation depending on the degree of fat malabsorption includes: 50,000 units of vitamin D_2 every week up to every day or up to 10,000 units of vitamin D_3 every day for up to 5 months. This may be followed by a maintenance dose of 50,000 units of vitamin D_2 every week. For children and adults without fat malabsorption, the recommendation ranges from 400–1000 units of vitamin D_3 every day.[74]

Drug–nutrient interaction from the pharmacotherapy used in the treatment of IBD may negatively affect nutrition. Sulfasalazine (azulfidine) interferes with folate absorption.[75] Methotrexate is a folic acid antagonist, and supplementation of folic acid helps to reduce methotrexate's hepatic side effects.[76,77] Corticosteroid therapy interferes with absorption of calcium, phosphate, and zinc.

The use of a low-residue, high-fiber, or low-refined-sugar diet to maintain remission of Crohn's disease is not recommended.[78,79] Dairy products need not be restricted in patients with IBD unless lactose malabsorption is present. Lactose intolerance is often temporary during times of active disease. Advice concerning the intake of dairy products should be individualized to avoid unnecessary dietary restrictions.[80]

Nutrition support has both a primary and an adjunctive role in the treatment of IBD.[64] Primary nutrition therapy appears to be more effective in the treatment of Crohn's disease than of ulcerative colitis.[64,81] In general, corticosteroids are more effective than enteral feedings in inducing remission. The protein composition of the formulas does not cause any difference in the effectiveness of the enteral nutrition therapy.[82] However, for the maintenance of remission in Crohn's disease, enteral feeds were found to be beneficial in all age groups with no known side effects.[83]

Using enteral formulas that contain higher amounts of medium-chain triglycerides (MCT) result in remission rates comparable to low-fat formulas or steroid therapy.[84,85] There is presently inadequate evidence to support the use of omega-3 fatty acids for the induction or maintenance of remission of ulcerative colitis,[86,87] nor do they appear to be effective in the maintenance of remission in Crohn's disease.[88] Probiotics are not effective for the induction or maintenance of remission of Crohn's disease,[89,90] but when added to standard therapy for ulcerative colitis they may lead to a reduction in disease activity.[91]

In patients not treated with enteral nutrition therapy during periods of active disease and/or weight loss, oral nutritional beverages in addition to food can be useful. Because protein composition does not affect rates of remission or disease improvement, formula choice should be based on palatability and patient tolerance. If voluntary intake is insufficient, nasogastric enteral supplementation may be considered. Parenteral nutrition (PN) should be reserved for patients who have bowel obstructions or short bowel syndrome or who are unable to tolerate a sufficient quantity of enteral nutrition because of active disease.

Pancreatitis

Pancreatitis can be divided into two groups: mild and severe. Most cases are mild and will often resolve within 5 to 7 days.[92,93] The remaining cases are severe and require medical and nutritional therapy. Severe pancreatitis creates a state of hypermetabolism and catabolism with significant nitrogen losses and results in an elevated systemic inflammatory response with infectious complications.[92,93]

Patients with mild pancreatitis who resume oral intake of liquids and solid foods prior to the resolution of pain may be able to advance to a solid food diet sooner than those on bowel rest.[94] Oral feeds, both liquids and solids, should be supported during the first few days with the benefit of improved nutrient intake.

Traditionally, severe pancreatitis has been treated with bowel rest and parenteral nutrition. However, PN increases the pro-inflammatory response and contributes to gut atrophy, likely leading to bacterial translocation and increased infection rates.[95,96] Outcomes are better with enteral feedings compared to parenteral nutrition.[97] If PN must be used, it should not be initiated within the first 5 days of admission due to the higher inflammatory response that is present in the beginning of the disease process.[98]

The timing of the start of nutrition support, either parenteral or enteral, varies widely in clinical practice. Initiation of enteral nutrition within the first 48 hours of admission has showed significant benefits over the use of PN.[96,99]

The feasibility of placing a nasogastric versus nasojejunal tube is important when considering the route of enteral feeding. Either a nasogastric, or nasojejunal feeding can be used with either a polmeric or semi-elemental formula in patients with severe pancreatitis. No data support the use of immunonutrition and probiotics.[100] As the patient improves clinically, low-fat oral feeds are initiated, and slowly advanced, as enteral feeds are weaned to a normal diet.

Liver Disease

Biliary atresia is one of the more common chronic cholestatic liver diseases that presents in infants and requires surgical intervention. Alagille syndrome, Byler syndrome, primary biliary cirrhosis, and primary sclerosing cholangitis are cholestatic liver diseases seen in childhood. Long-term use of PN nutrition can lead to cholestasis (see Chapter 20). In cholestatic disease, a decrease in biliary bile acids results in fat and fat-soluble vitamin malabsorption. As liver damage progresses, leading to cirrhosis, synthesis of albumin and transport proteins decreases, which causes laboratory protein markers to become low. Nutritional concerns progress from fat malabsorption to protein-energy malnutrition.[101]

Patients with chronic cholestasis/cirrhosis can present with ascites and/or organomegaly, which will falsely elevate the patient's weight. Weights are not reliable in assessing nutrition status on a growth chart. These measurements can underestimate the degree of malnutrition.[102] Tricep skinfold thickness and mid-arm circumference results can also be skewed by edema.[101]

Chronic cholestasis in infancy and early childhood leads to increased calorie needs. Calorie needs have been suggested to be 125–150% of the RDA for ideal body weight in children.[103] Infants with biliary atresia require 120–200 kcal/kg/day.[104] Protein requirements should focus on providing equal to or greater than the RDA for protein in the nonencephalopathic patient. Recommendations for protein in infants are 2–3 g/kg/day.[103] With encephalopathy, protein should be temporarily restricted below the RDA until mental status returns to normal.[105]

Cholestatic liver disease leads to decreased biliary bile acids, resulting in malabsorption of LCT. Bile is not required for solubilization of MCT, and thus formulas containing a high percentage of MCT oil or supplementing foods with MCT oil are often recommended to provide fat and calories.[103] MCTs do not, however, provide essential fatty acids,[106] and a source of linoleic acid is essential. Due to malabsorption with hepatobiliary disease, infants should receive well above 3% of calories from linoleic acid to prevent a deficiency.[107] Infants and older children with biliary atresia should consume formulas containing 40–60% of the fat from MCT.[108] In liver disease, the prevalence of fat-soluble vitamin deficiencies correlates with increasing bilirubin levels.[105] It is important to remember that the degree of fat malabsorption is unique to each patient's disease state and can change as treatments or medications are changed.

Vitamin A is stored in the liver, and requires retinol-binding protein to circulate throughout the body. As liver disease progresses, synthesis of retinol-binding protein is impaired, which leads to low vitamin A levels without a true deficiency. Clinical judgment needs to be used in the review of both serum retinol and retinol-binding protein laboratory results. Supplementation recommendations range from

5000–15,000 international units (IU)/day orally. For severe deficiency, intramuscular injections may be used.[101,103]

Vitamin E is stored in the liver and transported via lipoproteins. In patients with high triglycerides and cholesterol levels, the vitamin E level may be falsely elevated. It is best to check serum vitamin E levels in conjunction with total serum lipids to assess for deficiency. In children younger than 12 years of age a ratio of less than 0.6 mg vitamin E/g total serum lipids and in children older than 12 years of age a ratio less than 0.8 mg/g are indicative of a deficiency. Supplementation recommendations in pediatrics range from 20–25 IU/kg/day of vitamin E or 10–200 IU/kg/day of alpha-tocopherol or intramuscular injections. The use of D-alpha-tocopheryl polyethylene glycol 1000 succinate TPGS vitamin E enhances the absorption of other fat-soluble vitamins.[101,103]

In cholestatic and noncholestatic liver disease, metabolic bone disease has a multifactorial etiology that includes a decrease in insulin-like growth factor 1, hypogonadism, malnutrition, low BMI, loss of muscle mass, low calcium, and vitamin D deficiency. Vitamin D is hydroxylated in the liver. Increased vitamin D levels lead to increased calcium and phosphorus absorption in the intestine. In cholestatic patients with fat malabsorption, less vitamin D is absorbed, which decreases calcium and phosphorus absorption. The nonabsorbed fatty acids bind to calcium in the intestine, further decreasing calcium absorption. Absorption of calcium is also reduced by corticosteroid therapy.[109,110] A 25-OH vitamin D level shows the pool of both dietary and endogenous vitamin D. DEXA scans are the gold standard for assessing bone density, and all patients at risk should be screened. Vitamin D should be periodically evaluated and supplemented as needed.

Vitamin K deficiency is due to fat malabsorption and decreased absorption from gut flora alterations. This deficiency, as well as impaired hepatic synthesis of clotting factors, leads to prolonged prothrombin time (PT). If the abnormal PT is thought to be related to a vitamin K deficiency, the medical team can prescribe oral or intravenous supplementation. Zinc, magnesium, and calcium are also lost in the presence of fat malabsorption. Supplementation should be given, and adjusted as necessary to maintain adequate levels.

Liver Transplant

The most common disease requiring liver transplantation in childhood is biliary atresia. Other less prominent causes include inherited metabolic disorders (e.g., alpha-1-antitrypsin deficiency, urea cycle defects), intra-hepatic cholestasis syndromes (e.g., Alagille syndrome), chronic hepatitis with cirrhosis, and acute liver failure. Indications for transplantation include hepatic failure, complications of portal hypertension (e.g., variceal bleeding, ascities), specific metabolic disorders, and malignancy.

The patient with end-stage liver disease awaiting transplantation presents a formidable challenge. The particular liver disease involved, the magnitude of liver dysfunction, the presence of complications, and the transplantation procedure itself combine to present a complex treatment process, including meeting nutritional needs for healing and growth. Pretransplant nutritional care involves assessment of the current status and development of a therapeutic nutritional plan tailored to the liver disease and degree of debilitation. Patients with chronic cholestasis/cirrhosis can present with ascites and/or organomegaly, which will falsely elevate the patient's weight.

End-stage liver disease creates a hypermetabolic state where lean body mass and proteins are broken down for gluconeogenesis once the body's glucose supply is exhausted.[111] Protein should not be restricted and is often provided at levels above the RDA, unless encephalopathy is present.[103,104] If the end-stage liver disease is related to a cholestatic liver disease, then the decreased pool of bile acids will result in malabsorption of long-chain triglycerides. MCTs and essential fatty acids should be used to provide calories and minimize steatorrhea.[103] See the section on cholestatic liver disease.

Preoperative malnutrition negatively affects the outcome of liver transplant. Height Z-score is a good indicator of pretransplant malnutrition. Severe growth retardation is linked to increased length of stay and increased hospital costs after transplant.[112] Post-transplant mortality and graft failure risks include weight/height that is below two standard deviations at the time of listing.[113] Close nutrition monitoring in end-stage liver disease and optimizing nutritional intake will maximize growth potential and nutritional status going into transplant.

In many cases, the underlying disease is corrected by transplant; therefore, energy and protein needs should be individualized to the patient's specific postoperative needs and nutritional status. Immediately after transplant, early nutritional support should be implemented due to preoperative malnutrition, surgical stress, and postoperative catabolism.[114] Nutrition support should be initiated and slowly advanced to meet calorie and protein needs. The enteral formula should be chosen based on each patient's protein and fat composition needs.

The nutritional goal is catch-up growth to achieve an age-appropriate weight and height. Many growth-retarded children transplanted after 2 years of age continue to have some linear growth retardation.[115,116] If transplanted prior to 2 years of age, patients may be able to catch up in height.[115] Patients with biliary atresia and alpha-1-antitrypsin achieve better linear growth post-transplant than patients with fulminant liver failure or chronic hepatitis.[117]

Drug–nutrient interactions are key considerations post-transplant. Steroids affect linear growth and bone health, and contribute to hyperglycemia and diabetes mellitus.[118]

Immunosuppressive medications also contribute to electrolyte and magnesium losses.

Concern regarding metabolic bone disease continues after liver transplant. Bone loss is greatest in the first year after transplant.[119] Patients with cholestatic liver disease who undergo liver transplant improve their bone mineral density.[120]

Another concern that the dietitian and medical transplant team must keep in mind is transplant-acquired food allergies (TAFA). A food allergy can be passed from a donor to the liver recipient. If allergy symptoms occur, an elimination diet may be needed, and the food allergen(s) avoided in the diet. Risk factors for developing food allergies post-transplant include patients who:

- Are younger than 1 year of age
- Have hypereosinophilia
- Have Epstein-Barre virus (EBV) viremia[121]

Short Bowel Syndrome

Short bowel syndrome (SBS) is a condition in which the patient has an anatomic or functional loss of more than 50% of the small intestine.[122] SBS results from necrotizing enterocolitis (NEC), volvulus, intestinal atresias, gastroschisis, ruptured omphalocele, or vascular infarct.[122-124] The result of the injury and/or resection is decreased small intestine surface area, which leads to malabsorption and large-volume watery diarrhea.[125] The degree of malabsorption is dependent on the extent of missing or injured bowel; most affected individuals have difficulty sustaining appropriate growth and development without nutritional support. Growth is a major concern in this population.

Intestinal adaptation is the process by which the remaining intestine grows, dilates, and changes via cellular hyperplasia and villous hypertrophy in order to compensate for its loss of surface area or function. Adaptation is the ultimate goal of treatment and is the key to successful withdrawal of parenteral nutrition (PN). Adaptation begins soon after resection and continues for the first few years postresection.[2,124] The ability of the intestine to adapt is largely dependent on how much intestine remains, the health of the remaining intestine, the presence or absence of the ileocecal valve (ICV), and whether the colon is in continuity with the small bowel. In infants, it is possible to survive with 20–40 cm of small bowel if the colon is present. Without a colon, at least 40 cm of small bowel is needed to survive.[2]

Absorption of fluids and nutrients occurs throughout the small intestine and colon. Half of the mucosal surface is contained within the proximal one-fourth of the small intestine.[125] Figure 12-1 illustrates sites of nutrient absorption in the small intestine and colon and the possible implications of intestinal resections of these areas.

The duodenum and jejunum are the primary sites of digestion and absorption of proteins, carbohydrates, lipids, and most vitamins and minerals. Resections in these areas result in decreased surface area for absorption, causing increased osmotic diarrhea and loss of water-soluble vitamins.[126] Loss of calcium, iron, and magnesium can occur as well as losses of trace minerals such as copper. Decreased secretin, cholecystokinin, and pancreatic/biliary secretions result in decreased digestion and absorption of fats, proteins, and fat-soluble vitamins. Decreased disaccharidase secretion allows increased the risk for bacterial overgrowth.

Decreased surface area from ileal resection results in decreased vitamin B_{12} absorption. Decreased bile salt reabsorption in the ileum increases bile acid in the stool and decreases enterohepatic circulation.[126] This causes decreased bile acid pools and decreased micelle formation. Decreased absorption of long chain fats and fat-soluble vitamins result. There is increased steatorrhea, and the potential for cholelithiasis and renal oxalate stones. Many gut hormones that affect GI motility are produced in the ileum, including enteroglucagon and peptide YY. Resection of the ileum can impair the nutrient-regulated gut motility.[127]

With jejunal resection, the ileum can assume the place of the jejunum in some ways to absorb less site-specific nutrients such as electrolytes and fluid, which the jejunum is responsible for when the bowel is intact.[128] However, the jejunum cannot assume the role of the ileum. For example, loss of the terminal ileum requires B_{12} provision via intramuscular or nasal route for absorption because there are no other sites for B_{12} absorption in the proximal ileum, duodenum, or jejunum.

The ileocecal valve (ICV) slows transit time and acts as a barrier to bacteria moving into the small bowel from the colon.[126] Resection of the ICV leads to vitamin B_{12} and possibly folate deficiency because sites for absorption often are lost with adjacent ileum resection. Combined ICV and ileum resections lead to decreased transit time and a large influx of nutrients into the large intestine. Bacterial overgrowth in the small bowel can be a major problem and lead to increased diarrhea and malabsorption.[122] Antibiotics may be used to treat bacterial overgrowth for varying amounts of time, depending on the child's response.

The colon absorbs water, salvages malabsorbed carbohydrate, and absorbs sodium. Colonic resection decreases water and sodium reabsorption and increases risk for dehydration.[126]

Growth and Nutritional Assessment

Growth is the ultimate measurement of nutritional adequacy. Caloric and protein needs are dependent on many variables, such as age, state of growth, degree of malabsorption, and site of resection. Clinical judgment along with known intake levels and growth outcomes for each child should be used. Growth and assessment of nutritional status should be monitored routinely and deficiencies such as vitamin B_{12} and zinc corrected as needed.

Nutritional management of the pediatric patient with short bowel syndrome (SBS) can be divided into four phases. The first phase involves fluid, electrolyte, and hemodynamic stability and PN initiation while the GI tract is recovering postoperatively. PN should be started as soon as possible via central line.[129] Initial PN macronutrient needs vary greatly:

- Initiation of dextrose should be at 5–7 mg/kg/min and advancement by 1–3 mg/kg/min to an endpoint goal of 12–14 mg/kg/min.[129]
- Lipid can begin at 1 g/kg/day advancing 1 g/kg/day to an endpoint of no more than 3 g/kg/day.[129]
- Protein is begun at 1–2 g/kg/day and advanced by 1–2 g/kg/day to an endpoint of 3–3.5 g/kg/day.[129]

Initial stool output, whether per rectum or ileostomy, typically increases needs for sodium, magnesium, and zinc to compensate for losses.[129,130] Monitoring trends in zinc status can be helpful. An infant not responding to adequate caloric and protein provision but with high-output stool volume may benefit from additional zinc supplementation. PN should be monitored carefully to minimize complications such as parenteral nutrition associated liver disease (PNALD).[131] See Chapter 20 for more on PN management.

EN is the next phase of nutrition therapy. It should be started as soon as the patient is stable and GI motility has returned.[2,124] EN should be infused continuous via the gastric route.[2,124,132] In some conditions, if infants have a proximal high ostomy and a mucous fistula connected to a substantial portion of the bowel, refeeding the mucous fistula with the proximal bowel content can be done to prevent diffuse atrophy.[133]

If available, breast milk should be used in infants with SBS to initiate EN. The abundance of growth factor and nucleotides available in breast milk makes it the ideal choice.[124,129] If breast milk is unavailable, an infant formula should be selected to start EN, depending on the patient's clinical situation.

In pediatrics, hydrolyzed and even amino acid formulas are often preferred over polymeric products. Mucosal breakdown, bowel dilation, and bacterial overgrowth all predispose the infants to higher rates of food allergies; thus, the provision of an amino acid formulation is a considerable advantage.[134] Some advocate amino acid formulations for infants and more intact formulations for toddlers and older children, whereas others recommend use of a protein hydrolysate formula.[2,132]

If fat malabsorption exists from bile acid hypersecretion, PNALD, or pancreatic insufficiency, use of a formula with a higher percentage of fat from MCTs is preferred.[134] If bilirubin levels are elevated, use of a very high MCT formula such as Pregestimil (55% MCT oil) is recommended.[134,135] Many advocate using a blend of both MCTs and LCTs.[134,135] In practice, amino acid formulations with higher MCT content are preferred over lower MCT oil formulations.

The third stage of nutritional management should be started while the infant is still hospitalized, if possible. PN should be weaned as EN and oral tolerance increases, stool output decreases, and growth is achieved. The ultimate goal is to wean off the PN as soon as possible to prevent cholestasis and liver failure.[136–138] Gradual advances in EN/oral intake are dependent on gastric tolerance, stool output (frequency and consistency), and rate of growth.[2] This stage can be quite lengthy. Stool should be monitored for frequency, acidosis, and reducing substances as EN and oral intake advances. PN should be cycled when 35–50% of EN goal has been achieved and if blood sugar levels are stable. Two to 6 hours off of PN each day allow for GI hormone release.[129,134] As PN is weaned, vitamin and mineral status should be closely monitored and supplemented, as needed.

Oral feedings, even the smallest of volumes, should be started as soon as the patient is clinically stable to prevent oral aversion.[2,124,132,134] Feeding aversions are common for many reasons. First and foremost, prematurity and severe illness delay oral attempts and result in immature feeding skills.[129] Furthermore, frequent vomiting and diarrhea prevent pleasurable associations with food.[124] Oral feeds can be introduced as developmentally appropriate, while monitoring for food allergies. If the infant is unable to take any oral feedings, an oral motor stimulation program should be in place to help develop feeding skills. Feeding aversion in patients with SBS is notoriously difficult to treat, and the focus is on prevention of aversion as feasible.[2,139,140]

The fourth phase of management is long-term advancement of EN, maximizing oral intake and monitoring growth. Once EN is at goal, it may be beneficial to start fiber therapy if the colon (or most of it) is present. The conversion of complex carbohydrate to short-chain fatty acids (SCFAs; acetate, propionate, and butyrate) in the colon can cause significant caloric reuptake by colonic cells.[2,138,139] Additionally, SCFAs also stimulate sodium and water reabsorption, which aids in fluid management. Addition of a 1–3% pectin solution can decrease reducing substances and improve pH to allow for more fermentation of carbohydrates.[129] In orally fed patients, use of guar gum fiber such as Nestlé's Resource Benefiber at 0.5 g/kg/day may be used as a more palatable replacement to pectin.

As the intestine adapts, the goal is to normalize the EN schedule while promoting oral intake and growth. If possible, EN should be cycled overnight to maximize oral intake during the day. Children must be given palatable beverages providing complete nutrition to help lessen EN dependence and increase oral intake. Higher calorie formulas typically have higher osmolality and may interfere with desired gain. Products such as Boost Kids Essentials 1.5 (Nestlé) provide a high percentage of calories from fat, with a lower osmolality.

Overly strict guidelines for oral intake should be discouraged. General guidelines include limiting simple sugars (juice, candy) in order to minimize osmotic diarrhea.[2,124,129,140,134,135,141]

Fat and protein should be adequate to support growth. Soluble fiber of at least 5–10 g/day as pectin/guar gum is beneficial to slow the gut transit time.[124,132,135] Those with a colon have an additional bonus of caloric reuptake from provision of soluble fiber in the diet. Lactose should be avoided only if symptoms are reported with ingestion.[2,135] Liberal salt intake at meals helps make the meal bolus isotonic in the gut.[135]

Guidelines for adults with SBS have been adapted to the child.[135] In adults with a colon, 50–60% of kcal from carbohydrates and 20–30% of kcal from fat is recommended as a balance of LCT and MCT. Those without a colon are encouraged to consume 40–50% kcal from carbohydrates and 30–40% of kcal from fat with more LCTs than MCTs. Isotonic fluids are always encouraged, regardless of the presence or absence of a colon. However, hypo-osmolar fluids and higher sodium-containing fluids are encouraged for those without a colon. Sometimes oral rehydration solutions (ORS) are recommended for those without a colon (see Table 12-3).

Increased renal oxalate stones occur with intestinal resections because of increased enteric absorption of oxalate (enteric hyperoxaluria).[143] Renal oxalate stones can develop but this is rare in children.[2,135,142,143] A low oxalate diet or provision of extra calcium is recommended if 24-hour urinary oxalate levels are elevated.[135] Urinary oxalate levels should be monitored annually in this population.

Alternative surgical procedures such as bowel lengthening, tapering enteroplasty, or intestinal transplant may be considered for those patients who are not making progress.[127,144–146]

Intestinal Transplantation

Small bowel transplantation may be indicated for patients who have failed standard management, especially in the setting of life-threatening liver dysfunction.[123,147] Surgical transplant can involve the isolated intestine or the liver and intestine, or it can be a multivisceral transplantation that includes stomach, pancreas, and the entire small bowel, which can include or preclude the liver as well.[123] Small bowel with a concurrent liver transplant is done in children due to the association of PNALD in children.[147] Management involves immunosuppression and nutritional rehabilitation with PN, EN, and oral feeding postoperatively.[123,147] Evaluation and monitoring similar to any transplant should occur in each child by an RD after transplant. Chronic rejection remains an issue.

Case Study

Nutrition Assessment of Adolescent with Chronic Diarrhea

Patient history: PL is a 14-year-old male who presents with diarrhea for 3 weeks that has recently become bloody. He now has more than five bowel movements per day. PL complains of fatigue and per mother has experienced an 8-pound weight loss since pediatrician's appointment 2 months prior.

Food/nutrition-related history: PL reports not feeling as hungry as usual. His mother states he is only eating about 50–75% of what he used to. PL does not take any vitamin, mineral, or herbal supplements. He also does not drink any oral nutritional supplements.

Biochemical data, medical tests, and procedures:

(↓= below normal)	Ca: 8.9 ↓	MCV: 74.1 ↓
Na: 142	H/H: 10.2 ↓/34.3 ↓	Albumin: 3.1
Cl: 102	K: 3.6 ↓	CRP: 5.9 ↑
BUN: 7	CO_2: 27 ↑	
Glucose: 82	Cr: 0.6	

Medical workup: EGD and colonoscopy: visual inflammation throughout small bowel and colon; biopsies pending. Findings consistent with Crohn's disease per attending. Plan to start Pentasa and enteral nutrition therapy to treat suspected disease and malnutrition.

Anthropometric Measures

Weight: 36.3 kg

BMI: 15.3 (< 5%)

Height: 154 cm

Std Ht for age: 164 cm

% of Std Ht for age: 94%

Estimated Nutrition Needs

Calories: REE (1286) × 1.7–1.9 = 2185–2445 per day

Protein: 1–1.8 g/kg/day

Fluid: 1825 mL/day

Assessment

Percentage of ideal body weight and percentage of standard height for age indicate mild wasting and mild stunting of growth. Significant weight loss of 9% of his usual body weight has been observed over the past 2 months. Per patient and family, his diet prior to admission was likely hypocaloric, with possible dehydration due to diarrhea. Labs reflect low potassium and albumin levels, elevated CO_2 and CRP levels, as well as microcytic anemia. Per hospital protocol, PL may benefit from receiving 80% of estimated total caloric goal via enteral nutrition because this is believed to induce remission of disease and to aid in the treatment of malnutrition.

Nutrition Diagnoses

Based on the above information, a nutritional problem or diagnosis can be made.

Interventions

Initiate EN: Recommend Peptamen 1.5 starting at 25 mL/hr, advancing by 25 mL every 5 hours, to a goal of 125 mL/hr × 10 hours per night, via nasogastric tube.

Initial/Brief Nutrition Education

Help patient to identify foods and nutritional supplement to meet 20% of estimated calorie needs orally. Outcome: patient will consume 20% of estimated calorie needs orally.

Coordination of Other Care During Nutrition Care

Discuss need for vitamin D and zinc levels on nutrition support rounds and signout to outpatient RD via email after patient's discharge. Outcome: labs ordered and evaluated, supplementation started if indicated. Outpatient appointment and email confirmed.

Questions for the Reader

1. What is the patient's IBW and percentage of IBW?
2. What is his estimated energy needs per kg?
3. Write at least one PES statement.
4. How many calories, how much protein, and how much free water are provided in this amount of tube feeding?
5. What would you want to monitor and evaluate during his hospitalization, and what are your plans for discharge?

REFERENCES

1. World Health Organization, Department of Child and Adolescent Health and Development. *The Treatment of Diarrhoea: A Manual for Physicians and Other Senior Health Care Workers,* 4th ed. rev. Geneva: World Health Organization; 2005.
2. Corkins MR, Scolapino J. Diarrhea. In: Merritt R (ed). *The ASPEN Nutrition Support Practice Manual,* 2nd ed. Silver Spring, MD: ASPEN; 2005:207–210.
3. American Academy of Pediatrics. Oral therapy for acute diarrhea. In: Kleinman RE (ed). *Pediatric Nutrition Handbook,* 6th ed. Elk Grove Village, IL: American Academy of Pediatrics; 2009:651–659.
4. Glass RI, Lew JF, Gangarosa RE, et al. Estimates of morbidity and mortality rates for diarrhea diseases in American children. *J Pediatr.* 1991;118:S27–S33.
5. King CK, Glass R, Breese JS, Duggan C. Management of acute gastroenteritis among children: oral rehydration, maintenance and nutritional therapy. *MMWR.* 2003;52:1–16.
6. American Academy of Pediatrics, Provisional Committee on Quality Improvement, Subcommittee on Acute Gastroenteritis. Practice parameter: the management of acute gastroenteritis in young children. *Pediatrics.* 1996;97:424–435
7. Brown KH. Appropriate diets for the rehabilitation of malnourished children in the community setting. *Acta Paediatr Scand.* 1991;374(Suppl):151.
8. Brown KH, Peerson JM, Fontaine O. Use of non-human milks in the dietary management of young children with acute diarrhea: a meta-analysis of clinical trials. *Pediatrics.* 1994;93:17–27.
9. Dai D, Walker WA. Protective nutrients and bacterial colonization in the immature human gut. *Adv Pediatr.* 1999;46:353–382.
10. Morrow AL, Ruiz-Palacios GM, Altaye M, et al. Human milk oligosaccharides are associated with protection against diarrhea in breast-fed infants. *J Pediat.* 2004;145:297–303.
11. Snyder JD, Merson MH. The magnitude of the global problem of acute diarrhea disease: a review of active surveillance data. *Bull World Health Organ.* 1982;60:605–613.
12. Bhutta ZA, Ghishan F, Lindley K, et al. Persistent and chronic diarrhea and malabsorption: working group report of the Second World Congress of Pediatric Gastroenterology, Hepatology, and Nutrition. *J Pediatr Gastroenterol Nutr.* 2004;39: S711–S716.
13. American Academy of Pediatrics. Chronic diarrhea disease. In: Kleinman RE (ed). *Pediatric Nutrition Handbook,* 6th ed. Elk Grove Village, IL: American Academy of Pediatrics; 2009: 637–649.
14. Klish WJ. Chronic diarrhea. In: Walker WA, Watkins JB (eds). *Nutrition in Pediatrics: Basic Science and Clinical Applications.* Hamilton, ON: Decker; 1997:603.
15. Chronic diarrhea in children: a nutritional disorder [editorial]. *Lancet.* 1987;1:143.
16. Lo CW, Walker WA. Chronic protracted diarrhea of infancy: a nutritional disorder. *Pediatrics.* 1983;72:786.
17. Evaluation of an algorithm for the treatment of persistent diarrhea: a multicentre study. *Bull World Health Organ.* 1996;74(5):479–489.
18. Baker SS, Davis AM. Hypocaloric oral therapy during an episode of diarrhea and vomiting can lead to severe malnutrition. *J Pediatr Gastroenterol Nutr.* 1998;27:1–5.
19. Burpee T. Diarrheal diseases. In: Duggan C, Watkins JB, Walker W (eds). *Nutrition in Pediatrics,* 4th ed. Hamilton, Ontario: BC Decker; 2008:631–640.
20. Solomon SM, Kirby KF. The refeeding syndrome: a review. *J Parenter Enteral Nutr.* 1985;85:28–36.
21. Stocks RJ, Davies DP, Allen F. Loss of breast milk nutrients during tube feeding. *Arch Dis Child.* 1985;60:164.

22. Greer FR, McCormick A, Loker J. Changes in fat concentration of human milk during the delivery by intermittent bolus and continuous mechanical pump infusion. *J Pediatr.* 1984;105:745.
23. Narayan I, Singh B, Harvey D. Fat loss during feeding of human milk. *Arch Dis.* 1984;59:475.
24. Lavin M, Clark RM. The effect of short-term refrigeration of milk and the addition of breast milk fortifier on the delivery of lipids during tube feeding. *J Pediatr Gastroenterol Nutr.* 1989;8:496.
25. WHO/UNICEF joint statement. Clinical management of acute diarrhea. 2004. Available at: http://www.unicef.org/publications/index_21433.html. Accessed August 9, 2011.
26. Lukacik M, Thomas L, Aranda JV. A meta-analysis of the effects of oral zinc in the treatment of acute and persistent diarrhea. *Pediatrics.* 2008;121(2):326–336.
27. Lazzerini M, Ronfani L. Oral zinc for treating diarrhea in children [review]. *Cochrane Library.* 2009;4:1–67.
28. Lee PC, Werlin SL. Carbohydrates. In: Baker RD Jr, Baker SS, Davis AM (eds). *Pediatric Parenteral Nutrition.* New York: Chapman and Hall; 1997:103.
29. Thobani S, Molla AM, Snyder JD. Nutritional therapy for persistent diarrhea. In: Baker SS, Baker RD Jr, Davis AM (eds). *Pediatric Enteral Nutrition.* New York: Chapman and Hall; 1994:291.
30. Sazawal S, Black RE, Bhan MK, et al. Zinc supplementation in young children with acute diarrhea in India. *N Engl J Med.* 1995;333:839–844.
31. Baker SS, Liptak GS, Colletti RB, et al. Constipation in infants and children: evaluation and treatment. A medical position statement of the North American Society for Pediatric Gastroenterology and Nutrition, *J Pediatr Gastroenterol Nutr.* 1999;29(5):612–626. Erratum in: *J Pediatr Gastroenterol Nutr.* 2000;30(1):109.
32. Goldberg D. Clinical assessment. In: Cox JH (ed). *Nutrition Manual for At-Risk Toddlers and Infants.* Chicago: Precept Press; 1997:59.
33. Dwyer JT. Dietary fiber for children: how much? *Pediatrics.* 1995;96(5):1019–1022.
34. Oski FA. Iron fortified formulas and gastrointestinal symptoms in infants: a controlled study. *Pediatrics.* 1980;66:168–170.
35. Reeves JD, Yip R. Lack of adverse side effects of oral ferrous sulfate therapy in 1 year old infants. *Pediatrics.* 1985;75:352–355.
36. Nelson SE, Ziegler EE, Copeland AM, et al. Lack of adverse reactions to iron fortified formula. *Pediatrics.* 1988;81:360–364.
37. American Academy of Pediatrics, Committee on Nutrition American Academy of Pediatrics. Iron fortified formulas. *Pediatrics.* 1999;104:119–123 (reaffirmed November 2002).
38. Sherman PM, Hassall E, Fagundes-Neto U, et al. A global, evidence-based consensus on the definition of gastroesophageal reflux disease in the pediatric patient. *Am J Gastroenterol.* 2009;104(5):1278–1295.
39. Vandenplas Y, Rudolph CD, DiLorenzo C, et al. Pediatric gastroesophageal reflux clinical practice guidelines: joint recommendations of the North American Society for Pediatric Gastroenterology, Hepatology, and Nutrition and the European Society for Pediatric Gastroenterology, Hepatology, and Nutrition. *J Pediatr Gastroenterol Nutr.* 2009;49(4):498–547.
40. Horvath A, Dziechciarz P, Szajewska H. The effect of thickened-feed interventions on gastroesophageal reflux in infants: systematic review and meta-analysis of randomized, controlled trials [review]. *Pediatrics.* 2008;122(6):e1268–e1277. Erratum in: *Pediatrics.* 2009;123(4):1254.
41. Heyman MB, Committee on Nutrition. Lactose intolerance in infants, children, and adolescents. *Pediatrics.* 2006;118:1279–1286.
42. Lifshitz CH. Breath hydrogen testing in infants with diarrhea. In: Lifshitz F (ed). *Carbohydrate Intolerance in Infancy.* New York: Marcel Dekker; 1982:31–42.
43. Nevin-Folino N, Pediatric Nutrition Practice Group. Lactose controlled diet. *Pediatric Manual of Clinical Dietetics,* 2nd ed. Chicago: American Dietetic Association, 2008:635–640.
44. Kretchmer N. Lactose and lactase: a historical perspective. *Gastroenterology.* 1971;61:805–813.
45. Sahi T. Genetics and epidemiology of adult-type hypolactasia. *Scand J Gastroenterol Suppl.* 1994;202:7–20.
46. Paige DM, Bayless TM, Mellitis ED, Davis L. Lactose malabsorption in preschool black children. *Am J Clin Nutr.* 1977;30:1018–1022.
47. Erasmus H, Ludwig-Auser H, Paterson P, et al. Enhanced weight gain in preterm infants receiving lactase-treated feeds: a randomized, double-blind, controlled trial. *J Pediatr.* 2002;141:532–537.
48. Mobassaleh M, Montgomery R, Biller J, Grand R. Development of carbohydrate absorption in the fetus and neonate. *Pediatrics.* 1985;75(1 Pt 2):160–166.
49. MacLean WC, Fink BB. Lactose malabsorption by premature infants: magnitude and clinical significance. *J Pediatr.* 1980;97:383.
50. Savilahti E, Launiala K, Kuitunen P. Congenital lactase deficiency: a clinical study on 16 patients. *Arch Dis Child.* 1983;58:246–252.
51. Torniainen S, Savilahti E, Jarvela I. Congenital lactase deficiency—a more common disease than previously thought. *Duodecim.* 2009;125(7):766–770.
52. Hill ID, Dirks MH, Liptak GS. Guidelines for the diagnosis and treatment of celiac disease in children: recommendations of the North American Society for Pediatric Gastroenterology, Hepatology and Nutrition. *J Ped Gastroenterol Nutr.* 2005;40(1):1–19.
53. Niewinski M. Advances in celiac disease and gluten free diet. *J Am Diet Assoc.* 2008;108(4):661–672.
54. Alehan F, Canan O, Cemil T, et al. Increased risk for coeliac disease in paediatric patients with migraine. *Cephalalgia.* 2008;28:945–949.
55. Lurz E, Scheidegger U, Schibli S, et al. Clinical presentation of celiac disease and the diagnostic accuracy of serologic markers in children. *Eur J Pediatr.* 2009;168:839–845.
56. Niewinski M. Advances in celiac disease and gluten free diet. *J Am Diet Assoc.* 2008;108(4):661–672.
57. Anderson R. Coeliac disease: current approach and future prospects. *Intern Med J.* 2008;38:790–799.
58. Murray J, See J. Gluten-free diet: the medical and nutrition management of celiac disease. *Nutr Clin Prac.* 2006;21:1–15.
59. Case S. *The Gluten Free Diet: Comprehensive Resource Guide.* Regina, Saskatchewan, Canada: Case Nutrition Consulting; 2006.

60. American Dietetic Association. Celiac disease. ADA Evidence Analysis Library. Available at: http://www.adaevidencelibrary.com. Accessed September 9, 2009.
61. Cammarota G, Danese S, DeLorenzo A, et al. High prevalence of celiac disease in patients with lactose intolerance. *Digestion.* 2005;71:106–110.
62. Pellerin G, Turner J. Prevalence of metabolic bone disease in children with celiac disease is independent of symptoms at diagnosis. *J Ped Gastroenterol Nutr.* 2009;49:1–5.
63. Motil KJ, Grand RJ. Inflammatory bowel disease. In: Walker WA, Watkins JB (eds). *Nutrition in Pediatrics: Basic Science and Clinical Applications.* Hamilton, ON: Decker; 1997:516.
64. Motil KJ, Grand RJ. Nutritional management of inflammatory bowel disease. *Pediatr Clin North Am.* 1985;32:447.
65. Motil KJ, Grand RJ, Davis-Kraft L, et al. Growth failure in children with inflammatory bowel disease: a prospective study. *United States Department of Agriculture/Agricultural Research Service Children's Nutrition Research Center, Houston, Texas Gastroenterology.* 1993;105(3):681–691.
66. Azcue M, Rashid M, Friffiths A, Pencharz PB. Energy expenditure and body composition in children with Crohn's disease: effect of enteral nutrition and treatment with prednisolone. *Gut.* 1997;41:203–208.
67. Stokes MA, Hill GL. Total energy expenditure in patients with Crohn's disease: measurement by the combined body scan technique. *J Parenter Enteral Nutr.* 1993;17:3–7.
68. Takeda H, Ishihama K, Fukui T, et al. Significance of rapid turnover proteins in protein-losing gastroenteropathy. *Hepatogastroenterology.* 2003;50(54):1963–1965.
69. Hartman C, Eliakim R, Shamir R. Nutritional status and nutritional therapy in inflammatory bowel diseases. *World J Gastroenterol.* 2009;15(21):2570–2578.
70. Parrish CR, Krenitsky J, Willcutts K, Radigan AE. Gastrointestinal disease. In: Gottschlich MM (ed). *The ASPEN Nutrition Support Core Curriculum.* Silver Spring, MD: ASPEN; 2007:508–539.
71. Vagianos K, Bector S, McConnell J, Bernstein CN. Nutrition assessment of patients with inflammatory bowel disease. *J Parenter Enter Nutr.* 2007;31(4):311–319.
72. Semeao EJ, Jawad AF, Stouffer NO, et al. Risk factors for low bone mineral density in children and young adults with Crohn's disease. *J Pediatr.* 1999;135(5):593–600.
73. Paganelli M, Albanese C, Borrelli O, et al. Inflammation is the main determinant of low bone mineral density in pediatric inflammatory bowel disease. *Inflamm Bowel Dis.* 2007;13(4):416–423.
74. Holick MF. Vitamin D deficiency. *N Engl J Med.* 2007;357(3):266–280.
75. Davis AM, Baker SS, Baker RD Jr, et al. Pediatric gastrointestinal disorders. In: Meritt RM (ed). *The ASPEN Nutrition Support Practice Manual.* Silver Spring, MD: ASPEN; 1998:27–30.
76. Prey S, Paul C. Effect of folic or folinic acid supplementation on methotrexate-associated safety and efficacy in inflammatory disease: a systematic review. *Br J Dermatol.* 2008;160(3):622–628.
77. Hyams JS. Crohn's disease. In: Hyams WS, Hyams JS (eds). *Pediatric Gastrointestinal Disease: Pathophysiology, Diagnosis, Management.* Philadelphia, PA: WB Saunders; 1993:750–764.
78. Levenstein S, Prantera C, Luzi C, et al. A low residue or normal diet in Crohn's disease: a prospective controlled trial of Italian patients. *Gut.* 1985;26:989.
79. Levi AJ. Diet in the management of Crohn's disease. *Gut.* 1985;26:985.
80. Mishkin S. Dairy sensitivity, lactose malabsorption, and elimination diets in inflammatory bowel disease. *Am J Clin Nutr.* 1997;65:564–567.
81. Siedman EG, Leliedo N, Ament M, et al. Nutritional issues in pediatric inflammatory bowel disease. *J Pediatr Gastroenterol Nutr.* 1991;12:424.
82. Zachos M, Tondeur M, Griffiths AM. Enteral nutritional therapy for induction of remission in Crohn's disease. *Cochrane Database of Systematic Reviews.* 2007;1:CD000542.
83. Akobeng AK, Thomas AG. Enteral nutrition for maintenance of remission of Crohn's disease. *Cochrane Database of Systematic Reviews.* 2007;3:CD005984.
84. Gassull MA, Fernandez-Banares F, Cabre E, et al. Fat composition may be a clue to explain the primary therapeutic effect of enteral nutrition in Crohn's disease: results of a double blind randomized multicentre European trial. *Gut.* 2002;51(2):164–168.
85. Sakurai T, Matsui T, Yao T, et al. Short-term efficacy of enteral nutrition in the treatment of active Crohn's disease: a randomized, controlled trial comparing nutrient formulas. *J Parenter Enteral Nutr.* 2002;26(2):98–103.
86. DeLey M, de Vos R, Hommes DW, Stokkers P. Fish oil for induction of remission of ulcerative colitis. *Cochrane Database of Systemic Reviews.* 2007;4:CD005573.
87. Turner D, Steinhart AH, Griffiths AM. Omega 3 fatty acids for maintenance of remission of ulcerative colitis. *Cochrane Database of Systemic Reviews.* 2007;3:CD006443.
88. Turner D, Zlotkin SH, Shah PS, Griffiths AM. Omega 3 fatty acids for maintenance of remission of Crohn's disease. *Cochrane Database of Systemic Reviews.* 2009;1:CD006320.
89. Butterworth AD, Thomas AG, Akobeng AK. Probiotics for induction of remission in Crohn's disease. *Cochrane Database of Systemic Reviews.* 2008;3:CD006634.
90. Rolfe VE, Fortun PJ, Hawkey CJ, Bath-Hextall F. Probiotics for maintenance of remission in Crohn's disease. *Cochrane Database of Systematic Reviews.* 2006;4:CD004826.
91. Mallon P, McKay D, Kirk S, Gardiner K. Probiotics for induction of remission in ulcerative colitis. *Cochrane Database of Systematic Reviews.* 2007;4:CD005573.
92. Abou-Assi S, O'Keefe SJ. Nutrition support during acute pancreatitis. *Nutrition.* 2002;18(11–12):938–943.
93. Frossard JL, Steer ML, Pastor CM. Acute pancreatitis. *Lancet.* 2008;371(9607):143–152.
94. Eckerwall GE, Tingstedt BB, Bergenzaun PE, Andersson RG. Immediate oral feeding in patients with mild acute pancreatitis is safe and may accelerate recovery—a randomized clinical study. *Clin Nutr.* 2007;26(6):758–763.
95. Marik PE, Zaloga GP. Meta-analysis of parenteral nutrition versus enteral nutrition in patients with acute pancreatitis. *BMJ.* 2004;328(7453):1407.
96. Marik PE. What is the best way to feed patients with pancreatitis? *Curr Opin Crit Care.* 2009;15(2):131–138.
97. Petrov MS, Pylypchuk RD, Emelyanov NV. Systematic review: nutritional support in acute pancreatitis. *Aliment Pharmacol Ther.* 2008;28(6):704–712.

98. McClave SA, Chang WK, Dhaliwal R, Heyland DK. Nutrition support in acute pancreatitis: a systematic review of the literature. *J Parenter Enteral Nutr.* 2006;30(2):143–156.
99. Petrov MS, Pylypchuk RD, Uchugina AF. A systematic review on the timing of artificial nutrition in acute pancreatitis. *Br J Nutr.* 2009;101(6):787–793.
100. Petrov MS, Loveday BP, Pylypchuk RD, et al. Systematic review and meta-analysis of enteral nutrition formulations in acute pancreatitis. *Br J Surg.* 2009;96(11):1243–1252.
101. Alnounou M, Munoz SJ. Nutrition concerns of the patient with primary biliary cirrhosis or primary sclerosing cholangitis. *Pract Gastroenterol.* 2006;37:92–100.
102. Sokol RJ, Stall C. Anthropometric evaluation of children with chronic liver disease. *Am J Clin Nutr.* 1990;52:203–208.
103. Ng VL, Balistreri WF. Treatment options for chronic cholestasis in infancy and childhood. *Curr Treat Options Gastroenterol.* 2005;8(5):419–430.
104. Baker A, Amoroso P, Wilson S, et al. Increased resting energy expenditure: a cause of undernutrition in pediatric liver disease. *J Pediatr Gastroenterol Nutr.* 1991;13:318.
105. Delich PC, Siepler JK, Parker P. Liver disease. In: Gottschlich MM (ed). *The ASPEN Nutrition Support Core Curriculum.* Silver Spring, MD: ASPEN; 2007:540–557.
106. Kleiman R, Warman KY. Nutrition in liver disease. In: Baker SS, Baker RD Jr, Davis AM (eds). *Pediatric Enteral Nutrition.* New York: Chapman and Hall; 1994:261.
107. Pettei MJ, Daftary S, Levine JJ. Essential fatty acid deficiency associated with the use of a medium-chain-triglyceride infant formula in pediatric hepatobiliary disease. *Am J Clin Nutr.* 1991;53:1217–1221.
108. Kelly DA, Davenport M. Current management of biliary atresia. *Arch Dis Child.* 2007;92:1132–1135.
109. Sanchez AJ, Aranda-Michel J. Liver disease and osteoporosis. *Nutr Clin Pract.* 2006;21(3):273–278.
110. O'Brien A, Williams R. Nutrition in end-stage liver disease: principles and practice. *Gastroenterology.* 2008;134(6):1729–1740.
111. Greer R, Lehnert M, Lewindon P, et al. Body composition and components of energy expenditure in children with end-stage liver disease. *J Pediatr Gastroenterol Nutr.* 2003;36(3):358–363.
112. Barshes NR, Chang IF, Karpen SJ, et al. Impact of pretransplant growth retardation in pediatric liver transplantation. *J Pediatr Gastroenterol Nutr.* 2006;43(1):89–94.
113. Utterson EC, Shepherd RW, Sokol RJ, et al. Biliary atresia: clinical profiles, risk factors, and outcomes of 755 patients listed for liver transplantation. *J Pediatr.* 2005;147(2):180–185.
114. Stickel F, Inderbitzin D, Candinas D. Role of nutrition in liver transplantation for end-stage chronic liver disease. *Nutr Rev.* 2008;66(1):47–54.
115. Renz JF, de Roos M, Rosenthal P, et al. Posttransplantation growth in pediatric liver recipients. *Liver Transpl.* 2001;7(12): 1040–1055.
116. McDiarmid SV, Gornbein JA, DeSilva PJ, et al. Factors affecting growth after pediatric liver transplantation. *Transplantation.* 1999;67(3):404–411.
117. Van Mourik ID, Beath SV, Brook GA, et al. Long-term nutritional and neurodevelopmental outcome of liver transplantation in infants aged less than 12 months. *J Pediatr Gastroenterol Nutr.* 2000;30(3):269–275.
118. Viner RM, Forton JT, Cole TJ, et al. Growth of long-term survivors of liver transplantation. *Arch Dis Child.* 1999;80(3): 235–240.
119. Sanchez AJ, Aranda-Michel J. Liver disease and osteoporosis. *Nutr Clin Pract.* 2006;21(3):273–278.
120. Gasser RW. Cholestasis and metabolic bone disease—a clinical review. *Wein Med Wochenschr.* 2008;158(19–20):553–557.
121. Ozbek OY, Ozcay F, Avci Z, et al. Food allergy after liver transplantation in children: a prospective study. *Pediatr Allergy Immunol.* 2009;20(8):741–747.
122. Ziegler MM. Short bowel syndrome in infancy: Etiology and management. *Clin Perinatol.* 1986;13:167.
123. Mazariegos GV, Squires RH, Sindhi RK. *Curr Gastroenterol Rep.* 2009;11(3):226–233.
124. King KL, Phillips SM. The ins and outs of pediatric short bowel. *Support Line.* 2009;31(3):18–26.
125. Taylor SF, Sokol RJ. Infants with short bowel syndrome. In: Hay WW (ed). *Neonatal Nutrition and Metabolism.* St. Louis, MO: Mosby Year Book; 1991;437.
126. Wessel JJ. Short bowel syndrome. In: Groh-Wargos S, Thompson M, Cox JH (eds). *Nutritional Care for High Risk Newborns,* 3rd ed. Chicago, IL: Precept Press; 2000:469–488.
127. Vanderhoof JA. Short bowel syndrome. In: Walker WA, Watkins JB (eds). *Nutrition in Pediatrics: Basic Science and Clinical Applications.* Hamilton, ON: Decker; 1997:610.
128. Klish WJ. The short gut. In: Walker WA, Watkins JB (eds). *Nutrition in Pediatrics.* Boston: Little, Brown; 1985:561.
129. Abad-Sinden A, Sutphen J. Nutritional management of pediatric short bowel syndrome. *Pract Gastro.* 2003;12:28–48.
130. Fleming CR, George L, Stoner GL, et al. The importance of urinary magnesium values in patients with gut failure. *Mao Clin Proc.* 1996;71:21–24.
131. Farrell MK. Physiologic effects of parenteral nutrition. In: Baker RD Jr, Baker SS, Davis AM (eds). *Pediatric Parenteral Nutrition.* New York: Chapman and Hall; 1997:36.
132. Abad-Jorge A, Roman B. Enteral nutrition management in pediatric patients with severe gastrointestinal impairment. *Support Line.* 2007;29(2):3–11.
133. Wong KY, Lan LC, Lin SC, et al. Mucous fistula refeeding in premature neonates with enterostomies. *J Pediatr Gastroenterol Nutr.* 2004;39:43–45.
134. Ching YA, Gura K, Modi B, Jaksic T. Pediatric intestinal failure: nutritional and pharmacological approaches. *Nutr Clin Pract.* 2007;22:653–663.
135. Matarese LE, O'Keefe SJ, Kandil HM, et al. Short bowel syndrome: clinical guidelines for nutrition management. *Nutr Clin Pract.* 2005;20:493–502.
136. Galea MH, Holliday H, Carachi R, et al. Short bowel syndrome: a collective review. *J Pediatr Surg.* 1992;27:592–596.
137. Cooper A, Floyd TF, Ross AJ. Morbidity and mortality of short bowel syndrome acquired in infancy: an update. *J Pediatr Surg.* 1984;19:711–717.
138. Linsheid TR, Tarnowski KJ, Rasnake LK, et al. Behavioral treatment of food refusal in a child with short gut syndrome. *J Pediatr Psych.* 1987;12:451.
139. Parekh NR, Seidner DL. Advances in enteral feeding of the intestinal failure patient. *Support Line.* 2006;28(3):18–24.

140. Nordgaard I, Hansen BS, Mortensen PB. Importance of colonic support for energy absorption as small-bowel failure proceeds. *Am J Clin Nutr.* 1996;64:222–231.
141. Byrne TA, Veglia L, Camelio M, et al. Clinical observations: beyond the prescription: optimizing the diet of patients with short bowel syndrome. *Nutr Clin Pract.* 2000;15:306–311.
142. Rahman N, Hitchcock R. Case report of paediatric oxalate urolithiasis and a review of enteric hyperoxaluria. *J Pediatr Urol.* 2010:6(2):112–116.
143. Chang-Kit L, Filler G, Pike J, Leonard MP. Pediatric urolithiasis: experience at a tertiary care pediatric hospital. *Can Urol Assoc J.* 2008;2(4):381–386.
144. Chaet MS, Warner BW, Farrell MF. Intensive nutritional support and remedial surgical intervention for extreme short bowel syndrome. *J Pediatr Gastroenterol Nutr.* 1994;19:295–298.
145. Thompson JS. Surgical management of short bowel syndrome. *Surgery.* 1993;113:4–7.
146. Warner BW, Chaet MS. Nontransplant surgical options for management of the short bowel syndrome. *J Pediatr Gastroenterol Nutr.* 1997;17:1–12.
147. Matarese LE, Costa G, Bond G, et al. Therapeutic efficacy of intestinal and multivisceral transplantation: survival and nutrition outcome. *Nutr Clin Pract.* 2007;22:474–481.

CHAPTER 13

Kidney Disease

Linda A. Phelan

Infants and children with chronic kidney disease (CKD) face many dietary manipulations throughout their course of treatment. Nutritional management is a key component with focus on normal growth and bone health.

Stages of CKD help identify the progression of the disease toward end-stage kidney failure. These stages progress from mild CKD (stages 1 and 2), to moderate (stage 3), severe (stage 4), and end stage (stage 5). At stage 5, the treatment options are dialysis (stage 5D) and transplant (stage 5T).[1] Diagnostic criteria used for placement in one of the CKD stages is based on presence of kidney damage (e.g., proteinuria) and functional impairment defined by the estimate of glomerular filtration rate (GFR).[2] Designation of a CKD stage is useful in estimating the degree of medical nutrition therapy necessary for controlling uremia, managing electrolyte balance, and setting goals for calorie, protein, and other nutrients.

CKD in infants and children is caused by acquired and congenital etiologies.[3] Acquired diseases, such as chronic glomerulonephritis, fortunately have less impact on growth, due to their more insidious onset. Congenital diseases, however, can result in early and severe growth retardation.

Infants and toddlers (ages birth to 4 years) presenting with CKD must be aggressively nourished in order to promote at least a normal growth rate, preferably greater than the fifth percentile of length for age.[4,5] The earlier the age of onset of renal failure (GFR less than 30% of normal), the more potentially severe its impact on growth.[6–9]

The consequences of chronic kidney disease and its treatments for infants and children all potentially influence growth (see **Table 13-1**). If any of these conditions are left inadequately managed, the child's linear growth will be delayed.[10,11] Medical nutrition therapy that includes adequate calories and protein for growth, interventions to control renal osteodystrophy, management of electrolyte balance via addition and/or restriction of minerals and fluid, and finally control of uremia and anemia play a vital role in the control and progression of CKD and the ability of the child to grow normally. Growth retardation can be arrested; however, catch-up growth is difficult to achieve.

The characteristic symptoms of CRF in children signaling increasing uremia are noted in **Table 13-2**. Several of those listed, including nausea and growth retardation, may respond favorably to some dietary modification(s). When, despite aggressive attempts at optimizing nutritional intake and preventing renal osteodystrophy, normal growth velocity is unattainable, the initiation of rhGH becomes necessary.[12,13] Adequate nutrition and control of renal bone disease continue to be significant therapies in the management of children with CKD.

Published guidelines include the following areas:

- Chronic kidney disease
- Hemodialysis
- Peritoneal dialysis
- Vascular access
- Nutrition
- Bone metabolism and disease
- Dyslipidemias[14,15]

These guidelines are meant to be used as a starting point for assessment and intervention steps of medical nutrition therapy. Adjustments in the recommendations set forth by these guidelines may be necessary, based on clinical judgment, to achieve the ultimate goals of normal growth and development and bone health.

The impact of CKD on growth in children depends on the severity and duration of the renal insufficiency, the diagnosis, and the age of onset. The treatments for CKD, namely dialysis and transplantation, will affect growth as well.

Nutrition Management

Treating children with CKD without dialysis requires judicious and frequent monitoring of diet intake, biochemical parameters, and growth.[15–17] In CKD, weight and weight-for-height are particularly difficult to assess given the accumulation of extracellular fluid not always apparent in

TABLE 13-1 Consequences of Chronic Kidney Disease

- Water/electrolyte imbalance
- Accumulation of endogenous/exogenous toxins
- Hypertension
- Acidosis
- Anemia
- Renal osteodystrophy
- Anorexia/undernutrition
- Need for steroid therapy

Source: Linda Phelan, RD

TABLE 13-2 Symptoms of Uremia in Children

- Nausea
- Weakness
- Fatigue
- Decreased school performance
- Loss of attention span
- Growth retardation
- Changes in urine output
- Shortness of breath
- Swelling of face/extremities/abdomen
- Amenorrhea in adolescent girls

Source: Linda Phelan, RD

children. Also, the normal ranges for a number of laboratory values are different for children of different ages and should be considered whenever assessing a child's metabolic status and whether the restriction and/or addition of minerals is warranted.

Breast milk is the preferred feeding for infants with CKD when available. Now that normal growth can be obtained in infants with CKD and waste products significantly reduced, formula choice does not need to be limited unless the infant has other intolerances or conditions, such as lactose intolerance or GI disorders. The infant should be transitioned to a standard infant formula once growth is evident and electrolytes are within normal ranges in order to provide an adequate intake of nutrients. This is particularly important to consider in fluid-restricted infants whose volume of formula may need to be reduced.[4]

Renal osteodystrophy contributes significantly to growth retardation in children with renal insufficiency.[18] Early in the course of renal disease, synthesis of 1,25-dihydroxycholecalciferol ($1{,}25(OH)_2D_3$) and the excretion of excessive dietary phosphate decrease lead to the development of renal osteodystrophy and secondary hyperparathyroidism if left untreated. This often occurs before derangements in calcium, phosphorous, and parathyroid hormone levels are detected.[19–21] Hyperphosphatemia is considered a late indicator of bone deformities. Vitamin D deficiency and insufficiency is commonly seen in children with CKD.[19,22] Insufficient vitamin D can exacerbate the suppression of calcitriol in CKD patients; therefore, vitamin D levels should be assessed early in the course of CKD and supplemented as needed.[15,23] Therapy may include any or all of the following:

- Dietary restriction of high-phosphorus foods and fluids (primarily dairy products, chocolate, nuts, and colas)
- Supplementation of vitamin D (1,25 $(OH)_2D_3$) and calcium
- Prescription of nonaluminum-, nonmagnesium-containing phosphate binders (calcium carbonate, acetate, glubionate, and/or sevelamer hydrochloride) to be taken with meals[24–28]

In infants, PM 60/40 may be the initial formula of choice; however, it contains less phosphorus than the more common infant formulas, and it may be inadequate in providing sufficient phosphorus for the growing infant.[4] Changing formula to one containing more phosphorous or starting a phosphorous supplement may be necessary in infants with CKD who exhibit lower-than-normal phosphorous levels.

Sodium and fluid restriction might be necessary to prevent or control the incidence of hypertension and edema commonly associated with CKD. Usually, a no-added-salt diet is sufficient. Limitation of fluid should be based on the child's urine output and insensible losses. Hyperkalemia is rarely a problem as long as kidney function is greater than 5% of normal. However, some children may be prescribed medications such as ACE (angiotensin-converting enzyme) inhibitors (used to reduce proteinuria), which cause a reduction in GFR and concomitant reduction in the excretion of potassium. Limiting high-potassium foods in the diet may be helpful.

For infants requiring sodium and/or potassium restriction, formulas such as PM 60/40 or Carnation Good Start are appropriate. If the volume of formula must be restricted, it is unlikely that any significant contribution of sodium or potassium will come from formula. Infants with increased urine losses of sodium and/or potassium will need supplementation to their usual diet. Attention to the causes of CKD is particularly important in infants and young children. Obstructive uropathy and renal dysplasia are often accompanied with defects in the kidney tubule's ability to concentrate the urine. This results in increased excretion of water and sodium chloride. Careful attention to providing increased fluid and salt supplementation may be necessary. Infants and young children with excessive losses of fluid and salt experience growth retardation and vomiting due to dehydration.[29]

Energy needs are at least 80% of the RDA for height age and may be greater than 100%, depending on activity level.[30] Protein should be provided at 100% of the DRI for chronological age.[15,17] Monitoring of energy intake over the course of CKD should be ongoing with the goal of providing the DRI for chronological age, sex, and physical activity. Equations to adjust calorie needs for normal weight and obese children are available. These equations should be implemented in calorie prescriptions for CKD children with BMI's above the 95th percentile (see Appendix G).

Children with CKD are at highest risk for pediatric CVD due to the frequency of dyslipidemia[30] and extra skeletal calcification, including vascular calcification.[19] Children with CKD need caloric guidelines that primarily allow for proper growth and control the uremia and/or electrolyte abnormalities, but the guidelines also reduce or limit the risk of CVD, which is the leading cause of mortality in children with CKD.

Anytime protein, phosphorous, and/or potassium is restricted in the diet it reduces sources of calories. If these restrictions must be in place and extra simple sugars and fat must be increased to provide adequate calories, then guidelines that advise on using heart-healthy fats may be the only dyslipidemic choice available to use.[15] However, if the child with CKD is growing well and is stable, the dyslipidemia guidelines may be appropriate to use.

Protein restriction much below the DRI for chronological age is contraindicated in growing children with CKD. With dietary phosphate restriction alone, a considerable limitation of protein intake could occur without restriction of protein per se. Protein is generally unrestricted at CKD stages 1 and 2, 100–140% of the DRI at CKD stages 3 and 4 and 100–120% of the DRI at CKD stages 4 and 5.[15] Restricting protein below the DRI will not slow down the progression of CKD in children; however, restricting protein below the DRI can cause growth failure. Routine nutritional assessment, including anthropometric measurements and dietary intake, will indicate whether the prescribed protein and calorie levels are adequate.[31]

Providing optimal nutrition within the limitations of fluid restriction is possible only by caloric supplementation of the formula to as much as 60 kcal/oz. Attempts should be made to maintain caloric distribution as follows, with the lower intakes of fat calories recommended for children older than age 2 years are 35–65% carbohydrate, 5–16% protein, and 30–55% fat.

Carbohydrate sources such as Polycose (Abbott Laboratories) and Moducal (Mead Johnson) are coupled with an oil (such as canola oil, or medium-chain triglyceride [MCT] oil for premature infants). Concentration of the formula with or without the addition of a protein supplement increases protein content. Caloric density can be advanced by 2 to 4 calories/day as tolerated.[4] Diluting adult renal formulas also has been done for CKD infants as young as 6.9 months.[32] Ensuring the consistent daily intake of a sufficient volume of formula to meet an infant's nutritional goals for growth most often can be achieved only after the initiation of enteral tube feedings.[31–35] The presence of gastroesophageal reflux in infants with CKD is a major factor contributing to feeding problems in this age group.[36] However, continuous nighttime infusions of formula via feeding pump allow maximum tolerance of formula.

Once nutritional goals are realized and a feeding regimen established, additional oral stimulation through nonnutritive sucking can begin.[37] Once children are successfully transplanted they eventually return to normal feeding practices.

A multivitamin should be routinely recommended. Additionally, 0.5–1 mg folic acid per day should be included. Iron supplementation may be indicated, especially if the child is receiving erythropoietin and ferritin and/or transferrin saturation levels are depressed.[38,39]

Dialysis

Dialysis is indicated once a child experiences symptoms that significantly interfere with activities of daily living. Peritoneal dialysis (continuous cycling or continuous ambulatory) is the preferred choice of dialytic care for young children. Hemodialysis and peritoneal dialysis are options for older children. Nutritional management is dictated by the type of dialytic therapy chosen. Nutrient losses via dialysate (in particular, protein, phosphorus, sodium, and potassium) must be considered when assessing nutritional adequacy of the diet.[40]

Management of calcium and phosphorus balance is necessary even while on dialysis. Serum levels should be checked periodically and supplemented, as needed. A child's recommended intake for sodium and potassium is directly related to his or her residual renal function and the type and effectiveness of dialysis. Likewise, the degree of ultrafiltration possible and the child's urine output will dictate an advisable fluid intake. If restriction of sodium and potassium is necessary, which usually happens with hemodialysis, the elimination or limitation of foods containing especially large amounts of sodium and potassium is generally sufficient. Severely restricted diets often result in noncompliance and dull a child's interest in food. Individualization of diet is essential to successfully control sodium, potassium, and fluid intake.[41] With peritoneal dialysis, restriction of potassium often is not necessary except with anuric children. Infants on peritoneal dialysis often require continued sodium supplementation and/or phosphorous supplementation. Indeed, an infant with CKD stages 1 to 5 on a low-mineral formula, such as PM 60/40, may be able to switch to a standard infant formula once started on peritoneal dialysis due to increased losses of sodium and phosphorous in the dialysate.

The exact nutritional requirements for protein and energy for patients undergoing peritoneal dialysis are not clear. It is known that some protein is lost to the dialysate, while glucose is absorbed from the dialysate. The degree to which these changes occur can be determined only through measurement of individual patients. Periodic calculations of urinary and dialysate urea nitrogen, dialysate protein and amino acids, and miscellaneous nitrogen losses are necessary.[42] For hemodialysis, the addition of 0.1 g protein/kg/day to the DRI for chronological age is recommended. For peritoneal dialysis, the addition of 0.15–0.35 g protein/kg/day to the DRI for chronological age is suggested. Diets can be developed and altered when measurements indicate the need while promoting growth and preventing obesity.[43] During periods of peritonitis, there is an increased loss of protein to the dialysate, and the child usually feels ill. Careful attention to dietary intake is important to prevent a potentially significant loss of lean body weight during this time of infection.

Protein and energy requirements for children on hemodialysis are 0.3 g/cm/day and 10 kcal/cm/day, respectively. The routine use of urea kinetic modeling is especially helpful in determining dialysis and nutritional adequacy in children.[44–46] Monthly monitoring of protein catabolic rates and urea generation provides insight into subtle changes in dialysis treatment and/or diet intake that otherwise might go unnoticed. Kinetic modeling, usually conducted by the dietitian, allows the dietitian access to the fundamental parameters and concepts of dialysis prescription.

Hyperlipidemia remains a problem in children on dialysis, particularly peritoneal dialysis.[47] Treatment in growing children is controversial.[41] Children on both hemodialysis and peritoneal dialysis should be provided water-soluble vitamins and folate, which are lost to dialysate.[48] Care should be taken not to exceed the tolerable upper intake (UL) levels of vitamins when dietary and supplement sources of vitamins are provided.[15] Specially formulated dialysis vitamin preparations such as Nephro-Vite Rx (R&D Laboratories) and Nephrocaps (Fleming & Co.) fulfill most patients' needs. Infants can be given less frequent dosing or partial dosing of the adult renal vitamin supplements on the market. Vitamin supplementations may not be needed if the dialysed child is receiving 100% of his or her nutritional needs by infant formula or adult renal formulas.

Secondary carnitine deficiency has been noted in patients receiving dialysis.[49] However, carnitine supplementation for children on dialysis is currently not recommended.[15]

Transplant

The ultimate goal of all pediatric end-stage renal disease programs is transplantation. This is the only treatment option that provides children with the opportunity for normal growth and development and potentially for catch-up growth.[50] Clinicians must be constantly vigilant for signs of rejection and infection, especially in the first postoperative year. Immunosuppression and antibiotic therapy result in side effects related to inefficient digestion and metabolism of nutrients, as well as to growth retardation.[51] New immunosuppressants that provide increased protection from rejection also increase the risk of the patient developing hyperglycemia (due to insulin resistance), hyperlipidemia, and hypercholesterolemia. Alternate-day steroid therapy may promote normal and, at times, catch-up growth.

For small children receiving adult kidneys, PN may be considered immediately postoperatively. Surgically implanting an adult-size kidney into a very small child usually requires significant bowel manipulation to make enough room for the organ, and an ileus may result.

Once oral feedings are resumed, the dietary recommendations are individualized. If kidney function is not normal, attention to sodium, potassium, phosphorus, and fluid will be necessary. A rise in blood urea nitrogen (BUN) level and a slow recovery to normal is usual even with normal kidney function due to the catabolic stress of surgery. Aggressive nutritional support of the patient should be started soon after transplant.[52]

With the attainment of normal kidney function, a no-added-salt diet is still advisable. Hypertension, a potential result of high-dose steroid therapy, is frequently seen after transplantation, and sodium restriction, at least during the acute phase (first 6 to 8 months after transplant), is helpful. Also, tubular loss of phosphate and magnesium is often present, requiring phosphorus and magnesium supplementation. Dietary phosphorus intake usually is not adequate to maintain blood levels above 3.0 mg/dL.

Education on appropriate portion sizes and a heart-healthy diet should be a focus because most children with CKD have never learned to eat nutritionally balanced meals. Additionally, the increased appetite accompanying steroid therapy should be managed in a positive fashion, before a taste develops for high-carbohydrate, high-fat foods.

Once steroids are tapered to levels where hypertension and hyperglycemia are no longer problematic, a diet appropriate for chronological age is indicated. Because of the hyperlipidemic side effects of immunosuppressive drugs and the already deranged lipid levels of children with CKD, a heart-healthy diet focusing on low saturated and *trans* fats, low simple sugar, and low cholesterol should be advised. There is insufficient evidence to recommend omega-3 fatty acids to treat children with CKD.[15,53] Continued assessment of nutritional adequacy of the diet is necessary even with normal kidney function.

TABLE 13-3 Major Nutritional Considerations

Nutrient	Indication for Treatment	Modification
Phosphorus	CKD, elevated parathyroid hormone level, with or without hyperphosphatemia	Phosphate binders; low-phosphate diet; calcium and vitamin D supplement
	Posttransplant tubular loss; hypophosphatemia	Add supplement
Sodium	Hypertension; fluid retention	No added salt
	Daily steroid therapy	No added salt
	Increased urine losses	Add supplement
	Increased peritoneal dialysate losses	Add supplement
Potassium	< 5% GFR; hyperkalemia	Restrict diet
	Diuretic therapy; hypokalemia; diarrhea	Add supplement
Protein	Infants with CKD (no dialysis)	DRI
	Children with CKD (no dialysis)	Limit to DRI
	Children on hemodialysis	DRI
	Infants/children on peritoneal dialysis	> DRI
	Posttransplant	
Energy	Undernutrition/anorexia	≥ DRI
	Infants with CKD (no dialysis)	≥ DRI
	Children on hemodialysis	≥ DRI
	Dextrose absorption from peritoneal dialysate	≤ DRI
	Posttransplant steroid therapy	Varies
	Steroid-induced hyperglycemia	No concentrated sweets

Abbreviation: GFR, glomerular filtration rate.
Source: Linda Phelan, RD

Conclusion

The nutritional intake of the child is especially important in order to ensure optimal growth and development during all stages of renal disease. The diet must be adequate and consistent. Diet modification (see **Table 13-3**) and implementation must be individualized for all age groups, taking into account developmental levels, growth potentials, and renal functional limitations. Frequent evaluation of food intake, growth, kidney function, and developmental stages is essential to adequate care.

Case Study

Nutrition Assessment of Child with Kidney Disease

JA is an 8-year-old girl who was referred to pediatric nephrology because of lack of weight gain for the previous 6 months, a poor appetite with some nausea and fatigue, and elevated blood pressures on two previous visits to her pediatrician. Labs were drawn at her initial visit, which included BUN 30, Cr 2.0, Ca 7.8, Phos 8.2, Na 139, K 4.9, albumin 2.3, and hematocrit 25. Anthropometric measurements included height of 120 cm, weight of 17 kg, and BMI of 11.8. Her blood pressure was checked and again found to be elevated at 130/92. Urinalysis showed proteinuria of 200 mg/dL. When asked if anyone in the family had high blood pressure or a kidney disease, the parents spoke of JA's grandfather, who was on dialysis before he died.

The dietitian was asked to meet with the family to assess JA's dietary intake. The RD reported that JA was described as a "picky" eater. She eats very small portions and often felt "full" before she finished a meal. Her typical calorie intake was estimated to be 1000 kcal/day. Her parents reported that over the past few months, JA tires easily and generally is not the active child they were used to when she was younger.

The nephrologist estimated JA to be in CKD stage 3 with an estimated GFR of 50. An ACE inhibitor was prescribed for hypertension and to control her proteinuria. The nephrologist also ordered a low phosphorous diet; the RD instructed patient and family. Plans were made to admit JA to the hospital in 2 weeks for a kidney biopsy and to recheck her labs including % iron saturation, ferritin, vitamin D_{25}, and PTH.

Labs upon admit to the hospital showed a BUN of 29, creatinine 1.8, Ca 8.0, phos 7.5, hct 25, and alb 2.5. Her vitamin D_{25} level was low at 20, PTH high at 250, and iron studies showed 18% iron saturation and a ferritin of 82.

The biopsy showed membroproliferative glomerulonephritis type 2. The nephrologist advised JA's parents to return to the clinic in 2 weeks to begin training for EPO injections, another lab check for a phosphorous level, and follow-up with the dietitian. A 3-day food record was to be brought to the visit. Upon evaluation of the food record, the RD learned that JA's calorie intake remained at an average of 1000 kcal/day. Looking at the K/DOQI guidelines, the protein needs for stage 3 CKD were estimated to be 1–1.2 g protein/kg/day. Her food records showed adequate protein intake but inadequate calorie intake. JA's phosphorous level that day was 7.6.

Questions for the Reader

1. What are JA's height, weight, and BMI percentiles on the growth chart?
2. What is JA's desirable weight-for-height?
3. What is JA's estimated energy requirement (EER) based on desirable body weight?
4. Give an example of a PES statement for this initial assessment of JA.
5. What other nutrition intervention(s) should the RD address at this time? Mark all that apply.
   a. Potassium-restricted diet
   b. Sodium-restricted diet
   c. Increased calorie intake
   d. Decreased protein intake
6. What specific vitamin and mineral supplements should the RD recommend upon hospital admission?
7. What recommendations should the RD make at the final clinic visit? Mark all that apply.
   a. Start an oral nutritional supplement to increase calorie intake.
   b. Start a potassium-restricted diet.
   c. Initiate phosphorous binders.
   d. Restrict protein.

REFERENCES

1. Hogg RJ, Furth S, Lemley KV, et al. National Kidney Foundation's kidney disease outcomes initiative clinic practice guidelines for chronic kidney disease in children and adolescents: evaluation, classification and stratification. *Pediatrics.* 2003;111:1416–1421.
2. Mahan JD, Warady BA. Assessment and treatment of short stature in pediatric patients with chronic kidney disease: a consensus statement. *Pediatr Nephrol.* 2006;21;917–930.
3. Fine RN. Growth in children with renal insufficiency. In: Nissenson A, Fine RN, Gentile D (eds). *Clinical Dialysis.* New York: Appleton-Century Crofts; 1984:661.
4. Spinozzi NS, Nelson P. Nutrition support in the newborn intensive care unit. *J Renal Nutr.* 1996;6:188–197.
5. Ellis EN, Yiu V, Harley F, et al. The impact of supplemental feeding in young children on dialysis: a report of the North American Pediatric Renal Transplant Cooperative Study. *Pediatr Nephrol.* 2000;16:404–408.
6. Betts PR, White RHR. Growth potential and skeletal maturity in children with chronic renal insufficiency. *Nephron.* 1976;16: 325–332.
7. Broyer M. Growth in children with renal insufficiency. *Pediatr Clin North Am.* 1982;29:991–1003.
8. Rizzoni G, Broyer M, Guest G. Growth retardation in children with chronic renal disease: scope of the problem. *Am J Kidney Dis.* 1986;7:256–261.
9. Seikaly MG, Salhab N, Gipson D, et al. Stature in children with chronic kidney disease: analysis of NAPRTCS database. *Pediatr Nephrol.* 2006;21:793–399.
10. Rizzoni G, Basso T, Setari M. Growth in children with chronic renal failure on conservative treatment. *Kidney Int.* 1984;26: 52–58.
11. Kleinknecht C, Broyer M, Hout D, et al. Growth and development of nondialyzed children with chronic renal failure. *Kidney Int.* 1983;24(S15):40–47.
12. Fine RN, Kohout EC, Brown D, Perlman AJ. Growth after recombinant human growth hormone treatment in children with chronic renal failure: report of a multicenter randomized double-blind placebo-controlled study. *J Pediatr.* 1994;124:374–382.
13. Berard E, Crosnier H, Six-Beneton A, et al. Recombinant human growth hormone treatment of children on hemodialysis. *Pediatr Nephrol.* 1998;12:304–310.
14. National Kidney Foundation. K/DOQI clinical practice guideline for nutrition in children with CKD: 2008 update. *Am J Kidney Dis.* 2000;35(6):S105–S136.
15. National Kidney Foundation. K/DOQI clinical practice guideline for nutrition in children with CKD: 2008 update. *Am J Kidney Dis.* 2009;53(3, Suppl 2):S1–S124.
16. Hellerstein S, Holliday MA, Grupe WE, et al. Nutritional management of children with chronic renal failure. *Pediatr Nephrol.* 1987;1:195–211.
17. Rock J, Secker D. Nutrition management of chronic kidney disease in the pediatric patient. In: Ham-Gray L, Wiesenk K (eds). *A Clinical Guide to Nutrition Care in Kidney Disease,* 3rd ed. Chicago: American Dietetic Association; 2004:127–149.
18. Salusky IB, Goodman WG. The management of renal osteodystrophy. *Pediatr Nephrol.* 1996;10:651–653.
19. Wesseling K, Bakkaloglu S, Saluskey I. Chronic kidney disease mineral and bone disorder in children. *Pediatr Nephrol.* 2008;23:195–207.
20. Martinez I, Saracho R, Montenegro J, Llach F. A deficit of calcitriol synthesis may not be the initial factor in the pathogenesis

of secondary hyperparathyroidism. *Nephrol Dial Transplant.* 1996;11(Suppl 3):22–28.

21. Levin A, Bakris GL, Molitch M, et al. Prevalence of abnormal serum vitamin D, PTH, calcium and phosphorus in patients with chronic kidney disease: results of the study to evaluate early kidney disease. *Kidney Int.* 2007;71:31–38.
22. Seeherunvong W, Abitbol CL, Chandar J, et al. Vitamin D insufficiency and deficiency in children with early chronic kidney disease. *J Pediatr.* 2009;154:906–911.
23. National Kidney Foundation. K/DOQI clinical practice guidelines for bone metabolism and disease in children with chronic kidney disease. *Am J Kidney Dis.* 2005;46:S1–S122.
24. Brookhyser J, Pahre SN. Dietary and pharmacotherapeutic considerations in the management of renal osteodystrophy. *Adv Renal Replace Ther.* 1995;2:5–13.
25. Tamanah K, Mak RH, Rigden SP, et al. Long-term suppression of hyperparathyroidism by phosphate binders in uremic children. *Pediatr Nephrol.* 1987;1:145–149.
26. Schiller LR, Santa Ana CA, Sheikh MS, et al. Effect of the time of administration of calcium acetate on phosphorus binding. *New Engl J Med.* 1989;320:1110–1113.
27. Schmitt J. Selecting an appropriate phosphate binder. *J Renal Nutr.* 1990;1:38–40.
28. Bleyer AJ, Burke SK, Dillon M, et al. A comparison of the calcium-free phosphate binder sevelamer hydrochloride with calcium acetate in the treatment of hyperphosphatemia in hemodialysis patients. *Am J Kidney Dis.* 1999;33:694–701.
29. Parekh RS, Flynn JT, Smoyer WE, et al. Improved growth in young children with severe chronic renal insufficiency who use specified nutritional therapy. *J Am Soc Nephrol.* 2001;12:2418–2426.
30. Betts PR, Macgrath G. Growth pattern and dietary intake of children with chronic renal insufficiency. *Br Med J.* 1974;2:189.
31. Nelson P, Stover J. Nutritional recommendations for infants, children and adolescents with ESRD. In: Stover J (ed). *A Clinical Guide to Nutrition Care in End Stage Renal Disease,* 2nd ed. Chicago: American Dietetic Association; 1994:79–97.
32. Hobbs DJ, Gast TR, Furguson KB, et al. Nutritional management of hyperkalemic infants with chronic kidney disease using adult renal formulas. *J Renal Nutr.* 2010;20(2):121–126.
33. Yiu VWY, Harmon WE, Spinozzi NS, et al. High-calorie nutrition for infants with chronic renal disease. *J Renal Nutr.* 1996;6:203–206.
34. Ledermann SE, Spitz L, Malony J, et al. Gastrostomy feeding in infants and children on peritoneal dialysis. *Pediatr Nephrol.* 2002;17:246–250.
35. Reed EE, Roy LP, Gaskin KJ, Knight JF. Nutritional intervention and growth in children with chronic renal failure. *J Renal Nutr.* 1998;8:122–126.
36. Ruley EJ, Boch GH, Kerzner B, Abbott AW. Feeding disorders and gastroesophageal reflux in infants with chronic renal failure. *Pediatr Nephrol.* 1989;3:424–429.
37. Bebaum JC, Pererra GR, Watkins JB, et al. Non-nutritive sucking during gavage feeding enhances growth and maturation in premature infants. *Pediatrics.* 1983;71:41–45.
38. Eschbach MD, Egrie JC, Downing MR, et al. Correction of the anemia of end-stage renal disease with recombinant human erythropoietin. *N Engl J Med.* 1987;310:73–78.
39. Van Wyck DB, Stivelman JC, Ruiz J. Iron status in patients receiving erythropoietin for dialysis-associated anemia. *Kidney Int.* 1989;35:712–716.
40. Wolfson M. Nutritional management of the continuous ambulatory peritoneal patient. *Am J Kidney Dis.* 1996;27:744–749.
41. Secker D, Pencharz MB. Nutritional therapy for children on CAPD/CCPD: theory and practice. In: Fine RN, Alexander SR, Warady BA (eds). *CAPD/CCPD in Children.* Boston, MA: Kluwer Academic; 1998:567–603.
42. Schleifer CR, Teehan BP, Brown JM, Raimondo J. The application of urea kinetic modeling to peritoneal dialysis: a review of methodology and outcome. *J Renal Nutr.* 1993;3:2–9.
43. Harvey E, Secker D, Braj B, et al. The team approach to the management of children on chronic peritoneal dialysis. *Adv Renal Replace Ther.* 1996;3:3–13.
44. Harmon WE, Spinozzi NS, Meyer A, Grupe WE. The use of protein catabolic rate to monitor pediatric hemodialysis. *Dial Transplant.* 1981;10:324.
45. Goldstein SL, Sorof JM, Brewer ED. Natural logarithmic estimates of Kt/V in the pediatric hemodialysis population. *Am J Kidney Dis.* 1999;33:518–522.
46. Juarez-Congelosi M, Orellana P, Goldstein SL. Normalized protein catabolic rate versus serum albumin as a nutrition status marker in pediatric patients receiving hemodialysis. *J Renal Nutr.* 2007;17:269–274.
47. Querfeld U, Salusky IB, Nelson P, et al. Hyperlipidemia in pediatric patients undergoing peritoneal dialysis. *Pediatr Nephrol.* 1988;2:447–452.
48. Warady BA, Kriley M, Alon U, Hellerstein S. Vitamin status of infants receiving long-term peritoneal dialysis. *Pediatr Nephrol.* 1994;8:354–356.
49. Matera M, Bellinghieri G, Costantino G, et al. History of L-carnitine: implications for renal disease. *J Renal Nutr.* 2003;13:2–14.
50. Fine RN. Renal transplantation for children—the only realistic choice. *Kidney Int Suppl.* 1985;17:515–517.
51. Neu AM, Warady BA. Dialysis and renal transplantation in infants with irreversible renal failure. *Adv Renal Replace Ther.* 1996;3:48–59.
52. Seagraves A, Moore EE, Moore FA, et al. Net protein catabolic rate after kidney transplantation: impact of corticosteroid immunosuppression. *J Parenter Enteral Nutr.* 1986;10:453–455.
53. Chronic Kidney Disease (CKD) evidence based nutrition practice guideline. Available at: http://www.adaevidencelibrary.com/topic.cfm?cat=3927. Accessed June 2, 2011.

CHAPTER 14

Cardiology

Melanie Savoca, Monica Nagle, and Susan Konek

Congenital Heart Disease

Congenital heart disease (CHD) is one of the most common congenital defects in the United States, with an incidence of approximately 8 per 1000 live births.[1] Malnutrition and growth disturbances are especially prevalent in this population. Failure to thrive in cardiac patients is attributed to a variety of factors, including inadequate energy intake, poor feeding skills, increased metabolic demands, and disturbances in gastrointestinal (GI) function as well as type and clinical impact of the cardiac lesion.[2] The combination of chronic disease and malnutrition can have a detrimental effect on growth, development, and disease-related morbidity and mortality.[3]

Nutrition support for infants and children with CHD covers a wide range of topics, from acute care in infancy to chronic care in childhood. The magnitude of the effect of the cardiac defect on growth, development, and nutritional status depends on the particular lesion and its severity.[4] Malnutrition and growth retardation are common in infants and children with CHD.[5–16] The majority of cardiac defects are diagnosed during routine prenatal care or soon after birth.[17]

Corrective surgeries for CHD are common at an early age and can improve the nutritional status of infants with CHD and prevent failure to thrive.[18] If early cardiac surgery is not an option for an infant, then aggressive nutrition intervention and special nutrition considerations are required to prevent unsuccessful outcomes associated with malnutrition. Despite improvements in surgical palliation, nutritional problems contributing to malnutrition often emerge shortly after surgery and persist throughout the first year or years of life. Failure to thrive in pediatric patients with CHD results in more frequent hospital admissions with longer lengths of stay.[19]

Malnutrition

Inadequate energy intake has been frequently cited as a component of the growth failure in infants and children with CHD.[18,20–27] Controversy exists concerning the etiology of growth failure and the role of inadequate energy intake, hypermetabolism, malabsorption, and cardiac anomaly. An increased basal metabolic rate is a contributing factor to failure to thrive in some infants and children with CHD.

The type of cardiac lesion also significantly impacts the pattern of growth failure. Cardiac lesions are designated as cyanotic or acyanotic (see **Table 14-1**), depending on the hemodynamic effect. Cyanotic heart diseases are characterized by insufficient pulmonary blood flow. Acyanotic heart diseases consist of lesions with left-to-right shunting, resulting in pulmonary overcirculation and signs of congestive heart failure. Other acyanotic lesions are those associated with compromised systemic output and include aortic stenosis, coarctation of the aorta, and interrupted aortic arch. Patients with cyanotic heart lesions usually exhibit reduced height and weight.[5–7,15,28,29]

Congestive heart failure (CHF) also may cause growth failure. Heart failure is thought to increase metabolic rate, therefore increasing the energy required for growth. Some cardiac diseases that may cause CHF include atrioventricular canal defects, cardiomyopathy, or CHD causing chronic hypoxemia. Additionally, patients with pulmonary hypertension in combination with CHD, particularly left-to-right shunts, have a higher risk for growth failure.[30] These children tend to weigh less than do children with cyanotic heart lesions.[25,27] Obstructive malformations, such as pulmonary stenosis and coarctation of the aorta, typically result in impaired linear growth, with linear growth more affected than weight.[5,30,31]

Nutrition Management

Nutrition is an integral component of care during all stages of treatment, including the acute phase when metabolic responses to stress are more profound.[32–34] Some infants with cardiac problems are admitted to the newborn or cardiac intensive care unit in an acutely ill state within the first days of life. Some can be stabilized and surgery may be deferred for weeks; others may need immediate surgery.

TABLE 14-1 Congenital Heart Defects

Cyanotic	Acyanotic
Ebstein's Anomaly of the Tricuspid Valve	Atrial Septal Defect (ASD)
Hypoplastic Left Heart Syndrome (HLHS)	Atrioventricular Septal Defect
Pulmonary Atresia with Intact Ventricular Septum (PA/IVS)	Patent Ductus Arteriosus (PDA)
Pulmonary Stenosis (PS)	Truncus Arteriosus
Tetralogy of Fallot (TOF)	Ventricular Septal Defect (VSD)
Total Anomalous Pulmonary Venous Return (TAPVR)	Aortic Stenosis (AS)
Transportation of the Great Arteries (TGA)	Coarctation of the Aorta (CoA)
Tricuspid Atresia	Interrupted Aortic Arch (IAA)

Source: George Ofori-Amanfo, MD, and Melanie Savoca, MS, RD, CNSC, LDN, Children's Hospital of Philadelphia.

Many infants with CHD require surgery before 1 year of age.[35] Depending on the type of cardiac defect, multiple surgeries may be planned for a staged palliation throughout childhood. As in any surgery, the best outcome is achieved in the patient who has a good nutritional status and positive nitrogen balance. The immediate goal for nutrition support in infants is to achieve the best nutritional status possible in preparation for surgery as well as during postoperative recovery.[36] Other less immediate nutrition support goals are to encourage normal growth velocity and support normal feeding skill development. Optimal nutrition support may be unattainable at times due to the many complicating factors in these patients in the acute care setting.[36] Nutrition goals should include adequate provision of nutrients for maintenance of lean body mass and wound healing.

For neonates diagnosed with CHD, the primary nutrition goal after birth is to minimize neonatal weight loss during the preoperative period. Enteral feedings may increase the risk of necrotizing enterocolitis (NEC) from cyanosis, prostaglandin (PGE) administration, or the presence of umbilical arterial catheters (UAC) prior to surgery. However, feeding of infants with cyanosis is not associated with elevated incidence of NEC, and in hemodynamically stable infants PGE administration has not been shown to be a risk factor for adverse events associated with enteral feeding.[37] Early initiation of minimal enteral nutrition in newborns appears to enhance functional maturation of the GI tract.[37]

During the immediate postoperative period, nutrition support should be initiated to promote wound healing, minimize loss of lean body mass, and support vital organ function. Barriers may preclude the delivery of adequate calories for growth at this time. These barriers include the following:

- Hemodynamic instability
- Hypotension
- Hyperglycemia
- Electrolyte derangements
- Fluid restrictions
- Impaired renal function
- Mechanical ventilation[36]

In infants with CHD, growth is not a critical priority during the immediate postoperative period. Growth cannot occur until the infant begins to recover from the postoperative stress response and positive nitrogen balance is achieved.[32] Additionally, overfeeding is associated with increased carbon dioxide (CO_2) production, difficulties weaning from ventilatory support, and impaired immune and organ function.[36] Nutrition support in the acutely ill infant typically involves the use of parenteral nutrition (PN) and intravenous (IV) fluids and requires careful attention. The infant may be fluid restricted; there may be multiple lines requiring 0.5–1 mL/hr each for patency. Medications and infusions may use a significant amount of fluid. It is not uncommon to have only 60–80 mL/kg of fluid allotted for nutrition support.

Laboratory values may be abnormal. The use of diuretics may deplete total body sodium and potassium; calcium, phosphorus, and magnesium levels may also be abnormal.[38] Due to the need for fluid restriction, the renal lab values may reflect some degree of dehydration, with elevated sodium and blood urea nitrogen. Acid–base status may also be altered, complicating electrolyte management.

Other end-organ dysfunction is often common. Renal problems, such as acute tubular necrosis or renal insufficiency, may develop. Some infants may temporarily need dialysis, further complicating nutrition support (see Chapter 13). For infants and children needing support prior to surgery or those unable to be weaned from the bypass pump after surgery, extracorporeal life support (ECLS) may be used.[39–41]

Enteral nutrition (EN) should be introduced as tolerated. PN and EN should be used simultaneously in the gradual transition to full enteral feedings. Once full EN is achieved, nutrition support should provide adequate calories and protein for optimal growth. Anthropometric measurements and growth trends should be regularly monitored. Development of feeding skills may also be an integral component of care at this point. A speech-language pathologist should be consulted if difficulties or concerns are noted with oral feeds.

Extracorporeal Life Support

Extracorporeal life support (ECLS), also called extracorporeal membrane oxygenation (ECMO), is an advanced form of cardiopulmonary support for acute reversible cardiac or respiratory failure that is unresponsive to conventional medical management. ECLS is a supportive intervention, not a therapeutic intervention. It allows for cardiopulmonary rest to support the resolution of a reversible lung and/or heart pathology. If function does not recover, ECLS may be used as a bridge to transplant. Indications for ECLS in the cardiac population include acute cardiac arrest or being unable to separate from cardiopulmonary bypass. The physiologic goal of ECLS is to improve systemic oxygen delivery and allow normal aerobic metabolism to continue while allowing the lungs and/or heart to "rest."[42] There is no difference in nutrition support for vein (veno-venous; VV) or artery (veno-arterial; VA) ECLS.[42]

Nutrition goals for patients on ECLS are to provide adequate calories and protein to minimize catabolism and promote wound healing. Although critically ill patients on ECLS are severely stressed, catabolic, and have an increased metabolic burden of wound healing,[43] caloric requirements are decreased as neonates use energy to fuel the stress response.[42] ECLS replaces native pulmonary function and approximately 80% of cardiac function. The majority of thermoregulation is also provided by the ECLS circuit.[43] Calorie needs for infants on ECLS range between 70–80 kcal/kg. For older children, estimated energy needs may be 70–90% of the REE.[42,44,45]

Nevertheless, provision of adequate caloric intake is paramount in this patient population. Fluid restriction, problems with glucose control, end organ dysfunction, and concerns of effects of IV lipids on the ECLS membrane pose challenges of meeting the calorie and protein needs. The key to nutritional management of the patient on ECLS is to provide optimal nutrition within the limits of restricted fluid intake. Total PN is initiated as early as possible with maximized caloric density. IV fat emulsion may be used to enhance caloric supply; however, fat emulsion should be administered through separate IV access during ECMO. Due to fluid restrictions, glucose infusion rate (GIR) should be calculated with each fluid change. A low-volume amount of 25% dextrose may yield a modest GIR; care should be taken if fluids are liberalized to adjust the dextrose percentage. GIR should be limited to approximately 7 mg/kg/min (~10 g/kg/day) because excess carbohydrate intake may increase CO_2 production and respiratory quotient. Due to renal dysfunction, fluid resuscitation, and endocrine problems, electrolyte derangements are frequent occurrences among patients on ECMO. Careful attention to electrolytes and appropriate supplementation is of prime importance to avoid dysrhythmias. The electrolyte composition of PN should be determined by the patient's current serum electrolytes, prior needs, and current clinical condition, particularly renal function. Problems have been noted with potassium, calcium, and magnesium. There may be an increased need for potassium in most infants and children undergoing ECLS, but vigilant monitoring of serum levels and urine output is needed. Sodium levels may initially be elevated secondary to sodium-containing resuscitation medications. Therefore, PN often is written with lower sodium and higher potassium amounts.

Multiple complications can arise after initiation of ECMO support. Capillary leak syndrome is caused by increased vascular permeability due to prolonged hypoxia and hypotension. This can cause severe edema, particularly in neonates, with as much as a 50–75% weight increase. A systemic inflammatory response syndrome most often occurs related to blood exposure to foreign material, but is self-limited to 24 to 72 hours after initiation of ECLS or after a circuit change. Hemorrhagic or bleeding complications can also occur and are related to systemic heparization, which makes the blood twice as thin as normal. Cholestasis may be seen, but often resolves without long-term hepatic complications.[46] Gastroesophageal reflux (GER), delayed gastric emptying, and reduced gut motility are also seen in critically ill patients.[47]

The early initiation of enteral feeds in patients on ECMO is associated with the following findings:

- Gut mucosal integrity and GI blood flow
- Secretion of GI hormones that enhances cell growth and development
- Improved glucose tolerance
- Stimulation of motor activity
- Improved GI mucosal immune function
- Reduced morbidity in critically ill patients[48–50]

EN may be instituted via the nasogastric route, initially as minimal or trophic feeds (10–15 mL/kg/day), and advanced slowly as tolerated.[51] Postpyloric feeding is suggested only if patients fail to tolerate gastric feeds. While on enteral nutrition, the patients should be monitored very closely for early signs of feeding intolerance.

Parenteral Nutrition Support

Parenteral nutrition (PN) support is driven by the total fluid limit of each patient. Laboratory tests, including basic metabolic and renal panels, glucose, and ionized calcium, should be monitored daily. Phosphorus and magnesium should be monitored daily until stable, and liver function should be checked weekly or as indicated. A bed scale should be used to obtain daily weights to evaluate fluid status. Any dextrose used in fluid administration should be counted toward the overall GIR and carbohydrate and calorie intake. Sodium used in these fluids should be calculated because it can represent a significant amount. Line patency fluids should be counted toward electrolyte, carbohydrate, calorie (if dextrose is a component), and fluid intake. PN fluids should be written last, accounting for the content of the other fluids. Because fluid is such an issue and may require altering in the course of the day, it may be helpful if total PN admixtures are not used and lipids run separately. PN is usually very concentrated in the cardiac infant due to fluid restrictions. Central lines are generally used with a maximum dextrose concentration of 25%. The risks and benefits of providing higher calories through a higher percentage of glucose should be considered carefully. GIR should be calculated daily or with every dextrose-containing fluid change. Postoperative infants may tolerate a GIR of only 10–12 mg glucose/kg/minute.

IV lipids are a concentrated source of calories and a source of essential fatty acids. (See Chapter 20.) Lipids should be used over the greatest amount of time possible (24-hour infusion, if not contraindicated by a lipid-incompatible medication). Triglyceride levels should be monitored to assess tolerance to this therapy.

Protein needs are important to consider in this stressed population. Starting PN with protein immediately postoperatively is warranted, even if only half of maintenance fluids can be used for this endeavor due to electrolyte fluctuations. Careful attention to limited dextrose, protein, and electrolytes should be made because renal output may be temporarily reduced after cardiopulmonary bypass. Hyperglycemia is common after infant cardiac surgery. Insulin is not often used because glucose levels usually improve within 24 to 48 hours. In addition, it may not be possible for mineral needs for bone development to be met in the short term due to the use of PN and fluid limitations. Diuretic use may alter calcium status. Premature and term infant calcium and phosphorus requirements for bone mineralization often cannot be met until later. The use of premature infant or premature follow-up formulas may be considered as a component of the nutrition support for a fluid-restricted infant with higher mineral needs. Signs of cholestasis and bone demineralization should be monitored closely for patients requiring long-term PN.[52]

Complications

Complications of hospitalized infants with CHD include inadequate enteral intake, GI morbidity, and feeding problems.[8] These affect growth and recovery and can influence short- and long-term outcomes.[30] A number of GI concerns are common in many of these infants. Malabsorption, including fat and/or protein malabsorption, is common.[18,53] Protein-losing enteropathy is a condition reported in patients with increased right-sided heart pressures, especially young children who have undergone the Fontan operation. Decreased cardiac output, in addition to causing early satiety and vomiting, may also cause decreased nutrient absorption.[27] Furthermore, some children with CHD have GI malformations that will affect their ability to be nourished. These may include pyloric stenosis, duodenal atresia, malrotation, and severe defects such as gastroschisis, all requiring surgical repair. Reduced gut perfusion is another factor recognized as a complication often present in infants with cardiac insufficiency. The risk of NEC is increased and care must be taken to avoid this serious condition.

Inadequate energy intake is the major cause of growth failure in infants with CHD. Achieving adequate calories through oral feedings is difficult. Oral feeding, even if the patient's condition allows, requires a great deal of energy expenditure and may result in tachypnea and fatigue. It is difficult to achieve adequate intake to support nutritional needs. Other factors contributing to inadequate intake include early satiety, decreased gastric capacity related to hepatomegaly, and delayed gastric emptying as a result of low cardiac output or medication side effect.

In planning for transition to enteral feeding, it is important to remember the impact of the cardiorespiratory system on the achievement of enteral nutrition support.[54] Infants with a history of cardiopulmonary bypass and prolonged respiratory support may have abnormalities in oromotor feeding skills. For pediatric patients intubated for more than 7 days, the risk of dysphagia increases, as does the inability to feed orally by hospital discharge.[55,56] Tachypnea may also cause an uncoordinated suck, swallow, and breathe pattern necessary for successful oral feeding. Fatigue is common in these infants. They often cannot feed long enough to support their nutritional needs.

Sluggish reflexes, decreased sensory input, hypoxemia, neurological insults, or bowel ischemia may impair the GI system. In the event of gut hypoperfusion, waiting for bowel recovery may cause delayed initiation of EN. GER may play a role in CHD. The use of a nasogastric tube may result in increased reflux symptoms.

Neurologic maturation is another key factor that should be considered for the infant to reach optimal intake.[57] Infants with CHD have higher risk for neurologic sequelae, including bleeds or strokes. Children with CHD are often found to have neurologic disabilities.[58] Although neurologic deficits result from a variety of causes, infants with these complications are most often supported by long-term tube feedings. An acquired neurologic complication in patients with hypoplastic left heart syndrome (HLHS) may have a profound effect on the ability to feed. During surgery, the recurrent laryngeal nerve is at risk for injury. Although injury to this nerve can be caused by a variety of operative events, the result is vocal cord paresis or paralysis and often

GER.[59] Laryngopharyngeal dysfunction presenting after the Norwood procedure is common in patients, with resultant dysphagia, aspiration, and left recurrent laryngeal nerve injury.[60] For these reasons, vocal cord dysfunction will often result in the need for gavage feedings to support nutrition.

Other complicating factors to achievement of EN goals include feeding difficulties. Risk factors include patients with a high risk-adjusted congenital heart surgery (RACHS) score[61] and those who require prolonged intubation. Premature infants with chronic hypoxia and poor pulmonary function also may have higher energy expenditure and greater caloric requirements, which affects the plan to support the CHD infant with enteral feedings.

Enteral Nutrition

Many factors necessitate the need for enteral nutrition support. GI function may not be optimal in some infants with cardiac anomalies, and a slow, cautious approach to enteral feeding may be needed.[39] PN can be the supplemental nutrition source until full volume enteral feeding has been established. In the transition from PN to EN, caution should be used with the addition of hyperosmolar medications.[62,63] NEC is associated with hyperosmolar formulas, and the addition of medications can make an isotonic feeding hypertonic.[64,65] Hyperosmolar medications have also been known to cause osmotic diarrhea.

Many infants with CHD will need additional calories, and often require 20–30 kcal/oz enteral feedings. Full volume of enteral feeds should be achieved first, followed by gradually increasing the caloric density.[63] The amount of fluid used is often related to the amount of diuretic therapy. Diuretics may be used to lessen the effects of high-volume feedings, although side effects of potassium wasting, acid-base problems, and altered calcium and magnesium excretion exist.[66] The enteral formulas used for infants and children with CHD are the same as for other children. To increase the caloric density of formulas, they can be made using less water with formula powder or liquid concentrate, which keeps the original proportion of carbohydrate, protein, and fat the same. However, when the caloric density of formulas is increased, the amount of electrolytes and minerals is also increased, and should be taken into consideration. Although this change does increase the osmolality of the formula, in practice, the medications added to formulas alter the osmolality to a much greater extent than the formula alone.[43]

Calorie needs of infants and children with CHD are usually greater than those without cardiac problems. The precise energy needs of infants with CHD are difficult to estimate, but many infants will need at least 120–150 kcal/kg. Toddlers and children may need 20–33% more than normal estimated needs. After cardiac surgical repair, the calorie needs will usually decrease[16] but may stay 10–15 kcal/kg above the average for some infants or children. Calorie needs also may remain increased for catch-up growth for patients malnourished prior to surgery. The best method is to set an estimated goal, assess growth parameters, and make adjustments as needed until appropriate growth velocity is achieved.

Cardiomyopathy

Pediatric cardiomyopathy is a serious disorder of the heart muscle that is responsible for significant morbidity and mortality among affected children. The estimated incidence is between 1.13 and 1.24 cases per 100,000 children 18 years of age and younger, with the highest incidence among children younger than 1 year of age.[67–69] Despite the low incidence, children with cardiomyopathy have some of the worst clinical outcomes compared to other heart diseases in children. Nearly one-third of all children diagnosed with pediatric cardiomyopathy prior to 1 year of age will die within 1 year of diagnosis, and approximately one-third will receive pediatric heart transplants.[70] Cardiomyopathy predominates as the most common indication for heart transplantation in older children.[70] Heart transplantation remains the standard of care for children who fail medical therapy.

Cardiomyopathy is classified into four distinct categories:[71]

1. Dilated cardiomyopathy is characterized by pathologic stretching of the myocardial fibers, causing dilatation of the ventricles and decreased contractility.
2. Hypertrophic cardiomyopathy is an abnormal growth or arrangement of myocardial fibers that leads to a thickening of the ventricular walls and reduction in size of the pumping chamber; it is often associated with obstruction of the left ventricular outflow tract.
3. Restrictive cardiomyopathy is stiffening of the walls of the ventricles and loss of ventricular compliance, resulting in decreased cardiac filling and hence decreased cardiac output.
4. Arrythmogenic right ventricular cardiomyopathy is characterized by the replacement of myocytes in the right ventricle with fatty, fibrous tissue.

Malnutrition is one of the most significant clinical problems in children with cardiomyopathy. The disease is associated with increased caloric demands of the failing heart, increased work of breathing, and a general catabolic state of chronic illness. The patients have decreased oral intake from decreased appetite, feeding intolerance, and poor gastrointestinal absorption. Many children with this disorder will manifest some degree of growth failure during the course of their illness.[71] The fundamental cause is primarily persistent CHF, which can result in increased metabolic demands, GI issues, malabsorption, and decreased food intake. Malnutrition may further lead to complications that may directly or indirectly impact heart function and overall clinical status.[71] Infants, children, and adolescents with cardiomyopathy also may need a ventricular assist device (VAD) as a bridge to transplantation. Little is known about VAD-related gastroenterologic complications; however, because of its intra-abdominal placement, the potential exists for major abdominal complications, including intra-abdominal infections, delayed gastric emptying, gastritis, and pancreatitis.[72,73]

Adequate nutrition forms an integral part of the management of heart failure associated with cardiomyopathy. Nutritional rehabilitation should be instituted early and aggressively to prevent a vicious downward cycle of growth failure and worsened clinical outcome. Optimal nutrition is critical in providing affected children the means to withstand the detrimental metabolic effects of the disease, participate in rehabilitation, and recover from their illness. The goal of therapy is adequate EN; however, the hospitalized acutely ill patient with decompensated heart failure may not tolerate enteral feeds. In such cases, PN should be instituted with transition to enteral feeds as soon as possible.

Chylothorax

Chylothorax is the presence of lymphatic fluid in the pleural space caused by a leak in the thoracic duct or because of lymphatic abnormalities. It is usually a result of iatrogenic complications of cardiac or thoracic surgery, commonly trauma to the thoracic duct or other surrounding vessels.[74,75] It occurs in children with syndromes associated with CHD, such as trisomy 21, Noonan's syndromes, and cardio-facio-cutaneous syndrome.[76–82] Sometimes chylothorax can result from high pressure within the superior vena cava (SVC), thereby affecting the pressure in the lymphatic system.[74,83] This is seen mainly in operations that cause increased SVC pressure, such as the hemi-Fontan, bidirectional Glenn, and Senning procedures, and also can be seen in patients with thrombus occluding the SVC or subclavian vessels.[83]

Chyle is a white, milky-appearing substance composed of chylomicrons and lymph, which is transported to the systemic circulation via the thoracic duct. The primary purpose of chyle is the absorption and transportation of long-chain triglycerides (LCT) in the intestines. Chyle is formed in the lacteals of the intestines during digestion in response to the presence of intraluminal fat. The chyle binds with LCT to form chylomicrons, which are then absorbed and transported by the intestinal lymphatics to the bloodstream. Chyle also contains protein and is responsible for absorption of fat-soluble vitamins; therefore, high losses are of great nutritional concern.[75] When a person is not being fed, the fluid can appear less white, and more yellowish or clear. Diagnosis of chylothorax can be made if there are elevated lymphocytes, triglycerides, and high total protein content in a sample of the pleural fluid.[75,83–85]

Treatment of chylothorax can be multifactorial. Pleural drainage, a very low-fat diet and/or a diet containing the majority of fats as MCT oil, gut rest, or PN are the main modalities used in treating chylous effusions.[86] MCTs are absorbed directly into the portal system and do not stimulate an increase in lymphatic flow. Nutritional management usually starts with trialing a low-fat or MCT-enriched formula, observing for a reduction in chylous output and, if ineffective, providing gut rest with PN.[75,87] Supplementation with small amounts of LCT to meet 2–4% of total calories may be necessary to prevent EFA deficiency in patients who are fed long term with high MCT oil containing specialty formulas.[75,87] An elevated triene-to-tetraene ratio is one clinical indicator of an EFA deficiency.[88] Formulas commonly used for the management of chylothorax are listed in **Table 14-2** for comparison purposes. Some patients are successfully fed using skimmed breast milk, which has been supplemented in calories using MCT, protein powder, and a source of EFA.[89,90]

Medical management of chylous effusions may include use of somatostatin and its analogue octreotide, which are known to reduce intestinal secretions and inhibit lymph

TABLE 14-2 Selected Formulas with High MCT Content for Chylothorax

Formula	Type	Calories per 100 g Powder	MCT:LCT Ratio	Fat % of Calories	Protein g per 100 g Powder	n6:n3 Ratio
Monogen (Nutricia)	Powder	470	87:13	40	16.5	40.5:1
Portagen* (Mead Johnson)	Powder	424	90:10	25	11.4	4.6:1
Vivonex Pediatric** (Néstle)	Powder	412	68:32	25	12.4	7.7:1

*Not intended as a sole source of nutrition. For chronic (long-term) use: supplementation of essential fatty acids and other nutrients should be considered [manufacturer's notation]. Only contains vitamins and minerals, no trace elements.

**1 packet of Vivonex Pediatric contains 48.5 g powder.

Abbreviations: MCT, medium chain triglycerides; LCT, long chain triglycerides; n6, omega-6; n3, omega-3; g, grams.

Source: Data from manufacturers' product labels.

excretion.[91] Caution must be used when enterally feeding patients receiving somatostatin or octreotide because splanchnic circulation may be diminished; GI side effects should be closely monitored.[91]

High losses of chylous pleural fluid can result in deficiencies in fat-soluble vitamins.[75,85,87] Large volume output from chylothorax can cause high protein losses, resulting in low albumin levels and losses of electrolytes and immunoglobulins. Sodium and calcium levels may be decreased, and metabolic acidosis may be seen in patients with high outputs. Hypovolemia also can occur, which can lead to hemodynamic instability.[75]

Genetic Syndromes and Chromosome Anomalies

Many genetic syndromes and chromosome anomalies are associated with congenital heart defects, such as Down syndrome (trisomy 21), trisomy 13 and 18, Turner's syndrome, William's syndrome, Marfan syndrome, and CHARGE syndrome (coloboma, heart defect, atresia choanae, retarded growth and development, genital hypoplasia, ear anomalies/deafness).

Within the spectrum of genetic syndromes, many of these infants and children are likely to have feeding difficulties and may be genetically prone to growth delays. Feeding in children with genetic and chromosomal anomalies can be a significant challenge for families and medical professionals. These children may require aggressive medical nutrition management, often requiring long-term enteral access via gastrostomy and jejunostomy feeding tubes. Gastroesophageal fundoplication may be indicated for GER that does not respond to conventional medical therapy.

Nutritional Care

Feeding methodology often becomes a concern in the follow-up care of infants and children with cardiac anomalies. In infancy, when caloric needs are very high, an infant may eat eagerly for a short time and then quit. Parents and caregivers may assume the infant is full, but it may be that the infant lacks the energy needed to adequately feed. Other infants and children may refuse to eat or feed very poorly.

Higher calorie formulas or supplements may be used to decrease the volume needed for optimal caloric intake. For infants who may orally feed, oral feedings should typically not exceed 30 minutes in length. If an infant is unable to take a desired volume within that time, an indwelling nasogastric tube may be used to give the remainder of the feed. If an infant is close to goal, he or she may be able to feed by mouth during the day and receive overnight tube feedings to make up the daytime deficit. Frequent follow-up care with an outpatient dietitian should be recommended to ensure projected goal volumes and rate of growth are still appropriate for age. For some infants, 24-hour infusions may be needed. Attempts can be made to compress feedings into a shorter infusion time, giving a few hours off for social and developmental purposes. For infants and children not able to take oral feeds, an oral stimulation program should be initiated, and oral motor therapies can be instituted.

For infants and children who are thought to need tube feeding assistance for more than 3 months, a gastric tube (G-tube) is a positive step toward simplifying the care. Without the pressure of forced or unpleasant mealtimes or around-the-clock marathons, feeding can be pleasurable, with the best possible behavioral and developmental outcome. Oral feedings should be a pleasant time for both the caregiver and the infant or child. Monitoring growth and preventing malnutrition are the goals for infants and children with CHD.

Pediatric Hyperlipidemia

Hyperlipidemia is an elevation of lipids in the bloodstream. These lipids include cholesterol, cholesterol esters, phospholipids, and triglycerides. They are transported in the blood as part of lipoproteins. The aim of nutrition support in pediatric hyperlipidemia is to provide nutrition for normal growth and development, as well as to normalize lipid levels as much as possible to decrease the risk of cardiovascular disease.[92] The Therapeutic Lifestyle Changes (TLC) diet macronutrient recommendations include the following:[93]

- 50–60% of total calories from carbohydrates
- 15% of total calories from protein
- Limiting total fat to 25–35% of total calories
- Limiting saturated fat and dietary cholesterol, which are LDL-raising nutrients, to less than 7% of total calories and 200 mg/day, respectively

Therapeutic options for lowering LDL cholesterol include consuming 2 g/day of plant stanols/sterols and increased viscous (soluble) fiber.[93] The dietary changes suggested for all individuals are similar to the TLC diet guidelines and can be incorporated into the use of the food pyramid.[93] Before the age of 2 years, restriction of fat intake may result in altered growth.[94] The American Academy of Pediatrics recommends that total fat intake should not fall below 20% of total calories for children and adolescents.[94]

The American Heart Association (AHA) heart-healthy dietary guidelines emphasize the importance of a diet low in saturated and trans fats and rich in fruits, vegetables, whole grains, fat-free and low-fat dairy products, and lean meat, fish, and poultry.[95] For children at higher risk, the new National Cholesterol Education Program (NCEP) TLC guidelines offer dietary therapy for subgroups of people with specific medical conditions and risk factors, which include high LDL cholesterol, dyslipidemia, coronary heart disease or other cardiovascular disease, diabetes mellitus, insulin resistance, or metabolic syndrome. If serum levels are not improved with dietary intervention alone, medication may be considered for children older than 10 years of age.[94]

Increasing fiber intake is advocated for all children older than 2 years of age. (See Chapter 12 and Appendix F.) Programs such as Healthy Start have been shown to reduce serum cholesterol in preschoolers. This program in a largely minority Head Start preschool population reduced the total and saturated fat content of snacks and meals.[96]

Nutrition education and dietary intervention can improve weight loss in obese children, reduce obesity-related health risks, and improve dyslipidemias.[96–100]

Case Study

Nutrition Assessment of Infant with CHD

Patient history: JT is a 1-day-old male delivered at an outside hospital by vaginal delivery at 38 weeks gestation and birth weight of 3200 grams (25th percentile). He had a prenatal diagnosis of congenital heart disease. He was transported to a pediatric tertiary care facility on the day of birth in anticipation of corrective cardiac surgery. He arrived intubated and mechanically ventilated. His echocardiogram upon arrival confirmed a diagnosis of hypoplastic left heart syndrome (HLHS). He underwent Norwood procedure on day of life (DOL) #2. JT initially came off cardiopulmonary bypass but had open sternum due to profound hypoxemia associated with chest closure. He underwent delayed sternal closure on post-operative day (POD) #4 after aggressive dieresis had been accomplished.

Food/nutrition-related history: No enteral feeds were started in the preoperative period because surgery was planned for the following day. Parenteral nutrition was started on POD#1. JT was to receive 45 kcal/kg/day, 2 g protein/kg/day, and 2 g fat/kg/day from TPN. This was advanced to 60 kcal/kg/day on POD#2 and POD#3. Once his chest was closed and urine output improved, fluids were liberalized and TPN was advanced to 75 kcal/kg/day, 3 g/kg/day of protein, and 3 g/kg/day of lipid on POD#4.

On POD#5, the patient was started on trophic nasogastric (NG) feedings of maternal breast milk at 2 mL/hr. On POD#6, his umbilical arterial catheter was removed and a peripheral arterial line was placed. Feeds were then advanced by 30 mL/kg/day over the next few days to a goal of 100 mL/kg. The parenteral nutrition was weaned as the enteral feeding was advanced. Lipids were maintained at 3 g/kg/day to support calorie needs as the team was made aware that the child would not meet calorie needs if he was only at 100 mL/kg of enteral feedings of breast milk (20 kcal/oz). JT was slowly weaned off the ventilator and extubated onto nasal continuous positive airway pressure (NCPAP). Patient was made NPO peri-extubation. Once respiratory status was stable, enteral nutrition was resumed and enteral feeds were increased to 150 mL/kg/day. At this point, maternal breast milk was fortified with a standard infant formula liquid concentrate to 24 kcal/oz and lipids were discontinued. As of POD#12, JT was receiving 120 kcal/kg/day of current body weight, which had increased to 3.25 kg, up 100 grams from birth weight. By POD#18, JT had weaned off NCPAP, and continuous enteral feedings were condensed to bolus feeds every 3 hours. Oral feedings were attempted by the speech therapist, but found to be inappropriate at this time secondary to his increased work of breathing and uncoordinated suck and swallow patterns.

Anthropometric Measures

	Weight	Length	Wt/length
Birth	3.20 kg	49 cm	50th–75th percentile
DOL#14	3.25 kg	50 cm	25th–50th percentile
DOL#28	3.45 kg	51 cm	25th–50th percentile
	Std Ht for age: 54.5 cm	% of Std Ht for age: 94%	

Estimated Nutrition Needs

Calories: WHO × 1.2–1.3 = 130–140 kcal/kg/day
Protein: 2–3 g/kg/day
Fluid: <150 mL/kg/day for enteral nutrition

Biochemical Data, Medical Tests, and Procedures

Labs on DOL#28: (↓ = below normal; ↑ = above normal)

Na: 134	Cl: 91 ↓	BUN: 17	Gluc: 98	Mg: 1.9	H/H: 14.5/42.2 ↓
K: 3.7 ↓	CO_2: 36 ↑	Creat: 0.4	Ca: 9.3	Phos: 5.7	Alb: 2.8 ↓

Gastroesophageal Reflux Study/ Gastric Emptying Study

Studies showed multiple episodes of gastroesophageal reflux to the level of lower to mid esophagus, no evidence of pulmonary aspiration, and the rate of gastric emptying was within normal limits.

Current medications: Captopril, furosemide, pantoprazole, aspirin, cholecalciferol 400 units/day

Assessment on DOL#28: Patient is currently receiving breast milk fortified to 24 kcal/oz at 60 mL every 3 hours. Current weight is 3.45 kg. Work of breathing has improved. Speech therapist continues to work with JT on oral feeding skills. Percentage of IBW indicates weight is within normal limits, but percentage of standard height for age indicates mild stunting of growth. JT may benefit from increasing total caloric intake to achieve optimal growth. JT is on a proton pump inhibitor for reflux precautions. Labs reflect low potassium, chloride, and albumin, and elevated CO_2 levels.

Nutrition Diagnosis

Based on the information detailed above, a nutritional problem or diagnosis is made.

Interventions

Because JT's weight gain has been suboptimal, recommend breast milk fortified to 27 kcal/oz and adjust volume to provide 150 mL/kg (65 mL every 3 hr) at JT's current body weight of 3.45 kg. Recommend limiting oral intake to ≤ 30 minutes, with the remainder of bolus feeds through the NG tube.

Questions for the Reader

1. What is JT's ideal body weight (IBW) and % of IBW on DOL#28?
2. How many calories and how much fluid per kilogram did JT's original regimen provide?
3. On average, how many grams per day of weight has JT gained over the past 14 days (between DOL#14 and DOL#28)?
4. Write one PES statement.
5. How many calories per kg are provided in his current feeding regimen?
6. What would you want to monitor?
7. What rate of weight gain would be ideal for an infant of this age?
8. What are your goals for nutrition before discharge?

REFERENCES

1. Kay JD, Colan SD, Graham TP. Congestive heart failure in pediatric patients. *Am Heart J.* 2001;142(5):923–928.
2. Nydegger A, Bines JE. Energy metabolism in infants with congenital heart disease. *Nutrition.* 2006;22:697–704.
3. Steltzer M, Rudd N, Pick B. Nutrition care for newborns with congenital heart disease. *Clin Perinatol.* 2005;32:1017–1030.
4. Carlson SJ, Ryan JM. Congenital heart disease. In: Groh-Wargo S, Thompson M, Cox J (eds). *Nutritional Care for High Risk Newborns,* rev ed. Chicago: Precept Press, Inc.; 2000:397–408.
5. Mehrizi A, Drash A. Growth disturbance in congenital heart disease. *J Pediatr.* 1962;61:418–429.
6. Glassman MS, Woolf PK, Schwarz SM. Nutritional considerations in children with congenital heart disease. In: Baker SB, Baker RD Jr, Davis A (eds). *Pediatric Enteral Nutrition.* New York: Chapman & Hall; 1994:340.
7. Venogopalan P, Akinbami FO, Al-Minai KM, et al. Malnutrition in children with congenital heart disease. *J Saudi Med J.* 2001;22:1964–1967.
8. Cameron JW, Rosenthal A, Olson AD. Malnutrition in hospitalized children with congenital heart disease. *Arch Pediatr Adolesc Med.* 1995;149:1098–1102.
9. Villasis-Keever MA, Aquiles Pineda-Cruz R, Halley-Castillo E, et al. Frequency and risk factors associated with malnutrition in children with congenital cardiopathy. *Saluda Publica Mex.* 2001;43:313–323.
10. Thompson Chagoyan OC, Reyes Tsubaki N, Rubiela Barrios OL, et al. The nutritional status of the child with congenital cardiopathy. *Arch Inst Cardiol Mex.* 1998;68:119–123.
11. Dimiti AI, Anabwani GM. Anthropometric measurements in children with congenital heart disease at Kenyatta National Hospital (1985–1986). *East Afr Med J.* 1991;68:757–764.
12. Leite HP, de Camargo-Carvalho AC, Fisberg M. Nutritional status of children with congenital heart disease and left-to-right shunt. The importance of the presence of pulmonary hypertension. *Arq Bras Cardiol.* 1995;65:403–407.
13. Miyague NI, Cardoso SM, Meyer F, et al. Epidemiological study of congenital heart defects in children and adolescents. Analysis of 4538 cases. *Arq Bras Cardiol.* 2003;80:269–278.
14. Jacobs EG, Leung MP, Karlberg JP. Postnatal growth in southern Chinese children with symptomatic congenital heart disease. *J Pediatr Endocrinol Metab.* 2000;3:387–401.
15. Tambic-Bukovac L, Malcic I. Growth and development in children with congenital heart disease. *Lijec Vjesh.* 1993;115:79–84.
16. Mitchell IM, Logan RW, Pollock JCS, et al. Nutritional status of children with congenital heart disease. *Br Heart J.* 1995;73(3):277–283.
17. Levey A, Glickstein JS, Kleinman CS, et al. The impact of prenatal diagnosis of complex congenital heart disease on neonatal outcomes. *Pediatr Cardiol.* 2010;31(5):587–597.
18. Leitch CA. Growth, nutrition and energy expenditure in pediatric heart failure. *Prog Pediatr Cardiol.* 2000;11:195–202.
19. Silberback M, Shumaker D, Menshe V, et al. Predicting hospital discharge and length of stay for congenital heart surgery. *Am J Cardiol.* 1993;72:958–963.
20. Krieger I. Growth failure and congenital heart disease. Energy and nitrogen balance in infants. *Am J Dis Child.* 1970;120:497–502.
21. Huse DM, Feldt RH, Nelson RA, et al. Infants with congenital heart disease. *Am J Dis Child.* 1975;129:65–69.
22. Yahav J, Avigad S, Frand M, et al. Assessment of intestinal and cardiorespiratory function in children with congenital heart disease on high calorie formulas. *J Pediatr Gastroenterol Nutr.* 1985;4:778–785.

23. Hansen SR, Dorup I. Energy and nutrient intakes in congenital heart disease. *Acta Paediatr.* 1993;82:166–172.
24. Barton JS, Hindmarsh PC, Scrimgeour CM, et al. Energy expenditure in congenital heart disease. *Arch Dis Child.* 1994;70:59.
25. Van Der Kuip M, Hoos MB, Forget PP, et al. Energy expenditure in infants with congenital heart disease, including a meta-analysis. *Acta Paediatr.* 2003;92:921–927.
26. Davis D, Davis S, Cotman K, et al. Feeding difficulties and growth delay in children with hypoplastic left heart syndrome versus d-transposition of the great arteries. *Pediatr Cardiol.* 2008;29(2):328–333.
27. Kelleher D, Lauseen P, Teixeira-Pinto M, Duggan C. Growth and correlates of nutrition status among infants with hypoplastic left heart syndrome (HLHS) after stage 1 Norwood procedure. *Nutrition.* 2006;22:237–244.
28. Forchielli ML, McColl R, Walker WA, et al. Children with congenital heart disease: a nutrition challenge. *Nutr Rev.* 1994;52:348–353.
29. Cheung MMH, Davis AM, Wilkinson JL, Weintraub RG. Long term somatic growth after repair of tetralogy of Fallot: evidence for restoration of genetic growth potential. *Heart.* 2003;89:1340–1343.
30. Varan B, Tokel K, Yilmaz G. Malnutrition and growth failure in cyanotic and acyanotic congenital heart disease with and without pulmonary hypertension. *Arch Dis Child.* 1999;81(1):49–52.
31. Stranway A, Fowler R, Cunningkam K, et al. Diet and growth in congenital heart disease. *Pediatrics.* 1976;57:75–86.
32. Agus MS, Jaksic T. Nutritional support of the critically ill child. *Curr Opin Pediatr.* 2002;14:470–481.
33. Wang KS, Ford HR, Upperman JS. Metabolic response to stress in the neonate who has surgery. *Neoreviews.* 2006;7:410–418.
34. Madhok AB, Ojamaa K, Haridas V, et al. Cytokine response to children undergoing surgery for congenital heart disease. *Pediatr Cardiol.* 2006;27:408–413.
35. Roth SJ, Adatia I, Pearson GD, Members of the Cardiology Group. Summary proceedings from the cardiology group on postoperative cardiac dysfunction. *Pediatrics.* 2006;117:S40–S46.
36. Owens JL, Musa N. Nutrition support after neonatal cardiac surgery. *Nutr Clin Pract.* 2009;24:242–249.
37. Bellander M, Ley D, Polberger S, Hellström-Westas L. Tolerance to early human milk feeding is not compromised by indomethacin in preterm infants with persistent ductus arteriosus. *Acta Paediatrica.* 2003;92(9):1074–1078.
38. Pronsky ZM. *Food-Medication Interactions,* rev ed. Birchrunville, PA: Food-Medication Interactions; 2004.
39. Walters HL III, Hakimi M, Rice MD, et al. Pediatric cardiac surgical ECMO: multivariate analysis of risk factors for hospital death. *Am Thorac Surg.* 1995;60:329–336.
40. Ishino K, Wong Y, Alexi-Meskishvili V, et al. Extracorporeal membrane oxygenation as a bridge to cardiac transplantation. *Artif Organs.* 1996;30:728–732.
41. Keckler SJ, Laituri CA, Ostlie DJ, Peter SD. A review of venovenus and venoarterial extracorporeal membrane oxygenation in neonates and children. *Eur J Pediatr Surg.* 2010;20(1):1–4.
42. Jaksic T, Shew SB, Keshen TH, et al. Do critically ill surgical neonates have increased energy expenditure? *J Pediatr Surg.* 2001;36(1):63–67.
43. Gravlee GP, Davis RF, Stammers AH, Ungerleider RM. *Cardiopulmonary Bypass: Principles and Practice.* Philadelphia, PA: Lippincott, Williams & Wilkins; 2008:155–171.
44. Brown RL, Wessel J, Warner BW. Nutrition considerations in the neonatal extracorporeal life support patient. *Nutr Clin Pract.* 1994;9(1):22–27.
45. Keshen TH, Miller RG, Jahoor F, Jaksic T. Stable isotopic quantitation of protein metabolism and energy expenditure in neonates on- and post-extracorporeal life support. *J Pediatr Surg.* 1997;32(7):958–962.
46. Abbasi S, Stewart DL, Radmacher P, Adamkin D. Natural course of cholestasis in neonates on extracorporeal membrane oxygenation (ECMO): 10-year experience at a single institution. *Am Soc Artif Org J.* 2008;54(4):436–438.
47. Ukleja A. Altered GI motility in critically ill patients: current understanding of pathophysiology, clinical impact, and diagnostic approach. *Nutr Clin Pract.* 2010;25:16–25.
48. Tyson JE, Kennedy KA. Trophic feedings for parenterally fed infants. *Cochrane Database Syst Rev.* 2005;3:CD000504.
49. Okada Y, Klein N, van Saene HK, et al. Small volumes of enteral feedings normalise immune function in infants receiving parenteral nutrition. *J Pediatr Surg.* 1998;33:16–19.
50. Hadfield RJ, Sinclair DG, Houldsworth PE, Evans TW. Effects of enteral and parenteral nutrition on gut mucosal permeability in the critically ill. *Am J Respir Crit Care Med.* 1995;152:1545–1548.
51. Mishra S, Agarwal R, Jeevasankar M, et al. Minimal enteral nutrition. *Indian J Pediatr.* 2008;75(3):267–269.
52. Hartl WH, Jauch KW, Parhofer K, Rittler P. Working group for developing the guidelines for parenteral nutrition of the German Association for Nutritional Medicine. Complications and Monitoring—Guidelines on Parenteral Nutrition, Chapter 11. *GMS Ger Med Sci.* 2009;7.
53. Vaisman N, Leigh T, Voet H, et al. Malabsorption in infants with congenital heart disease with diuretic treatment. *Pediatr Res.* 1994;36:545–549.
54. Jadcherla SR, Vijayapal AS, Leuthner S. Feeding abilities in neonates with congenital heart disease: a retrospective study. *J Perinatol.* 2009;29:112–118.
55. Einerson KD, Arthur HM. Predictors of oral feeding difficulty in cardiac surgical infants. *Pediatr Nurs.* 2003;29:315–319.
56. Kohr L, Dargan M, Hauge A, et al. The incidence of dysphagia in pediatric patients after open heart procedures with transesophageal echocardiography. *Ann Thorac Surg.* 2003;76:1450–1456.
57. Medoff-Cooper B, Irving SY. Innovative strategies for feeding and nutrition in infants with congenitally malformed hearts. *Cardiol Young.* 2009;19(Suppl 2):90–99.
58. Maher KO, Giddings SS, Baffa JM, et al. New developments in the treatment of hypoplastic left heart syndrome. *Minerva Pediatr.* 2004;56(1):41–49.
59. Daya H, Hosni A, Bejar-Solar J, Evans M. Pediatric vocal fold paralysis: a long-term retrospective study. *Arch Otolaryngol Head Neck Surg.* 2000;126:21–25.
60. Skinner ML, Halstead LA, Rubinstein CS, et al. Laryngopharyngeal dysfunction after Norwood procedure. *J Thoracic Cardiovasc Surg.* 2005;130:1293–1301.
61. Jenkins KJ, Gauvreau K, Newburger JW, et al. Consensus-based method for risk adjustment for surgery for congenital heart disease. *J Thorac Cardiovasc Surg.* 2002;123(1):110–118.

62. Pereira-da-Silva L, Henriques G, Videira-Amaral JM, et al. Osmolality of solutions, emulsions and drugs that may have a high osmolality: aspects of their use in neonatal care. *J Matern Fetal Neonatal Med.* 2002;11(5):333–338.
63. Sapsford A. Enteral nutrition products. In: Groh-Wargo S, Thompson M, Cox J (eds). *Nutritional Care for High Risk Newborns*, rev ed. Chicago: Precept Press; 1994:176.
64. White KC, Harkavy KL. Hypertonic formula resulting from added oral medications. *Am J Dis Child.* 1982;136:931.
65. Zenk L, Hutzable R. Osmolality of infant formulas, tube feedings, and total parenteral solutions. *Hosp Form.* 1978;577:8.
66. Cavell B. Gastric emptying in infants with congenital heart disease. *Acta Paediatr Scand.* 1981;70:517–520.
67. Nugent AW, Daubeney PE, Chondros P, et al. The epidemiology of childhood cardiomyopathy in Australia. *N Engl J Med.* 2003;348(17):1639–1646.
68. Lipchultz SE, Sleeper LA, Towbin JA, et al. The incidence of pediatric cardiomyopathy in two regions of the United States. *N Engl J Med.* 2003;348(17):1647–1655.
69. Grenier MA, Osganian SK, Cox GF, et al. Design and implementation of the North American Pediatric Cardiomyopathy Registry. *Am Heart J.* 2000;129:S86–S95.
70. Kirk R, Edwards LB, Aurora P, et al. Registry of the International Society for Heart and Lung Transplantation: twelfth official pediatric heart transplantation report—2009. *J Heart Lung Transplant.* 2009;28(10):993–1006.
71. Miller TL, Neri D, Extein J, et al. Nutrition in pediatric cardiomyopathy. *Prog Pediatr Cardiol.* 2007;24(1):59–71.
72. Costantini TW, Taylor JH, Beilman GJ. Abdominal complications of ventricular assist device placement. *Surg Infect (Larchmt).* 2005;6(4):409–418.
73. Arabía FA, Tsau PH, Smith RG, et al. Pediatric bridge to heart transplantation: application of the Berlin Heart, Medos and Thoratec ventricular assist devices. *J Heart Lung Transplant.* 2006;25(1):16–21.
74. Beghetti M, La Scala G, Belli D, et al. Etiology and management of pediatric chylothorax. *J Pediatr.* 2000;136:653–658.
75. Spain DA, McClave SA. Chylothorax and chylous ascites. In: Gottschlich MM (ed). *The ASPEN Nutrition Support Core Curriculum: A Case Based Approach—The Adult Patient.* Silver Spring, MD: ASPEN; 2007:477–486.
76. Prasad R, Singh K, Singh R. Bilateral congenital chylothorax with Nona syndrome. *Indian Pediatr.* 2002;39:975–976.
77. Lanning P, Simia S, Saramo I, et al. Lymphatic abnormalities in Noonan's syndrome. *Pediatr Radiol.* 1978;7:106–109.
78. Munoz Conde J, Gomez de Terroros I, Sanchez Ruiz F. Chylothorax associated with Turner's syndrome in a child. *An Esp Pediatr.* 1975;8:449–454.
79. Goens MB, Campbell D, Willins JW. Spontaneous chylothorax in Noonan syndrome. *Am J Dis Child.* 1992;146:1453–1456.
80. Hamada H, Fujita K, Kubo T, et al. Congenital chylothorax in a trisomy 21 newborn. *Arch Gynecol Obstet.* 1992;252:55–58.
81. Chan PC, Chiu HC, Hwu WL. Spontaneous chylothorax in a case of cardio-facio-cutaneous syndrome. *Clin Dysmorph.* 2002;11:297–298.
82. Bellini C, Mazzella M, Arioni C, et al. Hennekam syndrome presenting as non immune hydrops fetalis, congenital chylothorax, and congenital lymphangiectasis. *Am J Med Genetics.* 2003;120A:92–96.
83. Suddaby E, Schiller S. Management of chylothorax in children. *Pediatr Nurs.* 2004;30(4):290–295.
84. Büttiker V, Fanconi S, Burger R. Chylothorax in children: guidelines for diagnosis and management. *Chest.* 1999;116:662–687.
85. Winkler MF. Nutrition management of the patient with chylous fistula. *Support Line.* 2003;25:8–13.
86. Chan EH, Russell JL, Williams WG, et al. Postoperative chylothorax after cardiothoracic surgery in children. *Ann Thorac Surg.* 2005;80:1864–1871.
87. Parrish C, McCray SR. When chyle leaks: nutrition management options. *Pract Gastroenterol.* 2004;26(5):60–76.
88. Sardesai VM. The essential fatty acids. *Nutr Clin Pract.* 1992;7(4):179–186.
89. Lessen R. Use of skim breast milk for an infant with chylothorax. *Infant Child Adolesc Nutr.* 2009;1(6):303–310.
90. Chan GM, Lechtenberg E. The use of fat-free human milk in infants with chylous pleural effusion. *J Perinatol.* 2007;27:434–436.
91. Roehr CC, Jung A, Proquitté H, et al. Somatostatin or octreotide as treatment options for chylothorax in young children: a systematic review. *Intensive Care Med.* 2006;32:650–657.
92. American Academy of Pediatrics Committee on Nutrition. Statement on cholesterol. *Pediatrics.* 1992;90:469–473.
93. National Cholesterol Education Program Expert Panel Detection, Evaluation, and Treatment of High Blood Cholesterol in Adults (Adult Treatment Panel III). Third report of the National Cholesterol Education Program (NCEP) Expert Panel on Detection, Evaluation, and Treatment of High Blood Cholesterol in Adults (Adult Treatment Panel III): final report. *Circulation.* 2002;106:3143–3421.
94. NCEP Expert Panel on Blood Cholesterol Levels in Children and Adolescents. National cholesterol education program (NCEP). Highlights of the report of the Expert Panel on Blood Cholesterol Levels in Children and Adolescents. *Pediatrics.* 1992;89:525–527.
95. Krauss RM, Eckel RH, Howard B, et al. AHA dietary guidelines: revision 2000: a statement for healthcare professionals from the Nutrition Committee of the American Heart Association. *Circulation.* 2000;102(18):2284–2299
96. Williams CL, Stobino BA, Bollella M, et al. Cardiovascular risk reduction in preschool children: the "Healthy Start" project. *J Am Coll Nutr.* 2004;23:117–123.
97. Wabitsch M, Hauner H, Heinze E, et al. Body fat distribution and changes in atherogenic risk factor profile in obese adolescent girls during weight loss. *Am J Clin Nutr.* 1994;60:54–60.
98. Sothern MS. Obesity prevention in children: physical activity and nutrition. *Nutrition.* 2004;20(7–8):704–708.
99. Cotts TB, Goldberg CS, Palma Davis LM, et al. A school-based health education program can improve cholesterol values for middle school students. *Pediatr Cardiol.* 2008;29(5):940–945.
100. Bond M, Wyatt K, Lloyd J, Taylor R. Systematic review of the effectiveness of weight management schemes for the under fives. *Obes Rev.* 2011;12(4):242–253.

CHAPTER 15

Diabetes

Laurie Anne Higgins

Introduction

Diabetes management tools include intensive insulin therapy, medications, blood glucose self-monitoring devices, continuous blood glucose monitoring, psychological intervention, inclusion and education for family and support persons, insulin/food adjustment for exercise, and medical nutrition therapy. The challenge to the dietitian on the diabetes team is to support the family's efforts and to help promote healthy eating habits.

Meal planning is one of the most important tools of diabetes self-management. Unfortunately, diet is overwhelmingly the number one problem in diabetes care.[1] Many factors associated with poor adherence to diabetes-related meal planning are psychosocial in nature (e.g., anger, denial, frustration, poor understanding, social pressures, restriction of favorite foods).[1] Food provides more than nutrients, especially for children. Changes in eating should not be viewed as restrictions and losses but rather as a healthful way for the whole family to eat. To be successful, the meal plan must not only meet nutritional requirements but also be realistic and workable, without requiring major routine changes from those involved. Every attempt should be made to establish a meal plan that reflects the youth's food preferences and the family's social and cultural attitudes. Flexibility and goal setting are important keys to success, increasing the chances of the youth's achieving optimal management and decreasing the development of complications. The goals for medical nutrition therapy are listed in **Table 15-1**.

Management of diabetes requires teamwork. The ultimate therapeutic diabetes team consists of the patient and family as the primary players, along with the diabetes nurse educator, dietitian, behaviorist, and diabetologist. Nutrition guidelines are focused on an "individualized approach to nutrition self-management that is appropriate for the personal lifestyle and diabetes management goals of the individual with diabetes."[2]

Pediatric diabetes centers often include pediatric phlebotomists, child-life specialists, and care ambassadors. Often the last part of an office visit is having the blood drawn, which leaves the child very upset. The pediatric phlebotomist and child-life specialist can work with the family to reduce a child's anxiety. A child-life specialist can be instrumental in providing the family with therapeutic play and techniques to help them with the often-difficult task of blood glucose checks and insulin injections. The care ambassador is usually a college graduate or a child-life specialist who is assigned to a family to help them navigate the healthcare system. The care ambassador will make sure the family has regular scheduled appointments and contacts the family between visits to assist them with whatever they need for their child's care,[3] such as making appointments with members of the diabetes team.

Nutrition Management

A positive approach to meal planning is to encourage family members and other support persons to follow the same lifestyle recommendations as the child with diabetes. It is essential that the nutrition recommendations promote "normal" healthy eating and prevent isolating and dividing the child and family in their food choices. The nutrition needs of children with diabetes are the same as for those without diabetes and should follow the Dietary Guidelines for Americans.[4] The current nutrition recommendations can only be defined as a nutrition prescription based on assessment, individual treatment goals, and outcomes (see **Table 15-2**).[5,6]

The meal plan should include enough calories to maintain consistent growth and to achieve and/or maintain a desirable body weight. In growing children, caloric intake should not be restricted. Energy needs vary during periods of growth, so calorie needs should be compared and validated based on age, height, ideal body weight (IBW), activity, and average energy allowance per day. See Appendix F for methods of estimating energy needs for an individual child and for the recommended dietary allowance (RDA). In general, nutrition management for children with diabetes continues to require carbohydrate counting and healthy eating.

TABLE 15-1 Goals of Medical Nutrition Therapy for Children and Adolescents

- To provide adequate nutrition to maintain normal growth and development based on child's appetite, food preferences, and family lifestyle
- To maintain near-normal blood glucose levels and reduce/prevent the risks of short- and long-term diabetes
- To achieve optimal serum lipid levels
- To preserve social and psychological well-being
- To improve overall health through optimal nutrition
- To provide a level of information that meets the interest and ability of the family
- To provide information on current research to help the family make appropriate nutrition decisions

Carbohydrate and Sweeteners

The percentage of calories ingested from carbohydrate will vary and is individualized based on nutritional assessment and treatment goals. Many factors influence the glycemic response to foods, including the following:

- Total amount of carbohydrate
- The type of carbohydrate (i.e., glucose, sucrose, fructose, lactose, starch)
- Degree of processing
- Glycemic index
- Glycemic load
- Combination with other foods and ingredients

A strong relationship exists between the total carbohydrate intake and the premeal insulin dose.[7] Therefore, adjustment of the premeal insulin dose can allow a person with diabetes to incorporate most carbohydrates into the meal plan and still maintain appropriate blood glucose control. The family is encouraged to provide rapid insulin 20 to 30 minutes before the meal, especially when the meal is composed primarily of carbohydrates.

The glycemic index (GI) is the ranking of the glucose response after ingesting a 50-gram portion of a food and comparing it to the glucose response of an index food.[8] The GI is not a precise tool, because there are many variables.[2] However, it can be used as an indicator of the general glucose response of an individual food. It can be a helpful tool when encouraging children and adolescents to increase the amount of whole-grain products and fresh fruits and vegetables in their meal plan because these foods tend to demonstrate a slower glucose response and are healthier choices.

The glycemic load (GL) takes the GI into account but also uses the quantity of the carbohydrate eaten. This again can be used as a teaching tool to educate the youth and his or her family that when choosing a food with a high GI, having a smaller portion might be more manageable to cover with insulin.

Flexibility in allowing some sucrose into the meal plan may lead to better adherence. Sucrose can be incorporated into a child's meal plans on a regular basis, assuming that overall dietary intake is adequate and consists of foods from all of the essential food groups. To moderate the impact of these food choices on blood glucose levels, sucrose and sucrose-containing foods should be substituted for other carbohydrates in the diet and not simply added to the meal plan.[9] Because most sources of sugar for children younger than 10 years are from milk and milk products, fruit drinks, and carbonated soft drinks, it is important to promote overall healthy eating and optimal dental health by limiting empty-calorie foods. Added sucrose-containing foods should be related to extra activity and special occasions. These foods should be promoted as a special "treat" or "once in a while" foods.

Sweeteners other than sucrose also contain large amounts of carbohydrate and calories and can impact glycemic control. Common sweeteners such as fructose, corn syrup, honey, molasses, carob, dextrose, lactose, and maltose offer no significant advantage over foods sweetened with sucrose.[5]

Commonly used sugar alcohols such as sorbitol, mannitol, xylitol, erthritol, lactitil, isomalt, maltitol, and hydrogenated starch hydrolysate may produce less of a glycemic response and average about 2.4–3.0 kcal/g, compared with 4 kcal/g

TABLE 15-2 Nutrition Recommendations Redistributed the Calories from Macronutrients

Acceptable Macronutrient Distribution Range (% of energy)			
	Children 1–3 Years	Children 4–18 Years	Adults
Protein	5–20	10–30	10–35
Carbohydrate	45–65	45–65	45–65
Fat	30–40	25–35	20–35
Fiber	1–3 years of age		19 g/day
	4–8 years of age		25 g/day
	9–13 years of age Males Females		 31 g/day 26 g/day
	14–50 years of age Males Female		 38 g/day 26 g/day
Calories	Requirements for growth, based on nutrition assessment		

Fiber dietary reference intake = 14 g fiber/1000 kcal after 12 months of age
Source: Institute of Medicine of the National Academies. *Dietary Reference Intakes: The Essential Guide to Nutrient Requirements*. Washington, DC: National Academies Press; 2006.

from other carbohydrates.[10] However, gastrointestinal side effects such as stomach distress or diarrhea are noted when sugar alcohols are ingested in large amounts (e.g., 50 g/day for sorbitol, 20 g/day for mannitol for an adult). Children may be more sensitive and can have diarrhea with intake as little as 0.5 or less g/kg body weight.[11]

The FDA determines an acceptable daily intake (ADI) for noncaloric sweeteners. ADI is defined as the amount of a food additive that can be safely consumed on a daily basis over a person's lifetime without any adverse effects and includes a 100-fold safety factor (see **Table 15-3**). Aspartame, acesulfame K, neotame saccharin, sucralose, and steviol glycosides are the most common noncaloric sweeteners used in the United States.

- *Aspartame* provides 4 kilocalories per gram but is 160 to 220 times sweeter than sucrose. Aspartame is rapidly metabolized in the gastrointestinal tract and does not accumulate in the system at recommended intakes. Aspartame is not heat stable and may decompose on long exposure to high temperatures. Because aspartame is composed of phenylalanine and aspartic acid, it should be restricted in those with phenylketonuria (PKU). The FDA requires all products containing aspartame to display the words "Phenylketonurics: Contains Phenylalanine."
- *Acesulfame K* has no caloric value and is 200 times sweeter than sucrose. It is not metabolized by the body and is eliminated unchanged in the urine. Acesulfame K is heat stable and blends well with other sweeteners. The amount of potassium (K) in this sweetener is minimal, with only 10 mg of potassium in one packet. Acesulfame K is safe for all individuals.[2,10]
- *Saccharin* is 200 to 700 times sweeter than sucrose and has no caloric value. Saccharin is heat stable, is not metabolized by the body, and is excreted unchanged in the urine.
- *Sucralose* is 600 times sweeter than sugar, is the only low-calorie sweetener made from sugar, and is excreted in the urine essentially unchanged.[10] Sucralose is not recognized by the body as either sugar or carbohydrate because it is not broken down or metabolized by the body. It does not affect blood glucose levels. Sucralose is marketed as *Splenda,* which contains a small amount of maltodextrin or dextrose. It does provide some carbohydrate and calories. Individual packages contain less than 1 gram of carbohydrate, but 1 cup of Splenda granular contains 96 calories and 24 grams of carbohydrate. Sucralose is heat stable and may be used during cooking and baking. It is approved by the FDA.
- *Neotame* is 7000 to 13,000 times sweeter than sugar, partially digested in the small intestine, and excreted in the urine and feces. Neotame does have a small amount of phenylalanine, but, even when consumed at 90% of the estimated daily intake, it is not clinically significant for individuals with PKU.[10] It has a clean, sweet taste without the aftertaste associated with other noncaloric sweeteners and is used in beverages and a variety of other foods. It is heat stable and can be used in a variety of products, such as beverages, dairy products, and baked goods.

TABLE 15-3 FDA ADI Guidelines for Non-Nutritive Sweeteners

	ADI (mg/kg body wt)	Average Amount (mg) in 12-oz. Can of Soda*	Cans of Soda to Reach ADI for 45-kg (100-lb.) Child	Amount (mg) in a Packet of Sweetener	Packets to Reach ADI for a 45-kg (100-lb.) Child
Acesulfame K	15	40[+]	17	50	13
Aspartame	50	200	11	35	63
Neotame	18	6[a]	135	N/A	N/A
Saccharin	5	140*	1.6	36	6.25
Sucralose	5	70	3.2	5	45
Stevioside (steviol glycosides)	4[b]	56	10	28	20

These recommendations are set by the Food and Drug Administration (FDA) for Acceptable Daily Intake (ADI) and include a 100-fold safety factor. The World Health Organization's Joint Expert Committee of Food Additives has set the ADI for saccharin. Use these as guidelines.[10]

*This number represents an average; different brand names and fountain drinks may have varied amounts of sweeteners.

[+]Based on the most common blend with 90 mg aspartame.

[a]http://www.neotame.com/pdf/neotame_science_brochure_US.pdf

[b]ADI is translated to 12 mg/kg/day for Rubiana (Truvia) and RebA (PureVia)

Source: Copyright 1999 American Diabetes Association. From *American Diabetes Association Guide to Medical Nutrition Therapy for Diabetes.* Reprinted with permission from the American Diabetes Association. To order this book, please call 1-800-232-6455 or order online at http://shopdiabetes.org.

- *Stevioside* is 250 to 300 times sweeter than sucrose and comes from the stevia plant. It is extracted from the leaf of the plant and is used as a noncaloric sweetener. It has been approved by the FDA and is being used in a variety of foods.[12] Steviosides are marketed as Rubiana (Truvia) and RebA (PureVia), both of which have zero calories per serving.

Dietary Components

Total dietary fiber consists of structural and storage polysaccharides and lignin in plants that are not well digested in humans.[13] Soluble fiber is made up of pectins, gums, mucilages, and some hemicelluloses. Insoluble fiber is made up of noncarbohydrate components, which include cellulose, lignin, and many hemicelluloses. Fiber recommendations for children with diabetes are the same as for children without diabetes.

Dietary fiber may be useful in the treatment or prevention of constipation, gastrointestinal disorders, and colon cancer. However, a high-fiber diet for some very young children may result in an insufficient caloric intake necessary for growth due to the satiety value provided by fiber, as well as possible impairment of mineral absorption. Therefore, the amount of dietary fiber recommended for children should be based on individual eating habits and lipid goals. See Chapter 12, Gastrointestinal Disorders, for further details about fiber.

Current nutrition recommendations for children with diabetes include protein from both animal and vegetable sources comprising 5–30% of calories per day. Children with diabetes require the same amount of protein as the DRI (see Appendix F). Diabetic nephropathy occurs in 20–40% of individuals with diabetes and is the leading cause of end-stage renal disease (ESRD).[14] Therefore, protein intake should be carefully assessed with a focus on overall healthy protein intake. Children engaging in consistent competitive exercise may need some additional protein due to increased energy needs, which can be met by increasing consumption of low-fat, protein-rich foods.

The primary dietary fat goal in children with diabetes is a healthy fat intake that is sufficient to optimize growth and development. Unfortunately, some children and adolescents with diabetes consume fat levels well above what is recommended, and these individuals may be at an even greater risk for heart disease than children without diabetes. Guidelines for the management of dyslipidemia in children with diabetes are available (see **Table 15-4**).[15] Careful consideration should be given to providing enough fat in the diet for children younger than 2 years of age because the development of the brain and central nervous system are dependent on an adequate intake of fats.

TABLE 15-4 Management of Dyslipidemia in Children and Adolescents with Diabetes

Screening
After glycemic control is achieved:
Type 1
Obtain lipid profile at diagnosis and then, if normal, every 5 years
Begin at age 12 years (or onset of puberty, if earlier)
Begin prior to 12 years (if prepubertal) only if positive family history
Type 2
Obtain lipids profile at diagnosis and then every 2 years
Goals
Total cholesterol < 170 mg/dL
LDL < 100 mg/dL
HDL > 35 mg/dL
Triglycerides < 150 mg/dL
Treatment Strategies
Maximize glycemic control
Weight reduction, if necessary
Diet
< 7% of calories from saturated fat
< 200 mg cholesterol per day
Consider LDL-lowering dietary options
Increase soluble fiber
Limit intake of trans fatty acids
Emphasize weight management and physical activity
Medication in collaboration with a physician
Manage other cardiac disease risk factors
Blood pressure
Smoking
Obesity
Inactivity

Source: Adapted with permission from the American Diabetes Association. Management of dyslipidemia in children and adolescents with diabetes. *Diabetes Care.* 2003;26(7):2194–2197.

The majority of people with diabetes do not need additional vitamin and mineral supplements as long as their food intake is adequate and well balanced. However, a child's normal eating habits throughout the growth cycle may exclude or severely limit foods or food groups, and thus nutrient supplementation may be needed.

Vitamin D and calcium are both very important for bone health and should be evaluated by the dietitian. The main sources of vitamin D are fortified milk (100 IU/8 oz) and exposure to the sunlight (~20 to 30 minutes a day). The American Academy of Pediatrics (AAP) recommends 400 IU per day for all infants, children, and adolescents.[16] If a child is not consuming adequate fortified milk or milk substitute, supplementation might be necessary, especially during the winter months in northern areas. Many children do not consume calcium in adequate amounts, especially if they do not drink milk or consume any dairy products. If milk and milk products are not consumed in adequate amounts, supplementation should be considered. See Chapter 6 for a listing of calcium sources.

Chromium deficiency is associated with elevated blood glucose, cholesterol, and triglyceride levels and with reduction in body growth and longevity. Most people with diabetes are not chromium deficient, and chromium supplementation is not recommended unless a deficiency is documented.[5]

Magnesium deficiency has been associated with insulin resistance, carbohydrate intolerance, and hypertension, among other disorders. Only those patients at high risk should routinely be evaluated, such as those in poor glycemic control (e.g., diabetic ketoacidosis, prolonged glycosuria), on diuretics, or with intestinal malabsorption.

Sodium recommendations for children and adolescents with diabetes are the same as for the general population. The current recommendation for children between 4 and 8 years of age is 1.2 g/day; for older children it is 1.5 g/day. The effect of sodium on blood pressure varies greatly depending on a person's level of sodium sensitivity. Routine monitoring of blood pressure is important and will help identify children and adolescents who may benefit from a reduction in sodium intake. Because sodium intake recommendations are the same as for the general population, guidelines should be directed toward the entire family.[17]

Although insulin is stored as inactive zinc crystals in the beta cells and zinc is involved in insulin action, supplementation is only suggested in children with a zinc deficiency. Poor growth has been attributed to zinc deficiency in children with type 1 diabetes, and zinc supplementation in children with low zinc levels has been shown to increase their rate of linear growth.[10] Zinc is found in red meats, some seafood, whole grains, and fortified breakfast cereals.

Many children with diabetes may need vitamins E and C supplements and may benefit from an age-appropriate multivitamin. Families should be encouraged to improve the variety of fruits and vegetables in the youth's meal plan. However, additional supplementation may or may not be needed.[14,19]

Vitamin and mineral supplements should not be used in place of a varied, balanced meal plan to ensure that infants and children receive adequate nutrients. Inadequate nutrient intake is rare in children with diabetes as long as the child is eating a well-balanced diet, growing, gaining weight, and staying active. It is important that children with diabetes meet annually with a registered dietitian to ensure that their diet is nutritionally sound. Children at risk for nutrient deficiencies and who may benefit from a multivitamin supplement with antioxidants include those who are not consuming a variety of foods, are eliminating certain food groups, are strict vegetarians (vegans), are taking medications known to alter certain micronutrients, or who have consistently poor glycemic control, which can result in excess excretion of water-soluble vitamins.

Alcohol

Alcohol use and abuse should be discussed with the adolescent in an objective manner. Alcohol lowers the blood glucose level and blocks gluconeogenesis, possibly leading to erratic behavior, loss of consciousness, or seizures, particularly if food is not consumed with the alcohol.[20] In addition, the teen should understand that glucagon is not effective in treating alcohol-induced hypoglycemia because alcohol depletes glycogen stores. Alcohol also alters the ability to think clearly. Imparting this information about the negative effects of alcohol may cause the teen to be more cautious about drinking alcohol or to avoid it altogether. Those who do choose to drink alcohol should wear diabetes identification, because intoxication and symptoms of hypoglycemia can often be confused for one another.

If alcohol is consumed, it should be consumed in moderate amounts (no more than one drink per day for most females and no more than two drinks a day for most males) and only if diabetes is well managed. One drink or alcohol portion is defined as 12 ounces of beer or 5 ounces of wine. Each of these portions provides about 0.5 ounces of alcohol. As a general rule, it takes about 2 hours for the average 150-pound male to metabolize 1 ounce of alcohol.[21]

Meal Planning

The ultimate goals when designing a meal plan for a child recently diagnosed with type 1 diabetes (TD1) are to:

- Provide healthy eating guidelines for the youth and family
- Promote positive behavioral changes
- Provide healthy meals and snacks
- Focus on healthy eating habits of the entire family

The amount of time required by the family to learn meal planning depends on multiple factors, including family dynamics, emotional status, extended support system, preconceived ideas about the "diabetic diet," and the family's social and cultural attitudes. The child should participate in the initial visit and be reassured that he or she will not be put on a "diet" or have many favorite foods taken away. Rather, healthy guidelines (a meal plan) will be provided based on the child's usual eating pattern to help promote healthy food choices. Meal planning is simply a heart-healthy eating plan for both the child and the entire family.

Nutrition Therapy

At the time of diagnosis, the parent and/or child may be asked to keep a record of what is eaten at each meal and snack. This helps establish the amount of food that is currently needed to satisfy the child's appetite. An accurate measurement of weight and height (or length), information on recent weight loss, and a calculation of IBW are needed to estimate the child's current nutrient and caloric needs.

Determining the percentile of height (length), weight, and body mass index (BMI) and the range for IBW will identify the child's initial nutrition status and help guide the development of the meal plan. A newly diagnosed child is more likely to experience increased hunger due to glycosuria. It is important to respond to this stimulated appetite by providing sufficient food so that hunger and restriction are not associated with having diabetes. The appetite of most children will usually stabilize within the first few weeks after diagnosis. If the youth has lost weight or is not growing adequately, appetite may be higher than estimated needs. Within reason, the meal plan should reflect the amount of food the child desires and be readjusted once appetite decreases. The family should be told that the meal plan might need to be adjusted 2 or 3 weeks after diagnosis, once the child has returned to his or her growth potential.

Nutrition intervention at diagnosis should be based on the family's ability, interest, and readiness to learn. Attempts to present all concepts upon initial diagnosis may result in confusion and the family members' loss of confidence in their ability as caretakers. General guidelines should be provided, such as consistency with timing; amount and types of foods; and the relationship among food, insulin, and exercise and their effect on blood glucose. Many questions will arise when the child returns home and normal activity resumes. Above all, it should be stressed that:

- Parents should not limit food to maintain blood glucose control.
- Any changes associated with food choices should be made slowly.
- Ranges for food choices should be used with young children (i.e., 1–2 oz protein, ½–1 fruit), offering smaller amounts first and using the larger end of the range if more food is requested.
- During initial education, the length of time required to achieve nutrition management survival skills varies between families and may require 2 to 4 hours of education in addition to time for menu writing and food selection using the meal plan.
- After the initial education, additional outpatient nutrition visits will be necessary to achieve ultimate nutrition education goals.

The initial visit in the outpatient setting should lay the groundwork in nutrition basics and serve to develop a sound and trusting relationship with the child and family. The Children's Checklist (see **Exhibit 15-1**) offers a detailed analysis of the child's and family's eating habits and behaviors, food preferences, and family lifestyle. This will assist the registered dietitian in producing a realistic and workable meal plan for each child.

The following guidelines can be helpful in developing a positive working relationship with the youth and his or her caretakers:

- Include the youth in the interview to allow him or her to be part of the decision-making process. The youth will dictate the amount of food based on hunger, and the parent will dictate the food choices.
- Do not refer to or label a youth as a *diabetic* but rather as a *child or adolescent with diabetes.*
- Interview the adolescent separately and then together with the family to stimulate self-management.
- Provide reassurance that many of the youth's usual foods can be included in the meal plan.
- Describe the meal plan as a guideline for healthy eating rather than a diet.
- Stress healthy eating practices for the entire family rather than just focusing on the youth with diabetes.
- Avoid negative words when explaining meal planning such as *cannot, do not, never, should not, bad, restrict,* and especially the word *diet.* In a child's mind, *diet* connotes deprivation or a short-term process, rather than an ongoing process.
- Avoid using the terms *good* or *bad* for foods. Instead, use *healthy* and *not as healthy* to describe individual foods.
- Ask about favorite foods and avoid eliminating these foods. Instead, stress balance, moderation, and variety.
- Review the reality of special treats for birthday parties, holidays, and special occasions and relate "treat" foods with extra exercise and active days.
- Encourage the caregiver to include the youth in shopping and meal preparation.
- Revise or draft a realistic and workable meal plan with input from the parent and/or youth.
- Encourage the parents to always keep the lines of communication open so the youth can request special foods that he or she wants to eat and that can be worked into the meal plan. Avoid being the "food police." If the youth is always told "no," he or she may start to sneak food, which will cause unexplained high blood glucose levels.
- Advise the caregivers that it is not advisable to omit foods from the meal plan because of a single high blood glucose reading. An elevated blood glucose level caused by stress may decrease rapidly when the stress is reduced, and hypoglycemia may occur if food is omitted.
- Continued nutrition follow-up and education are required every 6 months to 1 year as the child grows and develops and as the family works to gain expertise in the nutrition management of diabetes.

Several effective methods are available for teaching patients about food. Any method can be equally effective when

EXHIBIT 15-1 Children's Checklist: Assessing the Child Newly Diagnosed with Diabetes

Growth (Anthropometrics):
- Height
- Weight
- BMI or weight-for-height
- History of growth pattern
- Recent weight changes

Biochemical Indices:
- Blood glucose
- Glycosylated hemoglobin (A1C) and estimated average glucose (eAG)
- Lipid profile
- Microalbumin
- Ketones

Psychosocial Information:
- Identify the family unit at home (two parents, separated or divorced parents, single parent, siblings, other family, friends, or caretakers).
- Evaluate emotional state of parents, child, siblings (anger, fear, guilt, denial, anxiety).
- Assess child's interactions with parents and siblings.
- Identify person(s) responsible for shopping/cooking.
- Evaluate knowledge/comprehension levels and literacy.
- Identify cultural/religious systems that influence attitudes.
- Identify family members or friends with diabetes.
- Assess parents and family beliefs about the "diabetic diet."

Child's Usual Food Intake Prior to Symptoms of Diabetes

Home:
- Eats scheduled meals/snacks
- Includes staple foods, such as milk, cheese, yogurt, bread
- Eats meats, fruit, and vegetables on a regular basis
- Consumes beverages at meals/snacks other than milk
- Drinks soda/juice/water for thirst
- Follows special diet

School:
- Brings lunch from home or has school lunch.
- Beverage at lunch/snacks.
- Scheduled snacks are part of regular class activities.
- Obtains snack at school or snack sent from home.
- Frequency, length, and time of day of gym class.
- Participates in school sports or activities after school.

Weekends:
- Evaluate meals prepared or eaten with others on weekends.
- Identify meal schedule if different from weekdays.
- Determine restaurant eating habits on weekends.
- Assess sports/activities scheduled on weekends.

Eating Behaviors

Child:
- Overeats or undereats
- Relies on convenience and fast foods
- Experiences food jags often
- Refuses many of the family foods offered
- Finishes meals in reasonable amount of time
- Respects limits set for acceptable eating behavior at the table
- Location where meals and snacks are consumed
- Food allergies or intolerances

Family:
- Evaluate parents as role models.
- Healthy eaters, structured meals, planned meals, limit junk food in home.
- Unhealthy eaters, overweight, chronic dieters.
- Identify supervision at meals/snacks.
- Evaluate limit-setting around food choices.
- Assess cultural/religious eating behaviors.
- Identify whether food is used as a reward.

"geared to the patient's intellectual level, repeated frequently, and evaluated."[22] The two most common approaches used with children are advanced carbohydrate counting and basic carbohydrate counting. On occasion, the family might request a food choice list (exchange list) for meal planning. These methods give structure to meal planning and provide the right balance among food, insulin, and exercise.

The standard of care for children with T1D is to manage their diabetes on multiple daily injections (MDI) or continuous subcutaneous insulin infusion (CSII) using pump therapy. Advanced carbohydrate (carb) counting allows users greater flexibility in the timing of meals, the amount of food eaten at the meal, and the selection of specific foods. The meal-planning objective is to coordinate food intake (carb) by matching the peak activity of insulin with the peak levels of glucose resulting from the digestion and absorption of food. Only the carb value of the food is counted, which allows more accurate adjustment of premeal, rapid-acting insulin using an insulin-to-carb ratio. The insulin-to-carb ratio is based on the assumption that carb intake is the main consideration in determining meal-related insulin requirements, together with self-monitored blood glucose (SMBG) values. Targeted blood glucose values are set by the diabetes team, the child, and the family. A general rule is that approximately 1 unit of rapid-acting insulin will be needed for every 10–15 grams of carbohydrate.[23] The child's insulin-to-carb ratio should be individually determined by the diabetes team based on the child's present insulin needs and meal plan. A youth's ratio can range from 1 unit of insulin for every 5–40 grams of carbohydrate, depending on age, activity, and insulin needs.

In addition to covering the carbs at a meal, the youth is given a sensitivity factor (SF) and a target blood glucose level. This allows one to adjust the dose based on the blood glucose level prior to the meal or snack. If the blood glucose level is higher than target, some additional insulin is added; if it is lower, some insulin is subtracted using the SF.

Special care must be given to prevent overeating, because increased availability of insulin and food may promote unwanted weight gain. A good understanding of how carbohydrate affects blood glucose, what food groups contain carbohydrates, and the importance of portion control is necessary for carbohydrate counting to be effective.

The lists of food choices (exchange lists) are based on the following food groups:

- *The carbohydrate group:* Starches (e.g., breads, cereals, grains, starchy vegetables), fruit, milk, nonstarchy vegetables, sweets, desserts, and other carbohydrates. One serving equals 15 grams of carbohydrate.
- *The meat and meat substitute group:* Protein (e.g., meat, poultry, fish, beans).
- *The fats group:* Vegetable oils, avocado, and regular salad dressings.

Examples of the specific amount of carbohydrate, protein, fat, or combination of these nutrients in each food group are available online at http://www.nhibi.nih.gov. Foods with similar nutrient values are listed together and may be exchanged or traded for any other food on the same list. Exchange lists are used to achieve a consistent timing and intake of carbohydrate, protein, and fat and provide needed variety when planning meals. Exchange lists and a meal plan can be a starting point for the patients on intensive insulin management and can help them to understand and learn the carbohydrate content of foods.

Insulin Therapy

The standard of care for managing diabetes in children is called *intensive management* and uses a basal/bolus insulin plan. Intensive insulin therapy can include multiple daily injections (MDI) using rapid-acting insulin with either an intermediate or long-acting insulin or CSII pump therapy. A basal/bolus regimen allows more flexibility in scheduling of meals and may eliminate the need for some snacks. Intensive insulin therapy does increase the risk of hypoglycemia. The insulin action (onset, peak, and duration) of the insulin available is listed in **Table 15-5**. It is important to consider that insulin action will differ from person to person and can be affected by the injection site, activity level before and after the injection is given, and time of day.

Conventional insulin therapy is no longer the standard of care but is still used in practice. This therapy may include two daily injections of intermediate-acting insulin (NPH) or one injection of NPH with a long-acting/basal insulin (glargine [Lantus] or detemir [Levemir]), possibly combined with a small amount of rapid-acting insulin (lispro [Humalog], aspart [Novolog], or glulisine [Apidra]).

Many circumstances require permanent or temporary insulin adjustments to be made. As a child grows and food intake increases, the insulin dose also increases. During brief periods of illness, times of stress, or decreased activity, insulin needs may also increase. A change in the child's level of activity, which may be especially dramatic at the beginning and end of the school year, usually requires an adjustment in the insulin dosage. When these events resolve or change, the child's insulin dose will need to be readjusted. Otherwise, an increase of food in response to the higher insulin levels may result in inappropriate weight

TABLE 15-5 Insulin Actions

Insulin	When to Take	Onset	Peak	Effective Duration
Rapid Acting Lispro (Humalog), Aspart (Novolog), Glulisine (Apidra)	0–15 minutes before the meal	10–30 minutes	30 minutes–3 hours	3–5 hours
Short Acting Regular (R)	30 minutes before the meal	30–60 minutes	2–5 hours	Up to 12 hours
Intermediate Acting NPH	Does not need to be given with food	90 minutes–4 hours	4–12 hours	Up to 24 hours
Long Acting Glargine (Lantus), Detemir (Levemir)	Does not need to be given with food	45 minutes–4 hours	Minimal	Up to 24 hours

gain or hypoglycemia, whereas too little insulin may result in hyperglycemia.

Snacks should be part of a healthy eating plan and may be needed, depending on the child's age. Snacks can help maintain blood glucose and provide adequate calories during the day for growth and development. Snacking during the day is more desirable and will hopefully eliminate hunger in the evening hours. If the child is on a basal/bolus regimen, then snacks before bedtime are not necessary unless the blood glucose is lower than desired or the child is hungry.

Conventional insulin therapy with NPH insulin has a peaking action. To prevent hypoglycemia, the youth is encouraged to eat snacks between meals and at bedtime. Typically, a snack of 15–20 g of carbohydrate is recommended for young children and a snack of 20–30 g of carbohydrate or higher is recommended for adolescents. Snacking may be necessary depending on the child's activity, such as length of time at recess and in physical education (PE) classes and the type and length of afterschool activities. For example, if PE is offered only on Monday and Wednesday at 10:00 am, the child may need a larger snack on those days, preferably a snack with 20–30 g of carbohydrate and 1–2 ounces of protein. For very active days and extended appetite control, a long-lasting snack (2 to 3 hours) containing carbohydrate, protein, and fat can be given. For inactive children, whose main activity only includes watching television and studying, snacks may contain only 10–20 g of carbohydrate.

Continuous subcutaneous insulin infusion (CSII) has many benefits, including improved glycemic control,[24,25] reduced episodes of hypoglycemia, improved linear growth, and decreased episodes of recurrent diabetic ketoacidosis (DKA).[26] Pumps are becoming more widely used even in children as young as 1 to 2 years of age. The advantage of the pump for the young child is that it offers the parents the ability to dose a very small amount of insulin and provide multiple doses throughout the day without having to give the child injections by syringe or pen.

Pump therapy provides rapid-acting insulin (Humalog, Novolog, or Apidra), which eliminates the unpredictable action of the longer-acting insulins. The pump delivers a small amount of insulin continuously (basal) and can be programmed to deliver boluses when eating a meal or snack or for correcting high blood glucoses. Pump therapy has its pros and cons, which should be considered very carefully prior to putting any youth on an insulin pump.

Long-acting insulins (basal) are becoming more popular in school-age children and adolescents in place of the intermediate insulin NPH. They offer the child the flexibility of the pump without the additional equipment that comes with the pump. Long-acting insulin is given in one or two injections daily to meet the child's background or basal insulin needs. Additional injections of rapid insulin are given at meals and snacks to cover the carbohydrate and to correct the blood glucose. The long-acting insulin can last up to 24 hours and is usually started with one injection a day, usually at dinner or bedtime. Some children have benefited from splitting the dose, due to the insulin possibly not lasting a full 24 hours or having some peaking action.

This insulin regimen includes at least four to five injections in an older child and as many as five to six in a younger child. To avoid additional insulin injections at school, NPH insulin can be added at breakfast with the rapid insulin to cover the morning snack and lunch. Long-acting insulin can be used at bedtime in place of NPH if there is concern of hypoglycemia in the middle of the night, and it will also give a little coverage in the late afternoon.

Before starting CSII or MDI, the child and the family must master advanced skills, including having a good understanding of advanced carbohydrate counting, which includes using insulin-to-carbohydrate ratios, understanding the sensitivity or correction factor to determine each insulin dose, and having the necessary math skills needed to calculate dosage.

Developmental Concerns

The most important psychosocial issues facing families with children with diabetes are:[27]

- Defining responsibilities and support for diabetes management within the family
- Sharing treatment responsibilities among family members
- Transferring these responsibilities from parent to child as the child develops

As the child with diabetes progresses through the different stages of development, it is important to address how these changes affect the parents and/or the child and focus on the normal developmental issues of each stage. Encouraging parental involvement throughout childhood and early adulthood can be beneficial in the youth's diabetes management. See **Table 15-6** for some of the development stages and how they relate to T1D.[28]

Initially, most infants consume 100% of their calories as breast milk or formula, eating every 3 to 4 hours. All infants should be breastfed for the first 6 to 12 months of life or fed iron-fortified infant formula. Solids should be introduced at 4 to 6 months and progress from cereal to fruits, meat, vegetables, and/or vegetable–meat dinners. Infants with diabetes do well following the same schedule. Eventually when the infant begins eating 2–3 tablespoons of baby foods and/or table food (other than low-calorie vegetables), basic carbohydrate counting can be introduced as a guideline. A feeding schedule should be established despite somewhat erratic eating behaviors in the infant.

Although whole cow's milk should not be given during the child's first year, after the first year cow's milk should

TABLE 15-6 Major Development Issues and Their Effect on Diabetes in Children and Adolescents

Developmental Stage (Approximate Ages)	Normal Developmental Tasks	T1D Management Priorities	Family Issues in T1D Management
Infancy (0–12 months)	Developing a trusting relationship/"bonding" with primary caretakers	• Preventing and treating hypoglycemia • Avoiding extreme fluctuations in the BG levels	• Coping with stress • Sharing the "burden of care" to avoid parent burnout
Toddler (13–36 months)	Developing a sense of mastery and autonomy	• Preventing and treating hypoglycemia • Avoiding extreme fluctuations in the BG levels due to irregular food intake	• Establishing a schedule • Managing the picky eater • Setting limits and coping with toddlers' lack of cooperation with regimen • Sharing the burden of care
Preschooler and early elementary age (3–7 years)	Developing initiative in activities and confidence in self	• Preventing and treating hypoglycemia • Unpredictable appetite and activity • Positive reinforcement for cooperation with regimen • Trusting other caretakers with diabetes management	• Reassuring the child that diabetes is no one's fault • Educating other caretakers about diabetes management
Older elementary school age (8–11 years)	• Developing skills in athletic, cognitive, artistic, and social areas • Consolidating self-esteem with respect to the peer group	• Making diabetes regimen flexible to allow for participation in school/peer activities • Child learning short- and long-term benefits of optimal control	• Maintaining parental involvement in insulin and BG monitoring tasks while allowing for independent self-care for "special occasions" • Continuing to educate school and other caretakers
Early adolescence (12–15 years)	Managing body changes Developing a strong sense of self-identity	• Managing increased insulin requirements during puberty • Diabetes management and blood glucose control become more difficult • Weight and body image concerns	• Renegotiating parents' and teen's role in diabetes management to be accepted by both • Learning coping skills to enhance ability to self-manage • Preventing and intervening with diabetes-related family conflict • Monitoring for signs of depression, eating disorders, and risky behaviors
Later adolescence (16–19 years)	Establishing a sense of identity after high school (decision about location, social issues, work, education)	• Begin discussion of transition to new diabetes team • Integrating diabetes into new lifestyle	• Supporting the transition to independence • Learning coping skills to enhance ability to self-manage • Preventing and intervening with diabetes-related family conflict • Monitoring for signs of depression, eating disorders, or risky behavior

Source: Reproduced with permission from the American Diabetes Association. Silverstein J, Klingensmith G, Copeland K, et al. Care of children and adolescents with type 1 diabetes: a statement of the American Diabetes Association. *Diabetes Care.* 2005;28(1):186–212.

not be removed from the diets of infants who have a family history of T1D.

Between 12 and 15 months of age, breast milk (or formula) intake may begin to decrease and the intake of solid food increases. A total revision of the meal plan is needed at this time. A child may begin to be more accepting of meat and cheese, which can be added to the meal plan. Although fruits are included in the meal plan, fruit juice should be limited or avoided due to its effect on appetite, weight, and blood glucose.

As the toddler develops more mobility, interest in the environment also increases, and interest in food may wane. In some instances, getting the toddler to eat anything at a meal is an accomplishment. Erratic eating behaviors in toddlers require careful monitoring. In some cases, insulin is given after the meal, when the toddler has consumed the food and the dose of insulin can be titrated based on the amount of food consumed. This also is a popular time for parents to transition their child to CSII, which will give them flexibility to split the insulin dose. For instance, they can give the amount of insulin to correct the blood glucose if higher than desired and some of the insulin to cover the food as much as they feel comfortable giving and then make up the difference at the end of the meal. Food-behavior guidelines for this young group, with or without diabetes, should be firmly established by caregivers at the time the child begins solid foods.

Adjusting diabetes around the school schedule rather than changing physical education classes or lunch periods to accommodate an insulin regimen communicates to the child that the child is more important than the diabetes. It is possible to arrange snacks and injections around most school schedules. Parents should be encouraged to address food and diabetes treatment issues with school personnel; however, some parents may require assistance from their diabetes care team. School-age children will ordinarily need three meals and two to three snacks a day, scheduled according to their insulin regimen. However, some children can omit the morning snack without creating a problem as long as lunch is not delayed. Children should be instructed to carry a fast-acting carbohydrate with them at all times in case of emergency. The use of chocolate candy bars or other high-fat items is discouraged as a treatment for hypoglycemia because fat ingestion slows the absorption of the carbohydrate needed to raise the blood glucose to a safe level. Most schools will offer lunch items appropriate to the needs of children following a meal plan, such as low-fat milk and fresh fruit.

The advent of adolescence may bring a great deal of conflict into the lives of family members. Adolescents strive for independence and expect parents to trust them to manage their own diabetes. During adolescence, they may vent their anger for the first time about having diabetes. The key to working successfully with adolescents is for the parents and the diabetes team to make every effort to provide positive reinforcement and negotiated support. Parents should continue their involvement and supervision of monitoring blood glucose and insulin administration at home. It often is more effective for team members to see adolescents and their parents individually, while at the same time respecting their confidentiality. More flexibility in food choices and an increase in calories during this period of growth are usually necessary. Food choices may improve in a nonjudgmental atmosphere and with assistance for the teen to work favorite foods into the meal plan. In clinic visits, teens should be routinely asked if they have any questions about their food choices. Focusing on the positive choices the adolescents are making and what they are doing right can lead to open discussion.

Growth and Weight Control

Routine charting of a child's height, weight, and BMI is an excellent way to monitor his or her growth pattern. Deviation from the child's normal growth curve (except for increased height or decreasing weight in a child who has reached full height potential) needs close monitoring. Achieving optimal height potential can be used to motivate children to strive for better blood glucose control. Adolescents are more likely to be interested in improved self-care when they understand the relationship between good control, appropriate weight gain, consistent height increase, and/or normal menses.

Weight control can become an important issue to children prior to and when entering adolescence. Parents and the diabetes team must take concerns about body image seriously. Some weight gain is usually seen prior to growth spurts. If a youth's weight is disproportionate to height, the weight should be kept stable until the height fits the weight. Calorie reduction and food restriction are not recommended for children at any time during growth and development. Rather, the child should be encouraged to become involved in active play and physical exercise and to incorporate more fresh fruits and vegetables into his or her daily intake.

Youth who are overly concerned about weight gain but who find it hard to reduce their intake may choose to skip insulin injections to promote quick weight loss. Eating disorders in youth with diabetes can include anorexia nervosa, bulimia nervosa, and eating disorder not otherwise specified (EDNOS).[29] Early identification of eating disorders by the diabetes team can help the individual to get the treatment necessary. Some of the signs are as follows:[30]

- Deterioration of psychosocial functions (school, work, interpersonal)
- Weight fluctuations of 10 pounds or more
- High glycosylated hemoglobin (A1C)
- Controlled diabetes only when hospitalized

- Unexplained diabetic ketoacidosis
- Reluctance or refusal to take more insulin or other medications
- Not checking blood glucose
- Blaming insulin for weight problems
- Preoccupation with body image
- Engaging in excessive exercise
- Bingeing
- Restricting food
- Depression with low self-esteem

Referral to a registered dietitian or certified diabetes educator is the first line of defense when a child or adolescent exhibits weight dissatisfaction but does not exhibit clinical eating pathology. Strict guidelines regarding food and blood glucose should not be implemented because this may actually promote binge eating or weight gain. Adolescents should be advised that glucose fluctuations could create increased hunger and result in weight gain. Education should also be provided about serious short- and long-term consequences of destructive food behaviors. Referral to a mental health professional who is knowledgeable about diabetes and disordered eating, or hospitalization, is often necessary to break the disordered eating cycle.

Type 2 Diabetes

Type 2 diabetes (T2D) is increasing in our population, especially in high-risk ethnic groups.[31] The increased incidence of T2D in children is proportional with the increased incidence of childhood obesity. T2D in children, as in adults, is due to the combination of insulin resistance and beta-cell failure. Incorporating physical activity and nutrition counseling to help the child or adolescent maintain or lose weight is often prescribed, coupled with either Metformin or insulin. Metformin is presently the only oral diabetes medication approved by the FDA for pediatric use.

Youth diagnosed with T2D have a greater incidence of comorbidities at diagnosis. These children should have blood pressure measurements, a fasting lipid profile, a microalbuminuria assessment, and a dilated eye examination at diagnosis.[14] Other comorbidities include polycystic disease and obesity.

The increased rate of children being diagnosed with T2D is a public health problem. Current recommendations include the following:

- Children of families at risk should be aware of the benefits of weight maintenance or moderate weight loss and regular physical activity.
- Intervention strategies should involve counseling on weight loss and physical activity, with follow-up.
- Drug therapy should not be routinely used to prevent diabetes.[32]

Pregnancy

To help ensure a healthy pregnancy and a positive outcome for the woman with diabetes, optimal medical care must begin before conception. However, many unplanned pregnancies occur shortly after puberty among adolescents and young women with and without diabetes, putting those with pregestational diabetes mellitus (PGDM) at a higher risk for early pregnancy loss or congenital malformations. The deterioration of metabolic control in combination with other obstetric and medical complications during an unplanned pregnancy can lead to serious complications of diabetes, such as retinopathy, nephropathy, hypertension, and neuropathy. The diabetes team needs to provide prepregnancy counseling, including information on the risk of congenital malformations, to those of childbearing age who have diabetes.

Unplanned pregnancies should be addressed immediately through a multidisciplinary team approach. The team should include a diabetologist, an obstetrician, and diabetes educators, such as a nurse, a registered dietitian, a social worker, and possibly an exercise physiologist. The team approach can guide the mother toward a goal of a healthy pregnancy and offspring.[33] Members of the adolescent or young adult's immediate family are encouraged to attend and participate in all learning sessions.

A preconception interactive care plan should incorporate the following:

- Patient education related to interaction of diabetes, pregnancy, and family planning
- Education in diabetes self-management skills
- Physician-directed medical care and laboratory testing
- Counseling by a mental health professional to reduce stress and improve adherence to the diabetes treatment plan

Nutrition management during pregnancy should begin at the earliest possible time. Caloric intake should be evaluated as soon as possible in the first trimester and at the start of each trimester thereafter to ensure adequate intake. Guidelines for medical nutrition therapy for pregnancy for preexisting diabetes are listed in **Exhibit 15-2**.

Breastfeeding

Breastfeeding is encouraged for mothers with diabetes. Breastfeeding has many advantages, as addressed in Chapter 5. Breastfeeding increases the need for fluids, and mothers should be encouraged to drink 2 to 3 liters (8 to 12 cups) of caffeine-free liquids per day to cover their fluid needs and replace what is used in breast milk. Meal planning during breastfeeding requires assistance from a dietitian and physician. Insulin requirements are usually reduced during breastfeeding; however, caloric intake requires an additional 500 calories per day above what was consumed before

EXHIBIT 15-2 Medical Nutrition Therapy Guidelines for Management of Diabetes in Pregnancy

Recommendations are the same for pre-existing diabetes and GDM except where noted.

Counseling and Education	• All pregnant women should receive MNT counseling by a registered dietitian (RD), Certified Diabetes Educator (CDE) preferred.
	• All pregnant women should receive SMBG training by a diabetes educator (DE), CDE preferred.
	• Daily food records and recorded SMBG are required to assess the effectiveness of MNT.
	• Carbohydrate counting skills are taught for either consistent carbohydrate intake or a personalized insulin-to-carbohydrate ratio so the patient can adjust insulin based on carbohydrate intake.
	• At least three encounters with a CDE are recommended:
	  • Visit 1 (60- to 90-minute individual or group visit with RD) for assessment and meal planning. This could be SMBG instruction if RD has received appropriate training.
	  • Visit 2 (30–45 min) with RD or RN in 1 week to assess and modify plan.
	  • Visit 3 (15–45 min) with RD or RN in 1–3 weeks to assess and modify plan as needed.
	• Additional visits every 2–3 weeks with RD or RN p.r.n. until delivery and one visit 6–8 weeks after delivery.

Calories	WHO BMI Range (kg/m^2)	Energy Needs (kcals/kg) Based on Pregravid kg	Total Weight Gain Range (lbs)	Twin	Rates of Weight Game (lb/week) in 2nd and 3rd Trimesters
	Underweight (< 18.5)	36–40	28–40		1.0 (1–3)
	Normal weight (18.5–24.9)	30	25–35	37–54	1.0 (0.8–1.0)
	Overweight (25.0–29.0)	24	15–25	31–50	0.6 (0.5–0.7)
	Obese (≥ 30.0)	**	11–20	25–42	0.5 (0.4–0.6)

For singleton pregnancy, add an additional 340 kcal/day to calculated needs in 2nd trimester and 452 kcal/day in 3rd trimester, or additional calories consistent with target weight gain. For twin pregnancy, add an additional 500 kcals to calculated needs after 1st trimester. For multiple pregnancies, add 500 kcal in the 1st trimester. (**Provisional guidelines for twin pregnancies per Institute of Medicine).

* Insufficient information was available to develop a provisional guideline for underweight women with multiple fetuses.

** Insufficient information to address energy needs (kcal/kg) in the obese category

Distribution of Calories	• Individualize based on usual intake, preferences, and medical regimen. • Six to eight small meals/snacks. More frequent meals decrease postprandial hyperglycemia. Weight should be monitored at each visit; track patient's weight gain on prenatal weight gain chart

	GDM	Preexisting Diabetes
Carbohydrate	40–45% total calories†	45–55% total calories
Breakfast	15–30 grams‡	Individualize as per usual intake and BG levels
Other Meals	45 grams lunch and dinner	Individualize as per usual intake and BG levels
HS Snack	15–30 grams carbs	15–30 grams carbs
Fiber	• Calculate 14 grams of fiber per 1000 kcals per day (25-30 grams/day) based on provider assessment.	
Protein	• Calculate 1.1 grams of protein per kg per day, based on provider assessment.	
Fat	• *Preexisting diabetes:* 30–40% total calories, with < 10% total calories from saturated fat. • *GDM:* 30–40% total calories, with 10% total calories from saturated fat. • Encourage use of polyunsaturated and monounsaturated fats instead of saturated fats.	

(continues)

EXHIBIT 15-2 *(Continued)*

Nutritive and non-nutritive sweeteners	• The safety of non-nutritive sweeteners has not been established.
Vitamin/mineral supplements	Prenatal multivitamin and mineral supplement including: • Iron (27 mg/day). • Folic acid (400 mcgs) to supplement average daily dietary intake of 400 mcgs for a total daily intake of 800 mcgs to 1 mg daily to decrease risk of neural tube defects. (Begin 400 mcgs prior to conception.) • Additional calcium supplementation may be needed to meet daily requirements of 1000 mg per day (1300 mg per day if under age 19). Begin prior to conception. • Vitamin D 600 IUs/day.
Caffeine	• Limit to <200 mg per day. Excess caffeine consumption during pregnancy may increase the risk of miscarriage.
Physical activity	• Regular physical activity is recommended after clearance by provider. • Benefits include reducing insulin resistance, postprandial hyperglycemia, and excessive weight gain. • Hypoglycemia is more likely with prolonged exercise (> 60 minutes). • Encourage activity after meals to reduce postprandial hyperglycemia.
Alcohol and tobacco use	• Alcohol and tobacco use should be avoided during pregnancy.

†Pregnant women should consume a minimum of 175 g carbohydrate per day.

‡May be increased if insulin is added.

Source: Adapted with permission from Joslin Diabetes Center and Joslin Clinic Guideline for Detection and Management of Diabetes and Pregnancy (Rev. June 2011). Joslin's Clinical Guidelines are reviewed periodically and modified as needed to reflect changes in clinical practice and available pharmacological information. Check Joslin's Website for the latest version (http://www.joslin.org).

the pregnancy. Extra calories may be added in the form of protein- and calcium-rich foods such as milk, yogurt, tofu, and cheese. The calcium requirement for lactating women younger than 18 years of age is 1300 mg per day.[6] Calcium intake should be routinely assessed by a dietitian to prevent calcium loss from the mother during breastfeeding. It is important to keep a carbohydrate food source (15–20 g) available while nursing because hypoglycemia may occur while breastfeeding. To prevent possible nocturnal hypoglycemia, an extra snack that has 20–30 g of carbohydrates and a source of protein may be added to the meal plan in the middle of the night.

Monitoring Blood Glucose

Glycosylated hemoglobin (A1C) measures the weighted average amount of glucose in the blood over a 2- to 3-month period. Used in conjunction with regularly monitored blood glucose, A1C levels can help evaluate the level of control. However, the A1C level reflects an average amount of glucose in the blood and can be the result of very high or low blood glucose levels, which is not indicative of good control. Although "excellent control" for an adult with diabetes is 6% or less, the activity levels and eating habits of children and adolescents vary, so even a level under 7% can be unsafe and difficult to achieve in children. A1C goals should be set by the child's diabetes team and tailored to each individual case. Age-appropriate A1C goals are shown in **Table 15-7**.[34]

Home blood glucose monitoring meters provide the child and family with immediate feedback on the effects of food, exercise, insulin, and stress on blood glucose levels, allowing for more flexibility in lifestyle and food intake.

A youth with diabetes has many self-care responsibilities. Checking and recording blood glucose levels may be one of the most bothersome responsibilities for a youth because it must be done so often and because others may inappropriately evaluate and judge the results. Blood glucose results are not totally reliable as a monitor of adherence to carb counting. If, by reporting a high blood glucose reading, a youth risks accusations of sneaking food or overeating, the youth may choose to record a more acceptable but false level. This practice may result in poor diabetes management. Establishing a nonjudgmental and honest atmosphere

TABLE 15-7 Age-Based A1C and eAG Goals

Age (years)	A1C	eAG (mg/dL)	Plasma BG Goal Range (mg/dL)*	
			Before Meals	Bedtime/Overnight
Toddlers and preschool (0–6)	< 8.5%	< 197	100–180	110–200
School age (6–12)	< 6–8%	< 126–183	90–180	100–180
Adolescents and young adults (13–19)	< 7.5%	< 169	90–130	90–150

*ADA goals

Estimated average glucose (eAG) is a new way to present the A1C. It is a number similar to the glucose meter readings. To determine average glucose the calculation is eAG = (28.7 × A1C) – 46.7. The American Diabetes Association has an eAG calculator available on its Website: http://www.diabetes.org/eag.jsp.

Source: Laffel LMB, Butler DA, Higgins LA, Lawlor MT, Pasquarello CA (eds). *Joslin's Guide to Managing Childhood Diabetes: A Family Teamwork Approach.* Boston, MA: Joslin Diabetes Center; 2009.

for the exchange of information is imperative for the parent as well as all healthcare providers. When monitoring blood glucose, the word *check* should be used instead of *test,* and positive words should be used to describe the results, such as *high* or *low* rather than *good* or *bad.* Any information received from monitoring provides information with positive feedback.[35]

High or low blood glucose levels will still occur in most children even when insulin, exercise schedules, and carb counting are followed closely. When a high or low level occurs, it is useful to review the day's activities to see if there is an obvious explanation. The extent to which children should monitor blood glucose levels is variable, depending on many factors, including the following:

- The type of insulin therapy
- Increased activity or exercise
- Sickness or infection
- New food choices
- Change in lifestyle
- Increased stress
- Change in insulin type or dose
- Episodes of hypoglycemia
- Overall control

A general guideline for blood glucose checking for most youth should be four checks daily, before each meal and before bedtime. Additional checks should be done before physical activity, if there is suspicion of hypoglycemia or hyperglycemia, or if the youth is ill.

Continuous glucose monitoring (CGM) is now widely available for the consumer, and some insurance companies are covering the system. The newer real-time CGM allows the person with diabetes to have a complete picture of his or her blood glucose activity in real time. The system has three components: the sensor, the transmitter, and the receiver. The sensor is a small flexible electrode that sits under the skin in the interstitial fluid, which is the liquid that surrounds our cells. It is introduced by a needle, and then the needle is removed and the sensor can be worn 3 to 7 days, depending on the CGM. The transmitter is a tiny computer attached to the sensor that sends the information from the sensor to a wireless receiver. The receiver is the size of a beeper or cell phone, and it will collect the information and display it on a screen. It will display a blood glucose reading every 1 to 5 minutes and provide a directional trend of where the glucose is going. There is a slight delay in the reading, however, and the finger stick is still the gold standard when treating hypoglycemia. The devices also have arrows and alarms that can be set to warn the individual if his or her blood glucose level is rising or falling quickly so action can be immediate. This technology enables educators to help youth cover meals (such as pizza, fast food, and Chinese food) that have been challenging in the past. Once the effect of the meal on the blood glucose level is viewed, the diabetes educator can help the youth determine the best way to cover the particular meal.

Exercise

Regular exercise or activity is an important element in controlling blood glucose, lowering lipid levels, and maintaining appropriate body weight. Aerobic exercise is necessary to maintain a healthy cardiovascular system and improve glucose control. To prevent obesity in children, emphasis should be placed on being physically active at least 30 minutes to 1 hour each day. However, exercising when ketones are present (i.e., when the blood glucose level is above 240 mg/dL) or when the blood glucose is 400 mg/dL or higher without ketones is not recommended.

To prevent hypoglycemia during activity, food intake may need to be increased or the dose of insulin decreased. Generally, children choose to increase food intake unless the activity occurs routinely, then the insulin can be adjusted accordingly. If the youth's overall activity increases and the youth is experiencing an increased number of hypoglycemic events, the diabetes team should be consulted for insulin adjustment. Older children and adolescents can be instructed on how to reduce their own insulin dose when participating in sports. Exercise should be avoided when insulin is peaking. However, if an unplanned activity occurs right after taking insulin, a larger snack, which includes carb as well as protein, may be needed.

Some children may find it difficult to eat a large volume of food prior to prolonged activity and will plan ahead to reduce their insulin dose. The amount of insulin reduction depends on the results of blood glucose checks done before and after the activity. Food adjustments will depend on the duration and intensity of the exercise and on the blood glucose level prior to the activity. A general rule is to add 10–15 g of carbohydrate for every 30 minutes of activity. Prolonged activity may utilize a majority of the glucose stores in the muscle. The body replaces these stores when blood glucose becomes available. An adequate snack, probably containing protein and carb, may be needed after prolonged exercise to avoid drops in blood glucose level, which may occur after the activity has stopped.

Hypoglycemia

The most common emergency in T1D is hypoglycemia. Hypoglycemia is defined for a child treated with insulin as a blood glucose level below 60 mg/dL, although some youth have symptoms at a higher number. Symptoms may occur when blood glucose levels are dropping rapidly, even when the level is still in the normal range. Youth with diabetes should be instructed to wear medical alert identification at all times to ensure proper treatment of hypoglycemic reactions because the child may be unable to communicate.

Treatment of mild hypoglycemia involves the 15–15 rule: Treat the low blood glucose level with 15 grams of fast-acting carbohydrate, wait 15 minutes, and then recheck. One gram of carbohydrate will bring the average adult's blood glucose up ~3 mg/dL; younger children tend to be more sensitive, as 1 gram could bring their blood glucose up 3–5 mg/dL. Because younger children are more sensitive to the fast-acting carbs, it is very easy to overtreat. Families are encouraged whenever possible to check the child's blood glucose before treating so they can determine how much to treat.

Illness

Illness in the child with diabetes always presents a challenge. Insulin must always be given and may need to be increased during periods of illness. Blood glucose should be monitored every 3 to 4 hours during illness. Parents need to know when to call the doctor for assistance in managing illness, because certain symptoms, such as prolonged vomiting and fever, can lead to rapid dehydration and diabetic ketoacidosis. During a brief illness, the child's normal eating pattern should be maintained, using foods that can be tolerated. Liquids also help to prevent dehydration, so the youth should have 6–8 ounces of fluids every 1 to 2 hours. If the child cannot tolerate food, it is important to replace some of the carb normally consumed with sugar-containing liquids that the body can easily use for energy. Some examples of easily tolerated liquids that contain 15 g of carbohydrate include 8 oz of a regular carbonated beverage (with sugar), 4 oz of fruit juice, a frozen fruit bar, or ½ cup of regular flavored gelatin. Room temperature liquids should be sipped at a rate of about 15 g of carbohydrate per hour.

Case Study

Nutrition Assessment of Child with Type 1 Diabetes

Patient history: JH, an 11-year-old male, visited his pediatrician for a sick visit. The family had just returned from a 5-day vacation at Disney World, and the parents noticed while on the trip that JH was going to the bathroom often and had nocturnal enuresis the last 2 nights in Florida. They also reported that he had not been eating very well, had been drinking a lot of water, and had no energy. In the pediatrician's office, it was noted that he had lost 5 pounds since his last well visit 4 months ago. His urine analysis was positive for glucose and negative for ketones. The pediatrician checked his blood glucose, which was >500 mg/dL, and referred the family to the local diabetes outpatient clinic on Friday afternoon before a 3-day holiday weekend for education. Additional lab work was done, and it was determined that JH was not in diabetic ketoacidosis (DKA) and that it was not necessary to admit him to a hospital.

Family history: No family history for diabetes, autoimmune diseases, hyperlipidemia, hypertension, cardiac disease, or renal disease. Mom's family has history of breast cancer.

Nutrition history: JH has no food allergies or intolerances. He typically eats breakfast at home, brings his lunch to school, and eats his afternoon snack and dinner at home. JH and his parents provided a typical day dietary recall and daily schedule.

- *Breakfast, 7–7:30 am on weekdays:* 1½ cups cold cereal (Fruit Loops, Multigrain Cheerios), ½ cup 1% milk, and lately 6–8 oz orange juice
- *Weekends, 8–8:30 am:* Bagel (large), scrambled egg, and milk (6–8 oz)
- *Morning snack at school, 11 am:* Kellogg's blueberry bar
- *Lunch, 12 pm:* Usually brings raisin bagel, grape juice pouch, raisins or a piece of fresh fruit (does not like school milk)

- *School lunch:* Usually once a week, Domino's pizza (one slice), juice box
- *Afternoon snack, 3 pm:* Apple or grilled cheese sandwich or frozen pizza, water or milk to drink
- *Dinner, 5:30–6:30 pm:* ~3 oz chicken, ¼–½ cup green beans, ~3/4–1 cup rice, pasta, or mashed potato. Mom tries to have 1–2 nights a week vegetarian, which is usually pasta ~1¼ cup with cheese, milk, or water, ½–¾ cup of chopped fruit or ice cream
- *Evening snack:* Usually none

Anthropometrics

Weight: 30.2 kg
Height: 143.4 cm
BMI: 14.66
BMI goal: 17.01
Other labs: A1C 10.8, Cholesterol 133, HDL 34, LDL 39, Trig 501

Insulin Plan

Basal insulin: 7 units at 9 am
Insulin-to-carbohydrate ratio (I:Carb): 1:30
Sensitivity factor (SF): 100
Target blood glucose: 150 mg/dL

Nutrition Diagnosis/Problem

1. Weight loss
2. Food and nutrition-related knowledge deficit related to new diagnosis of T1D

Nutrition Intervention

1. Comprehensive nutrition education:
   a. Review advance carbohydrate counting.
   b. Review label reading.
   c. Show how to weigh and measure food.
   d. Introduce calculating insulin doses using insulin-to-carbohydrate ratio.
2. Provide basic meal plan for weekend for family to use as a guide until they return at their next nutrition visit.
3. Reinforce education at following visit and build on the survival skills.
4. Goals of nutrition therapy:
   a. Impart advanced carb count skills.
   b. Gain back lost weight and continue to grow along growth parameters.
   c. Maintain blood glucose between 80–180 mg/dL.
   d. Reinforce healthy eating.

Questions for the Reader

1. What percentile on a growth chart are JH's weight, height, and BMI?
2. What are JH's estimated energy needs per day?
3. Write one PES statement.
4. What survival skills does the family have to learn to get them through the first weekend of diabetes?
5. Does JH need any further vitamin or mineral supplementation?

REFERENCES

1. Lockwood D, Frey ML, Gladish NA, Hiss RG. The biggest problem in diabetes. *Diabetes Educ.* 1986;12(1):30–33.
2. Franz MJ, Horton ES Sr, Bantle JP, et al. Nutrition principles for the management of diabetes and related complications. *Diabetes Care.* 1994;17(5):490–518.
3. Butler DA, Lawlor MT. It takes a village: helping families live with diabetes. *Diabetes Spectrum.* 2004;17(1):26–31.
4. Dietary Guidelines Advisory Committee. Dietary guidelines for Americans 2005. 2005. Available at: http://www.health.gov/dietaryguidelines/dga2005/document/default.htm. Accessed August 12, 2010.
5. Bantle JP, Wylie-Rosett J, Albright AL, et al. Nutrition recommendations and interventions for diabetes: a position statement of the American Diabetes Association. *Diabetes Care.* 2008;31(Suppl 1):S61–S78.
6. Institute of Medicine of the National Academies. *Dietary Reference Intakes: The Essential Guide to Nutrient Requirements.* Washington, DC: National Academies Press; 2006.
7. Sheard NF, Clark NG, Brand-Miller JC, et al. Dietary carbohydrate (amount and type) in the prevention and management of diabetes: a statement by the American Diabetes Association. *Diabetes Care.* 2004;27(9):2266–2271.
8. Jenkins DJ, Wolever TM, Taylor RH, et al. Glycemic index of foods: a physiological basis for carbohydrate exchange. *Am J Clin Nutr.* 1981;34(3):362–366.
9. Gillespie S. Implementing liberalized carbohydrate guidelines: nutrition free-for-all or a more rational approach to carbohydrate consumption? *Diabetes Spectrum.* 1996;9:165–167.
10. Position of the American Dietetic Association: use of nutritive and nonnutritive sweeteners. *J Am Diet Assoc.* 2004;104(2):255–275.
11. Payne ML, Craig WJ, Williams AC. Sorbitol is a possible risk factor for diarrhea in young children. *J Am Diet Assoc.* 1997;97(5):532–534.
12. Chatsudthipong V, Muanprasat C. Stevioside and related compounds: therapeutic benefits beyond sweetness. *Pharmacol Ther.* 2009;121(1):41–54.
13. Marlett JA, McBurney MI, Slavin JL. Position of the American Dietetic Association: health implications of dietary fiber. *J Am Diet Assoc.* 2002;102(7):993–1000.

14. American Diabetes Association. Standards of medical care in diabetes—2010. *Diabetes Care.* 2010;33(Suppl 1):S11-S61.
15. American Diabetes Association. Management of dyslipidemia in children and adolescents with diabetes. *Diabetes Care.* 2003;26(7):2194–2197.
16. Wagner, CL, Greer FR. Prevention of rickets and vitamin D deficiency in infants, children, and adolescents. *Pediatrics.* 2008;122(5);1142–1152.
17. National High Blood Pressure Education Program Working Group on High Blood Pressure in Children and Adolescents. The fourth report on the diagnosis, evaluation, and treatment of high blood pressure in children and adolescents. *Pediatrics.* 2004;114(Suppl 2):555–576.
18. Nakamura T, Higashi A, Nishiyama S, et al. Kinetics of zinc status in children with IDDM. *Diabetes Care.* 1991;14(7):553–557.
19. Mayer-Davis EJ, Nichols M, Liese AD, et al. Dietary intake among youth with diabetes: the SEARCH for Diabetes in Youth Study. *J Am Diet Assoc.* 2006;106(5):689–697.
20. Madison LL, Lochner A, Wulff J. Ethanol-induced hypoglycemia. II. Mechanism of suppression of hepatic gluconeogenesis. *Diabetes.* 1967;16(4):252–258.
21. American Diabetes Association. Nutrition principles and recommendations in diabetes. *Diabetes Care.* 2004;27(Suppl 1):S36–S46.
22. Arky RA. Current principles of dietary therapy of diabetes mellitus. *Med Clin North Am.* 1978;62(4):655–662.
23. Grinvalsky M, Nathan DM. Diets for insulin pump and multiple daily injection therapy. *Diabetes Care.* 1983;6(3):241–244.
24. Tamborlane WV, Sherwin RS, Genel M, Felig P. Outpatient treatment of juvenile-onset diabetes with a preprogrammed portable subcutaneous insulin infusion system. *Am J Med.* 1980;68(2):190–196.
25. Tamborlane WV, Sherwin RS, Koivisto V, et al. Normalization of the growth hormone and catecholamine response to exercise in juvenile-onset diabetic subjects treated with a portable insulin infusion pump. *Diabetes.* 1979;28(8):785–788.
26. Steindel BS, Roe TR, Costin G, et al. Continuous subcutaneous insulin infusion (CSII) in children and adolescents with chronic poorly controlled type 1 diabetes mellitus. *Diabetes Res Clin Pract.* 1995;27(3):199–204.
27. Anderson BJ. Diabetes and adaptations in family systems. In: Holmes C (ed). *Neuropsychology and Behavioral Aspects of Diabetes.* New York: Springer-Verlag; 1990:85–101.
28. Silverstein J, Klingensmith G, Copeland K, et al. Care of children and adolescents with type 1 diabetes: a statement of the American Diabetes Association. *Diabetes Care.* 2005;28(1):186–212.
29. Colton P, Rodin G, Berenstal R, Parkin C. Eating disorders and diabetes: introduction and overview. *Diabetes Spectrum.* 2009; 22(3):138–142.
30. Criego A, Crow S, Goebel-Fabbri AE, et al. Eating disorders and diabetes: screening and detection. *Diabetes Spectrum.* 2009;22(3):143–146.
31. Dabelea D, Bell RA, D'Agostino RB Jr, et al. Incidence of diabetes in youth in the United States. *JAMA.* 2007;297(24):2716–2724.
32. American Diabetes Association. The prevention or delay of type 2 diabetes. *Diabetes Care.* 2002;25(4):742–749.
33. American Diabetes Association. Gestational diabetes mellitus. *Diabetes Care.* 2004;27(Suppl 1):S88–S90.
34. Laffel LMB, Butler DA, Higgins LA, et al. (eds). *Joslin's Guide to Managing Childhood Diabetes: A Family Teamwork Approach.* Boston: Joslin Diabetes Center; 2009.
35. Lawlor MT, Anderson B, Laffel L. *Blood Sugar Monitoring Owner's Manual Booklet.* Boston: Joslin Diabetes Center; 2007.

CHAPTER 16

HIV and AIDS

Jill Rockwell

Human immunodeficiency virus (HIV) is a sexually transmitted and blood-borne disease. Modes of transmission include exposure to blood and body fluids through sexual contact, breastfeeding, sharing of contaminated needles, or transmission from mother to child during the perinatal period or during labor and delivery. The greatest impact of the acquired immune deficiency syndrome (AIDS) epidemic is among men who have sex with men (MSM); racial and ethnic minorities, with a growing number of infected minority women; and cases attributed to heterosexual transmission.[1] Nearly all transfusion-associated cases occurred prior to screening of the blood supply in 1985.[1]

The prognosis of children with HIV and AIDS has improved tremendously in much of the developed world. Once a fatal disease, HIV can now be described as a chronic, manageable disease. Where treatment is available and affordable, most children are maintaining healthy states and thriving.

The medical, nutritional, and social implications of pediatric HIV and AIDS are numerous and complex. Effective management of the disease requires a coordinated and comprehensive approach that involves early diagnosis and aggressive medical, nutritional, and psychosocial intervention. This chapter gives a brief overview of pediatric HIV infection and AIDS and an in-depth description of the goals and strategies of nutritional management of the pediatric patient with HIV infection and AIDS.

HIV is a retrovirus that primarily infects cells of the immune system, a system composed of lymphocytes and other white blood cells. The lymphocytes are divided into two types:

- T-cells are responsible for cellular immunity, or fighting off invading antigens.
- B-cells are responsible for humoral immunity, or antibody (immunoglobulin) production.

T-cells express different antigens; HIV targets T-cells expressing the CD4 antigen (referred to as CD4 cells). HIV integrates itself into the host CD4 cell's DNA and then replicates itself, creating additional viruses that ultimately cause the immune cell's destruction and death, which leads to a weakened immune system because there are not enough immune cells to fight infections.[2]

AIDS is an advanced disease caused by acquisition of HIV-1 or HIV-2 and subsequent destruction of the immune system. This decrease in cellular immunity impairs the host's ability to fight off infection and results in the host acquiring opportunistic infections and malignancies. Untreated HIV infection allows for the continued destruction of CD4 cells, resulting in a progression of HIV disease. When the immune system deteriorates to specified and measurable levels, the disease is termed AIDS.

Individuals with HIV disease range from healthy to seriously ill. The term *AIDS* is employed by the Centers for Disease Control and Prevention (CDC) to refer to those individuals who typically display specific "indicator" diseases as a result of HIV infection.[3]

As shown in **Table 16-1**, the current CDC definition criteria for children younger than 13 years of age are based on clinical disease conditions/diagnoses and laboratory criteria. Only those children who meet the strict diagnostic criteria are classified as having AIDS. The classification categories include a letter designation (i.e., N, A, B, C) indicative of the presence of clinical conditions and a number designation indicative of immune status, which is based on CD4 T-cell counts and the CD4 percentage of total lymphocytes. The immune categories (see **Table 16-2**) are further delineated by age groups because CD4 T-cell norms differ according to age, usually being higher in younger children at baseline.[3]

As the immune system declines, the likelihood of symptomatic HIV infection increases. The AIDS diagnosis is reserved for those patients in category C: severely symptomatic. An undiagnosed infant may present to the medical system with *Pneumocystis carinii* pneumonia (PCP), an AIDS-defining illness. With the advent of medical therapies, that same child may have immune reconstitution (recovery of the CD4 T-cell number and percentage), which places the child in category A

TABLE 16-1 Clinical Manifestations/Categories for Children with HIV Infection and AIDS

Category N: Not Symptomatic

Children who have no signs or symptoms considered to be the result of HIV infection or who have only one of the conditions listed in Category A.

Category A: Mildly Symptomatic

Children with two or more of the conditions listed below but none of the conditions listed in Categories B and C.

- Lymphadenopathy (≥ 0.5 cm at more than two sites; bilateral = one site)
- Hepatomegaly
- Splenomegaly
- Dermatitis
- Parotitis
- Recurrent or persistent upper respiratory infection, sinusitis, or otitis media

Category B: Moderately Symptomatic

Children who have symptomatic conditions other than those listed for Category A or C that are attributed to HIV infection. Examples of conditions in clinical Category B include but are not limited to:

- Anemia (< 8 g/dL), neutropenia (< 1000/mm^3), or thrombocytopenia (< 100,000/mm^3) persisting ≥ 30 days
- Bacterial meningitis, pneumonia, or sepsis (single episode)
- Candidiasis, oropharyngeal (thrush), persisting > 2 months in children over 6 months of age
- Cardiomyopathy
- Cytomegalovirus infection, with onset before 1 month of age
- Diarrhea, recurrent or chronic
- Hepatitis
- Herpes simplex virus (HSV) stomatitis, recurrent (more than two episodes within 1 year)
- HSV bronchitis, pneumonitis, or esophagitis with onset before 1 month of age
- Herpes zoster (shingles) involving at least two distinct episodes or more than one dermatome
- Leiomyosarcoma
- Lymphoid interstitial pneumonia (LIP) or pulmonary lymphoid hyperplasia complex
- Nephropathy
- Nocardiosis
- Persistent fever (lasting > 1 month)
- Toxoplasmosis, onset before 1 month of age
- Varicella, disseminated (complicated chickenpox)

Category C: Severely Symptomatic

Children who have any condition listed in the 1987 surveillance case definition for acquired immune deficiency syndrome, with the exception of LIP.

Source: Data from Centers for Disease Control and Prevention. Revised classification system for human immunodeficiency virus infection in children less than 13 years of age. *MMWR.* 1994;43(RR-12):1–10.

TABLE 16-2 Immunologic Categories Based on Age-Specific CD41 T-Cell Counts and Percentage of Total Lymphocytes

Immunologic Category	< 12 Months μL (%)	1–5 Years μL (%)	6–12 Years μL(%)
1: No evidence of suppression	≥ 1500 (≥ 25)	≥ 1000 (≥ 25)	≥ 500 (≥ 25)
2: Evidence of moderate suppression	750–1499 (15–24)	500–999 (15–24)	200–499 (15–24)
3: Severe suppression	< 750 (<15)	< 500 (< 15)	< 200 (< 15)

Source: Data from Centers for Disease Control and Prevention. Revised classification system for human immunodeficiency virus infection in children less than 13 years of age. *MMWR.* 1994;43(RR-12):1–10.

(no immune suppression), and remain quite healthy. The clinical category provides a snapshot for categorizing the historical "sickest" that the child has been. The immune category is a reflection of the child's current immune status.

Diagnosis

Ideally, pregnant women are screened for HIV infection as part of routine prenatal care. This screening provides for antenatal, peripartal, and neonatal HIV treatment that significantly decreases the rate of perinatal transmission to infants (approximately 1–4% versus 15–30% transmission without treatment).[4]

Infants are screened and diagnosed with laboratory testing that can usually confirm or exclude infection by 6 months of age. The DNA and RNA polymerase chain reaction (PCR) tests are used to determine an infant's HIV infection status. Children older than 18 months can be tested using the enzyme-linked immunosorbent assay (ELISA) and Western Immunoblotting (Western Blot) methods that screen for the presence of antibodies to HIV. This is the same test utilized for adult HIV testing. The ELISA and Western Blot cannot be used on children younger than 18 months because they give false positive readings by detecting maternal antibody that is passed to the infant in utero.[5] The index of suspicion should be high when the mother's HIV status is unknown. Infants born to high-risk mothers or with symptoms as described in the clinical categories for children with HIV should be tested for HIV infection.

Clinical Features and Treatment

Children with HIV infection display a wide array of clinical features. Some untreated children have rapid disease progression, whereas others appear quite healthy and present after many years of immune decline. Presenting symptoms include lymphadenopathy, hepatosplenomegaly, failure to thrive, diarrhea, and multiple bacterial infections. As the clinical course progresses, the child may have severe cases of common childhood infections such as varicella (chicken pox), herpes simplex, and cytomegalovirus. With profound immunosuppression, severe infections such as disseminated mycobacterium avium complex (MAC/MAI), cryptococcal meningitis, and esophageal candidiasis may occur. Many of these infections and/or conditions are found in the description of the clinical categories, as described in Table 16-1.[3,5]

In untreated children or children with advanced HIV disease or AIDS, conditions such as oral or esophageal candidiasis, diarrhea, severe bacterial infections, MAI, tuberculosis (both pulmonary and extrapulmonary), and encephalopathy can severely affect enteral intake and/or absorption of nutrients. Failure to thrive is a common issue in the untreated child, compounding the disease's effects on the immune system.[3,5]

HIV treatment also can negatively impact the child's nutritional intake. Frequent doctor visits, blood draws, tests, and hospitalizations may result in emotional upset and decreased appetite. Medication regimens used to treat HIV infection and prophylactic medications used to prevent opportunistic infections may consist of several pills taken two to three times per day and may have gastrointestinal side effects such as nausea, vomiting, indigestion, and diarrhea. Some of the more severe medication side effects that can severely compromise intake include anemia, pancreatitis, and liver steatosis.[5]

Highly active antiretroviral therapy (HAART) is the hallmark of current treatment for HIV infection. HAART consists minimally of a three-drug regimen utilizing drugs from two different HIV drug classes. Antiretroviral drug classes include six major categories, with the following five used in pediatrics:[5]

- Nucleoside/nucleotide analogue reverse transcriptase inhibitors (NRTIs/NtRTIs)
- Non-nucleoside analogue reverse transcriptase inhibitors (NNRTIs)
- Protease inhibitors (PIs)
- Entry inhibitors
- Integrase inhibitors

These drugs work on specific areas of the cell targeted by HIV and must be taken consistently and in combination to be effective. Efficacy of drug therapies is measured by clinical assessment, rebound, and/or maintenance of the CD4+ lymphocyte counts and on the amount of HIV virus in the blood, commonly referred to as *viral load*. Effective medication therapy decreases the patient's viral load, allowing the CD4 cell counts to increase and be maintained. Common drug combinations include a protease inhibitor and two drugs from the NRTI class, NNRTI and two drugs from the NRTI class, or three NRTI drugs.[5] All of the drugs have significant side effects (see **Table 16-3**). Many are available in liquid and tablet/capsule formulation. The fusion inhibitors are injectable only. Rarely, patients may be on suboptimal therapy, such as one or two drugs from the same class. This can be seen with patients with medication-related side effects or with poor adherence while medical, behavioral, psychiatric, and/or psychosocial interventions can be instituted. Monotherapy (the use of one drug) is utilized with neonates. Zidovudine (AZT/ZDV) is administered to a mother during labor and delivery and then to the neonate for 6 weeks to decrease the risk of perinatal transmission.

In addition to HAART, the pediatric patient may be taking medications regularly for prophylaxis or prevention of opportunistic infections. Many of the drugs used to treat HIV and prevent opportunistic infection have significant side effects and interactions. Foods, herbal treatments, and home remedies can significantly affect drug levels, leading

TABLE 16-3 Antiretrovirals and Common Side Effects (Nutritional Implications)

Class	Drug/Formulation	Side Effects
NRTI/NtRTI	Zidovudine (ZVD/AZT) capsule/liquid/tablets	Anemia, granulocytopenia, malaise, headache, nausea, vomiting, anorexia, myopathy, myositis, fat redistribution, lactic acidosis, liver toxicity
	Didanosine (ddI) capsule/liquid	Diarrhea, abdominal pain, nausea, vomiting, peripheral neuropathy, electrolyte abnormalities, hyperuricemia
	Lamivudine (3TC) tablet/liquid	Headache, fatigue, nausea, decreased appetite, diarrhea, skin rash, abdominal pain, pancreatitis, peripheral neuropathy, anemia, fat redistribution, lactic acidosis, hepatic steatosis
	Stavudine (d4T) capsule/liquid	Headache, GI disturbances, skin rashes, pancreatitis, peripheral neuropathy, lipodystrophy/lipoatrophy, lactic acidosis, hepatic steatosis
	Abacavir (ABC) tablet/liquid	Potentially lethal hypersensitivity reaction, nausea, vomiting, diarrhea, fever, rash, anorexia, headache
	Emtricitabine (FTC) capsule	Headache, insomnia, diarrhea, nausea, rash, skin discoloration, neutropenia, lactic acidosis, hepatic steatosis
	Tenofovir (TDF) tablet	Nausea, diarrhea, vomiting, flatulence, lactic acidosis, hepatic steatosis
NNRTI	Nevirapine (NVP) tablet/liquid	Skin rash, fever, nausea, headache, abnormal transaminase levels, hepatotoxicity
	Efavirenz (EFV) capsule/tablet	Skin rash, increased transaminase levels, central nervous system effects
	Etravirine (ETR) tablets	Nausea, rash, hypersensitivity reaction
PI	Nelfinavir (NFV) tablet/liquid	Diarrhea, asthenia, abdominal pain, rash, lipid abnormalities, fat redistribution
	Ritonavir (RTV) capsule/liquid	Nausea, vomiting, diarrhea, headache, abdominal pain, anorexia, circumoral paresthesias, lipid abnormalities, fat redistribution
	Lopinavir/ritonavir (LPV/RTV) tablet/liquid	Diarrhea, headache, asthenia, nausea, vomiting, rash, fat redistribution, lipid abnormalities
	Indinavir (IDV) capsule	Nausea, abdominal pain, headache, metallic taste, dizziness, hyperbilirubinemia, pruritis, rash, nephrolithiasis, fat redistribution
	Saquinavir (SQV) capsule/tablet	Diarrhea, abdominal discomfort, headache, nausea, paresthesias, skin rash, fat redistribution, lipid abnormalities
	Atazanavir (ATV) capsule	Elevation of indirect bili, jaundice, headache, fever, arthralgia, depression, insomnia, dizziness, nausea, vomiting, diarrhea, paresthesias, prolongation of PR interval (EKG changes)
	Fosamprenavir (f-APV) tablet/liquid	Vomiting, nausea, diarrhea, headache, perioral parasthesias, rash, lipid abnormalities, fat redistribution, neutropenia
	Darunavir (DRV) tablets	Diarrhea, nausea, vomiting, abdominal pain, headache, fatigue, skin rash, lipid abnormalities
	Tipranavir (TPV) capsule, liquid	Diarrhea, nausea, fatigue, headache, rash, vomiting, lipid abnormalities, fat redistribution
Entry inhibitor	Maraviroc (MVC) tablet	Cough, fever, upper respiratory tract infections, rash, musculoskeletal symptoms, abdominal pain, dizziness
Fusion inhibitor	Enfuvirtide (T-20) injection	Local injection site reactions
Integrase inhibitor	Raltegravir (RGV) tablet	Nausea, headache, dizziness, diarrhea, fatigue, itching, abdominal pain, vomiting

Use of antiretrovirals in pediatric patients is evolving rapidly. These guidelines are updated regularly to provide current information. The most recent information is available at http://aidsinfo.nih.gov.

Source: Adapted from Working Group on Antiretroviral Therapy and Medical Management of HIV-Infected Children. Guidelines for the use of antiretroviral agents in pediatric HIV infection. February 23, 2009; 1–139. Available at: http://aidsinfo.nih.gov/ContentFiles/PediatricGuidelines.pdf. Accessed February 21, 2010.

to suboptimal drug levels or severe side effects. A thorough assessment of nutritional adjuncts is essential to optimize medical therapy.

Growth and Nutritional Concerns

The growth and cellular immune function of HIV-infected children is impacted by their nutritional state. The majority of children infected with HIV will experience nutritional deficits during the course of their illness.[6] Pre-HAART nutritional issues affecting growth deficits and malnutrition include impaired absorption,[7] decreased dietary intake,[8] increased nutrient requirements, and the disease itself (see **Table 16-4**). Malnutrition has a deleterious effect on immune function, compromising the ability to produce effective antibodies; thus, it increases risks of life-threatening infections.[9]

In the current era of HIV and HAART, children in developed countries are living longer with fewer opportunistic infections. When seen, malnutrition is more likely associated with drug-resistant virus, noncompliance with therapy, and/or end-stage viral disease. Nutritional issues have become further complicated by potent drug therapies and possibly by the consequences of living longer with the disease itself. Some of the clinical and metabolic complications seen in adult HIV populations are now being seen in children. These include body fat redistribution, altered serum lipid levels, insulin resistance, and decreased bone mineral density.

The growth patterns in HIV-infected children are quite variable, reflecting a broad spectrum of clinical course and disease activity. Growth can be an important prognostic indicator for children with HIV.[10–12] In particular, height velocity is an independent predictor of survival when controlling for age, viral load, and CD4+ count.[12] The presence of wasting syndrome classifies a child in clinical category C of the CDC criteria discussed earlier, which indicates that a child is severely symptomatic.[5] Growth failure can occur early in life and continue over time. Insulin-like growth factor-1 (IGF-1) levels have been found to be low in children with HIV who have impaired growth. Effective antiretroviral therapy, leading to an increase in the percentage of lymphocytes that are CD4 cells (CD4%), appears to have an association with an improvement in IGF-1 levels.

TABLE 16-4 Causes of Malnutrition

Causes	Etiology
Decreased intake	Nausea, anorexia, oral ulceration, esophagitis, chewing difficulties, pain, dementia, depression
Increased losses	Lactose intolerance, pancreatic insufficiency, malabsorption
Increased requirements	Fever, opportunistic infections, metabolic abnormalities
Psychosocial barriers	Inadequate access to food, unsafe food practices, caretaker substance abuse

Lipodystrophy syndrome in HIV-positive adults is characterized by several changes in body composition. Classifications of lipodystrophy include the following:

- Lipoatrophy, or arm, leg, buttock, and/or facial wasting
- Lipohypertrophy, or truncal obesity
- Mixed lipodystrophy, including a combination of peripheral wasting and truncal obesity

In addition, affected individuals may exhibit metabolic complications, including hypercholesterolemia, hyperlipidemia, and/or insulin resistance. Many, but not all, of these features have recently been described in children using various methods of diagnosis including, DXA (dual energy X-ray absorptiometry), magnetic resonance imaging (MRI), and clinical assessment.[13–18] This may be due to drug therapies, particularly those containing protease inhibitors. Development of symptoms may be related to duration of HAART therapy and increasing doses of medications.[13,14] Chemical abnormalities, including high cholesterol and triglycerides, can occur in children with or without clinical features of lipodystrophy.[17] Thus serial anthropometry, clinical assessment, and laboratory values can provide valuable information about a child tending toward lipodystrophy.

HIV-infected adults have increased rates of osteoporosis and osteopenia that may also be a side effect of HAART therapy. Lower bone mineral densities have also been found in HIV-positive children.[19–21] Thus, dietary prevention of osteopenia and osteoporosis should be a treatment goal.

Caloric requirements of HIV-infected children are not completely known. Weight loss in HIV-positive children can be linked to inadequate intake, increased requirements imposed by opportunistic infections, or malabsorptive losses.[22] Caloric requirements should be calculated according to additional needs subsequent to stress, fever, increased respiratory needs, and careful monitoring of serial growth measures.

The most appropriate nutrition plan for HIV-infected children is one tailored to their clinical manifestations, growth, dietary history, gastrointestinal function, and social situation (see **Table 16-5**). The child's caretakers should receive ongoing education to optimize growth, ensure access to food, promote safe food handling, and accommodate any necessary dietary modifications. Because of the risk of micronutrient deficiency in the HIV-infected child, a complete multivitamin/mineral supplement should be considered that provides one to two times the dietary reference intakes (DRIs).[23,24]

If an HIV-infected child is exhibiting slow growth, a high-calorie, high-protein, nutrient-dense diet is indicated early on. If enhancement of the typical diet is not sufficient to promote desired growth, oral nutritional supplementation,

TABLE 16-5 Nutritional Evaluation and Management of the HIV-Infected Child

Nutritional Assessment

Dietary intake and nutrient analysis

- 24-hour diet recall or 3-day food diary
- Access to food
- Stability of home environment/caretakers

Anthropometry and body composition measurements

- Four-site skinfolds (if possible)
- Serial height (length), weight, and head circumference (until 36 months)
    - Z-scores (particularly with measurements < 3rd percentile)
    - BMI and BMI percentage

Biochemical evaluation

- Albumin, lipid profile (fasting, if possible), fasting glucose/insulin, iron, other vitamin/mineral levels as indicated by degree of malnutrition and malabsorption

Drug–nutrient interactions

- Amprenavir: Avoid excess vitamin E supplementation because it contains ~100 IU/pill.

Nutritional Intervention

Diet modifications and education (based on growth, gastrointestinal function, and lipid abnormalities)

- Nutrient-dense with supplements as needed to optimize growth
- Lactose-free (if evidence of diarrhea/malabsorption)
- High fiber or low fiber
- Heart healthy, balanced with adequate calories for growth

Food safety assessment and counseling

Vitamin and mineral supplementation

- Multivitamin: 1 to 2 times RDA/DRI depending on diet
- Calcium and vitamin D supplement to achieve at least DRI

Tube feedings/total parenteral nutrition (when enteral diet alone fails)

including shakes, puddings and commercial formulas, should be considered. When oral measures alone cannot meet the nutritional goals, enteral tube supplementation should be administered. Gastrostomy (g) tubes are beneficial in providing both complete and supplemental feedings as well as medication administration. Children with anorexia, neurological impairment, swallowing difficulty, or those taking a significant number of pills may benefit from a g-tube.

Nocturnal tube feedings are often preferred to daytime feedings because they can allow the child to eat normally during the day without interrupting daily activities. Formula selection should be determined based on the child's need for any modification from a polymeric formula. This may include fiber-containing, lactose-free, or more elemental formulas for the patient with enteropathy. Improvements in weight gain (primarily as increased fat mass) in response to the increased caloric provisions can occur and suggest improvements in morbidity and mortality.[25]

Parenteral nutrition (PN), despite its associated infection risks, may be warranted if hydration, electrolyte balance, or weight gain cannot be achieved through the enteral route. Candidates for PN include children with intractable diarrhea with accompanying weight loss or severe recurrent or chronic pancreatic or biliary tract dysfunction.[4,25] For children experiencing oroesophageal ulcers, soreness, or inflammation, care should be given to selecting foods that are soft and nutrient dense, and not highly spiced or acidic. Drug side effects (see Table 16-3) may lead to anorexia, nausea/vomiting, epigastric distress, diarrhea, and/or glossitis affecting the child's intake. Appetite stimulants such as megestrol acetate (Megace) increase oral intake in some anorectic children.

Dysphagia, developmental delay, and poor gross motor control secondary to neurologic complications associated with HIV may also contribute to poor intake. Neurologically impaired children should be closely monitored to ensure adequate intake and to prevent aspiration.

Case Study

Nutrition Assessment of HIV-Positive Adolescent

Patient history: The patient is a 15-year-old female recently diagnosed with HIV and started on HAART therapy. She has no past medical history.

Food/nutrition-related history: The patient had a good appetite and intake until HAART therapy was started. She has been experiencing nausea and anorexia since starting on HAART therapy and estimates that she has lost 10 pounds over the past 3 weeks. Her usual weight is 105 pounds. She consumed three meals and one or two snacks per day prior to starting HAART therapy. She reports she has been unable to eat breakfast in the morning due to nausea and often does not eat lunch at school. Her symptoms usually improve in the afternoon, and she is able to eat dinner with her family. She is not currently taking any vitamin, mineral, or herbal supplements.

Anthropometric Measurements

Weight: 43 kg (10th percentile)
Height: 162 cm (50th percentile)
BMI: 16.4 kg/m^2 (5th percentile)
Medications: Efavirenz, lamivudine, zidovudine
Labs: CD4 250 cells/mm^3
Diet order: High calorie, high protein

Nutrition Diagnoses

Based on the information provided, the following nutritional diagnosis is made: inadequate oral food/beverage intake.

Intervention Goals

Goals are to promote weight gain to restore the patient's normal body weight of 105 pounds and to improve oral intake to a minimum of three meals and two snacks per day.

Nutrition Interventions

Initial/brief nutrition education:

- Counsel to consume three meals and two snacks daily.
- Review sources of nutrient-dense foods.
- Review nutrition interventions for nausea.

Vitamin/mineral supplement: Start multivitamin to meet one to two times RDA/DRI for age.

Medical food supplements: Start one to two cans adult oral supplement to promote weight gain.

Monitoring and Evaluation

Weight change: Monitor for improvement back to usual weight of 105 pounds.

Meal/snack pattern: Goal of minimum three meals and two snacks per day.

Questions for the Reader

1. What are the patient's estimated energy needs?
2. What are the patient's estimated protein needs?
3. Write at least one PES statement.
4. What will you do during the follow-up visit 2 months later:
   a. If the patient has not gained weight since her last visit?
   b. If the patient develops diarrhea?

REFERENCES

1. Centers for Disease Control and Prevention. HIV/AIDS—United States, 1981–2000. *MMWR.* 2001;50:430–433.
2. Weiss RA. Gulliver's travels in HIV land. *Nature.* 2001;410:963–967.
3. Centers for Disease Control and Prevention. Revised classification system for human immunodeficiency virus infection in children less than 13 years of age. *MMWR.* 1994;43(RR-12):1–10.
4. Centers for Disease Control and Prevention. U.S. Public Health Service task force recommendations for use of antiretroviral drugs in pregnant HIV-1 infected women for maternal health and interventions to reduce perinatal HIV-1 transmission in the United States. *MMWR.* 2002;51:1–38.
5. Working Group on Antiretroviral Therapy and Medical Management of HIV-Infected Children. Guidelines for the use of antiretroviral agents in pediatric HIV infection. February 23, 2009; 1–139. Available at: http://aidsinfo.nih.gov/ContentFiles/PediatricGuidelines.pdf. Accessed February 21, 2010.
6. Miller TL. Nutritional aspects of pediatric HIV infection. In: Walker WA, Watkins JB (eds). *Nutrition in Pediatrics,* 2nd ed. Hamilton, Ontario, Canada: B. Dekker; 1996:534–550.
7. Miller TL, Orav EJ, Martin SR, et al. Malnutrition and carbohydrate malabsorption in children with vertically transmitted human immunodeficiency virus 1 infection. *Gastroenterology.* 1991;100:1296–1302.
8. Arpadi SM. Growth failure in children with HIV infection. *J Acquir Immune Defic Syndr.* 2000;25(Suppl 1):S37–S42.
9. Chandra RK. Mucosal immune responses in malnutrition. *Ann NY Acad Sci.* 1983;409:345–352.
10. Benjamin DK Jr, Miller WC, Benjamin DK, et al. A comparison of height and weight velocity as a part of the composite endpoint in pediatric HIV. *AIDS.* 2003;17:2331–2336.
11. Carey VJ, Yong FH, Frenkel LM, McKinney RE Jr. Pediatric AIDS prognosis using somatic growth velocity. *AIDS.* 1998;12:1361–1369.
12. Chantry CJ, Byrd RS, Englund JA, et al. Growth, survival and viral load in symptomatic childhood human immunodeficiency virus infection. *Pediatr Infect Dis J.* 2003;22:1033–1039.
13. Amaya RA, Kozinetz CA, McMeans A, et al. Lipodystrophy syndrome in human immunodeficiency virus-infected children. *Pediatr Infect Dis J.* 2002;21:405–410.
14. Vigano A, Mora S, Testolin C, et al. Increased lipodystrophy is associated with increased exposure to highly active antiretroviral therapy in HIV-infected children. *J Acquir Immune Defic Syndr.* 2003;32:482–489.
15. Arpadi SM, Cuff PA, Horlick M, et al. Lipodystrophy in HIV-infected children is associated with high viral load and low CD41-lymphocyte count and CD41-lymphocyte percentage at baseline and use of protease inhibitors and stavudine. *J Acquir Immune Defic Syndr.* 2001;27:30–34.
16. Lainka E, Oezbek S, Falck M, et al. Marked dyslipidemia in human immunodeficiency virus-infected children on protease inhibitor-containing antiretroviral therapy. *Pediatrics.* 2002;110:E56.
17. Jaquet D, Levine M, Ortega-Rodriguez E, et al. Clinical and metabolic presentation of the lipodystrophic syndrome in HIV-infected children. *AIDS.* 2000;14:2123–2128.
18. Beregszaszi M, Jaquet D, Levine M, et al. Severe insulin resistance contrasting with mild anthropometric changes in the adipose tissue of HIV-infected children with lipohypertrophy. *Int J Obes Relat Metab Disord.* 2003;27:25–30.
19. Mora S, Sala N, Bricalli D, et al. Bone mineral loss through increased bone turnover in HIV-infected children treated with highly active antiretroviral therapy. *AIDS.* 2001;15:1823–1829.
20. Arpadi SM, Horlick M, Thornton J, et al. Bone mineral content is lower in prepubertal HIV-infected children. *J Acquir Immune Defic Syndr.* 2002;29:450–454.
21. O'Brien KO, Razavi M, Henderson RA, et al. Bone mineral content in girls perinatally infected with HIV. *Am J Clin Nutr.* 2001;73:821–826.
22. Coodley GO, Loveless MO, Merrill TM. The HIV wasting syndrome: a review. *J Acquir Immune Defic Syndr.* 1994;7:681–694.
23. Heller LS, Shattuck D. Nutrition support for children with HIV/AIDS. *J Am Diet Assoc.* 1997;97:473–474.
24. Galvin T. Micronutrients: implications in human immunodeficiency virus disease. *Top Clin Nutr.* 1992;7:63–73.
25. Miller TL, Awnetwant EL, Evans S, et al. Gastrostomy tube supplementation for HIV-infected children. *Pediatrics.* 1995;96:696–702.

CHAPTER 17

Oncology and Sickle Cell Disease

Paula Charuhas Macris and Kathryn Hunt

Cancer is the fourth overall leading cause of death in children younger than age 20, ranking behind only unintentional injury, homicide, and suicide.[1,2] Leukemia constitutes the highest percentage of pediatric cancers, followed by children with central nervous system malignancies and lymphoma. Over the past three decades, the medical community has made tremendous improvements in both short- and long-term survival rates of children with cancer.

The incidence of malnutrition in children with newly diagnosed cancer is highly variable and dependent on factors such as advanced or metastatic disease, the degree of tumor burden, histology, and treatment protocols. Certain types of treatment procedures promote the development of malnutrition:

- Major abdominal surgery
- Radiation to the head, neck, esophagus, abdomen, or pelvis
- Frequent (compressed) courses of chemotherapy (3-week intervals or less)[3]

Approximately 40–80% of children become malnourished during intensive cancer treatment due to the aggressive nature of treatment protocols and the negative implications of therapy.[4] Characteristics of childhood malnutrition may include tissue wasting, anorexia, weakness, anemia, hypoalbuminemia, and skeletal muscle atrophy.[4] Malnutrition is clearly associated with increased infection rates, decreased tolerance of chemotherapy, delays in treatment, and diminished quality of life.[5] Childhood cancers associated with high nutrition risk are presented in **Table 17-1**.[1,2,4–7]

Infants (birth to 12 months) with leukemia, hepatoblastoma, or brain tumors are highly vulnerable to malnutrition and chemotherapy-related toxicities, as are young toddlers, whose development of self-feeding skills is often interrupted. Children often suffer from pain, mucositis, and vomiting and are therefore unable to accept breastmilk, infant formula, or solid foods at sufficient energy and protein levels needed to sustain growth and weight gain.

Adolescent cancer patients are equally vulnerable to therapy-induced malnutrition, because adolescence is the second period in the human life cycle where significant gains in growth and development occur. Cancers that develop during the second decade of life (10 to 20 years), such as Ewing's sarcoma and osteosarcoma, pose special challenges for the adolescent patient and the care team.

Childhood obesity presents its own set of risks during treatment. Obese children with cancer, especially those with acute leukemias, may suffer increased toxicities from chemotherapy. The cause of increased morbidity is likely multifactorial, including altered drug clearance due to increased body fat and comorbidities associated with obesity, such as obstructive sleep apnea and glucose intolerance.[5]

Nutritional Concerns

Children with cancer often are treated with multimodal therapies, depending on the type and stage of the malignancy. Cancer therapies may produce only mild, transient nutrition issues or they may lead to severe, permanent problems that impact nutritional status. The four main treatments are chemotherapy, surgery, radiation therapy, and hematopoietic cell transplantation (HCT).

Chemotherapeutic agents work by inhibiting DNA synthesis of both normal tissues and malignant cells. Most of the adverse effects associated with chemotherapy stem from damage to rapidly proliferating cells, including the epithelial cells of the gastrointestinal (GI) tract. The degree of the GI alterations depends on the specific medication, dosage, duration, rate of metabolism, and the child's susceptibility.[8]

Nutritional and medical complications associated with chemotherapy are outlined in **Table 17-2**.[9–11] Nausea and vomiting, which are associated with chemotherapy, are the most common problems interfering with adequate oral intake. Complications of chemotherapy-induced emesis include weight loss, dehydration, fluid and electrolyte imbalances, and metabolic alkalosis.[11] Management of chemotherapy-induced nausea and vomiting includes the judicious use of

TABLE 17-1 Common Childhood Cancers, Standard Treatment Plans, and Factors Affecting Nutritional Status

Childhood Cancer	Factors Affecting Nutritional Status	5-Year Relative Survival Rates (1999–2005)
Acute lymphocytic leukemia High-risk categories: • White blood cell count ≥ 50,000 mm^3 and/or age ≥ 10 years • Infants < 12 months of age • Chromosomal abnormalities (Philadelphia+) • T-cell phenotype • Relapsed Lymphoblastic lymphoma	• Need for cranial radiation • Treatment with highly emetogenic and mucosal toxic chemotherapy • Asparaginase-induced pancreatitis • Steroid-induced hyperglycemia requiring insulin • Frequent NPO status for procedures and intrathecal chemotherapy • HCT often necessary for cure	83.8% Infant < 1 year: 51.7% Lymphoblastic lymphoma: 65–85%
Acute myelogenous leukemia • Newly diagnosed • Relapsed disease	• Prolonged immunosuppression • At risk for fungal infections • Prolonged hospitalizations ("same old food" burn-out); HCT may be necessary	56.7%
Brain tumors • Medulloblastoma • Ependymoma/choroid plexus (PNET) • Astrocytoma • Other gliomas	• Treatment consists of 6 weeks of radiation therapy • Younger children require sedation for radiation (prolonged NPO status) • Hypogeusia • Nausea, vomiting, fatigue • Increased risk for dysphagia	Medulloblastoma: 85% Ependymoma/choroid plexus (PNET): Metastatic: < 60%; localized, nonmetastatic: 69.6% Astrocytoma: 82.6% Other gliomas: 52.8%
Hepatic tumors Hepatoblastoma • High risk: unresectable, metastatic, and prematurity	• Prematurity • Young age (< 2 years) • Liver transplant	69.2%
Neuroblastoma • High risk: stage III and IV • MYCN* amplification • Relapsed disease	• Young age (average age at diagnosis: 3.1 years) • Interruption in baseline feeding pattern • Significant nausea and vomiting • High need for enteral tube feeding • Postsurgery complication: high-output diarrhea • HCT • Prolonged transition to baseline oral intake after treatment	73.2% (also includes low risk)
Non-Hodgkin's lymphoma • Burkitts • Anaplastic large cell • Diffuse large B-cell	• Mucosal toxic chemotherapy (mouth and GI tract) • Frequent NPO status for intrathecal chemotherapy • Lack of interest in eating due to GI mucosal damage • Major nausea • At risk for infection	Burkitts: 80–90% Anaplastic large cell: 60–75% Diffuse large B-cell: 80–90%
Sarcomas • High risk: stage III and IV • Rhabdomyosarcoma (RMS) (especially parameningeal RMS) • Ewing's • Osteosarcoma • Metastatic disease	• Compressed chemotherapy cycles • Treatment with highly emetogenic and mucosal toxic chemotherapy • Lack of recovery time between chemotherapy cycles to regain lost weight • High energy and protein requirements	Osteosarcoma: 67.1% Ewing's: 63.1% Soft tissue and extraosseous sarcomas: 9.9% Rhabdomyosarcoma: 61.4%

TABLE 17-1 *(Continued)*

Childhood Cancer	Factors Affecting Nutritional Status	5-Year Relative Survival Rates (1999–2005)
Wilms' tumor • High risk: stage III and IV • Unfavorable resection • Relapsed/metastatic disease	• Surgical resection of tumor and kidney • Postoperative ileus requiring PN support • Radiation therapy: younger patients often NPO several hours prior to treatment	87.1% (also includes low risk)
Other, rare childhood malignancies • Chronic myelogenous leukemia (CML) • Juvenile chronic myelogenous leukemia (JCML)	• Treatment for both CML and JCML is HCT	CML:70–75% JCML: 50%

*MYCN: An oncogene present on chromosome 2. The MYCN gene is amplified (has more than 10 copies instead of 2 copies) in a subset of neuroblastoma tumors; this amplification is associated with poor outcome.

Abbreviations: GI, gastrointestinal; HCT, hematopoietic cell transplantation; NPO, non per os (nothing by mouth); PN, parenteral nutrition.

Sources: Ries LAG, Smith MA, Gurney JG, et al. (eds). *Cancer Incidence and Survival among Children and Adolescents: United States SEER Program 1975–1995.* Bethesda, MD: National Cancer Institute; 1999; Gurney JG, Bondy ML. Epidemiology of childhood cancer: general principles of chemotherapy. In: Pizzo PA, Poplac D (eds). *Principles and Practice of Pediatric Oncology,* 5th ed. Philadelphia: Lippincott Williams & Wilkins; 2006:1–13; Mauer AM, Burgess JB, Donaldson SS, et al. Special nutritional needs of children with malignancies: a review. *J Parenter Enteral Nutr.* 1990;14:315–324; Ladas EJ, Sacks N, Meacham L, et al. A multidisciplinary review of nutrition considerations in the pediatric oncology population: a perspective from Children's Oncology Group. *Nutr Clin Pract.* 2005;20:377–393; Williams DM, Hobson R, Imeson J, et al. Anaplastic large cell lymphoma in childhood: analysis of 72 patients treated on the United Kingdom Children's Cancer Study Group chemotherapy regimens. *Br J Haematol.* 2002;117:812–820; and Cairo MS, Raetz E, Lim MS, et al. Childhood and adolescent non-Hodgkin lymphoma: new insights in biology and critical challenges for the future. *Pediatr Blood Cancer.* 2005;45:753–769.

TABLE 17-2 Nutritional Implications of Chemotherapeutic Agents

Drug	Antitumor Spectrum	Nutritional Implications
Alkylating Agents		
Busulfan	Leukemias (HCT)	Nausea and vomiting, mucositis, hepatic (high dose)
Carboplatin	Brain tumors, germ cell tumors, neuroblastoma	Nausea and vomiting, hepatic (mild)
Cisplatin	Testicular and other germ cell tumors, brain tumors, osteosarcoma, neuroblastoma	Nausea and vomiting, renal
Cyclophosphamide	Lymphomas, leukemias, sarcomas, neuroblastoma	Nausea and vomiting, fluid retention
Ifosfamide	Sarcomas, germ cell tumors	Nausea and vomiting, renal
Lomustine	Brain tumors, lymphomas, Hodgkin's disease	Nausea and vomiting, renal
Melphalan	HCT	Nausea and vomiting, mucositis, diarrhea (high dose)
Procarbazine	Hodgkin's disease, brain tumors	Nausea and vomiting, mucositis
Temozolomide	Brain tumors	Nausea and vomiting
Antimetabolites		
Cladaribine	AML, CLL, indolent lymphomas	Mild nausea and vomiting
Cytarabine	Leukemia, lymphomas	Nausea and vomiting, mucositis, flu-like syndrome
Fludarabine phosphate	AML, CLL, indolent lymphomas	Mild nausea and vomiting
Fluorouracil	Carcinomas, hepatic tumors	Nausea and vomiting, mucositis, diarrhea
Mercaptopurine	ALL, CML	Hepatic, mucositis
Methotrexate	Leukemia, lymphomas, osteosarcoma	Mild mucositis, hepatic, renal
Thioguanine	ALL, AML	Nausea and vomiting, mucositis, hepatic (VOD)

(continues)

TABLE 17-2 *(Continued)*

Drug	Antitumor Spectrum	Nutritional Implications
Antitumor Antibiotics		
Bleomycin	Lymphoma, testicular and other germ cell tumors	Nausea and vomiting, mucositis
Dactinomycin	Wilms', sarcomas	Nausea and vomiting, mucositis, hepatic (VOD)
Daunomycin	ALL, AML, lymphomas	Nausea and vomiting, mucositis, diarrhea
Doxorubicin	ALL, AML, lymphomas, most solid tumors	Nausea and vomiting, mucositis, diarrhea
Idarubicin	ALL, AML, lymphomas	Nausea and vomiting, mucositis, diarrhea
Mitoxantrone	ALL, AML, lymphomas	Nausea and vomiting, mucositis
Plant Product		
Etoposide	ALL, AML, lymphomas, neuroblastoma, sarcoma, brain tumors	Nausea and vomiting, mucositis, diarrhea
Irinotecan	Rhabdomyosarcomas	Nausea and vomiting, diarrhea, hepatic, dehydration, ileus
Topotecan	Neuroblastoma, rhabdomyosarcoma	Nausea and vomiting, mucositis, diarrhea
Vincristine	ALL, lymphoma, most solid tumors	SIADH, constipation
Vinblastine	Histiocytosis, Hodgkin's disease, testicular	Mucositis, constipation
Miscellaneous		
All-trans retinoic acid	Acute promyelocytic leukemia	Hypertriglyceridemia
Dexamethasone	Leukemia, lymphomas, brain tumors	Highly variable*
Imatinib mesylate	Ph+ CML	Nausea and vomiting, fatigue, hepatic
Native asparaginase	ALL, lymphoma	Pancreatitis, hepatic
PEG-asparaginase	ALL, lymphoma	Pancreatitis, hepatic
Prednisone	Leukemia, lymphomas	Highly variable*
13-cis-retinoic acid	Minimal residual disease neuroblastoma	Xerostomia, hypertriglyceridemia, hypercalcemia

*Refer to Table 17-4, section on corticosteroids.

Abbreviations: ALL, acute lymphoblastic leukemia; AML, acute myelogenous leukemia; CLL, chronic lymphoblastic leukemia; CML, chronic myelogenous leukemia; HCT, hematopoietic cell transplantation; SIADH, syndrome of inappropriate antidiuretic hormone; VOD, veno-occlusive disease.

Sources: Adamson PC, Balis FM, Berg S, Blaney SM. General principles of chemotherapy. In: Pizzo PA, Poplac D (eds). *Principles and Practice of Pediatric Oncology,* 5th ed. Philadelphia: Lippincott Williams & Wilkins; 2006:290–365; Chu E, DeVita VT. *Physicians' Cancer Chemotherapy Drug Manual.* Burlington, MA: Jones & Bartlett Learning; 2006; and Charuhas PM, Aker SN. Nutritional implications of antineoplastic chemotherapeutic agents. *Clin Appl Nutr.* 1992;2:20–33.

antiemetics. Single-agent or combination antiemetics are frequently used and can decrease the child's discomfort. Nonpharmacologic interventions such as music therapy, hypnosis, and muscle relaxation may be effective techniques for treating nausea and vomiting.[12] Acupuncture, acupressure, and aromatherapy also may help to prevent and treat chemotherapy-induced nausea and vomiting.[13]

Alterations in taste and smell as a result of chemotherapy may persist well beyond periods of nausea and vomiting and result in prolonged anorexia.[14] In addition, children may develop food aversions that can limit oral intake.

Mucositis is a major GI complication and is usually intensified by concurrent radiation therapy.[15] Mucositis may affect any part of the GI tract and can lead to ulceration, bleeding, and malabsorption. Chemotherapy-induced neutropenia accentuates these complications. Diligent mouth care may help to prevent additional oral breakdown.

Certain chemotherapy and antibiotic agents may cause malabsorption and alterations in the gut flora, with subsequent weight loss and diarrhea.[11] Children who experience diarrhea either due to chemotherapy or from an infectious cause may benefit from probiotic replacement therapy in the setting of multiple antibiotic coverage.[16] Constipation related to the use of vincristine or narcotics or due to inactivity may result in significant abdominal discomfort and loss of appetite.

Treatment

Surgery is often the preferred method of therapy for solid tumors and tumors in the GI tract. Surgical removal of a tumor may lead to insufficient oral intake over several days during a time of increased energy and protein requirements. Depending on the surgical site, nutrient intake and absorption may be significantly affected. Surgery involving the head or neck area or the GI tract may result in profound nutritional implications, including chewing and swallowing issues, diarrhea, malabsorption of vitamins and minerals, and fluid and electrolyte imbalances.

Radiation therapy is a primary treatment modality for many brain tumors and is used in combination with surgery and chemotherapy to treat other cancers, including unresectable tumors. The nutritional implications of radiation depend upon many factors, including:

- The region of the body radiated
- Dose, fractionation, length of time, and field size of the radiation administered
- Concurrent use of other antitumor therapy, such as surgery or chemotherapy
- The child's initial nutritional status

As with chemotherapy, radiation destroys malignant cells as well as rapidly replicating normal tissues, including the GI tract. Nutritional sequelae associated with radiation therapy are detailed in **Table 17-3.**[8]

Treatment with HCT is an established therapeutic modality for certain pediatric hematologic and malignant disorders, such as acute leukemia, advanced-stage neuroblastoma, Fanconi anemia and many other disorders, solid tumors, and hematologic malignancies.[17] Children receiving a traditional myeloablative regimen are prepared with high doses of chemotherapy and possibly total body and local irradiation. In recent years, nonmyeloablative conditioning regimens, which deliver lower dose chemotherapy and radiation, have also been developed. Children with relapsed malignancy following myeloablative HCT or those with nonmalignant disorders may be candidates for the nonmyeloablative regimens. The intense conditioning regimen is designed to eliminate active and residual malignant cells or a defective hematopoietic system to restore normal hematopoiesis and immunologic function.[18] An intravenous infusion of autologous (child's own), syngeneic (identical twin), or allogeneic (from a histocompatible related or unrelated donor) stem cells follows conditioning. The source of the stem cells may be bone marrow, peripheral blood, or umbilical cord blood.

TABLE 17-3 Nutritional Implications of Radiation Therapy

Radiation to the central nervous system
• Anorexia
• Nausea and vomiting
Radiation to the head and neck
• Nausea
• Mucositis, esophagitis
• Altered taste and smell
• Tooth decay
• Altered salivation (saliva becomes thick and viscous)
• Dysphagia
Radiation to the gastrointestinal system
• Nausea and vomiting
• Diarrhea
• Steatorrhea and malabsorption
• Fluid and electrolyte imbalances
Total body radiation
• Nausea, vomiting, diarrhea
• Mucositis, esophagitis
• Altered taste acuity and salivation
• Anorexia
• Delayed growth and development

Source: Barale KV, Charuhas PM. Oncology and hematopoietic cell transplantation. In: Samour PQ, King K (eds). *Handbook of Pediatric Nutrition,* 3rd ed. Burlington, MA: Jones & Bartlett Learning; 2005:459–481.

Posttransplant Course

Severe pancytopenia (low blood counts) lasts from 2 to 6 weeks posttransplant. Children are at the greatest risk for bacterial and fungal infections until the stem cells engraft. During this period, supportive care, including frequent red blood cell and platelet transfusions, systemic antibiotic therapy, and parenteral nutrition (PN) support, are instituted.

Nutrition effects of HCT are due to the conditioning therapy, infections, graft-versus-host disease (GVHD), and medications, including anti-infectious and immunosuppressive agents.[18] Complications interfering with nutrient intake include the following:

- Mucositis
- Esophagitis
- Dysgeusia (impaired taste)
- Xerostomia (oral dryness)
- Thick, viscous saliva
- Nausea
- Vomiting
- Anorexia
- Diarrhea
- Steatorrhea
- Multiple-organ dysfunction[18]

The duration and intensity of symptoms, as well as the stress of treatment, preclude oral intake for a minimum of 3 to 4 weeks posttransplant and necessitate the use of PN. Oral intake is encouraged as soon as tolerated. Calorie, protein, and fluid goals should be defined for each child.

At hospital discharge, some children are still unable to eat an adequate amount of nutrients, and partial PN and/or enteral tube feeding may be prescribed, especially for children with chronic food aversions and long-term anorexia. Supplemental intravenous hydration may also be necessary. Follow-up nutrition counseling and assessment are imperative throughout the child's posttransplant course to ensure provision of adequate nutrition support.

Graft-Versus-Host Disease

Children who receive allogeneic transplants are at risk for the development of GVHD, an immunologic reaction in which the newly engrafted stem cells react against the host's tissue antigens following engraftment. The ensuing immunologic response can cause multiple-organ damage.[19] The GVHD may occur as an acute reaction early posttransplant or progress to a chronic condition. Because of its potentially devastating effects, efforts are directed at prevention of GVHD. Medications and therapy used for prophylaxis and treatment of GVHD are presented in **Table 17-4.**[20]

Acute GVHD can affect the skin, liver, or GI tract. Clinical symptoms include a maculopapular rash, cholestatic liver dysfunction, and nausea, vomiting, and diarrhea. Intestinal GVHD can involve either the upper or lower GI tract.[19] Upper intestinal GVHD symptoms include early satiety, anorexia, nausea, and vomiting. In lower intestinal GVHD, diarrhea may be severe and, at its worst, associated with crampy abdominal pain and bleeding. Children with severe disease often require a period of bowel rest with PN support. Refeeding guidelines include slow diet progression and feeding one new food at a time, gradually advancing to a regular diet.[21]

Nutrition Assessment

Nutritional status at diagnosis has been associated with treatment outcome in children with cancer.[22,23] Nutrition assessment should begin at diagnosis and continue throughout treatment.[8] A clear understanding of the specific type and stage of cancer, treatment protocol, and effects of therapy are necessary to better formulate an appropriate nutrition care plan.

Initial measurements should include age, height/length, weight, and, in children younger than 2 years of age, occipital frontal head circumference (see Appendix B). Any measurement below the 10th percentile should be investigated as a sign of growth impairment due to inadequate nutrition. Weight-for-height percentile is believed to be the most reliable anthropometric indicator of nutrition status in the child with cancer.[4] In the pediatric cancer patient, current or previous chemoradiotherapy may depress growth. Catch-up growth has been observed in these children; however, children who receive cranial irradiation may develop long-term growth disturbances.[24,25] Children receiving long-term therapy or those post-HCT should have their growth velocity

TABLE 17-4 Therapies Used for Prophylaxis and Treatment of GVHD

Therapy	Nutritional Effects
Antithymocyte globulin	Nausea and vomiting, diarrhea, stomatitis
Azathioprine	Nausea and vomiting, anorexia, diarrhea, mucosal ulceration, esophagitis, steatorrhea
Beclomethasone dipropionate	Xerostomia, dysgeusia, nausea
Budesonide	None known
Corticosteroids	Sodium and fluid retention resulting in weight gain or hypertension, hyperphagia, weight gain, hypokalemia, skeletal muscle catabolism and atrophy, gastric irritation and peptic ulceration, osteoporosis, growth retardation in children, decreased insulin sensitivity and impaired glucose tolerance, hyperglycemia or steroid-induced diabetes, hypertriglyceridemia
Cyclosporine	Nausea and vomiting, renal insufficiency, magnesium wasting, potassium wasting
Extracorporeal photopheresis	Intravenous fluid may be necessary to maintain adequate hydration status; monitor calcium status if citrate anticoagulant is used because it may bind calcium and induce hypocalcemia
Methotrexate	Nausea and vomiting (mild to moderate); anorexia; mucositis and esophagitis; diarrhea; renal and hepatic changes; decreased absorption of vitamin B_{12}, fat, and D-xylose; hepatic fibrosis; change in taste acuity
Methoxsalen (in conjunction with Psoralen 1 ultraviolet A light)	Nausea, hepatotoxicity
Monoclonal antibodies	Nausea and vomiting
Mycophenolate mofetil	Nausea and vomiting, diarrhea
Sirolimus	Hypertriglyceridemia
Tacrolimus	Nephrotoxicity, hyperglycemia, hyperkalemia, hypomagnesemia
Thalidomide	Constipation, nausea, xerostomia
Ursodeoxycholic acid	Nausea and vomiting, diarrhea, dyspepsia

Source: Hematopoietic Stem Cell Transplantation, *Nutrition Care Criteria*. Seattle, WA: Seattle Cancer Care Alliance, 2002.

plotted yearly to detect deviations from normal growth patterns.[18] From the baseline anthropometry information, the child's body surface area and ideal weight, which are often used to calculate medication dosages, can be determined.

For prepubertal children, ideal weight is determined by matching the weight at the 50th percentile for height on the age- and gender-specific CDC growth charts. For postpubertal children, an estimation of the ideal weight is determined using the body mass index (BMI) CDC growth charts for age. If the child's BMI is between the 25th and 75th percentiles, this may be considered an ideal weight. An adjusted weight is calculated for children greater than 120% ideal weight using the following equation:[26]

$$\text{Adjusted weight} = [\text{actual weight (kg)} - \text{ideal weight (kg)}] \times 0.25 + \text{ideal weight (kg)}$$

It is important to assess both growth history and the current height for age, weight for age, and weight for length or BMI. Arm anthropometry, to determine somatic muscle protein and adipose reserves, also may be assessed.

Finding reliable measures to detect malnutrition in the pediatric cancer patient can be challenging. Both the disease itself and the treatment can affect laboratory data used for nutrition assessment. Hematologic parameters, such as hemoglobin and hematocrit, often reflect the disease state and treatment with blood transfusions, rather than nutritional status. Many chemotherapy agents will suppress bone marrow production and lower lymphocyte counts; therefore, the complete blood count must be interpreted cautiously once therapy begins. Biochemical indices on renal and hepatic function as well as serum lipids, glucose, and electrolytes should always be reviewed for detection of nutrient deficiencies.

Serum albumin is used to evaluate internal protein status. A low serum albumin measurement does not necessarily establish malnutrition, because infection, excessive GI or renal losses, impaired liver function, certain chemotherapy agents, and overhydration each depress serum albumin levels.[27] Furthermore, serum albumin levels may not be as clinically useful as prealbumin, which has a half-life of approximately 2 days. Prealbumin is less influenced by changes in body fluids than serum albumin is, making it a more reliable test to evaluate nutritional status. Like albumin, however, prealbumin measurements may also be influenced by infection and fever. Nevertheless, prealbumin is the best available marker of nutritional status.

The nutrition history should include a comprehensive assessment of current oral and GI symptoms, including the following:

- Chewing or swallowing difficulties
- Mucositis and esophagitis
- Taste alterations
- Xerostomia
- Heartburn
- Nausea and vomiting
- Early satiety
- Changes in appetite
- Altered bowel habits

Current dietary modifications, including the use of special diets; presence of food allergies, food aversions, or intolerances; and use of vitamin, mineral, and herbal supplements, also should be included in the initial evaluation. Stage of eating development (e.g., self-feeding skills, puree versus table food, bottle versus cup) and use of infant formulas or breastfeeding should also be assessed.

Careful clinical observation is valuable to detect the presence of obesity, emaciation, dehydration, or edema. The child's medical history, physical strength, activity level, organ function, and level of pain and pain control, which may interfere with oral intake, should also be evaluated.

Nutrient and Energy Requirements

Nutrient requirements during childhood cancer are described in **Table 17-5**. The goals are to:

- Provide adequate nutrition to preserve lean tissue and promote growth and development.
- Identify and prevent or correct protein-energy malnutrition.
- Prevent or correct metabolic abnormalities.
- Maximize quality of life.

Energy requirements should be based on age, weight, gender, therapy, and growth needs.[18] The DRI for energy and protein may not be appropriate in this population. Factors affecting nutrient needs include inactivity, bacterial sepsis, fever secondary to neutropenia, and secondary complications, such as neutropenic enterocolitis. Basal metabolic rate with additions for growth, infection, and stress can be used to determine energy needs.[28] Multiplying the basal metabolic rate by a factor of 1.6 to 1.8 for very young or malnourished children will allow for growth, stress, and light activity.[18] The Harris-Benedict formula and other equations can be used to estimate calorie needs in older children who have completed their growth.[29]

Vitamin and mineral requirements have not been determined for children with cancer. Recommendations are based on the DRI (see Appendix F). Extensive radiation or surgical damage to the GI tract and treatment with long-term antibiotic therapy for chronic infections may increase the child's need for vitamins and minerals. Most children receiving cancer treatment benefit from taking an age-specific multivitamin/mineral supplement without iron, to prevent iron overload, which may develop due to red cell transfusions during therapy.

Children diagnosed with ALL, non-Hodgkin's lymphoma, or those who develop GVHD following HCT are especially at risk for developing osteopenia and fractures due to the use

TABLE 17-5 Nutrient Requirements During Childhood Cancer

Nutrient Requirements	Recommendations

Calories	• Infants: Birth to 12 months: Use RDA for age for appropriate weight infants. Use catch-up growth calculation if underweight: (Kcal/kg/day = Kcal/kg/day for weight age × ideal weight age [kg] ÷ actual weight in kg)
	• Older children (> than 1 year): Use BMR table multiplied by additional factors:
	  • Appropriate weight for height: BMR × 1.6
	  • Obese: BMR × 1.3
	  • Sedentary with 5% weight loss: BMR × 1.4–1.6
	  • 10% weight loss from usual weight or weight is 90% or less of usual or ideal weight: BMR × 1.8–2.0
	• Use adjusted weight calculation for obese children; BMI weight at the 75th percentile may also be used to calculate energy needs in obese children
	• HCT: BMR × 1.6 during immediate posttransplant course; BMR × 1.4 following engraftment and medically stable

Protein	• Infants birth to 6 months: 3 g/kg/day • Infants 6 to 12 months: 2.5–3 g/kg/day • Children: 2–2.5 g/kg/day (in most cases) • Adolescents with increased lean body mass: 1.5–1.8 g/kg/day
Fat	• 10–30% total calories
Fluid	• 1–10 kg: 100 mL/kg/day • 11–20 kg: 1000 mL plus 50 ml for every kg > 10 per day • 21–40 kg: 1500 mL plus 20 mL for every kg > 20 per day • > 40 kg: 1500 mL/m^2 body surface area
Vitamins	• Use ASPEN[44] parenteral vitamin guidelines for age • After PN discontinued, oral multiple vitamin/mineral without iron, during antineoplastic therapy • Provide additional vitamin C during HCT: < 31 kg, additional 250 mg vitamin C per day > 31 kg, additional 500 mg vitamin C per day
Minerals and electrolytes	• Iron supplementation contraindicated during oncologic therapy and HCT • Eliminate copper and manganese from PN in presence of hepatic dysfunction (i.e., serum bilirubin > 10.0 mg/dL) • Closely monitor serum electrolytes during therapy

Abbreviations: ASPEN, American Society for Parenteral and Enteral Nutrition; BEE, basal energy expenditure; BMI, body mass index; BMR, basal metabolic rate; CDC, Centers for Disease Control and Prevention; PN, parenteral nutrition; RDA, recommended dietary allowance.

of corticosteroids during treatment.[9,30] Corticosteroids disrupt calcium absorption,[31] and the natural intake of calcium and vitamin D from the child's own diet is often insufficient to meet increased needs. Therefore, calcium and vitamin D supplementation, in addition to the multivitamin/mineral supplement, is often necessary to maintain bone health.

Children undergoing HCT require additional vitamin C to promote tissue recovery via collagen biosynthesis after cytoreductive therapy.[18] Some chemotherapies, as well as medications used to treat fungal and viral infections, are nephrotoxic and may cause increased losses of certain minerals. Children undergoing cancer treatment with nephrotoxic chemotherapy agents may require long-term supplementation of these nutrients, such as zinc.

Vitamin D deficiency is pandemic across all age groups in industrialized countries.[32] Although determining a clear relationship between vitamin D deficiency and the development of certain diseases is unknown,[33] practitioners who care for children with cancer should routinely measure the serum 25-OH vitamin D level to evaluate for deficiency.

Certain medications, including tacrolimus, corticosteroids, and all-trans retinoic acid, are known to cause a fluctuation and possible increase in serum triglyceride levels.[34] Fish oil (omega-3 fatty acids, including docosahexaenoic and eicosapentaenoic acid) supplementation can improve hypertriglyceridemia (≥500 mg/dL) in adults. This is currently[35] an accepted practice among pediatric practitioners for children with cancer when the child is tolerating oral medications.

Nutrition Therapy

The primary goal of nutrition therapy for the pediatric oncology population is to sustain and promote normal growth and development while undergoing necessary anticancer therapy. Suboptimal oral intake of short duration during treatment is of less concern if the child is initially well nourished and can compensate or eat more when feeling well. These children may benefit from high-density foods that increase energy and other nutrient levels of the diet. **Table 17-6** offers suggestions for boosting the nutrient density of foods consumed. Dietary guidelines for managing common nutrition problems seen during and following therapy are addressed in **Table 17-7**.

Refeeding a child following intensive cancer therapy may be a slow process, because the child's appetite and tolerance for food fluctuate widely. Young children with preexisting delays in feeding development should have intervention from a feeding team. Determination of feeding skills in the young child will facilitate choices for self-feeding, because many young children's feeding skills will regress during intense oncologic therapy.

Individualizing the child's diet by including frequent servings of foods enjoyed (in the absence of oral and GI symptoms) may enhance oral intake. Although many commercial liquid medical nutritional supplements designed for pediatric patients are currently available, taste acceptance may be a limiting factor. Nutritional supplements are often acceptable if offered in an unobtrusive manner as part of the regular meal or snack pattern. For the lactose-intolerant

TABLE 17-6 Guidelines for Increasing Nutrient Density

Butter, margarine, and oils • Add to soup, mashed and baked potatoes, hot cereal, grits, rice, noodles, and cooked vegetables.	• Stir into sauces and gravies.
Cream • Use on desserts, gelatin, pudding, fruit, pancakes, waffles, and mashed potatoes. • Use in soups, sauces, egg dishes, batters, puddings, and custards; put on cereals.	• Mix with pasta, mashed potatoes, and rice. • Substitute for milk in recipes. • Make cocoa with cream and add marshmallows.
Sour cream • Add to soups, baked potatoes, vegetables, sauces, salad dressings, gelatin desserts, bread, and muffin batter.	• Use as dip for raw fruits and vegetables.
Mayonnaise • Add to salad dressing. • Spread on sandwiches and crackers.	• Use in sauces and gelatin desserts.
Honey (use in children over 1 year of age) • Add to cereal, milk drinks, fruit desserts, smoothies, or yogurt.	• Use as a glaze for meats such as chicken.
Granola • Use in cookie, muffin, and bread batters. • Sprinkle on vegetables, yogurt, ice cream, pudding, custard, and fruit.	• Mix with dried fruits and nuts for a snack. • Substitute for bread or rice in pudding recipes.
Dried fruits and nuts • Cook and serve dried fruits for breakfast or as dessert. • Add to muffins, cookies, breads, cakes, rice and grain dishes, cereals, puddings, and stuffing.	• Bake in pies and turnovers. • Combine with cooked vegetables such as carrots, sweet potatoes, or acorn and butternut squash.
Milk and cheese • Mix one cup dry milk powder in four cups of liquid milk; use this milk for cooking and baking. • Add milk powder directly to hot or cold cereals, scrambled eggs, soups, gravies, casserole dishes, and desserts.	• Add grated cheese or chunks of cheese to sauces, vegetables, soups, salads, and casseroles. • Spread cream cheese on hot buttered bread.
Eggs • Add eggs to soups and casseroles.	• Slice boiled eggs in sauces and serve over rice, cooked noodles, buttered toast, or hot biscuits.
Peanut butter • Add peanut butter to sauces; use on crackers, waffles, or celery sticks.	• Spread peanut butter on hot buttered bread.

Source: Medical Nutrition Therapy Services Program, Seattle Cancer Care Alliance, Seattle, Washington.

TABLE 17-7 Dietary Guidelines for Managing Common Nutrition Problems of Children with Cancer

Oral and esophageal mucositis (inflammation of the oral and esophageal mucosa) • Try soft or pureed foods or a blenderized liquid diet. • Offer soft, nonirritating, cold foods (popsicles, ice cream, frozen yogurt, slushes) and smooth, bland, moist foods (custard, cream soups, mashed potatoes).	• Encourage frequent mouth rinsing to remove food and bacteria and promote healing.
Xerostomia (oral dryness) • Offer moist foods (stews, casseroles, canned fruit) and liquids. • Add sauce, gravy, margarine, butter, or broth to dry foods.	• Drink liquids with meals. • Offer sugar-free lemon-flavored candy to help stimulate saliva. • Encourage good oral hygiene.
Thick, viscous saliva and mucous • Try club soda, hot tea with lemon, or a beverage with citric acid. • Encourage adequate fluid intake.	• Encourage good oral hygiene.
Dysgeusia (impaired taste) • Enhance food taste with herbs, spices, flavor extracts, and marinades. • Offer cold foods. • Offer fruit-flavored beverages.	• Try tart foods like oranges or lemonade, which may have more taste. • Encourage good oral hygiene. • Offer fluids with meals to help take away a bad taste in the mouth.
Nausea and vomiting • Try high carbohydrate foods and fluids (crackers, toast, gelatin) and nonacidic juices. • Try small, frequent feedings. • Offer cold, clear liquids and solids. • Avoid overly sweet or high fat foods. • Avoid feeding in a stuffy, too-warm room or one filled with cooking odors or other odors that might be disagreeable.	• Encourage drinking or sipping liquids frequently throughout the day; using a straw may help. • Encourage rest periods after meals. • Avoid offering favorite foods when nauseated; it may cause a permanent dislike of the food.
Diarrhea • Try a low-fat, low-fiber, low-lactose diet. • Avoid caffeine.	• Eat warm or room temperature foods because hot foods may increase bowel motility • Encourage adequate fluids to prevent dehydration.
Constipation • Encourage fluids. • Drink hot liquids to increase bowel activity.	• Offer high-fiber foods.
Other helpful hints • Take the child's sports bottle filled with a favorite beverage when going shopping or to a clinic appointment. • If lack of appetite is a problem at mealtimes, limit snacks and fluids for 1 to 2 hours before the meal. • Serve food "family style" to allow the child to dish out his or her own food portions.	• Serve very small servings on a large dinner plate so that portions will not look as overwhelming. • Arrange foods creatively on plates. • Serve brightly colored foods and different food shapes together. • Offer new foods along with favorite foods. • Allow the child to help prepare the food.

Source: Medical Nutrition Therapy Services Program, Seattle Cancer Care Alliance, Seattle, Washington.

child, lactose-free or soy-based products (e.g., soy milk, soy-based or milk-based lactose-free commercial medical nutritional supplements) can be useful. Oral and esophageal lesions may limit tolerance for oral supplements. Hyperosmolar or lactose-containing products may aggravate diarrhea.

For a thorough evaluation of the child's intake, daily food intake records provide a basis for decisions regarding supplemental or nonvolitional feeding. Parenteral or enteral nutrient solutions, other intravenous fluids, and oral intake must all be included when evaluating intake. Older children and family members may assist with record keeping and provide valuable intake information.

Enteral tube feeding is the primary nutrition intervention strategy for children undergoing cancer treatment. Such children already require placement of a central line for chemotherapy, intravenous fluids, medications, and the administration of blood products. Because tube feeding maintains the function and integrity of the GI tract, its other benefits include reduced risk for infection and that it is a more cost-effective therapy than PN. For children who have difficulty taking oral medications, enteral tube feeding provides a safe route for administration. Finally, feeding tubes can help reduce anxiety in children, parents, and providers from failing to meet nutrient and fluid goals via oral feeding.

Overcoming barriers to successful nasogastric (NG) tube placement requires skilled pediatric oncology dietitians, dedicated oncology nurses, nurse practitioners, and an educated medical staff. The necessity for NG tube placement must be presented to the child and family in a positive manner to restore the malnourished child back to normal weight and health or to prevent further nutrition deficits in at-risk children.

The following criteria may be useful when considering enteral tube feeding candidates:

- Interval or total weight loss is >5% of pre-illness body weight (usual weight).
- Weight for height reaches ≤90% of ideal weight for height, adjusted for height and age.
- BMI falls to or below the 10th percentile.
- Repeated attempts to meet nutrient needs orally have failed.
- Child or adolescent has functioning GI tract.
- Lowest weight threshold: an agreed upon weight, determined by healthcare providers and parents that, if reached, is unsafe for the child or adolescent to proceed with therapy without enteral nutrition support intervention. This can be based on the above criteria.

NG tubes can be placed in children whose weight decreases to or below 90% of ideal weight for height for age. Malnutrition during intensive chemotherapy for pediatric sarcomas can usually be prevented with aggressive enteral nutrition support, which has proven feasible and well tolerated for extended durations.[36]

Complications such as dislodgement of nasoenteral tubes; delayed gastric emptying; inadequate electrolyte and mineral intake, specifically calcium, magnesium, phosphorus, and zinc; and inadequate energy intake can occur.[37–42] The combined use of enteral feedings with PN during HCT is an acceptable and cost-effective alternative.[43] Candidates for enteral nutrition during HCT include children who:

- Receive a nonmyeloablative or reduced-intensity conditioning regimen
- Fail to recover appetite and resume eating after engraftment and resolution of conditioning-related mucositis and esophagitis
- Have chronic GVHD (i.e., oral, esophageal, liver, pulmonary, weight loss, quiescent phases of GI)
- Have neurological complications that preclude safe swallowing
- Are ventilated[44,45]

During cancer therapy, the child's GI tract may not be usable for oral diet or enteral feedings due to complications associated with surgery, nausea and vomiting, diarrhea, colitis, pancreatitis, intestinal GVHD, ileus, or radiation enteritis. In these situations, PN is indicated. The decision to use PN is often based on the child's nutritional status, type of therapy, expected oral and GI complications associated with the chosen treatment, and availability of peripheral veins. Multiple-lumen central venous catheters are often placed at the start of treatment for delivery of medications and blood products, so access is available for PN and hydration fluids. Cyclic or home PN can be used to provide nutrition support while allowing the child time out of the hospital. A home health agency can work with caregivers to provide PN solutions, education, and monitoring.

Children maintained on PN support must be closely monitored to ensure that nutrient and fluid requirements are met and that any serum electrolyte alterations, especially as a result of medications and/or GI losses, are corrected promptly. In addition to ongoing monitoring and assessment throughout the child's treatment course, the pediatric oncology dietitian also must be aware of special considerations that may impact the child's nutritional status.

Due to intensive treatment regimens, PN is the standard nutrition support therapy for children undergoing HCT.[45] PN therapy results in improved visceral protein status, maintenance of body weight, and earlier engraftment following cytoreductive therapy.[46–48]

Long-Term Nutritional Sequelae

Chronic complications associated with cancer therapy may impact a child's nutritional status and require intervention for several years. Endocrine and growth disorders (e.g., thyroid disease, obesity, alterations in pubertal development), osteonecrosis, cardiopulmonary disease, and neurologic or neurosensory disorders can occur.[25]

Growth hormone deficiency with decreased growth velocity and delayed onset of puberty can occur in children following HCT.[49] Children who have received cranial irradiation prior to HCT show growth hormone deficiency with deceleration of normal growth rates.[49] Regular evaluations to determine occurrence of endocrine gland dysfunction are recommended. Medical complications of long-term survivors of HCT include chronic GVHD, osteoporosis, hyperlipidemia, hyperglycemia, and infection.[30,50–53]

Complementary Therapies

The use of complementary or integrative therapies by the pediatric oncology population has become more prevalent. Parents seek out these therapies for their children undergoing conventional cancer treatments for many reasons, including a desire to relieve the burden of side effects caused by chemotherapy, motivation to find a cure, pursuit of greater control over their child's disease, improved quality of life, and hope.[54] Parents often choose nonconventional therapies such as herbs, high-dose antioxidants, homeopathy, and botanicals that they feel may help their child, but are unaware of their potential harmful effects or the possibility that they may interfere with conventional treatments. Acupuncture and massage may help alleviate treatment side effects, including nausea, vomiting, pain, and anxiety.[13]

The use of herbals and megavitamin therapy in the treatment of childhood cancer raises several concerns, including:

- Unexpected or undesirable interactions between preparations and prescribed medications may affect the action of drugs routinely used during the course of chemotherapy and HCT.
- Potential contamination of preparations derived from plants poses the risk of bacterial, fungal, or parasitic infections. A few specific preparations have been associated with serious toxic side effects or infections.[20]
- Alternative nutrition therapy may be chosen as the sole source of treatment.

Some herbals are contraindicated in children with cancer because of their association with serious side effects. Garlic and gingko biloba may reduce blood-clotting factors.[55,56] Other botanicals containing pyrrolizidine alkaloids, such as comfrey and maté tea, may induce hepatotoxicity.[57] Herbal preparations should be discontinued during HCT. The pediatric oncology dietitian must be sensitive to the family's views and biases and educate the healthcare team appropriately.

Feeding the Immunosuppressed Child

The goal of the diet for the immunosuppressed child is to maximize healthy food options while minimizing GI exposure to pathogenic organisms resulting in increased morbidity and mortality.[58] Most cancer facilities place restrictions ranging from no raw fresh fruits or vegetables to a specific low microbial diet.[58-60] **Table 17-8** shows an example of diet restrictions for immunosuppressed children. High-risk foods, identified as potential sources of organisms known to cause infection during immunosuppression, are restricted. In recent years, many transplant centers have liberalized their diets to allow well-washed raw fruits and vegetables. Recommendations on the duration of the diet are based on treatment and type of HCT.

TABLE 17-8 Diet Guidelines for Immunosuppressed Patients

These guidelines are intended to minimize the introduction of pathogenic organisms into the GI tract by food while maximizing healthy food options for immunosuppressed children. These guidelines should be coupled with food safety education to assume proper food preparation and storage in the home and hospital kitchen. High-risk foods, identified as potential sources of organisms known to cause infection in immunosuppressed children, are restricted.

In general, these guidelines should be followed by children who have an absolute neutrophil count of below 1×103 μl. Children receiving an autologous transplant should follow the diet for the first 3 months after HCT; children receiving an allogeneic transplant should follow the diet until off all immunosuppressive therapy (i.e., cyclosporine, tacrolimus, prednisone).

Food Restrictions

Contraindicated:

- Raw and undercooked meat (including game), fish, shellfish, poultry, eggs, sausage, and bacon
- Raw tofu, unless pasteurized or aseptically packaged
- Luncheon meats (including salami, bologna, hot dogs, ham, and others) unless heated until steaming
- Refrigerated smoked seafood typically labeled as lox, kippered, nova-style, or smoked or fish jerky (unless contained in a cooked dish); pickled fish
- Nonpasteurized milk and raw milk products, nonpasteurized cheese, and nonpasteurized yogurt
- Blue-veined cheeses, including blue, Gorgonzola, Roquefort, and Stilton
- Uncooked soft cheeses including brie, camembert, feta, and farmer's
- Mexican-style soft cheese, including queso blanco and queso fresco
- Cheese containing chili peppers or other uncooked vegetables
- Fresh salad dressings (stored in the grocer's refrigerated case) containing raw eggs or contraindicated cheeses
- Unwashed raw and frozen fruits and vegetables and those with visible mold; all raw vegetable sprouts (alfalfa, mung bean, all others)
- Raw or unpasteurized honey
- Unpasteurized commercial fruit and vegetable juices

Source: Medical Nutrition Therapy Services Program, Seattle Cancer Care Alliance, Seattle, Washington.

Providing education on food safety may be more important in reducing food-borne illness than extensive diet restrictions.[61] Education should emphasize hand washing; high-risk foods; proper temperatures for storage, defrosting, handling, and cooking; cross-contamination issues; correct cooling and reheating procedures; and sanitation.

Several infections are of particular concern with the pediatric oncology population, including *Salmonella enteritis, Campylobacter jejuni, E. coli* 0157:H7, and *Listeria monocytogenes.* See the CDC website for the diagnosis and management of food-borne illness.[62]

The food service for pediatric oncology patients should be able to provide a variety of foods served at frequent intervals to meet the child's tolerance. A flexible food service, such as hotel-style room service with extended hours, unit nourishment centers, or satellite kitchens, will provide opportunities for improving a child's oral intake.[63]

An often overlooked and unintended consequence of pediatric cancer therapy is the disruption to the relationship between parents and their children in the area of food and nutrition. Because anticancer therapy often causes nausea, vomiting, loss of appetite, and taste alterations, children lose the pleasure of eating. By nature, children look to their parents for their daily food intake, and parents instinctively assume and guard their nurturing role as the primary food provider. The potential disruption to eating patterns and habits can be a source of stress and anxiety for the child and can lead to a family that becomes overly focused on food. It is essential that the pediatric oncology dietitian understand and appreciate the parent–child–food relationship and support both the parent's role and the child's need for his or her parent to continue as the food provider. Such family-centered care, including respect for the feeding dynamics between parents and children, is an essential component of pediatric cancer treatment.

Encouraging oral intake in a young child with cancer is challenging. Anxious, scared, or depressed children do not feel like eating. Chronic pain may also decrease the child's interest in eating. Providing a calm, relaxed hospital atmosphere for eating, with uninterrupted time for feeding (e.g., door closed, sign posted) may improve intake. Small children require a secure feeding position (e.g., high chair, toddler feeding table), a bib, towel, and covered floor area to limit anxiety over spills.

Children should not be forced to eat. A maximum mealtime of 20 to 30 minutes should be adequate, and the child should be provided with food textures and portion sizes that are age appropriate. Older children may benefit from group eating situations and by knowing their oral intake goals for hospital discharge. Food from home may be allowed, as long as the food conforms to the medical diet order. Perishable foods must be consumed immediately. Family education in food safety is vital.

For children who refuse to eat, behavior modification techniques may be necessary.[64] Children transitioning from tube feeding may exhibit oral, motor, sensory, and developmental feeding problems that make weaning difficult. A weaning process based on developmental stages is recommended.[65]

Sickle Cell Disease

Sickle cell disease (SCD) is a genetic disorder characterized by the production of abnormal hemoglobin, which causes red blood cells to become sickle shaped. Sickle-shaped red blood cells trigger inflammation, coagulation, and platelet aggregation, resulting in inadequate tissue blood flow and chronic anemia. Clinical manifestations of SCD include the following:

- Severe, painful crises
- Acute chest syndrome
- Splenic sequestration
- Stroke
- Chronic pulmonary and renal dysfunction
- Delayed growth
- Neuropsychological deficits
- Premature death[66]

The prevention of pain crises is key. Chronic blood transfusions, pain management, antibiotics to prevent infections, and immunizations are also necessary. The only curative treatment for SCD is HCT.[67] Children receiving a matched sibling HCT have a greater than 80% overall disease-free survival rate.[67]

Children with SCD may be at risk for deficiencies in vitamin A, vitamin B_6, red blood cell folate, and vitamin D.[68-71] Regular monitoring and supplementation is needed. Most children with SCD require folic acid supplementation. Hepatic iron overload is another serious complication of SCD due to chronic transfusion therapy.[72] Treatment for iron overload includes chelation therapy, which may cause depletion of divalent cations, such as calcium and magnesium. Delayed growth may or may not occur in children with SCD.

Oral intake may be compromised during acute pain crises, so a diet emphasizing nutrient-dense foods with provision of adequate calories and protein should be emphasized. Maintaining adequate hydration status is important because dehydration may cause sickling of red blood cells. An iron-free multivitamin/mineral supplement is recommended for all children with SCD.

Case Study

Nutrition Assessment of Child with Leukemia

A previously healthy 7-year-old female presented to her primary care physician for a well-child visit. During the appointment, it was observed that the child was pale. Parents gave a history of easy bruising, which had persisted for the past 2 months. A complete blood count with differential showed anemia, thrombocytopenia, and a white blood cell count of 65,000 thou/μL (normal: 4500–13,500 thou/μL). The family history is negative for cancer.

The patient was referred to the hospital for further evaluation. A diagnosis of acute myelogenous leukemia (AML)-M4 (select marker) was confirmed by bone marrow biopsy.

Anthropometry

Height: 128.1 cm

Weight: 24.2 kg

Ideal weight for height: 26 kg (50th percentile CDC height)

Nutrition History

No known allergies.

Typical daily intake:

- *Breakfast:* Pancakes or cereal with 2% milk or yogurt and cheese
- *Lunch:* Sandwich (ham or turkey with cheese and butter) or Caesar salad with ranch dressing or macaroni and cheese
- *Dinner:* Chicken or pasta with butter (no sauce) or steak or pizza, vegetables
- *Snacks:* Carrots, broccoli, bananas, apples, melon, grapes, strawberries

Patient is currently taking a pediatric multivitamin supplement.

During the first round of induction chemotherapy, the patient's weight decreased to a nadir of 22.2 kg 6 days into treatment (85% of ideal weight for height). Patient had symptoms of nausea, vomiting, and increased stooling.

A nasogastric (NG) enteral tube was placed for initiation of a 1 kcal/mL pediatric elemental formula; however, due to mucositis and bloody stools, she did not tolerate NG feeds well. Computed tomography (CT) scan confirmed typhilitis and pancolitis. Patient was placed on NPO and maintained on full total parenteral nutrition (TPN) support.

Nutrition Diagnosis/Problem

The nutrition diagnosis is inadequate energy intake related to altered gastrointestinal function and increased energy needs, as evidenced by bloody diarrhea and weight loss of more than 8% of usual body weight in 1 week.

Nutrition Intervention

Goal: Patient will be able to regain weight lost and maintain an acceptable weight throughout therapy.

Food/nutrient delivery: Patient to be placed NPO and TPN instituted.

Nutrition education: Educate patient/caregivers on need to remain NPO to allow for gut rest for healing of current gastrointestinal symptoms.

Nutrition counseling: Patient to remain NPO with TPN support until resolution of typhilitis and pancolitis. When symptoms have resolved, reinstitute NG feeds as tolerated and educate patient/caregivers on appropriate food/fluid choices.

Coordination of nutrition care: Work regularly with medical team (e.g., primary provider, team nurse) following patient.

Nutrition Monitoring and Evaluation

After placing patient NPO for 12 days, a low-lactose, low-fiber, low-acid diet with three to four foods per tray was instituted. NG feeds were reinitiated with a 1 kcal/mL pediatric elemental formula at an infusion rate of 10 mL/hour. Feeds were slowly advanced over 1 week until a goal of 65 mL/hour × 24 hrs was achieved, at which point TPN was discontinued.

Questions for the Reader

1. What is this patient's energy and protein needs per kg?
2. What is this patient's BMI, height, and weight percentiles on the growth chart?
3. Write one PES statement for this patient.
4. What was the total number of calories once the full tube feeding goal was achieved?

REFERENCES

1. Ries LAG, Smith MA, Gurney JG, et al. (eds). *Cancer Incidence and Survival among Children and Adolescents: United States SEER Program 1975–1995.* NIH Pub. No. 99-4649. Bethesda, MD: National Cancer Institute; 1999:1–15.
2. Gurney JG, Bondy ML. Epidemiology of childhood cancer. General principles of chemotherapy. In: Pizzo PA, Poplac D (eds). *Principles and Practice of Pediatric Oncology,* 5th ed. Philadelphia: Lippincott Williams & Wilkins; 2006:1–13.

3. Sala A, Pencharz P, Barr RD. Children, cancer, and nutrition—a dynamic triangle. *Cancer.* 2004;100:677–687.
4. Mauer AM, Burgess JB, Donaldson SS, et al. Special nutritional needs of children with malignancies: a review. *J Parenter Enteral Nutr.* 1990;14:315–324.
5. Ladas EJ, Sacks N, Meacham L, et al. A multidisciplinary review of nutrition considerations in the pediatric oncology population: a perspective from Children's Oncology Group. *Nutr Clin Pract.* 2005;20:377–393.
6. Williams DM, Hobson R, Imeson J, et al. Anaplastic large cell lymphoma in childhood: analysis of 72 patients treated on the United Kingdom Children's Cancer Study Group chemotherapy regimens. *Br J Haematol.* 2002;117:812–820.
7. Cairo MS, Raetz E, Lim MS, et al. Childhood and adolescent non-Hodgkin lymphoma: new insights in biology and critical challenges for the future. *Pediatr Blood Cancer.* 2005;45:753–769.
8. Barale KV, Charuhas PM. Oncology and hematopoietic cell transplantation. In: Samour PQ, King K (eds). *Handbook of Pediatric Nutrition,* 3rd ed. Burlington, MA: Jones & Bartlett Learning; 2005:459–481.
9. Adamson PC, Balis FM, Berg S, Blaney SM. General principles of chemotherapy. In Pizzo PA, Poplac D (eds). *Principles and Practice of Pediatric Oncology,* 5th ed. Philadelphia: Lippincott Williams & Wilkins; 2006:290–365.
10. Chu E, DeVita VT. *Physicians' Cancer Chemotherapy Drug Manual.* Burlington, MA: Jones & Bartlett Learning; 2006.
11. Charuhas PM, Aker SN. Nutritional implications of antineoplastic chemotherapeutic agents. *Clin Appl Nutr.* 1992;2:20–33.
12. Keller VE. Management of nausea and vomiting in children. *J Pediatr Nurs.* 1995;10:280–286.
13. Ladas EJ, Post-White J, Hawks R, Taromina K. Evidence for symptom management in the child with cancer. *J Pediatr Hematol Oncol.* 2006;28:601–615.
14. Sherry VW. Taste alterations among patients with cancer. *Clin J Oncol Nurs.* 2002;6:73–76.
15. Kennedy L, Diamond J. Assessment and management of chemotherapy-induced mucositis in children. *J Pediatr Oncol Nurs.* 1997;4:164 174.
16. Lipkin AC, Lenssen P, Dickson BJ. Nutrition issues in hematopoietic stem cell transplantation: state of the art. *Nutr Clin Pract.* 2005;20:423–439.
17. Locatelli F, Giorgiani G, Di-Cesare-Merlone A, et al. The changing role of stem cell transplantation in childhood. *Bone Marrow Transplant.* 2008;41:S3–S7.
18. Charuhas PM. Pediatric hematopoietic stem cell transplantation. In: Hasse JM, Blue LS (eds). *Comprehensive Guide to Transplant Nutrition.* Chicago, IL: American Dietetic Association; 2002:226–247.
19. Vogelsang GB, Lee L, Bensen-Kennedy DM. Pathogenesis and treatment of graft-versus-host disease after bone marrow transplant. *Annu Rev Med.* 2003;54:29–52.
20. Charuhas PM (ed). *Nutrition Care Criteria.* Seattle, WA: Seattle Cancer Care Alliance; 2002.
21. Gauvreau JM, Lenssen P, Cheney CL, et al. Nutritional management of patients with intestinal graft-versus-host disease. *J Am Diet Assoc.* 1981;79:673–677.
22. Deeg HJ, Sediel K, Bruemmer B, et al. Impact of patient weight on non-relapse mortality after marrow transplantation. *Bone Marrow Transplant.* 1995;15:461–468.
23. Murry DJ, Riva L, Poplack DG. Impact of nutrition on pharmacokinetics of anti-neoplastic agents. *Int J Cancer Supp.* 1998;11:48–51.
24. Katz JA, Chambers B, Everhart C, et al. Linear growth in children with acute lymphoblastic leukemia treated without cranial irradiation. *J Pediatr.* 1991;118:575–578.
25. Diller L, Chow EJ, Gurney JG, et al. Chronic disease in the childhood cancer survivor study cohort: a review of published findings. *J Clin Oncol.* 2009;14:2339–2355.
26. Wiggins KL (ed). *Guidelines for Nutrition of Renal Patients,* 3rd ed. Chicago, IL: American Dietetic Association; 2001:13.
27. Elhasid R, Laor A, Lischinsky S, et al. Nutritional status of children with solid tumors. *Cancer.* 1999;86:119–125.
28. Altman PL, Dittmer DS. *Metabolism.* Bethesda, MD: Federation of American Societies for Experimental Biology; 1968:344.
29. Bechard LJ, Adiv OE, Jaksic T, Duggan C. Nutritional supportive care. In: Pizzo PA, Poplac D (eds). *Principles and Practice of Pediatric Oncology,* 5th ed. Philadelphia: Lippincott Williams & Wilkins; 2006:1330–1335.
30. Sanders JE, Hoffmeister PA, Storer BA. Treatment of osteopenia/osteoporosis in pediatric hematopoietic cell transplantation [abstract]. *Blood.* 2004;104:57.
31. Zeitler PS, Travers S, Kappy MS. Advances in the recognition and treatment of endocrine complications in children with chronic illness. *Adv Pediatr.* 1999;46:101–149.
32. Holick MF, Chen TC. Vitamin D deficiency: a worldwide problem with health consequences. *Am J Clin Nutr.* 2008;87(Suppl):1080S–1086S.
33. Lappe JM, Travers-Gustafson D, Davies KM, et al. Vitamin D and calcium supplementation reduces cancer risk: results of a randomized trial. *Am J Clin Nutr.* 2007;85:1586–1591.
34. Sadovsky R, Kris-Etherton P. Prescription omega-3-acid ethyl esters for the treatment of very high triglycerides. *Postgrad Med.* 2009;121:145–153.
35. Bays H. Clinical overview of omacor: a concentrated formulation of omega-3 polyunsaturated fatty acids. *Am J Cardiol.* 2006;98:71i–76i.
36. Hawkins DS, Ehling S, Gard K, et al. Nasogastric nutritional support is feasible in pediatric sarcoma patients receiving intensive chemotherapy. Poster presentation at Connective Tissue Oncology Society. 12th Annual Meeting, November 2–4, 2006. Venice, Italy.
37. Sefcick A, Anderton D, Byrne JL, et al. Naso-jejunal feeding in allogeneic bone marrow transplant recipients: results of a pilot study. *Bone Marrow Transplant.* 2001;28:1135–1139.
38. Lenssen P, Bruemmer B, McDonald GB, Aker SN. Nutrient support in hematopoietic cell transplantation. *J Parenter Enteral Nutr.* 2001;25:219–228.
39. Eagle DA, Gian V, Lauwers GY, et al. Gastroparesis following bone marrow transplantation. *Bone Marrow Transplant.* 2001;28:59–62.
40. Papadopoulou A, MacDonald A, Williams MD, et al. Enteral nutrition after bone marrow transplantation. *Arch Dis Child.* 1997;77:131–136.
41. Langdana A, Tully N, Molloy E, et al. Intensive enteral nutrition support in paediatric bone marrow transplantation. *Bone Marrow Transplant.* 2001;27:741–746.
42. Szeluga DJ, Stuart RK, Brookmeyer R, et al. Nutritional support of bone marrow transplant recipients: a prospective randomized clinical trial comparing total parenteral nutrition to an enteral feeding program. *Cancer Res.* 1987;47:3309–3316.

43. Hopman GD, Pena EG, Le Cessie S, et al. Tube feeding and bone marrow transplantation. *Med Pediatr Oncol.* 2003;40:375–379.
44. Charuhas PM, Lipkin A, Lenssen P, McMillen K. Hematopoietic stem cell transplantation. In: Merritt R (ed). *The American Society for Parenteral and Enteral Nutrition Support Practice Manual,* 2nd ed. Silver Spring, MD: ASPEN; 2006:187–199.
45. American Society for Parenteral and Enteral Nutrition. Guidelines for the use of parenteral and enteral nutrition in adult and pediatric patients. *J Parenter Enteral Nutr.* 2002; (1Suppl):1SA–138SA.
46. Uderzo C, Rovelli A, Bonomi M, et al. Total parenteral nutrition and nutritional assessment in leukaemia children undergoing bone marrow transplantation. *Eur J Cancer.* 1991;27:758–762.
47. Yokoyama S, Fujimoto T, Mitomi T, et al. Use of total parenteral nutrition in pediatric bone marrow transplantation. *Nutrition.* 1989;5:27–30.
48. Weisdorf S, Hofland C, Sharp HL, et al. Total parenteral nutrition in bone marrow transplantation: a clinical evaluation. *J Pediatr Gastroenterol Nutr.* 1984;3:95–100.
49. Sanders JE. Growth and development after hematopoietic cell transplant in children. *Bone Marrow Transplant.* 2008;41:223–337.
50. Flowers MED, Storer B, Carpenter P, et al. Treatment change as a predictor of outcome among patients with classic chronic graft-versus-host disease. *Biol Blood Marrow Transplant.* 2008;14:1380–1384.
51. Taskinen M, Saarinen-Pihkala UM, Hovi L, Lipsanen-Nyman M. Impaired glucose tolerance and dyslipidaemia as late effects after bone-marrow transplantation in childhood. *Lancet.* 2000;356:993–997.
52. Hoffmeister PA, Storer BE, Sanders JE. Diabetes mellitus in long-term survivors of pediatric hematopoietic cell transplantation. *J Pediatr Hematol Oncol.* 2004;26:81–90.
53. Nichols WG. Combating infections in hematopoietic stem cell transplant recipients. *Expert Rev Anti Infect Ther.* 2003;1:57–73.
54. Seely D, Stempak D, Baruchel S. A strategy for controlling potential interactions between natural health products and chemotherapy. A review in pediatric oncology. *J Pediatr Hematol Oncol.* 2007;29:32–47.
55. American Cancer Society. *American Cancer Society's Guide to Complementary and Alternative Cancer Methods.* Atlanta, GA: Author; 2000:204–205.
56. Gardiner P, Kemper KJ. Herbs in pediatric and adolescent medicine. *Pediatr Rev.* 2002;21:44–57.
57. McGee J, Patrick RS, Wood CB, Blumgart LH. A case of veno-occlusive disease of the liver in Britain associated with herbal tea consumption. *J Clin Pathol.* 1976;29:788–794.
58. Moody K, Finlay J, Mancuso C, Charlson M. Feasibility and safety of a pilot randomized trial of infection rate: neutropenic diet versus standard food safety guidelines. *J Pediatr Hematol Oncol.* 2006;28:126–133.
59. French MR, Levy-Milne R, Zibrik D. A survey of the use of low microbial diets in pediatric bone marrow transplant programs. *J Am Diet Assoc.* 2001;101:1194–1198.
60. Restau J, Clark AP. The neutropenic diet. Does the evidence support this intervention? *Clin Nurse Spec.* 2008;22:208–211.
61. Anderson JB, Shuster TA, Hanson KE, et al. A camera's view of consumer food-handling behaviors. *J Am Diet Assoc.* 2004;104:186–191.
62. Diagnosis and management of foodborne illnesses: a primer for physicians and other health care professionals. *MMWR.* 2004;53:1–33.
63. Lowe M, Mortensen S. "Room service"—feeding on demand succeeds for cancer patients. *J Am Diet Assoc.* 1995;95(Suppl):A82.
64. Handen BL, Mandell F, Russo DC. Feeding induction in children who refuse to eat. *Am J Dis Child.* 1986;140:52–54.
65. Schauster H, Dwyer J. Transition from tube feedings to feeding by mouth in children: preventing eating dysfunction. *J Am Diet Assoc.* 1996;96:277–281.
66. Bhatia M, Walters MC. Hematopoietic cell transplantation for thalassemia and sickle cell disease: past, present, and future. *Bone Marrow Transplant.* 2008;41:109–117.
67. Bolanos-Meade J, Brodsky RA. Blood and marrow transplantation for sickle cell disease: overcoming barriers to success. *Curr Opin Oncol.* 2009;21:158–161.
68. Schall JI, Zemel BS, Kawchak DA, et al. Vitamin A status, hospitalizations, and other outcomes in young children with sickle cell disease. *J Pediatr.* 2004;145:99–106.
69. Nelson MC, Zemel BS, Kawchak DA, et al. Vitamin B_6 status of children with sickle cell disease. *J Pediatr Hematol Oncol.* 2002;24:463–469.
70. Kennedy TS, Fung EB, Kawchak DA, et al. Red blood cell folate and serum vitamin B_{12} status in children with sickle cell disease. *J Pediatr Hematol Oncol.* 2001;23:165–169.
71. Buison AM, Kawchak DA, Schall J, et al. Low vitamin D status in children with sickle cell disease. *J Pediatr.* 2004;145:622–627.
72. Brown K, Subramony C, May W, et al. Hepatic iron overload in children with sickle cell anemia on chronic transfusion therapy. *J Pediatr Hematol Oncol.* 2009;31:309–312.

CHAPTER 18

Nutrition in Burns

Michele Morath Gottschlich and Theresa Mayes

Burn Injury Challenges

Burn injury poses a complex metabolic challenge that is directly related to subsequent morbidity and mortality. Pediatric burn injury has a high mortality rate.[1] The high incidence of complications in pediatric burn patients is partially attributable to the fact that the unique physical and metabolic features of infants and children are frequently overlooked.

Although the older child rapidly approaches the physical and metabolic makeup of the adult and responds to injury and treatment in a corresponding fashion, specialized nutritional care is required by younger age groups due to their anatomic and physiologic immaturity (see **Table 18-1**). All burned children, however, pose a special challenge to meet obligatory growth needs. Burn injuries represent a particular threat to growth through imposition of a catabolic state. Bone growth is slowed during the acute phase postburn.[2] Furthermore, height and weight gain velocities following the burn injury may not catch up.[3]

A burned child—because he or she has more limited endogenous reserves and greater caloric and protein requirements than an adult—quickly reaches negative nitrogen balance with a smaller area of burn. Furthermore, the functional immaturity of the infant's gastrointestinal (GI) tract and renal system poses a unique challenge to the child's ability to tolerate nonvolitional feeding regimens and nutrient-dense products.[4–6] Burned children are extremely susceptible to diarrhea, dehydration, and malnutrition, which only worsen the degree of catabolism.

Extensive burn injury initiates the most marked alterations in body metabolism that can be associated with any illness. The pattern of physiologic events following thermal injury falls into two phases: the ebb response and the flow response.[7,8] The initial, or ebb, response of the burn syndrome is short, lasting 3 to 5 days postinjury. This phase is characterized by general hypometabolism and is manifested by reductions in oxygen consumption, cardiac output, blood pressure, and body temperature. Fluid resuscitation is conducted during this time in response to the tremendous fluid losses that occur during the early postburn period.

With the resuscitative restoration of circulatory blood volume, the body advances to a prolonged state of hypermetabolism and increased nutrient turnover, termed the *flow phase.* This second phase is influenced by elevations in circulating levels of catecholamines, glucocorticoids, and glucagon.[9–18] Insulin levels are usually in the normal range or even elevated. However, the rise in the glucagon/insulin ratio in combination with other hormonal derangements, initiates gluconeogenesis, lipolysis, and protein degradation.[18] Hypermetabolism and hypercatabolism also vary with the time postburn. Following the ebb phase, catabolic hormone production and oxygen consumption increase dramatically, peaking between the 6th and 10th day following burns.[10,19] Thereafter, the metabolic rate slowly begins to decrease, and a gradual recession of catabolism occurs. These metabolic and hormonal sequelae have important implications from a nutritional perspective.

Fluid and Nutritional Needs

Altered capillary permeability results in the escape of fluid, electrolytes, and protein from the vascular compartment to the interstitial area surrounding the burn wound. The injured area also loses its ability to act as a barrier to water evaporation. In children, with their relatively larger surface area per weight, the insensible water loss is of critical magnitude. Infants and young children are particularly susceptible to a lack of sufficient water intake because of their considerably higher obligatory urinary and insensible water losses, compared with those of adults. Children require more fluid per square meter of body surface area than do adults with burns.[20]

The most popular pediatric fluid replacement formula is the Parkland formula,[21] modified for children (see **Table 18-2**). The modified Parkland formula includes a factor for basal fluid needs, in addition to compensation for losses from the

TABLE 18-1 Anatomic and Physiologic Immaturities of Children of Various Ages

System	Deficit	Clinical Implications	Age of Maturation
Temperature regulation	Labile system Surface area/body weight ratio greatly increased	Increased radiant and evaporative heat loss Increased metabolic rate in an attempt to maintain core temperature	10–12 years
Integument	Thin skin	Heat penetrates more rapidly, with resultant deeper burn	16–18 years
Gastrointestinal	Immature tract Limited surface area of the small intestinal mucosa Decreased gastric volume capacity	Limited capacity to digest or assimilate some nutrients Prone to antigen absorption High incidence of diarrhea	1–2 years
Renal	Glomerular immaturity Young kidneys inefficient in excretion of sodium chloride and other ions, as well as in water resorption	Renal concentrating ability low; therefore, more water required to excrete the renal solute load produced by the metabolism of protein and electrolytes	1–2 years

burn wound. The application of this formula should not replace assessment of the patient's vital signs, blood pressure, and urinary output because these are the ultimate determinants of the adequacy of fluid replacement.

Increased energy expenditure accompanies burn injury. The degree of hypermetabolism is generally related to the size of the burn, with burns of approximately 50% body surface area encountering a peak in energy expenditure.[2,19] Prevention of infection and reducing wound size are the primary means of decreasing metabolic rate. Sufficient pain and anxiety control are also crucial means of reducing metabolism. Application of a reliable pain scale index is vital so that severity of pain is treated appropriately. Children should be offered age-appropriate explanations of procedures and tests prior to their being performed in order to reduce anxiety.

The provision of sufficient calories to meet the increased metabolic expenditure is essential for nutrition management of the burned child. Energy needs may be estimated or measured. A number of pediatric energy equations have been applied successfully in burns (see **Table 18-3**). Energy needs for activity are also greatly reduced in the acute postburn phase.

The wide range of formulas for calculating energy needs is an indication of the uncertainties of this approach. Most mathematic derivations utilize body weight, age, and burn size as the only determinants of caloric requirements. Although these three factors predominately impact the metabolic rate, energy expenditure also is influenced by many other factors, including the following:

- Surgery
- Pain
- Anxiety
- Sepsis

Adequate energy intake is needed to compensate for hypermetabolism, growth, and development. Administering excessive calories should be avoided, because it may cause increased metabolic rate, hyperglycemia, and liver abnormalities and an increase in carbon dioxide production.[22,23]

Indirect calorimetry is a viable option in assessing energy expenditure in pediatric burn patients. In general, the patient's caloric goal should be calculated at 120–130% of the measured resting energy expenditure (REE).[24–26] Although some degree of error is possible with this extrapolation, it is more accurate than estimates based solely on weight, age, and burn size. To ensure the clinical validity of this goal, tests must be repeated at least twice weekly for proper adjustment of the nutritional support regimen.

Metabolic changes that occur following thermal injury include deranged carbohydrate metabolism. Early in the response to burns, glycosuria and hyperglycemia frequently occur. A predisposition to glucose intolerance correlates with the severity of the burn injury. Elevated blood glucose is also modulated by the phase of injury. During the shock phase, hyperglycemia is primarily caused by decreased peripheral tissue utilization in lieu of impaired tissue perfusion and low insulin levels.[27,28] Glucose intolerance typically persists during the flow phase.[27]

Carbohydrate is the most important nonprotein calorie source in terms of nitrogen retention in burned patients.[29] However, excessive glucose loads should be avoided, and all burn patients should be monitored for hypercapnia and hyperglycemia.[30–32] Exogenous insulin administration is often necessary to improve blood glucose levels and to achieve maximal glucose utilization. Intensive insulin therapy that maintains blood glucose levels significantly below previous thresholds correlates with reduced morbidity and mortality in

TABLE 18-2 Pediatric Fluid Calculations for Resuscitation and Maintenance

I. Resuscitation

A. Calculated resuscitation + basal requirement (less than 2 yrs: 2000 cc/m^2 BSA)

1. (4 cc × ____ kg × ____ % burn) + (1500 cc × _____ m^2 BSA)

   (_______) + (_______) = _____cc/24 hours

B. Resuscitation fluid per 8 hours

1. 1st 8 hours: give ½ of total calculated cc/24 hours
2. 2nd 8 hours: give ¼ of total calculated cc/24 hours
3. 3rd 8 hours: give ¼ of total calculated cc/24 hours

II. Maintenance Fluids

A. Basal fluid requirement: 1500 cc/m^2 BSA (less than 2 yrs: 2000 cc/m^2 BSA)

1. Total body surface area ________ m^2 BSA
2. 24 hours __________cc

B. Evaporative water loss

1. Adults: (25 + % burn) m^2 BSA = cc/hr
   Children: (35 + % burn) m^2 BSA = cc/hr
2. Calculated evaporative water loss
   a. (_____ + _____ % burn) _____ m^2 BSA = ______cc/hr; ________ cc/24 hours

C. Total maintenance fluids = basal requirement + evaporate water loss

1. 24 hours __________ cc
2. Hourly __________ cc

Example calculation for a 7-year-old patient weighing 25 kg, with a 45% TBSA burn, 0.95 m^2 BSA

I. Resuscitation

A. Calculated resuscitation + basal requirement

1. (4 cc × 25 kg × 45% burn) + (1500 cc × 0.95 m^2 BSA)

   (4500 cc) + (1425 cc) = 5925 cc/24 hours

B. Resuscitation fluid per 8 hours

1. 1st 8 hours: give ½ of total calculated cc/24 hours = 2962 cc, 370 cc/hr
2. 2nd 8 hours: give ¼ of total calculated cc/24 hours = 1481 cc, 185 cc/hr
3. 3rd 8 hours: give ¼ of total calculated cc/24 hours = 1481 cc, 185 cc/hr

II. Maintenance Fluids

A. Basal fluid requirement: 1500 cc/m^2 BSA

1. Total body surface area 0.95 m^2 BSA
2. 24 hours 1425 cc

B. Evaporative water loss

1. Adults: (25 + % burn) × m^2 BSA = cc/hr
   Children: (35 + % burn) × m^2 BSA = cc/hr
2. Calculated evaporative water loss
   a. (35 + 45% burn) × 0.95 m^2 BSA = 76 cc/hr; 1824 cc/24 hours

C. Total maintenance fluids = basal requirement + evaporate water loss

1. 24 hours: 1425 cc + 1824 cc = 3249 cc/24 hours
2. Hourly: 3249 cc/24 hours = 135 cc/hr

Abbreviations: BSA, body surface area; TBSA, total body surface area.

Source: Courtesy of the Shriners Hospitals for Children, Cincinnati, Ohio.

TABLE 18-3 Formulas for Calculating Energy Requirements of Burned Children

Source	Age	%TBSA Burned	Calories/Day
Curreri	0–1 yr	< 50	Basal + (15 × % BSAB)
	1–3 yr	< 50	Basal + (25 × % BSAB)
	4–15 yr	< 50	Basal + (40 × % BSAB)
Davies and Liljedal	Child	Any	60W + (35 × % BSAB)
Hildreth	< 15 yr	> 30	(1800/m^2 BSA) + (2200/m^2 burn)
Hildreth	< 12 yr		(1800/m^2 BSA) + (1300/m^2 burn)
Mayes	0–3 yr	10–50	108 + 68W + (3.9 × % BSAB) 818 + 37.4W + (9.3 × % BSAB)

Abbreviations: W, weight in kg; BSA, body surface area burn; TBSA, total body surface area.

critical care.[33-36] As a result, insulin protocols are used in the burn intensive care unit and result in improved outcomes.[37-41]

The protein requirements of the burned infant and child are elevated because of accelerated tissue breakdown and exudative losses during a period of rapid repair and growth. Failure to meet heightened protein needs can result in delayed wound healing and resistance to infection. The infant and child further adapt to inadequate protein intake by curtailing growth of cells, conceivably sacrificing genetic potential.

Enteral fortification with large quantities of protein can accelerate the synthesis of visceral proteins and promote positive nitrogen balance and host defense factors.[24,42-47] Infants and children older than 6 months of age with burns in excess of 30% TBSA should receive 20–23% of calories as protein.[7,43,48] This translates to 2.5–4.0 g/kg, for a nonprotein calorie/nitrogen ratio of 80:1. Other factors that influence protein repletion, assuming an adequate intake of energy, include the quality of dietary protein. As a result intact, whey protein is encouraged.

Close monitoring of protein intake is necessary because excessive protein loads or amino acid imbalances may result in azotemia, hyperammonemia, or acidosis. Feeding high-protein formulas to infants younger than 1 year of age should be avoided, because excessive amounts can have adverse effects on immature or compromised kidneys. Ongoing assessment of fluid status, blood urea nitrogen (BUN), plasma proteins, and nitrogen balance is recommended for individual evaluation of tolerance and adequacy. However, a high-protein diet is usually well tolerated when fluid intake is adequate, renal or hepatic dysfunction does not exist, and pathways of intermediary metabolism are relatively mature.

During the flow phase, burn-mediated increases in catecholamine and glucagon levels stimulate an accelerated rate of fat mobilization and oxidation. Lipid is important to the diet of the burned child because of its high caloric density, its role in myelination of nerve cells and brain development, the palatability it imparts to food, and its role as a carrier for the fat-soluble vitamins.

Two to 3% of calories from linoleic acid are needed to prevent omega-6 fatty acid deficiency. This requirement is usually easy to achieve because most enteral feeding supplements and intravenous fat emulsions contain high levels of fat and linoleic acid.[24,48,49] An overabundance of dietary lipid, however, can be detrimental to recovery from burns.[50] Complications of excessive fat intake include lipemia, fatty liver, diarrhea, and decreased resistance to infection.[49-51] Lipid also appears to be an inefficient source of calories for the maintenance of nitrogen equilibrium and lean body mass following major injury.[52-54]

Conservative use of fat, particularly linoleic acid, given its immunosuppressive metabolites, is recommended for burned children older than 6 months of age.[3,24] Providing a source of omega-3 fatty acid is recommended.[24,51]

Vitamin and mineral requirements increase with the severity of thermal injury and are related to the following:

- Heightened protein synthesis
- Enhanced caloric expenditure
- Increased micronutrient losses

Individual vitamin and mineral needs also are dependent on preburn status.

Oral, tube feeding, and intravenous hyperalimentation regimens frequently do not meet the heightened needs for certain micronutrients. Thus, additional supplementation must be provided.[49,50,55-62] Thiamine, riboflavin, niacin, folate, biotin, vitamin K, magnesium, phosphorus, chromium, and manganese are all cofactors for energy-dependent processes. The requirement for pyridoxine is closely related to dietary protein intake and protein metabolism. Vitamin B_{12}, folate, and zinc are cofactors for collagen synthesis. Furthermore, inadequacy of many micronutrients, particularly vitamins A, C, E, and pyridoxine, as well as zinc, copper, and iron inadequacies, can adversely affect immune function. Iron supplementation may not be needed[24] because excessive iron also enhances susceptibility to infection.[63]

Hypovitaminosis D should be avoided in pediatric burn patients.[59,64] In the acute postburn phase, the rate of bone demineralization is high, resulting in increased risk of fractures.[65-67] Burn patients are at risk for bone disease for a variety of reasons, including extended bed rest, institutionalization, increased glucocorticoids, and decreased growth hormone. The most effective means to treat this acute deficiency is to supplement with vitamin D_3. In addition, vitamin D depletion can occur even during convalescence, potentially impacting long-term bone growth and development in pediatric burn patients.[68,69]

A daily intake of a multivitamin and supplemental vitamins A, C, and D as well as zinc are usually needed. Extensive bleeding following burns and burn surgeries is common. The provision of therapeutic levels of intravenous vitamin K may be helpful, specifically in the postoperative period or while on antibiotic therapy. Although select vitamin and mineral replacement in excess of the RDAs appears to be justified in burned children, some micronutrients, particularly fat-soluble vitamins, are toxic in large amounts. Thus, all micronutrients should be administered judiciously.

Nutritional Strategies

The goal of nutritional support for the pediatric burn patient is to provide adequate calories and nutrients to facilitate wound healing, maximize immunocompetence, maintain or improve organ function, and prevent loss of lean body mass. Special consideration is indicated whenever fluid restriction, organ failure, septicemia, mechanical ventilation, or any other presenting condition limits the body's ability to obtain vital nutrients.

Small burns (less than 20% surface area) not complicated by facial injury, psychologic problems, inhalation injury, or preburn malnutrition can usually be supported by an oral high-protein, high-calorie diet that includes between-meal snacks. Commercial meal-replacement beverages or the addition of nutrient modules to menu and snack selections may be helpful in boosting intake.

Children with burns covering a larger surface area (20% or more) generally cannot meet their nutrient requirements by oral intake alone. The enteral route is preferred over intravenous.[49,70,71] Gastric feedings are not used for many reasons, including postburn gastric ileus, which often inhibits the initial advancement and full-volume delivery of enteral feedings. In addition, nasogastric feeding increases the risk for aspiration due to the multiple position changes that patients undergo for dressing changes, physical therapy, and operative procedures. Gastric feedings also potentiate limited oral intake because the patient minimally experiences hunger.

Enteral alimentation that bypasses the stomach and uses the functional small intestine is desirable. Feeding tube placement into the third portion of the duodenum can be a safe means of providing enteral nutritional even during septic ileus.[72,73] Small bowel feedings permit minimal interruption of the nutrition regimen, thereby maximizing nutrient intake.

In general, enteral nutrition should commence as soon as possible postburn. Aggressive enteral support often results in improved tube-feeding tolerance and sustained bowel mucosal integrity.[49,71,74] Furthermore, the hypermetabolic response can be partially suppressed, as evidenced by decreased energy expenditure and improvements in measurements of nitrogen balance, visceral proteins, and catabolic hormones.[43,71,75,76] Early feeding reduces cumulative caloric deficits and potentially stimulates insulin secretion while conserving lean body mass.

Because burn patients usually have unscathed digestive and absorptive capabilities, products containing intact nutrients should be used. Elemental or dipeptide formulations are usually not indicated in burns.[77] Most tube feedings can be started at full strength. The initial hourly infusion rate should begin at approximately half of the final desired volume and be increased by 5 mL/hour in the infant and toddler, 10 mL/hour in the school-age child, and 20 mL/hour in the teenager, as tolerated, until the final hourly goal rate is achieved.

As oral intake improves and nutrient needs decrease, the child can be gradually weaned from the tube feeding regimen. Initially, tube feedings can be held at mealtime to stimulate appetite. Once the patient demonstrates the ability to consume 25–50% of caloric needs by mouth, tube feedings may be necessary only at night. Eventually, when the patient is able to meet approximately 75% or greater of caloric needs orally, tube feedings can be discontinued.

The composition of the enteral infusate should take into account the unique metabolic and age-related alterations in nutrient utilization that accompany an extensive burn injury. Tube feeding regimens for pediatric burn patients include the following:

1. Those appropriate for children younger than 6 months of age
2. Those for patients 6 months of age or older

Enteral protocols for infants younger than 6 months of age are generally conservative, relying on commercial infant formulas. The normal dilution of infant formula is 20 kcal/oz. Gradually advancing the concentration to 24 kcal/oz is routinely safe. Further progression to 27–30 kcal/oz to meet the infant's energy needs must be monitored carefully, due to the increased renal solute load.

The protein content of infant formulas ranges from 9–12% of total calories. This level is sometimes insufficient for those with large surface area burns. The addition of a protein module to the infant formula may be indicated with close monitoring. Soy formulas should not be used unless casein or whey intolerances have been confirmed. Reducing the fat content is not recommended during infancy because fat is an extremely important nutrient during the period of central nervous system maturation.

Tube-feeding products for children older than 6 months of age can generally be selected from adult formulas containing 30 kcal/oz. If the tube feeding product selected is low in protein,[6,50,56,78] products should be enriched with protein modules to yield 20–23% of their energy content as protein.

No commercially manufactured tube feeding formulas specifically designed for the burn patient are on the market. However, this patient population has atypical nutritional needs that transcend traditional recommendations for a high-calorie, high-protein solution. Modular tube feeding recipes offer the only means of incorporating findings regarding unique fat, amino acid, vitamin, and mineral requirements.[24,49,76,79] Use of modular tube feeding is correlated with reductions in infection rates and length of hospital stay.[24] However, because complex recipes are not always feasible, evaluation of available enteral products looking for a high-protein, low-fat, low-linoleic acid, omega-3 fatty acid–enriched product is recommended as a practical alternative.

Parenteral Nutrition

Although the GI tract is the preferred route of nutritional support, under certain circumstances intravenous feeding is a critical part of burn management. Appropriate indications for intravenous feeding in burns are listed in **Table 18-4**. If at all possible, however, at least some nutrients should be administered enterally via trophic feeds during episodes of diarrhea.

TABLE 18-4 Indications for Total Parenteral Nutrition in Burns

- Gastrointestinal trauma
- Curling's ulcer
- Severe pancreatitis
- Superior mesenteric artery syndrome
- Obstructions of the gastrointestinal tract
- Severe vomiting or abdominal distention
- Intractable diarrhea
- Adjunct to insufficient enteral support
- Necrotic bowel

Peripheral parenteral support does not provide adequate calories and nitrogen, and the delivery of intravenous nutrients via a central line is necessary.[80] Standard central venous regimens usually consist of a final concentration of 25% dextrose and 5% crystalline amino acids.

If essential fatty acid requirements are being met in the trophic enteral feeds, then additional intravenous fat may not be needed. Patients receiving 100% of their energy needs via the parenteral route require the administration of intravenous fat. Five hundred milliliters of 10% lipid emulsion (or 250 mL of 20% lipid emulsion) infused two to three times weekly will meet essential fatty acid requirements.

PN should be reserved for only those patients who cannot meet their nutritional needs enterally. This is due to the numerous metabolic and mechanical complications of parenteral hyperalimentation and the high incidence of septic morbidity. (See also Chapter 20 on parenteral nutrition.) Strict adherence to infection-control standards and continuous monitoring of tolerance are needed. Every attempt should be made to advance the enteral feeding rate with subsequent decrease in parenteral nutrition to minimize the risks of immunosuppression.

Nutrition Assessment

Nutritional assessment includes identifying each individual's energy and nutrient requirements and evaluating the adequacy of enteral or parenteral nutrition intakes. Assessment and monitoring of the patient's response to diet therapy is important so that treatment changes can be made to reduce the risk of complications. Unique components of a nutrition assessment and reassessment include: percent total body surface area burned, percent full thickness burn, indirect calorimetry, and 24-hour urine for nutrition balance determinations. Monitoring calorie and protein intake and laboratory data such as prealbumin is essential. Discharge planning should include an assessment of oral intake, the need for nutrition supplements, and outpatient follow-up.

Case Study

Nutrition Assessment of Infant Burn Patient

Nutrition Assessment

TD is a previously healthy, 11-month-old female admitted to the intensive care unit. She suffered 40% total body surface area (TBSA) burns, 35% full thickness, when she pulled on the electric cord of a frying pot, tipping the container. The hot liquid splattered over her face, head, neck, and right side of her upper body and thigh.

In anticipation of face and neck swelling over the course of the next few hours, TD is sedated and intubated to maintain oxygen and airway. A nasogastric tube is placed to low wall suction. Her abdomen is soft and nondistended. She is 9 kg in weight and 74 cm in length. Her intravenous resuscitative fluids are infusing to maintain a urine output of approximately 1.0 mL/kg/hour. Past medical history is noncontributory. Labs are initially monitored every 6 hours, and electrolyte adjustment, glucose management, blood product replacement, and ventilator therapies are coordinated with respective panel results. A nutrition history from the mother indicated that the baby is beginning to wean from the bottle and increasing her intake of baby foods and soft table foods. She accepts a pacifier at afternoon nap and bedtimes. The patient has no known food allergies or intolerances.

Nutrition Intervention

TD's initial goals for calorie, protein, and micronutrients were established. Within 6 hours of admission to the unit, feeding tube placement is confirmed in the upper portion of the duodenum. Given her adequate hydration status and hemodynamic stability (i.e., lack of vasopressor use), the tube feeding (TF) rate is initiated at 5 mL per hour and advanced every 2 hours by 5 mL to a goal of 35 mL per hour. The goal TF rate provides 95% of kcal and 103% of protein goals.

TD undergoes surgery six times. Each excision procedure is followed by a 24-hour period of stabilization prior to donor site harvest and skin grafting over the burned areas. Enteral feeds are continued through surgery to ensure adequate nutritional support throughout the perioperative period.[73]

While on mechanical ventilatory support, oral stimulation is provided during physical therapy sessions. As TD progresses and sedation is weaned, a pacifier is provided for comfort as well as oral stimulation. Given her young age, she maintains a high risk for subsequent oral feeding coordination deficiencies due to prolonged NPO status. The pacifier supports skills necessary for eventual oral feeding coordination.

The patient's endotracheal tube is uncuffed, so indirect calorimetry is not possible initially; however, once extubated, indirect calorimetry is performed biweekly. The TF rate is adjusted based on a 30% addition to the resting energy expenditure. This ensures sufficient calories to cover additional metabolic influences such as fever spikes, pain, anxiety, dressing changes, therapy sessions, and the like that are not an inherent component of the test.

Following extubation on postburn day 10, TD is permitted an oral diet. Clear liquids are provided via bottle and accepted well. Gastrointestinal tolerance is deemed appropriate and the diet is therefore advanced to regular, age-appropriate provision. As wounds are increasingly covered, appetite improves and tube feedings are tapered. When TD is consuming 20% of the calorie goal consistently for a period of 2 days, feeds are tapered to be held 2 hours at meal times. When her wounds are 95% covered and she is accepting 80% of her nutrition goal orally, the feeding tube is discontinued.

Nutrition Monitoring and Assessment

The enteral regimen is assessed daily for calorie and protein intake and gastrointestinal tolerance. TD's clinical course is evaluated daily for parameters related to nutritional status and regimen tolerance. These include surgery, labs including fluid and electrolytes, infection, antibiotic use, respiratory status, physical therapy gains (e.g., head control, sitting up independently in a high chair, feeding self), and wound status. BUN/creatinine levels are assessed daily to ensure proper balance of fluids/hydration status. Glucose levels and need for insulin supplementation are monitored daily; however, the enteral regimen is not changed when insulin needs are increased. The preference for carbohydrate versus fat calories for wound healing supersedes a regimen change to a higher fat formula in an effort to assist glucose management. As TD's clinical course progresses, the appropriateness of an enteral feeding taper is evaluated daily.

Discharge

On postburn day 39, TD is discharged to home. She has 98% wound coverage. TD is at 95% of her preburn weight. She is eating well, having improved to 90% of her estimated goal, and her diet is similar to that consumed prior to injury. TD does not require any nutritional supplementation at this time.

Questions for the Reader

1. What are the TD's energy, protein, and micronutrient supplementation needs upon admission to the burn unit (weight = 9 kg)?
2. What are TD's weight and height percentiles on the growth chart upon admission?
3. Complete a PES statement for this patient.
4. What type of tube feeding product was recommended for TD?
5. What other weekly assessment parameters were closely monitored in TD?
6. What type of nutritional follow-up will TD receive in the outpatient clinic?

REFERENCES

1. Sheridan RL, Remensnyder JP, Schnitzer JJ, et al. Current expectations for survival in pediatric burns. *Arch Pediatr Adolesc Med.* 2000;154:245–249.
2. Klein GL, Herndon DN, Rutan TC, et al. Bone diseases in burn patients. *J Bone Miner Res.* 1993;8(3):337–345.
3. Rutan RL, Herndon DN. Growth delay in postburn pediatric patients. *Arch Surg.* 1990;125:392–395.
4. Grybowski JD. Gastrointestinal function in the infant and young child. *Clin Gastroenterol.* 1977;6:253–265.
5. Lebenthal E, Lee PC. Development of functional response in human exocrine pancreas. *Pediatrics.* 1980;66:556–560.
6. Spitzer A. The role of the kidney in sodium homeostasis during maturation. *Kidney Int.* 1982;21:539–545.
7. Gottschlich M, Alexander JW, Bower RH. Enteral nutrition in patients with burns or trauma. In: Rombeau JL, Caldwell MD (eds). *Enteral and Tube Feeding,* 2nd ed. Philadelphia: WB Saunders; 1990:306–324.
8. Cuthbertson DP, Zagreb H. The metabolic response to injury and its nutritional implications: retrospect and prospect. *J Parenter Enteral Nutr.* 1979;3:108–130.
9. Aikawa N, Caulfield JB, Thomas RJS, et al. Post burn hypermetabolism: relation to evaporative heat loss and catecholamine level. *Surg Forum.* 1975;26:74–76.
10. Wilmore DW, Long JM, Mason AD, et al. Catecholamines: mediators of the hypermetabolic response to thermal injury. *Ann Surg.* 1974;180:653–669.
11. Bane JW, McCaa RE, McCaa CS. The pattern of aldosterone and cortisone blood levels in thermal burn patients. *J Trauma.* 1974;14:605–611.
12. Jeshke MG, Chinkes D, Finnerty C, et al. Pathophysiologic response to severe burn injury. *Ann Surg.* 2008;248:387–401.
13. Vaughn GM, Becker RA, Allen JP, et al. Cortisol and corticotrophin in burned patients. *J Trauma.* 1982;22:263–273.
14. Wilmore DW, Lindsey CA, Moylan JA, et al. Hyperglucagonemia after burns. *Lancet.* 1974;1:73–75.
15. Johoor F, Herndon DH, Wolfe RR. Role of insulin and glucagon in the response of glucose and alanine kinetics in burn-injured patients. *J Clin Invest.* 1986;78:807–814.
16. Orton CI, Segal AW, Bloom SR, et al. Hypersecretion of glucagon and gastrin in severely burned patients. *Br Med J.* 1975;2:170–172.

17. Nygren J, Sammann M, Malm M, et al. Disturbed anabolic hormonal patterns in burned patients: the relation to glucagons. *Clin Endocrinol.* 2008;43:491–500.
18. Nair KS, Halliday D, Matthews DE, Welle SL. Hyperglucagonemia during insulin deficiency accelerates protein catabolism. *Am J Physiol Endocrinol Metab.* 1987;253:E208–E213.
19. Wilmore DW. Nutrition and metabolism following thermal injury. *Clin Plast Surg.* 1974;1:603–619.
20. Barrow RE, Jeschke MG, Herndon DN. Early fluid resuscitation improves outcomes in severely burned children. *Resuscitation.* 2000;45:91–96.
21. Baxter CR, Shires T. Physiological response to crystalloid resuscitation of severe burns. *Ann NY Acad Sci.* 1968;150:874–894.
22. Klein CJ, Stanek GS, Wiles CE. Overfeeding macronutrients to critically ill adults. *Metab Complications.* 1998;98:795–806.
23. Aarsland A, Chinkes D, Wolfe RR. Hepatic and whole-body fat synthesis in humans during carbohydrate overfeeding. *Am J Clin Nutr.* 1997;65:1774–1782.
24. Gottschlich MM, Jenkins M, Warden GD, et al. Differential effects of three enteral regimens on selected outcome parameters. *J Parenter Enteral Nutr.* 1990;14:225–236.
25. Kagan RJ, Gottschlilch MM, Mayes T, Warden GD. Estimation of calorie needs in the thermally injured child. *Proc Am Burn Assoc.* 1995;27:283.
26. Wilmore DW, Goodwin CW, Aulick LH, et al. Effect of injury and infection on visceral metabolism and circulation. *Ann Surg.* 1980;192:491–500.
27. Gauglitz GG, Herndon DN, Jeschke MG. Insulin resistance postburn: underlying mechanisms and current therapeutic strategies. *J Burn Care Res.* 2008;29:683–694.
28. McGowen KC, Malhotra A, Bistrian BR. Stress-induced hyperglycemia. *Crit Care Clin.* 2001;17:107–124.
29. Hart DW, Wolf SE, Zhang X-J, et al. Efficacy of a high-carbohydrate diet in catabolic illness. *Crit Care Med.* 2001;29:1318–1324.
30. Barrocas A, Tretola R, Alonso A. Nutrition and the critically ill pulmonary patient. *Respir Care.* 1983;28:50–61.
31. Askanazi J, Rosenbaum SH, Hyman AI, et al. Respiratory changes induced by large glucose loads of total parenteral nutrition. *JAMA.* 1980;243:1444–1447.
32. Young VR, Motil KJ, Burke JF. Energy and protein metabolism in relation to requirements of the burned pediatric patient. In: Suskind RM (ed). *Textbook of Pediatric Nutrition.* New York: Raven Press; 1981:309–340.
33. Van den Berghe G, Wouters P, Weekers F, et al. Intensive insulin therapy in critically ill patients. *N Engl J Med.* 2001;345:1359–1367.
34. Van den Berghe G, Wouters P, Bouillion R, et al. Outcomes benefit of intensive insulin therapy in the critically ill: insulin dose versus glycemic control. *Crit Care Med.* 2003;31:359–366.
35. Van den Berghe C, Wilmer A, Hermans G, et al. Intensive insulin therapy in the medical ICU. *N Engl J Med.* 2006;354:449–461.
36. Collier BC, Diaz J, Forbes R, et al. The impact of a normoglycemic management protocol on clinical outcomes in the trauma intensive care unit. *J Parenter Enteral Nutr.* 2005;29:353–359.
37. Cochran A, Davis L, Morris SE, Saffle JE. Safety and efficacy of an intensive insulin protocol in a burn-trauma intensive care unit. *J Burn Care Res.* 2008;29:187–191.
38. Hemmila MR, Taddonio MA, Arbabi S, et al. Intensive insulin therapy is associated with reduced infectious complications in burn patients. *Surg.* 2008;144:629–635.
39. Pham TN, Warren AJ, Phan HH, et al. Impact of tight glycemic control in severely burned children. *J Trauma.* 2005;59:1148–1154.
40. Thomas SJ, Morimoto K, Herndon DN, et al. The effect of prolonged euglycemic hyperinsulinemia on lean body mass after severe burn. *Surg.* 2002;132:341–347.
41. Jeschke MG, Klein D, Herndon DN. Insulin treatment improves the systemic inflammatory reaction to severe trauma. *Ann Surg.* 2004;239:553–560.
42. Alexander JW, MacMillan BG, Stinnett JD, et al. Beneficial effects of aggressive protein feeding in severely burned children. *Ann Surg.* 1980;192:505–517.
43. Dominioni L, Trocki O, Mochizuki H, et al. Prevention of severe postburn hypermetabolism and catabolism by immediate intragastric feeding. *J Burn Care Rehabil.* 1984;5:106–112.
44. Serog P, Baigts F, Apfelbaum M, et al. Energy and nitrogen balances in 24 severely burned patients receiving 4 isocaloric diets of about 10 MJ/m^2/day (2392 kcal/m^2/day). *Burns.* 1983;9:422–427.
45. Saito H, Trocki O, Wang S, et al. Metabolic and immune effects of dietary arginine supplementation after burn. *Arch Surg.* 1987;122:784–789.
46. Dominioni L, Trocki O, Fang CH, et al. Nitrogen balance and liver changes in burned guinea pigs undergoing prolonged high-protein enteral feeding. *Surg Forum.* 1983;34:99–101.
47. Dominioni L, Trocki O, Fang CH, et al. Enteral feeding in burn hypermetabolism: nutritional and metabolic effects of different levels of calorie and protein intake. *J Parenter Enteral Nutr.* 1985;9:269–279.
48. Gottschlich MM. Acute thermal injury. In: Lang CE (ed). *Nutritional Support in Critical Care.* Gaithersburg, MD: Aspen Publishers; 1987:159–181.
49. Gottschlich MM, Warden GD, Michel MA, et al. Diarrhea in tube-fed burn patients: incidence, etiology, nutritional impact and prevention. *J Parenter Enteral Nutr.* 1988;12:338–345.
50. Mochizuki H, Trocki O, Dominioni L, et al. Optimal lipid content for enteral diets following thermal injury. *J Parenter Enteral Nutr.* 1984;8:638–646.
51. Gottschlich MM, Alexander JW. Fat kinetics and recommended dietary intake in burns. *J Parenter Enteral Nutr.* 1987;11:85–89.
52. Long JM, Wilmore DW, Mason AD, et al. Effect of carbohydrate and fat intake on nitrogen excretion during total intravenous feeding. *Ann Surg.* 1977;185:417–422.
53. Souba WW, Long JM, Dudrick SJ. Energy intake and stress as determinants of nitrogen excretion in rats. *Surg Forum.* 1978;29:76–77.
54. Freund H, Yoshimura N, Fischer JE. Does intravenous fat spare nitrogen in the injured rat? *Am J Surg.* 1980;140:377–383.
55. Gottschlich MM, Warden GD. Vitamin supplementation in the burn patient. *J Burn Care Rehabil.* 1990;11:275–279.
56. Gamliel Z, DeBiasse MA, Demling RH. Essential microminerals and their response to burn injury. *J Burn Care Rehabil.* 1996;17:264–272.
57. Jenkins ME, Gottschlich MM, Kopcha R, et al. A prospective analysis of serum vitamin K and dietary intake in severely burned pediatric patients. *J Burn Care Rehabil.* 1998;19:75–81.
58. Gottschlich MM, Mayes T, Khoury J, Warden GD. Hypovitaminosis D in acutely injured pediatric burn patients. *J Am Diet Assoc.* 2004;104:931–941.
59. Pochon JP. Zinc and copper replacement therapy: a must in burns and scalds in children? *Prog Pediatr Surg.* 1981;14:151–172.

60. King N, Goodwin CW. Use of vitamin supplements for burned patients: a national survey. *J Am Diet Assoc.* 1984;84:923–925.
61. Council on Scientific Affairs. Vitamin preparations as dietary supplements and as therapeutic agents. *JAMA.* 1987;257: 1929–1936.
62. Shippee RL, Wilson SW, King N. Trace mineral supplementation of burn patients: a national survey. *J Am Diet Assoc.* 1987;87:300–303.
63. Weinberg ED. Iron and susceptibility to infectious disease. *Science.* 1974;184:952–956.
64. Klein GL, Langman CB, Herndon DN. Vitamin D depletion following burn injury in children: a possible factor in post-burn osteopenia. *J Trauma.* 2002;52:346–350.
65. Klein GL, Herndon DN, Langman CB, et al. Long term reduction in bone mass after severe burn injury in children. *J Pediatr.* 1995;126:252–256.
66. Klein GL, Herndon DN, Rutan TC, et al. Bone disease in burn patients. *J Bone Miner Res.* 1993;8:337–345.
67. Mayes T, Gottschlich MM, Scanlon J, Warden GD. Four year review of burns as an etiologic factor in the development of long bone fractures in pediatric patients. *J Burn Care Rehabil.* 2003;24:279–284.
68. Klein GL. The interaction between burn injury and vitamin D metabolism and consequences for the patient. *Curr Clin Pharmacol.* 2008;3:204–210.
69. Klein GL, Chen TC, Holick MF, et al. Synthesis of vitamin D in skin after burns. *Lancet.* 2004;363:291–292.
70. Saito H, Trocki O, Alexander JW, et al. The effect of route of nutrient administration on the nutritional state, catabolic hormone secretion, and gut mucosal integrity after burn injury. *J Parenter Enteral Nutr.* 1987;11:1–7.
71. Saito H, Trocki O, Alexander JW. Comparison of immediate postburn enteral versus parenteral nutrition. *J Parenter Enteral Nutr.* 1985;9:115.
72. Gottschlich MM. Early and perioperative nutrition support. In: Matarese L, Gottschlich MM (eds). *Contemporary Nutrition Support Practice.* Philadelphia: WB Saunders; 1998:265–278.
73. Jenkins M, Gottschlich M, Baumer T, et al. Enteral feeding during operative procedures. *J Burn Care Rehabil.* 1994;15:199–205.
74. Mochizuki H, Trocki O, Dominioni L, et al. Mechanism of prevention of postburn hypermetabolism and catabolism by early enteral feeding. *Ann Surg.* 1984;200:297–310.
75. Jenkins M, Gottschlich M, Waymack JP, et al. An evaluation of the effect of immediate enteral feeding on the hypermetabolic response following severe burn injury. *Proc Am Burn Assoc.* 1988;112.
76. Jenkins M, Gottschlich MM, Alexander JW, et al. Enteral alimentation in the early postburn phase. In: Blackburn GL, Bell SJ, Mullen JL (eds). *Nutritional Medicine: A Case Management Approach.* Philadelphia: WB Saunders; 1989:1–5.
77. Trocki O, Mochizuki H, Dominioni L, et al. Intact protein versus free amino acids in the nutritional support of thermally injured animals. *J Parenter Enteral Nutr.* 1986;10:139–145.
78. Gottschlich MM, Alexander JW, Jenkins M, et al. Burns. In: Blackburn GL, Bell SJ, Mullen JL (eds). *Nutritional Medicine: A Case Management Approach.* Philadelphia: WB Saunders; 1989:6–9.
79. Bell SJ, Molnar JA, Carey M, et al. Adequacy of a modular tube feeding diet for burned patients. *J Am Diet Assoc.* 1986;86: 1386–1391.
80. Gottschlich MM, Warden GD. Parenteral nutrition in the burned patient. In: Fischer JE (ed). *Total Parenteral Nutrition.* Boston: Little Brown & Co.; 1991:270–298.

CHAPTER 19

Enteral Nutrition

Lisa Simone Sharda

Enteral nutrition (EN), or enteral nutrition support (ENS), is the delivery of nutrition in the form of glucose, protein, and/or lipid directly into the gastrointestinal (GI) tract via a tube, catheter, or stoma. Indications for EN are a functioning GI tract of sufficient length and absorptive capacity. Infants and children meeting these criteria who possess the inability to consume adequate nutrition via the oral cavity are candidates for EN.[1,2]

EN often is preferred over parenteral nutrition (PN) because it is associated with fewer complications and is less expensive.[3–5] Advances in commercial formulas and equipment for the delivery of EN have made enteral feeding safe and efficacious to administer to pediatric patients in either the hospital or home setting.

This chapter provides practical guidelines for:

- Selecting appropriate pediatric candidates for EN
- Selecting specific products
- Administering and monitoring enteral feedings
- Considering specific factors of the pediatric population

Note that enteral feeding of the premature infant is addressed in Chapter 4 of this book.

Patients can receive EN in hospitals, rehabilitation facilities, and at home. The healthcare team should establish inpatient and outpatient criteria for consideration of EN. Nutrition screening should identify patients who are failing to thrive from either inorganic or organic sources or those who possess feeding disorders that affect their ability to ingest adequate nutrition. Factors to evaluate include:[3,5]

- Usual caloric intake of less than 80% of needs
- Weight maintenance or loss
- Weight-to-length or weight-to-height ratio below the 5th percentile
- Excessive feeding time
- Oral and/or texture aversion
- Mechanical problems with mastication, swallowing, or peristalsis

Pediatric patients with a variety of diseases who are at nutritional risk have been shown to benefit from EN (see **Exhibit 19-1**). Specific screens can be developed for a particular disease state or condition, as the need arises.[6–9] When EN is contraindicated due to severe intestinal dysfunction (see **Exhibit 19-2**), PN constitutes the appropriate route for specific nutritional support (see Chapter 20).

Enteral Products

Enteral formulas are classified by the U.S. Food and Drug Administration (FDA) as medical foods. *Medical foods* are defined as "a food which is formulated to be consumed or administered enterally under the supervision of a physician."[1] Medical foods are not regulated as either conventional foods or drugs.[10] Infant formula must meet FDA assurances of nutrition quality, as well as labeling criteria, nutrient content standards, and manufacturers' quality control procedures.

A wide variety of commercially prepared infant, pediatric, and adult enteral formulas can be utilized for pediatric patients requiring EN. The proper product selection is contingent on a number of factors related to the specific medical and nutritional status of the patient. Patient-specific factors include:

- Age
- Gastrointestinal function
- History of feeding tolerance
- Nutrient requirements
- Feeding route

Several formula-specific factors also must be considered prior to choosing an enteral formula, including osmolality, renal solute load, nutrient complexity, product availability, cost, and caloric density.

Age Considerations

Human milk and/or commercial infant formulas constitute the most appropriate feedings for infants younger than 1 year

EXHIBIT 19-1 Indications for Enteral Nutrition in the Pediatric Patient

Functional
1. Neurologic disorders
2. Neuromuscular disorders
3. Prematurity
4. Inability to take in adequate nutrition
5. Genetic/metabolic disorders

Structural
1. Congenital anomalies
   a. Tracheoesophageal fistula
   b. Esophageal atresia
   c. Cleft palate
   d. Pierre Robin syndrome
2. Obstruction
   a. Cancer of head/neck
   b. Intubation
3. Injury
   a. Ingestions
   b. Trauma
   c. Sepsis
4. Surgery

EXHIBIT 19-2 Potential Complications for Enteral Nutrition in Pediatric Patients

- Acute pancreatitis
- Gastrointestinal obstruction
- Inflammatory bowel disease
- Intestinal atresia
- Limited or impaired absorptive surface
- Necrotizing enterocolitis
- Overwhelming sepsis
- Side effects of cancer therapy

of age. (See also Chapters 4 and 5.) Human milk provides the optimal food for infants and offers many immunologic and nutritional benefits.[3] Infants who are unable to nurse at the breast can receive pumped breast milk through a feeding tube. However, the mother must be taught safe methods for the collection and storage of her milk.[11] Breast milk administration techniques also should be devised and implemented.

Continuous drip feedings of human milk have been associated with appreciable fat losses, which result in a significant reduction of energy delivered to the infant.[12] These losses occur because the fat in human milk separates and collects in the infusion system. A caloric loss of approximately 20% is typical. The delivery of essential fatty acids, phospholipids, cholesterol, and associated fat-soluble vitamins also may be diminished. It should be noted that when residual milk is flushed from the tubing, a large fat bolus may be delivered to the patient. Patients with impaired gastrointestinal function may not tolerate a fat bolus.

When delivering a continuous feeding of breast milk, the use of refrigerated milk may be advantageous.[13] Unfortunately, significant fat losses still occur. If continuous feedings of expressed breast milk are required, combining the expressed breast milk with a liquid fortifier or other liquid formulas can promote more efficient delivery of breast milk nutrients via tube.[11] Use of a syringe pump helps to decrease the adherence of fat to the feeding pump bag and tubing. It is also advantageous to invert the syringe pump to encourage any separation of fat to be pushed through the pump first.

Intermittent bolus feeding of human milk does not result in a significant loss of fat in the tubing or the terminal delivery of a large fat bolus. Therefore, intermittent bolus feeding is the preferred method of delivery for the tube feeding of human milk, whenever possible.

Iron-fortified infant formulas are an appropriate substitute for infants who are not able to receive breast milk. Concentrated or powdered infant formulas should be reconstituted with sterile water. When available, the use of a nutritionally appropriate sterile liquid infant formula is preferred, such as liquid-concentrated formulas or ready-to-feed formulas.[1]

A broad range of tube feeding products are available and are listed in **Table 19-1**. Most manufacturers' product guides have detailed information about the indicated use of formulas and their absorption/utilization routes.[14–19]

The standard dilution for infant formulas is 20 kcal/oz. In many cases, a more concentrated formula may be needed. As described in Chapter 5, infant formulas can be concentrated cautiously to a maximum of 30 kcal/oz (without modular additives) by adding less water to a concentrated liquid or powdered formula base.[20] If human milk is used, it can be "concentrated" with the addition of powdered infant formula. When this formula base (or human milk) is concentrated, the infant's water balance in relation to renal solute load should be monitored. Patients on formulas concentrated to more than 120% (24 kcal/oz)[21] should be monitored frequently for signs of dehydration, as noted by irregular output of urine, stool, or emesis; high urine specific gravity; or nutrient imbalances.

Guidelines for fluid needs are as follows:

- Use 100 mL/kg for the first 10 kg of body weight.
- For weights of 10–20 kg, use 1000 mL plus 50 mL/kg for each kg over 10 kg.
- For weights over 20 kg, use 1500 mL plus 20 mL/kg for each kg over 20 kg.[22,23]

TABLE 19-1 Characteristics of Selected Enteral Formulas

Formula Classification	Product Classification	Possible Indications for Use	Infant Formula up to 12 Months	Pediatric Formula 1 to 10 Years	Adult Formula 10+ Years
Standard milk-based (SMB)	Intact protein Contains lactose Long-chain triglycerides Moderate residue Low to moderate osmolality	Normally functioning GI tract Lactose tolerance	Human milk Abbott Laboratories Similac Advanced Mead Johnson Enfamil Lipil Nestle Good Start Bright Beginnings Gentle		
Standard milk-based altered	Intact protein Electrolyte manipulation (low iron, altered calcium, phosphorous) Low renal solute load Lactose free Added starch	Renal, endocrine conditions Lactose intolerant Mild reflux	Abbott Laboratories PM 60/40 Mead Johnson Enfamil AR Abbott Labs Similac Sensitive RS	Abbott Laboratories Pediasure‡ Nestle Compleat Pediatric‡ Resource Boost Nutren Junior‡ Kid Essentials	Abbott Laboratories Ensure Products Jevity‡ Osmolite‡ Nestle Compleat‡ Boost Nutren‡ Carnation Instant Breakfast Impact
Standard soy lactose free	Intact protein Low-moderate residue Low-moderate osmolality	Primary lactose deficiency Secondary lactose deficiency (intestinal injury or PEM) Galactosemia	Abbott Laboratories Isomil Products Mead Johnson Prosobee Nestle Good Start Soy Plus	Bright Beginnings Soy Pediatric Drink	
Standard added fiber	Intact protein Lactose free 4.3–14 g fiber/1000 mL Low-moderate osmolality	Constipation Diarrhea Normal digestive/absorptive capacity	Abbott Labs Isomil DF	Abbott Laboratories Pediasure with fiber‡ Nestle Nutrition Compleat Pediatric‡ Nutren Jr with fiber‡ Bright Beginnings Soy drink with fiber	Abbott Laboratories Ensure with fiber Jevity‡ Osmolite Nestle Nutrition Compleat‡ Boost Nutren‡ Impact with fiber
Lactose free/ modified fat	Intact protein Fat content 88% MCT 12% long-chain triglycerides	Chylothorax Intestinal lymphangiectasia, severe steatorrhea, cholestasis, liver disease	Nutricia North America Monogen‡	Mead Johnson Portagen‡ Nestle Nutrition Vivonex Pediatric‡	Mead Johnson Portagen‡

(continues)

TABLE 19-1 (Continued)

Formula Classification	Product Classification	Possible Indications for Use	Infant Formula up to 12 Months	Pediatric Formula 1 to 10 Years	Adult Formula 10+ Years
Semi-elemental	Hydrolyzed protein Lactose free Low-moderate osmolality Partial MCT content	Steatorrhea Intestinal resection Cystic fibrosis Chronic liver disease Inflammatory bowel disease Diarrhea associated with hypoalbuminemia Allergy to cow's milk and soy proteins Not needed for jejunal feedings in patients with normal GI function	Abbott Laboratories Alimentum Advanced‡ Mead Johnson Pregestimil Lipil‡ Nutramigen Lipil	Abbott Laboratories Vital Junior‡ Nestle Nutritionals Peptamen Junior‡	Abbott Laboratories Vital HN‡ Nestle Nutritionals Peptamen‡
Elemental	Protein as free amino acids Lactose free High osmolality Low fat Carbohydrate in form of glucose oligosaccharides	Intestinal fistula Glycogen storage disease Chylothorax, intestinal lymphangiectasia not responsive to Monogen Short gut syndrome HIV + inflammatory bowel disease	Mead Johnson Nutramigen AA Nutricia Neocate Infant‡ Neocate Nutra‡ Abbott Laboratories Elecare‡	Nestle Nutrition Vivonex Pediatric‡ Nutricia Neocate One Plus‡ Neocate Junior‡ Pediatric E028‡ Pepdite Junior‡ Abbott Laboratories Elecare‡	Nestle Nutrition Vivonex Plus‡ Vivonex RTF‡ Vivonex TEN‡ Tolerex
Calorically dense	Intact protein Lactose free High renal solute load High osmolality 1.5–2.0 kcal/mL	Fluid restriction Increased metabolic needs Not recommended for transpyloric feeds		Nestle Nutrition Boost Kid Essentials	Abbott Laboratories Oxepa Pulmocare TwoCal HN Nestle Nutritionals Boost High Protein Fibersource HN Isosource HN Isosource 1.5 Nutren Replete‡ Nutren 1.5 ‡ Nutren 2.0‡ Resource 2.0‡ Impact 1.5

Premature	Increased calories Increased calcium, phosphorous, protein	Premature infants for first year of life	Abbott Laboratories Similac Neosure‡ Similac Special Care‡ Mead Johnson Enfamil Enfacare‡ Bright Beginnings NeoCare	
Follow-up	Over 1 year of age iron fortified Balanced nutrition with vitamins, minerals			Mead Johnson Enfamil Next Step Enfamil Next Step Soy Abbott Laboratories Similac Advanced-2 Bright Beginnings Follow-On Formula Nestle Nutrition Good Start 2

‡ Contains medium-chain triglycerides (MCT) as part of total fat.

Source: Mead Johnson, referenced on December 20, 2009, http://www.enfamil.com; Abbott Laboratories, referenced on December 20, 2009, http://www.abbott.com; Nestle Nutrition, referenced on December 20, 2009, http://www.nestle-nutrition.com; Bright Beginnings, referenced on December 20, 2009, http://www.brightbeginnings.com; Nutricia North America, referenced on December 20, 2009, http://www.nutricia.com.

Fluid should be adjusted frequently based on weight changes. Insensible water loss should be factored in, as well as additional needs caused by any medical condition.

If insensible water losses are high, it is advisable to concentrate the base formula (or human milk) to 24 kcal/oz. The caloric density can be further increased by using modular additives of carbohydrate (glucose polymers) or fat (e.g., vegetable oil, medium-chain triglycerides [MCT]). Carbohydrate and fat additives do not increase the renal solute load; however, carbohydrate additives can cause a moderate increase in osmolality. With the addition of a long-chain triglyceride, gastric emptying time may be decreased. This effect may be clinically significant for those patients who are at risk for aspiration and already have delayed gastric emptying.

Increases in caloric density of the tube feeding are best tolerated by the patient when advanced gradually in increments of 2–4 kcal/oz/day.[20] Formulas that consist of a base concentration of 24–26 kcal/oz and also contain modular additives of fat (e.g., 0.25–0.50 g corn oil/oz, 2.5–5.0 kcal/oz, respectively) and/or carbohydrates (e.g., 0.5–1.0 g glucose polymer/oz, 2–4 kcal/oz, respectively) are generally tolerated by infants. The change in the percentage of calories from carbohydrate and fat and the ratio of protein/100 calories by the addition of modulars must be taken into account when offered to infants.

Table 19-2 contains three comparisons of nutrient percentages and the percentage change with modulars. Patients on concentrated formulas should be monitored closely and changed to a more appropriate distribution of macronutrients, as tolerated.

The distribution of calories in breast milk is approximately 6–7% calories from protein, 50–52% calories from fat, and 40–43% from carbohydrate. In infant formulas, it is 8–12% calories from protein, 45–50% calories from fat, and 40–45% calories from carbohydrate.[14,15,24–26]

Protein intakes accounting for more than 16% of calories could contribute to azotemia and negative water balance if associated fluid intakes are low. Established protein needs are 2.5–3.3 grams per 100 calories. A minimum of 2.2 g/kg is recommended for infants younger than 3 months and a minimum of 1.8 g/kg for infants older than 3 months.[27] Additionally, high carbohydrate intakes may contribute to osmotic diarrhea, and fat intakes that exceed 60% of the formula calories could lead to ketosis.

Diluting formula to less than 20 kcal/oz should be done only with careful consideration and monitoring because of the risk of hyponatremia, diluted or insufficient nutrients, and/or excess fluid.[21,28]

Feedings for children between 1 and 10 years of age include a choice of pediatric follow-up formulas, pediatric enteral formulas, and/or various homemade blenderized feedings. The caloric density of feedings utilized for children in this age group can range from 30–60 kcal/oz. The caloric density of an enteral formula may need to be increased with the use of a modular if the patient has increased metabolic needs and/or decreased fluid tolerance.

Formulas designed for pediatric enteral feedings must meet the daily recommended dietary allowances (RDAs) or the adequate intakes (AIs) in a volume of 900–1300 mL per day (see Appendix F).[24–26] These enteral products are isotonic and lactose free, with a partial MCT content to facilitate absorption.

Under specific conditions, infant formulas can be continued through 4 years of age. Additional vitamin or mineral supplementation may also be needed, depending on the specific volume provided. Infant formulas have a lower renal solute load than do products designed for patients who are older than 1 year of age. These formulas may be more appropriate for malnourished toddlers who may actually be infant size.

Standard milk-based, lactose-free, elemental, fiber-containing, and calorically dense formulas are commercially

TABLE 19-2 Nutrients in Different Concentrations and Formula Recipes

+ 4 kcal/oz Formula	24 kcal/oz from Standard Dilution	24 kcal/oz from Liquid Concentrates	20 kcal/oz Formula Powder or 20 kcal/oz Corn Oil
Oz per 100 calories	5	4.16	3.57
Cholesterol (g/oz)	2.4	2.5	2.5
% calories	43	43	36
Protein (g/oz)	0.43	0.51	0.51
% calories	9	9	7
Fat (g/oz)	1.08	1.3	1.82
% calories	48	48	57
Protein (g per 100 kcal)	2.14	2.14	1.82

available for children between the ages of 10 and 18 years. For these children, many factors must be considered, such as maturation level, physical ability or limitations, calorie requirements, and volume tolerance. Adolescent nutrient needs increase with the last growth phase. A pediatric formula may meet an adolescent's calorie and protein needs, but it will not satisfy other nutrient needs, such as those for calcium, sodium, and iron. It is important to assess the adequacy of the micronutrients provided by the volume of formula, particularly when assessing the intake of a child who requires low volumes to promote growth.

Tube Feeding Products

Blenderized feedings consist of a mixture of various meats, fruits, vegetables, milk (or formula), carbohydrates, fats, water, vitamins, and minerals that have been blenderized and strained. Blenderized feedings are moderate in residue and moderate to high in osmolality and viscosity. Because their high viscosity hinders flow through small feeding tubes, these feedings are most often administered as gastrostomy tube feedings. Other disadvantages of blenderized feedings include a potentially high bacteria count[11–13,29] and the additional labor required for preparation. Homemade blenderized feedings:

- Provide a more variable nutrient content than do commercially manufactured products
- Are not emulsified
- Can be used only when enteral feeding is delivered into the stomach
- May not provide all essential nutrients in the level required by a pediatric patient

Blenderized feedings can be used when third-party reimbursement or support is not provided. Because inappropriate homemade tube feedings can result in hypernatremic dehydration[20] and a number of nutrient deficiencies, it is important to perform a periodic analysis of the recipe, including verification of how the family is making the formula at home, the adequacy of the nutrients, and the associated fluids. It is equally important to monitor the intake of protein and electrolytes because excess may lead to a negative water balance in the patient.[23,29]

A large variety of adult enteral products are commercially available. As with adolescent formulas, they can also be divided into several general categories: standard milk-based, lactose-free, elemental, fiber-containing, and calorically dense. General characteristics of selected adult enteral products with possible indications for use are provided in Table 19-1. This list is not inclusive of all products that are commercially available, and information regarding the complete nutrient composition is readily available from various manufacturers (e.g., Abbott, Mead Johnson, Novartis).

It should be noted that adult enteral products are not designed for use in children. Specific concerns regarding the use of these products in children include issues such as renal solute load, osmolality, and nutrient requirements.

Tube Feeding Considerations

The renal solute load (RSL) of a formula consists primarily of electrolytes and metabolic end products of protein metabolism that the kidneys must excrete in the urine.[21] These solutes require water for urinary excretion and therefore have a major effect on water balance. Infants are at particular risk for negative water balance and subsequent dehydration. Potential renal solute load (PRSL) does not need to be calculated routinely, but is important to determine with patients who have medical problems or formula prescriptions that would influence renal metabolism. Equations for PRSL vary in the units of measurement for solute load.[3] An example of an equation for determining the PRSL:

$$\text{PRSL (mOsm/L)} = \text{mEq sodium/L} + \text{mEq potassium/L} + \text{mEq chloride/L} = [4 \times \text{protein g/L}]$$

The RSL and fluid balance should be closely monitored when infants have a low fluid intake, are receiving calorically dense feedings, or have increased extrarenal fluid losses (i.e., fever, diarrhea, sweating) and/or impaired renal concentrating ability.[21] Neurologically impaired infants and children who are unable to indicate thirst may also be at risk for dehydration.

Infant formulas at standard dilution contain approximately 90% free water[14–16,25] (preformed water plus water of oxidation). In contrast, standard pediatric and adult enteral formulas contain approximately 85% free water. Adult formulas are higher in protein and electrolytes and RSL. As a result, when administering adult products to infants and toddlers, additional water may be required and can usually be given while flushing the feeding tube.

Osmolality refers to the number of active particles in a kilogram of solution. The osmolality of a formula may affect tolerance. Feeding a hyperosmolar formula may result in delayed gastric emptying, abdominal distention, vomiting, or diarrhea. Carbohydrates, electrolytes, and amino acids are the major factors that determine the gastrointestinal osmotic load of a formula. Smaller particles, such as glucose and free amino acids, contribute more to a higher osmolality than do larger particles, such as polysaccharides or intact protein molecules. Thus, formulas that contain hydrolyzed protein and monosaccharides will have a higher osmolality than will formulas with intact protein and glucose polymers.

Osmolality recommendations for infant formulas are less than 460 mOsm/kg.[21] The osmolality in formulas for infants and children younger than 4 years should be less than

400 mOsm/kg and for older children under 600 mOsm/kg.[30] The osmolality of infant formulas at a caloric density of 20 kcal/oz generally falls below this suggested limit (range of 200–380 mOsm/kg). Several pediatric and adult enteral products exceed this limit at a caloric density of 30 kcal/oz and may require a dilution to two-thirds strength prior to use in infants. Medications can also increase osmolality significantly and should be evaluated prior to selecting a formula.[23] The osmolality of Pregestimil, for example, concentrated to 27 kcal/oz is approximately 446 mOsm/kg, whereas a multivitamin with iron (Poly-Vi-Sol with Iron) at 10 mg/mL Fe is 10,683 mOsm/kg.[23]

Nutrient Requirements

Nutrient adequacy depends on the enteral feeding being used and other factors. In certain circumstances, both infant and adult formulas may require vitamin and/or mineral supplementation. Supplements may not be absorbed or utilized in the body as desired and should be evaluated frequently. Infant formulas generally provide adequate amounts of vitamins and minerals with a volume of 1 quart. However, infants who have restricted fluid intakes (e.g., infants with congenital heart disease) may require vitamin and mineral supplementation.

Adult enteral formulas are designed to provide the adult RDAs for vitamins and minerals when a volume of 1500–2000 mL/day is administered. However, when these adult enteral products are administered to children at lower volumes, some nutrients may not be adequate. A micronutrient analysis may be warranted.

Product Selection

The cost of commercial enteral formulas may exceed the financial resources of some families. Therefore, whenever medically possible, the least specialized enteral product should be considered. The more specialized the feedings are (e.g., hydrolyzed protein, MCT oil), the higher will be the cost.

Formula costs do not necessarily constitute a socioeconomic barrier. Infants and children who range in age from birth to 5 years may be enrolled in the Women, Infants, and Children (WIC) nutrition program if their family income falls below a certain level. A variety of infant and pediatric formulas are available through this program. The Medicaid program and private insurance companies may cover enteral formulas and needed supplies, such as tubes, bags, or pumps. Coverage varies, and the healthcare team should work closely with home care companies and insurers to ensure that the patient obtains the best coverage possible. Letters of medical necessity are sometimes helpful in obtaining coverage for a specific enteral feeding product.

Feeding Routes

Common routes for EN in pediatric patients include nasogastric, nasoduodenal, nasojejunal, gastrostomy, and jejunostomy feedings. The risk of aspiration becomes a major consideration when determining whether the tube should be placed in the stomach or small intestine. If the patient is determined to have a high risk of aspiration due to GER, a gastrostomy tube is placed surgically. Fundoplication (surgical repair for GER) can sometimes be beneficial in reducing GER; however, postoperative complications can range from retching to dumping syndrome, swallowing problems, impaired esophageal emptying, slow feeding, and abdominal distention. **Figure 19-1** gives criteria for making a decision as to whether to use a nasogastric or enterostomy feeding route.[31]

A direct gastric feeding is preferable to an intestinal feeding because it allows for a more normal digestive process. This is generally true because the stomach serves as a reservoir and provides for a gradual release of nutrients into the small bowel. Gastric feedings are associated with a larger osmotic and volume tolerance, a more flexible feeding schedule, easier tube insertions, and a lower frequency of diarrhea and dumping syndrome. In addition, gastric acid has a bactericidal effect that may be an important factor in decreasing the patient's susceptibility to various infections.

Nasogastric (NG) feeding tubes are used for the short term (4 to 6 weeks). Patients requiring long-term EN should be evaluated to determine the best enteral device to meet their needs (such as a gastrostomy [g] tube). Nasogastric feeding is contraindicated in patients with severe esophagitis or who have an intestinal obstruction between the nose and stomach. In addition, nasogastric tubes may not be tolerated in neonates, who are obligate nose breathers. To prevent airway occlusion in this instance, orogastric tubes are often used when tube feeding is indicated.

Nasoduodenal, nasojejunal, or gastrojejunal feeding is desirable for patients who are at risk of aspiration or who are unable to tolerate feedings into the stomach. These tubes, however, may fail secondary to tube occlusion or tube dislodgement and interrupt tube feeding and medication schedule.[31,32]

Nasojejunal feeding may be more efficacious than nasoduodenal feeding in preventing aspiration.[33] Nasojejunal tubes are less likely than nasoduodenal tubes to become dislodged in children with cystic fibrosis, who may experience severe coughing episodes. This is also true for children with cancer, who may have vomiting associated with chemotherapy. A potential complication of transpyloric feeding is intestinal perforation with use of stiff, large-bore tubes.[34] Use of small-bore tubes made of polyurethane or silicone might decrease the incidence of this complication; however, it may increase the incidence of tube clogging.

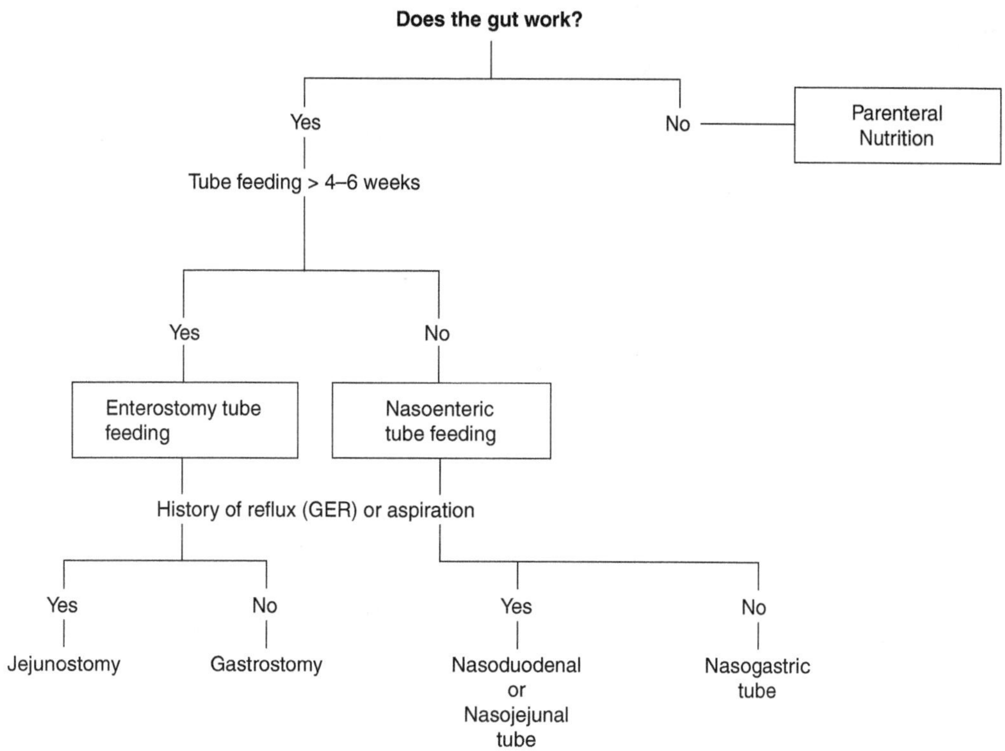

FIGURE 19-1 Decision Making for Selecting the Feeding Site

Source: Adapted with permission from Enteral and tube feedings, Figure 16-1, page 263. In: Rombeau JL, Caldwell MD, eds., *Clinical Nutrition*, vol. 1. © 1984, WB Saunders Co.

Endoscopically placed gastrostomies or jejunostomies (PEG/PEJ) are less invasive and require less time under anesthesia. Enteral feedings, although safer than parenteral nutrition, are not without complications (see **Table 19-3**).[35]

Tube Feeding Delivery

The enteral feeding delivery is contingent on the patient's clinical condition and the anatomic location of the tube (gastric or transpyloric). Continuous drip and intermittent bolus administration are the two methods most often used for delivery of enteral feedings to infants and children. Intermittent bolus feedings are generally delivered to the stomach by gravity over 15 to 30 minutes on a schedule of every 2 to 4 hours or via pump over a 1-hour period several times during 24 hours. Bolus feeding more closely mimics a normal oral feeding pattern and is often preferred for this reason. Bolus feeds are typically used during the day as opposed to overnight because of the increased likelihood of GER with bolus feeds.[31,36] Intermittent feedings better facilitate transition to a home setting and eventual weaning off of enteral feeds.

In contrast, the continuous drip method provides an infusion of nutrients at a constant rate over several hours. Continuous drip feedings are beneficial for patients who cannot tolerate bolus feedings or those with altered gastrointestinal function and are essential for those receiving enteral transpyloric or nocturnal feedings. Continuous feedings require the use of a feeding pump to deliver formula at a consistent rate.

In many cases, a combination of intermittent bolus feeds during the day and a continuous drip overnight is used. Each delivery method provides a number of specific advantages and disadvantages (see **Exhibit 19-3**).

Enteral feeding pumps are typically used to control the rate of delivery of continuous drip feedings and bolus feedings. A number of enteral feeding pumps are available for use in pediatric patients.[37] Portable enteral pumps or backpack pumps allow for greater patient mobility during enteral feeding.

Important features of enteral pumps for use in the pediatric population include the ability to provide low delivery rates (less than 5 mL/hour) and to advance in small increments

TABLE 19-3 Complications of Enteral Feeding

Complication	Possible Causes	Management/Prevention
Gastrointestinal		
Aspiration pneumonia	Aspiration of feedings	Confirm placement of tube prior to administration of feeds.
	Emesis	
	Displacement or migration	
	Supine position during feeds	Elevate head 30–45 degrees.
	Gastrointestinal reflux	
	Presence of nasogastric tube preventing complete closure of esophagus	Tube placement into the duodenum.
	Delayed gastric emptying	Use prokinetics.
Bloating/cramps, gas	Air in tubing	Remove as much air as possible when setting up feed.
Diarrhea	Bacterial contamination of formula	Proper storage, preparation and administration of feeds. Change feeding bag daily. Limit hang time to 4 hours for commercially prepared formula. Undiluted "ready to feed" products minimize risk.
	Food allergies	Consider changing to a lactose-free formula.
	Hyperosmolar formula	Consider changing formula to an isotonic formula.
	Too rapid infusion	Decrease rate of infusion to previously tolerated rate.
	Low fiber intake	Consider using formula containing fiber.
	Fat malabsorption	Consider changing formula to a product with partial MCT content.
	Medications (antibiotics), antacids, sorbitol, magnesium, antineoplastic agents	
Dumping syndrome	Cold formula	Administer formula at room temperature.
	Rapid feeding	Decrease infusion rate.
Vomiting	Hyperosmolar formula	Consider changing formula to an isotonic product.
	Delayed gastric emptying	Consider transpyloric route. Consider continuous infusion. Elevate head of bed 45 degrees during feeding. Check for residuals prior to feedings.
	Obstruction	Consider utilizing prokinetics. Discontinue feedings.
	Too rapid advancement of volume/concentration	Return to previously tolerated strength/volume, and advance more slowly.
Mechanical		
Clogged tubing	Inadequate flushing	Flush tube before and after aspirating residuals, after bolus feedings, and every 4–8 hours during continuous feedings.
	Inadequate crushing of medications	Dissolve crushed tablets in warm water. Use liquid form of medications when available.
	Formula and medication residual	Flush tube before and after medication administration. Avoid mixing formula with medication.
	Kinking of tubing	Replace feeding tube.
	Highly viscous fiber rice formulas	

Tube displacement	Coughing Vomiting Inadvertent dislodgment Removal of tube by patient	Replace feeding tube.
Metabolic		
Dehydration	Inadequate free water Hyperosmolar formulas	Monitor intake and output. Monitor hydration status routinely. Assess renal solute load of formula.
Overhydration	Excessive fluid administration Too rapid refeeding of patients with moderate to severe PEM	Advance feedings slowly. Allow a 5- to 7-day period to reach nutritional goals.
Electrolyte imbalance	Formula components Medical condition/diagnosis	Evaluate electrolyte adequacy of specific formula and appropriateness of formula dilution. Monitor electrolytes, phosphorus, BUN, creatinine, and glucose.
Failure to achieve appropriate weight gain	Inadequate nutrient intake	Evaluate adequacy of nutrient intake. Perform routine nutritional assessments.
Psychologic		
Fear of tube insertion	Psychologic trauma associated with insertion of nasogastric tube/gastrostomy	Utilize relaxation techniques. Medical play: allow child to handle tube and insert tube in doll. Comfort child after insertion. Consider sedation prior to replacement of tube.
Altered body image	Visible presence of nasogastric tube or gastrostomy tube	Consider nocturnal feedings and removal of tube during the day. Consider use of low-profile gastrostomy device.
Food refusal	Deprivation of normal oral feeding experiences	Initiate oral feedings when medically possible. Provide positive oral experience during tube feedings. Refer to speech therapist.

Source: Data from Grumow JE, Al-Hafidh AS, Tunell WP. Gastroesophageal reflux following percutaneous endoscopic gastrostomy in children. *J Pediatr Surg*. 1989;24:44–45.

EXHIBIT 19-3 Methods of Delivering Enteral Feedings

Continuous Drip Feedings

Advantages:

1. Ability to increase volume of formula more rapidly
2. Improved absorption of major nutrients in infants with intestinal diseases
3. Reduced stool output in hypermetabolic patients
4. Associated with a reduced incidence of vomiting in infants with gastroesophageal reflux
5. Greater caloric intake when volume tolerance may be a problem

Disadvantages:

1. More expensive feeding method because a pump is required for delivery
2. Restricts patient ambulation
3. Less physiologic

Intermittent Feedings

Advantages:

1. More physiologic because a normal feeding schedule is mimicked
2. Less expensive because an enteral pump is not required
3. Greater flexibility in feeding schedule
4. Freedom from infusion equipment
5. Improved nitrogen retention with less fat and fluid accumulation

Disadvantages:

1. Associated with a longer time to reach nutritional goals
2. Reduced weight gain and nutrient absorption in infants with malabsorption
3. Larger-bore tube may be required for gravity administration
4. More time required for administration than for pump-delivered feedings

(1–5 mL/hour). This, and many other features, contribute to the safe and efficient delivery of continuous tube feedings for the pediatric population.

Because the required volumes of human milk are often low, particularly with continuous infusions, a syringe pump is typically used to deliver human milk via an enteral feeding system. The use of the syringe pump also helps to avoid the adherence of fat to the feeding bag.[1]

In cases where enteral feeding pumps are not used, enteral formula can be delivered by gravity infusions either as intermittent or continuous drip. The feeding bag is suspended on a bedside pole, and the rate depends on the height of the feeding bag. The delivery rate is not precise and often predisposes the patient to gastroesophageal reflux or aspiration.[38]

The rate of advancement of a feeding regimen (see **Exhibit 19-4**) is contingent on the structure and function of the patient's gastrointestinal tract and should be guided by the patient's age, underlying disease, nutrition status, and nutritional requirements as well as the enteral access device.[24,33]

Isotonic formulas should be used initially at a rate of 1–2 mL/kg/hour for children < 35 kg and at a rate of 1 mL/kg/hour for children > 35 kg. Changes in volume and concentration should never be made simultaneously. Stable and/or older patients may be able to tolerate a rapid increase in the enteral feedings rate, generally reaching the nutritional goal within a 24- to 48-hour time frame.[1,36]

Diluting enteral feedings in the initial stages is not necessary and may increase the risk of microbial contamination.[37,39] However, diluted formulas can be considered for patients with altered gastrointestinal function or when transitioning to enteral feeding from parenteral nutrition. Volume of the tube feeding should be increased before its concentration is increased when administering transpyloric feedings. Advance concentration before volume when delivering gastric feedings. If feeding intolerance develops, return to the previously tolerated concentration and volume and advance at a slower rate with caution.

For intermittent feedings, determine the total volume of a full strength, isotonic formula needed to provide the nutritional goal. A volume of 2.5–5 mL/kg (or 25% of goal volume for day 1) can be given over five to eight bolus feedings per day. Feedings can be gradually advanced by 25% per day to reach the desired goal volume. Bolus feeds may be further increased in volume to reduce the number of feedings per day. Feedings can be administered via pump over 1 hour or by gravity over 15 to 30 minutes.[11] Bolus feedings should be given during the same period of time as it would take the child to consume the same volume orally.

EXHIBIT 19-4 Initiation and Advancement of Feedings

*Continuous Drip Feeding**

Age	Weight Maximum Range (kg)	Volume Range (mL/kg/d)	Initial Rate (mL/h)	Advancement Rate (mL/h)	Rate (mL/h)
Infant	3–10	125–160	1	1.5–3	25–50
Toddler/preschool	10–20	110–130	1	5–10	60–70
School age	20–40	70–110	2	5–10	80–100
Teenage	> 40	60–80	2	20–100	100–150

*Intermittent Feedings***

			Suggested Advancement***	
Age	Weight (kg)	Kcal/kg	1st day (mL)	Advance to and Evaluate for Tolerance (mL)
Infant	3–10	98–108	250	1000
Toddler/preschool	10–20	70–100	450	1800
School age	20–40	60–90	675	2700
Teenage	> 40	40–55	700	2800

*Adjust per needs, tolerance, and medical condition

**Adjust to needs and intake by mouth

***Divided over number of feeds

Sources: Data from Texas Children's Hospital. *Pediatric Nutrition Reference Guide*, 8th ed. Houston, TX: McGraw-Hill Professional; 2008; and American Academy of Pediatrics. *Pediatric Nutrition Handbook*, 6th ed. Elk Grove, IL: American Academy of Pediatrics: 2009:552–554.

For continuous feedings, the total volume of a full strength, isotonic formula needed to meet nutritional needs must be determined. Feedings should be initiated at 1–2 mL/kg/hour and advance by 0.5–1 mL/kg/hour every 6–12 hours as tolerated until the goal volume is reached. Maximum volumes for continuous or bolus feeds are determined by the individual child's tolerance.

Infants and children who are being weaned from parenteral nutrition and/or who are malnourished generally require a more conservative feeding progression than what is typically administered to children who have normal gastrointestinal function. (See also Chapter 20 on parenteral nutrition.)

Potential complications are generally classified into gastrointestinal, mechanical (tube-related), metabolic, and psychologic categories. A summary of the most common complications and associated management suggestions is presented in Table 19-3.

Formulas that require reconstitution or manipulation (dilution or additives) are at the greatest risk for bacterial contamination.[41] In contrast, the use of sterile, undiluted, ready-to-feed products minimizes the risk of contamination (see **Exhibit 19-5**).[4,24,33,39] Precautions to guard against the contamination of enteral feedings include frequently changing the feeding bag tubing, paying careful attention to clean technique during handling of the feedings, and limiting hang time of the formulas. Specific recommendations for preparation, administration, and monitoring of enteral feedings to maximize bacteriologic safety are available, and disposable enteral feeding bags should not be reused.[40,41] When nutritionally appropriate, sterile liquid formulas are recommended for all enteral feedings. Breast milk and all formulas either decanted, with modular additives, reconstituted, or diluted should hang no longer than 4 hours.[1,14] Enteral formula in a closed system is safe for a 24-hour hang time.[38,39]

Transition to Oral Intake

Many factors must be considered before weaning the patient off a tube feeding. Typically, the transition is done slowly

EXHIBIT 19-5 Guidelines for Storage and Administration of Enteral Feedings (in hours)*

Product	Storage Time Room Temp	Storage Time in Refrigerator	Hang Time[1]	Bag Change	Tubing Change
EBM/EBM with fortifiers[2]	2	24	2/2–4[5]	4	4
Sterile formula,[3] nonsterile with additives, or powdered formula[4]	< 4	24	4	4	4
Infant, pediatric, and adult sterile, canned/bottled liquid products	8	48	4	8	Infant 8 Pediatric 24
Closed system formula	24	48	24	24	24

*See references for neonates and immune-compromised patients. Manufacturer's guidelines and/or hospital policy should be followed for any manipulation of enteral nutrition products. Equipment with ice packs may be used in overnight delivery, but temperatures must be checked routinely to ensure safety. All enteral nutrition products should be placed in food-grade containers.

1. Hang time includes all periods of time that the product is not refrigerated below 45°F (i.e., transport time; tubing or equipment setup).
2. For hospitalized infants.
3. Sterile feeds include industrially produced, prepacked liquid formulas that are "commercially sterile."
4. Nonsterile feedings are those that may contain live bacteria and include hospital- or home-prepared formulas, reconstituted powdered feedings, and commercial liquid formulas to which nutrients and/or other supplements have been added in the hospital kitchen, pharmacy, unit, school, or home. Powdered formula is not recommended for neonates or immune-compromised patients, unless there is no alternative available.
5. One manufacturer recommends 2 hours and other companies recommend 4 hours.

Sources: Data from Lavine M, Clark RM. The effect of short-term refrigeration of milk and addition of breast milk fortifier on the delivery of lipids during tube feeding. *J Pediatr Gastroenterol Nutr.* 1989;8:496–499; Texas Children's Hospital. *Pediatric Nutrition Reference Guide*, 8th ed. Houston, TX: McGraw-Hill Professional. 2008; and American Academy of Pediatrics. *Pediatric Nutrition Handbook*, 6th ed. Elk Grove, IL: American Academy of Pediatrics; 2009:552–554.

with the incorporation of oral feedings used to replace nutrition previously provided by the enteral feedings.

When the patient's medical condition allows for normal oral feedings, weaning from tube feedings can be initiated. The management of the transition to oral feedings is multifaceted and involves the medical team, the patient, and the caregivers.[42] A complete weaning from EN should only be considered when the patient has achieved a satisfactory nutritional status.

The weaning time may vary from a few days to several months. Records of the patient's oral intake should be kept during this time. The tube feedings should be continued until the patient can demonstrate that nutrient requirements can be met consistently by oral intake. Some patients use EN in combination with PN and/or oral intake.[43] The combination of enteral and cycled parenteral nutrition is controlled on the basis of patient tolerance. Monitoring for intolerance or complications would be completed similarly to any nutrition delivery that is provided and not patient initiated.

A combination of enteral and oral feedings is more difficult to project. A guideline is to begin with a 25% decrease in the caloric intake by tube, then start to offer oral feeds. This transition will require frequent evaluation because of the risk of decrease in growth with a lower caloric intake or if the child has trouble or delay in progressing. If the oral intake varies from day to day, a sliding scale for supplemental enteral feeds should be created. The tube feeding schedule can be normalized to approximate the timing of meals and snacks, altering the feeding schedule to promote hunger, reducing the calories from tube feedings, providing adequate fluids, and, as oral intake increases, adjusting the tube feedings accordingly.

Formula Challenges and Disorders

As infant formulas become more elemental, the taste becomes less sweet and more bitter or sour. Partially hydrolyzed and elemental formulas often also have a less pleasant odor and an unpleasant aftertaste.[44] Amniotic fluid and breast milk are sweet and vary in flavor based on the mother's diet.[45] Infants accept a hydrolysate formula much easier than an older infant who is changed to the formula. Infants will readily drink hydrolyzed formulas if introduced before 4 months of age. If required after this age, it should be mixed with a formula that is already accepted while gradually increasing the proportion of hydrolysate.[44] The parent needs to work closely with a dietitian to make this transition acceptable to the child.

Infant and toddler feeding disorders constitute a tube feeding complication that is unique to the pediatric population. Many times, when chronically ill infants or toddlers are medically ready to begin oral feedings, they may display no interest in eating or may respond with manifested oral aversion when food, liquid, or utensils are near the face. In this situation, the child typically refuses, cries, gags, or vomits when offered feedings. This oral aversion can occur in children with or without mechanical eating problems.

Due to the emotional component of eating/feeding, a dysfunctional or uninformed family may further the trauma of eating by force feeding. Children who have been given EN often do not have normal hunger cycles, normal eating experiences at a table, or a mealtime routine. All of these points should be addressed when the transition to oral feeding occurs. Severe cases of oral aversion require intervention and behavior modification from pediatric psychologists, as well as other health professionals, such as speech pathologists, dietitians, and occupational therapists.[46]

Resistant feeding behavior may be due to missing a "critical period" in the development of the child's feeding skills. The critical period for the development of chewing skills is 6 to 7 months of age. If solids are not introduced during this time, the child typically will have difficulty accepting them later.[47]

Other important oral experiences during the first year of life include the development of the rooting and sucking reflexes, the oral exploration of objects, and the association of hunger with feeding. When a child is deprived of these normal oral feeding experiences during the first year of life, he or she may subsequently experience feeding difficulties that last throughout the toddler and preschool years. These children may also demonstrate significant delays in gross motor and personality development.[48] Daily oral therapy or "mouth play" can help to eliminate or reduce the problems that typically occur in the patient with nonoral nutrition support. Most feeding problems can be resolved or improved through medical, oral motor, and behavioral therapy.[49,50]

Initiating oral feedings as soon as medically possible can minimize feeding disorders. Concomitant speech or feeding therapy with EN can help to alleviate oral aversion.[51] Nonnutritive sucking during tube feedings in infancy can help to stimulate oral sucking and swallowing behavior. Intervention should be considered during enteral feeding rather than at its termination. Textured foods ideally should be offered, if medically feasible, when the infant is at a developmental age of 6 to 7 months. Positive caregiver–child mealtime interactions are critical for achieving feeding success.[52]

Eating/swallowing disorder therapy often includes recommendations to thicken liquids for therapy in the management of an infant or child who has been diagnosed with misswallowing by modified barium swallow studies using videofluoroscopy. This diagnosis means that on regular fluid consistency the patient is at risk for aspiration or actually aspirates. Several disease states or conditions contribute to misswallowing.[53]

Swallowing dysfunction is compounded in infants or young children who have not learned the act of swallowing. A behavioral eating plan is a complicated process because the family and/or medical team are often trying to avoid an alternative feeding delivery. Developmental progress, therapy, and nutrition all must be considered as the patient's plan is developed.[54]

Adding a thickening agent or food to the formula or liquid thickens the fluid so that the patient can swallow liquid with decreased risk of aspiration. If at all possible, a gel thickener should be considered. They are made from gum substances and contribute no calorie or carbohydrate value.[55] Powdered thickeners have nutritional consequences. The more thickener that is required, the more effect this will have on the nutrition content of the intake. Available powdered commercial thickening agents are carbohydrate based, with few or no other nutrients. Adding a carbohydrate product will skew the nutrients, add calories, and increase free water needs in a medically unstable patient or one who is at risk for dehydration. The recipe for thickened consistency is included with the package label, and the categories for thickening generally are nectar, honey, and pudding consistencies.

Baby rice cereal can be used a thickener, and it will provide some nutrients other than carbohydrate. Dehydrated baby cereal flakes are difficult to blend with the formula in a liquid form, do not thicken evenly, are not an exact measured substitute for thickener, and vary in the amount of time they take to thicken. Crushing the rice cereal prior to its addition to the formula creates a more uniform thickness and allows for easier passage through the opening of the nipple.[3]

In all situations, there may be an increased need for fluid or free water with no method of delivery unless EN is considered as a means of alternative delivery. Because of these factors, judicious prescription and follow-up must be made. Time frames for trial therapy should be established. A well-developed behavioral and skill progression feeding plan is helpful and should include a multidisciplinary team familiar with pediatric dysphagia. Oral intake is important to encourage—as much as is medically safe. At the conclusion of the trial therapy, the patient should be evaluated for progress and/or level of rehabilitation. If there has been no change in ability, a different modality for fluid delivery should be established, with swallowing therapy to work with oral skills.

In summary, the management plan for dysphagia should focus on the reduction or elimination of factors that potentially contribute to airway compromise, provide adequate nutrition and hydration, and facilitate a workable interaction between the caregiver and the child.[53]

Home Enteral Support

Whenever possible, EN should be provided in the home rather than in the hospital. A patient who is a candidate for home enteral feedings should be evaluated based on the following criteria:[56]

- The patient must be medically stable and have demonstrated a tolerance to the feeding regimen in the hospital.
- A safe home environment is required, with available running water, electricity, refrigeration, and adequate storage space.
- The family (or patient) must be educated and capable of administering the feedings at home.
- A payment source is needed for the formula and tube feeding equipment.
- A home care agency should be available to service the patient in his or her home locale. If an agency is not available, a hospital team that takes responsibility for home monitoring must be identified (e.g., pediatric nurse, dietitian, pharmacist).
- A physician must be willing to assume responsibility for following the patient after discharge from the hospital.
- Supplies and equipment must be available.
- Patient/caregiver education must be arranged.
- A nutrition plan must be established.
- A social support system must be identified.
- Outpatient follow-up must be established.

Monitoring forms should be used for these patients to document data collected between medical evaluations (see **Exhibit 19-6**). Any forms used or developed should allow for quality improvement monitoring or the collection of data to measure outcomes.[57] Lastly, arrangements should be made for outpatient follow-up.

EXHIBIT 19-6 Pediatric Home Care Monitoring Form

Date ______

Patient ______ DOB ______ Primary Care Physician ______
Caregiver ______ Hospital RD ______
Address ______ Monitoring Comments ______

Phone no. ______ Nutrition Support Contact Person ______

Age ______ Last measurements ______ Last nutrition Rx: Date ______
Wt ______ Wt ______ Formula ______
Ht ______ Ht ______ Total Volume ______
OFC ______ OFC ______ Delivery Schedule ______

Procurement Enteral ☐ Parenteral ☐ Supporting Medical Equipment ______
Formula ______ Provider ______ Monitor ☐ provider ______
Equipment ______ Provider ______ Oxygen ☐ provider ______
Supplies ______ Provider ______ Other ☐ provider ______
Problems ______ Problems ______

Formula and Delivery ☐ Same ☐ Change to

Formula ______ Concentration ______
Vol/day ______ Substitute Formula ______

Infusion and Schedule
☐ By mouth (PO)—attach diet history
☐ PO in combination with—attach diet history
☐ Intermittent Infuse ______ mL over ______ minutes ______ times per day
☐ Continuous Infuse ______ mL/hr for ______ hours from ______ to ______
☐ Parenteral Infuse ______ mL/hr for ______ hours from ______ to ______

EXHIBIT 19-6 *(Continued)*

Feeding Tube __________ Type __________ Size __________
☐ Nasogastric ☐ PEG ☐ Gastrostomy ☐ Jejunostomy ☐ Other

Water Flushes: Vol/day __________ mL __________ mL water per flush ______ flushes/day

Medications and Methods of Delivery: ____________________

Monitoring Instructions (e.g., labs, anthropometrics, nutrition, specialists) ____________________

Referral Recommendations ____________________

Caregiver Issues ____________________

Home Nutrition Support Information Given To ____________________

Signature ____________________

Home Care Staff ____________________
Telephone ____________________
Comments ____________________
____
____

Problems: ☐ Vomiting ☐ Reflux ☐ Aspiration ☐ Gagging ☐ Diarrhea ☐ Illness ☐ Constipation
☐ Weight Loss ☐ Behavioral ☐ Sepsis ☐ Equip. Malfunction ☐ Other ______________

PLAN OF CARE

Signature ____________________

Parenteral Rx Date ________
Dextrose ________
Amino Acid ________
NaCl ________
KCl ________
Kphos ________
CaGlu ________
Mg ________
Na Acetate ________
Other ________
____
____
____

Calories Provided ________
Amt. Protein ________

Case Study

Nutrition Assessment of Infant with Failure to Thrive

Patient history: AP, a 21-month-old female, presented with failure to thrive. AP was born full term with an uncomplicated pregnancy and birth history. Her birth weight was 2.96 and her length was 2.96 kg.

Patient has an unremarkable past medical history. Her family history is positive for diabetes in her paternal aunt. She is not presently taking medications or vitamins.

Parents report that AP eats a good variety of foods. Mom reports that AP drinks three cans of Pediasure per 24-hour period. Meals are offered in a high chair at the table, without distractions. Mom reports meal times take 45 minutes to 1 hour. Mom reports occasional coughing with meals, but denies gagging. AP has been evaluated for delayed speech; however, therapy has not yet started. Mom denies any swallow studies or oral motor assessments have been completed.

Weight history:

Age	*Weight*	*Height*
15 months	8 kg	73 cm
17 months	8.2 kg	74.5 cm
18 months	8.5 kg	75.2 cm
19 months	8.7 kg	76 cm

Pertinent labs: Hgb: 9 (L), Hct 12.5 (L), MCV 85.5, prealbumin 15 (L), albumin 3.2

Current weight: 8.97 kg, < 5th percentile

Height: 76 cm, 50th percentile

IBW: 11.6 kg

%IBW: 77%

Weight/height: < 5th percentile

Expected height for age: 83 cm

(Percentile, IBW, and weight/height determined using CDC growth charts)

Typical intake:

- *Wakes at 6 am:* Patient drinks 6 oz Pediasure. Patient typically returns to sleep following bottle.
- *10 am:* 3 tbsp tilapia, 2 strawberries, 3 oz water
- *12 pm:* 4 oz Pediasure. Patient then takes 1- to 2-hour afternoon nap.
- *5 pm:* ¼ cup chicken soup, grapes, 2 oz juice
- *7 pm:* 4 oz Pediasure
- *10 pm:* 4 oz Pediasure
- *1 am:* 6 oz Pediasure

Patient is 77% of IBW and 92% expected height for age. This places her in moderate chronic malnutrition and mild acute malnutrition based on the Waterloo Criteria.

Nutrition Diagnosis

Based on the above information, a nutrition diagnosis or problem is determined.

Nutrition Intervention

Patient is to be admitted to an inpatient hospital for nasogastric tube placement and teaching. The goal is for her to receive overnight feedings of currently tolerated formula.

Nocturnal feed of Pediasure should run at 60 mL/hour × 12 hours (run from 7 pm to 7 am). While on the inpatient unit, AP is assessed by a speech therapist for oral motor function and to rule out aspiration secondary to the reports of coughing during feeds as well as prolonged feeding time. Patient received clearance from the speech therapist to continue oral feeds of age-appropriate solids and nectar-thickened liquids.

Nutrition Education

1. Provide nutrition education on high-calorie and high-protein age-appropriate foods.
2. Limit oral feeds to 30 minutes.
3. Initiate nocturnal feed of Pediasure at 7 pm at 60 mL/hr × 12 hours.

Nutrition Monitoring and Evaluation

It is recommended that the patient continue to follow nutrition services monthly for assessment of anthropometrics until catch-up growth has been established. A 10% increase in total calories provided by enteral nutrition is recommended to achieve adequate weight gain. As patient's oral ability improves, a shift may be likely from nocturnal NG feeds to oral daytime feeds of Pediasure. Once the patient has exhibited good catch-up growth, follow-up should be shifted to once every 3 to 4 months. Adjustments to nocturnal feeds will be made to maintain adequate weight gain and linear growth. The patient should continue to receive regular speech therapy for continued monitoring of oral motor function.

Questions for the Reader

1. What are the patient's estimated energy and protein needs per kg?
2. What percentage of the patient's total energy needs and protein needs are provided by the Pediasure?
3. Write one PES statement for this patient.

REFERENCES

1. ASPEN Board of Directors. Enteral nutrition practice recommendations. *J Parenter Enteral Nutr.* 2009;33(2):122–167.
2. Joffe A, Anton N, Lequier L, et al. (ed). *Nutritional Support for Critically Ill Children.* Hoboken, NJ: Wiley; 2009:1–29.
3. Klawitter BM. Pediatric enteral nutrition support. In: Nevin-Folino NL (ed). *Pediatric Manual of Clinical Dietetics,* 2nd ed. Chicago: American Dietetic Association; 2003.
4. ASPEN Board of Directors. Clinical Guidelines for the use of parenteral and enteral nutrition in adult and pediatric patients, 2009. *J Parenter Enteral Nutr.* 2009;26(1 Suppl):1SA–138SA.
5. Schwart DB. Enhanced enteral and parenteral nutrition practice and outcomes in an intensive care unit with a hospital-wide performance improvement process. *J Am Diet Assoc.* 1996;96:484–489.
6. Cox JH (ed). *Nutrition Manual for At-Risk Infants and Toddlers.* Chicago: Precept Press; 1997:183–186.
7. Theriot L. Routine nutrition care during follow-up. In: Groh-Wargo S, Thompson M, Cox JH (eds). *Nutritional Care for the High Risk Newborn,* 3rd ed. Chicago: Precept Press; 2000:457–583.
8. Campbell MK, Kelsey KS. The PEACH survey: a nutrition screening tool for use in early intervention programs. *J Am Diet Assoc.* 1994;94(10):1156–1158.
9. Feldhausen J, Thomson C, Duncan B, Taren D. *Referral Criteria in Pediatric Nutrition Handbook.* New York: Chapman & Hall; 1996:65.
10. Food and Drug Administration. Regulation of infant formula. Available at: http://www.fda.gov/Food/GuidanceCompliance RegulatoryInformation/GuidanceDocuments/InfantFormula/ucm056524.htm. Accessed August 24, 2010.
11. Wessel JJ. Feeding methodologies. In: Groh-Wargo S, Thompson M, Cox JH (eds). *Nutritional Care for the High Risk Newborn,* 3rd ed. Chicago: Precept Press; 2000:321–339.
12. Greer FR, McCormick A, Loker J. Changes in fat concentration of human milk during delivery by intermittent bolus and continuous mechanical pump infusion. *J Pediatr.* 1984;105:745–749.
13. Lavine M, Clark RM. The effect of short-term refrigeration of milk and addition of breast milk fortifier on the delivery of lipids during tube feeding. *J Pediatr Gastroenterol Nutr.* 1989;8:496–499.
14. Ross Products Division, Abbott Laboratories. Available at: http://www.rosspediatrics.com. Accessed November 4, 2009.
15. Mead Johnson & Company. Available at: http://www.meadjohnson.com. Accessed November 4, 2009.
16. Nestle Clinical Nutrition. Available at: http://www.nestle-nutrition.com/Public/Default.aspx. Accessed August 24, 2010.
17. Novartis Nutrition Corporation. Currently Nestle Clinical Nutrition. Available at: http://www.novartis.com. Accessed August 24, 2010.
18. Scientific Hospital Supplies. Available at: http://www.shsna.com. Accessed November 4, 2009.
19. Wyeth-Ayerst Labs. Available at: http://www.parentschoiceformula.com. Accessed November 4, 2009.
20. Sapsford AB. Human milk and enteral nutrition products. In: Groh-Wargo S, Thompson M, Cox JH (eds). *Nutritional Care for the High Risk Newborn,* 3rd ed. Chicago: Precept Press; 2000:286–287.
21. Fomon SJ. *Nutrition of Normal Infants.* St. Louis, MO: Mosby-Year Book; 1993:100.
22. Cowen SL. Feeding gastrostomy: nutritional management of the infant or young child. *J Pediatr Perinat Nutr.* 1987;1:51.
23. Jew RK, Owen D, Kaufman D, Balmer D. Osmolality of commonly used medications and formulas in the neonatal intensive care unit. *Nutr Clin Pract.* 1997;12:158–163.
24. Texas Children's Hospital. *Pediatric Nutrition Reference Guide,* 8th ed. Houston, TX: McGraw-Hill Professional; 2008.
25. Gerber Good Start. Gerber Products. Available at: http://www.gerber.com/Products. Accessed December 2, 2009.
26. Joeckel RJ, Phillips SK. Overview of infant and pediatric formulas. *Nutr Clin Pract.* 2009;24:356–362.
27. Denne SC. Protein requirements. In: Polin RA, Fox WW (eds). *Fetal and Neonatal Physiology,* 2nd ed. Philadelphia: Sanders; 1998:315–325.
28. Fuentebella J, Kerner JA. Refeeding syndrome. *Pediatr Clin N Am.* 2009;56:1201–1210.
29. Santos VF, Morais TB. Nutritional quality and osmolality of home-made enteral diets, and follow-up growth of severely disabled children receiving home enteral nutrition therapy. *J Trop Pediatr.* 2010;56(2):127–128.
30. Rombeau JL, Jacobs DO. Nasoenteric tube feeding. In: Rombeau JL, Caldwell MD (eds). Clinical nutrition volume 1: Enteral and tube feeding. Philadelphia: Sanders; 1984:263.
31. American Academy of Pediatrics. *Pediatric Nutrition Handbook,* 6th ed. Elk Grove, IL: Author. 2009:108–554.
32. Delegge MH. Enteral access: the foundation of feeding. *J Parenter Enteral Nutr.* 2000;25:S8–S13.
33. Cone LC, Gilligan MF, Kagan RJ, et al. Enhancing patient safety. the effect of process improvement on bedside fluoroscopy time related to nasoduodenal feeding tube placement in pediatric burn patients. *J Burn Care Res.* 2009;30(4):606–611.
34. Wesley JR. Special access to the intestinal tract. In: Balistreri WF, Farrell MK (eds). *Enteral Feeding: Scientific Basis and Clinical Applications.* Report of the 94th Ross Conference on Pediatric Research. Columbus, OH: Ross Products; 1988:57–62.
35. Grunow JE, Al-Hafidh AS, Tunell WP. Gastroesophageal reflux following percutaneous endoscopic gastrostomy in children. *J Pediatr Surg.* 1989;24:44–45.
36. American Society for Parenteral and Enteral Nutrition Board of Directors. Clinical guidelines for the use of parenteral and enteral nutrition in adolescent and pediatric patients, 2009. *J Parenter Enteral Nutr.* 2009;33:255.
37. Walker WA, Hendricks KM (eds). Enteral nutrition support of the pediatric patient. In: Kerner J (ed). *Manual of Pediatric Nutrition.* Philadelphia: WB Saunders; 1985.
38. American Gastroenterological Association. American Gastroenterological Association Medical Position Statement: Guidelines for the Use of Enteral Nutrition. http://www3.us.elsevierhealth.com/gastro/policy/v108n4p1280.html. Accessed August 31, 2010.
39. Vanek VW. Closed versus open enteral delivery systems: a quality improvement study. *Nutr Clin Pract.* 2000;15:234–243.
40. Hutsler D. Delivery and bedside management of infant feedings. In: Robbins S, Beker L (eds). *Infant Feedings: Guidelines for Preparation of Formula and Breast Milk in Health Care Facilities.* Chicago: American Dietetic Association; 2003:1–10.

41. Arnold LDW. *Recommendations for Collection, Storage, and Handling of a Mother's Milk for Her Own Infant in the Hospital Setting.* Denver, CO: Human Milk Banking Association of North America; 1999.
42. Forchielli ML, Bines J. Enteral Nutrition. In: Walker WA, Watkins JB, Duggan C (eds). *Nutrition in Pediatrics,* 4th ed. Hamilton, Ontario, Canada: BC Decker; 2008:765–775.
43. Issacs JS, Lucas BL, Feucht SA, Grieger LE. Nutritional care for the gastrostomy-fed child with neurological impairments. *Top Clin Nutr.* 1993;8(4):58–65.
44. Mennella JA, Griffin CE, Beauchamp GK. Flavor programming during infancy. *Pediatrics.* 2004;113:840–845.
45. Mennella JA, Johnson A, Beauchamp GK. Garlic ingestion by pregnant women alters the odor of amniotic fluid. *Chem Senses.* 1995;20:207–209.
46. Stein, K. Children with feeding disorders: an emerging issue. *J Am Diet Assoc.* 2000;100(9):1000–1001.
47. Illingsworth RS, Lister J. The critical or sensitive period, with special reference to certain feeding problems in infants and children. *J Pediatr.* 1964;65:8.
48. Rommel N, DeMeyer A, Feenstra L, Veereman-Wauters G. The complexity of feeding problems in 700 infants and young children presenting to a tertiary care institution. *J Pediatr Gastroenterol Nutr.* 2000;37:75–84.
49. Rudolph CD, Link D. Feeding disorders in infants and children. *Pediatr Gastroenterol Nutr.* 2002;49:97–112.
50. Burklow KA, McGrath AM, Allred KE. Parent perceptions of mealtime behaviors in children fed enterally. *Nutr Clin Pract.* 2002;17:291–295.
51. Camp KM, Kalscheur MC. Nutritional approach to diagnosis and management of pediatric feeding and swallowing disorders. In: Tuchman DN, Walter RS (eds). *Disorders of Feeding and Swallowing in Infants and Children: Pathophysiology, Diagnosis, and Treatment.* San Diego, CA: Singular Publishing Group; 1994:153–185.
52. Manikam R, Perman JA. Pediatric feeding disorders. *J Clin Gastroenterol.* 2000;30:34–46.
53. American Academy of Pediatrics. *Pediatric Nutrition Handbook,* 6th ed. Elk Grove, IL: Author; 2009:108–554.
54. Lefton-Grief MA. Diagnosis and management of pediatric feeding and swallowing disorders: role of the speech-language pathologist. In: Tuchman DN, Walter RS (eds). *Disorders of Feeding and Swallowing in Infants and Children: Pathophysiology, Diagnosis, and Treatment.* San Diego, CA: Singular Publishing Group; 1994:97–113.
55. Phagia-GelTechnologies. Available at: http://www.simplythick.com. Accessed May 29, 2004.
56. Vanderhoff JA, Young RJ. Overview of considerations for the pediatric patient receiving home parenteral and enteral nutrition. *Nutr Clin Pract.* 2003;18:221–226.
57. Gallagher AL, Onda RM. Using quality assurance procedures to improve compliance with standards to nutrition care for patients receiving isotonic tube feeding. *J Am Diet Assoc.* 1993;93:678–679.

CHAPTER 20

Parenteral Nutrition

Janice Hovasi Cox and Ingrida Mara Malbardis

Parenteral nutrition (PN) is the intravenous delivery of nutrients, including water, carbohydrates, fat, protein, electrolytes, vitamins, minerals, and trace elements. The proportions of these nutrients are individualized, based on an assessment of the child's clinical and nutritional needs. The goal of PN is to support normal growth and development as well as to promote tissue repair and maintenance while oral/enteral feedings are precluded.

PN in pediatrics is commonly used for the treatment of a wide variety of conditions in both the hospital and home settings.[1–4] This chapter summarizes the complexities of pediatric PN as it is utilized in the hospital and in the home.

It is important to ensure that PN is used appropriately and that the infants and children who receive PN are managed effectively to support the best outcome at the lowest cost. Policies and decision trees can help practitioners choose the most suitable form of nutrition support.[5] Conditions that may require PN are listed in **Exhibit 20-1**. Some hospitals utilize interdisciplinary nutrition support teams (physicians, dietitians, nurses, and pharmacists)[6] and clinical pathways[7,8] to help evaluate and manage patients requiring enteral nutrition or PN.[9]

Gastrointestinal (GI) tract dysfunction can occur at any age due to disease, injury, or radiation/chemotherapy.[10,11] Although PN may help bring about disease remission in children with irritable bowel disease (IBD), ulcerative colitis, or Crohn's disease, relapse occurs soon after a normal diet is resumed.[12] PN should be reserved only for those children who are unable to tolerate enteral feedings. Gastrointestinal disorders requiring nutritional support are discussed in detail in Chapter 12.

The child with cancer may have an improved quality of life with PN.[13–16] Helping children maintain optimal nutrition during therapy may promote improved growth and better tolerance of therapies.[17] Some children may be able to tolerate small gastric feedings along with PN to meet nutrition needs. Most practitioners agree that children receiving aggressive cancer therapy should also receive supportive nutrition therapy, but the benefits of PN should be weighed against the potential risks, which include increased infection rates and metabolic abnormalities.[18,19]

PN may be used in the refeeding process for children with anorexia nervosa simply because it has less resemblance to food than the enteral feeding. The use of PN in these patients depends on the severity of malnutrition and on the patient's tendency to interfere with the infusion apparatus.[20,21]

Access

Use of central versus peripheral venous access is an important factor to consider when providing PN to the patient. PN may be delivered through a peripheral or central venous catheter, depending on the anticipated length of therapy, nutrition needs, and fluid tolerance. Peripheral parenteral nutrition (PPN) is used when the anticipated length of therapy is less than 2 weeks, PN is needed to maintain rather than replete nutrition status, and fluid tolerance is ample. Because PPN solutions are not as calorie dense as total PN (TPN) solutions, greater fluid volumes are required to provide comparable nutrition.

The peripheral delivery route is more restrictive than central venous access as it restricts normal movement and activity, depending on the site and stability of the venous access. The major complications associated with PPN are soft tissue sloughs and phlebitis, which are more likely to occur if the infused solution has an osmolality greater than 900 mOsm/L. A final concentration of no more than 12.5% dextrose with a maximum solution osmolality less than 900 mOsm/L with lipids, or less than 600 mOsm/L without lipids, is recommended in the administration of PPN.[4] A simple equation can be used to estimate osmolality.[22] Using g/L for glucose and amino acids, mg/L for phosphorus, and mEq/L for sodium, the equation is:

$$\text{Osmolality (mOsm/L)} = (\text{amino acid} \times 8) + (\text{glucose} \times 7) + (\text{sodium} \times 2) + (\text{phosphorus} \times 0.2) - 50$$

EXHIBIT 20-1 Conditions that May Require Parenteral Nutrition

GI Conditions		*Other Circumstances*
Bowel obstruction	Meconium ileus	Anorexia nervosa
Crohn's disease	Necrotizing enterocolitis	Bronchopulmonary dysplasia
Diaphragmatic hernia	Neuromuscular intestinal disorders	Cancer cachexia
Gastroschisis	Omphalocele	Chylothorax
High-output fistulas	Radiation enteritis	Low-birth-weight neonate (< 1500 g)
Intestinal atresia	Severe Hirschsprung's disease	
Intractable diarrhea	Short bowel syndrome	
Intussusception	Ulcerative colitis	
Malrotation/volvulus		

Limiting calcium to a maximum of 8 mEq/L also may help decrease the risk of phlebitis.[4]

Providing TPN through a central vein is indicated when an infant or child requires fluid restriction or long-term nutrition therapy or when an infant or child is a candidate for home PN. Infusion of TPN into a central vein allows the high blood flow to rapidly dilute the hypertonic solution. Central venous catheters (CVCs) also are used to provide chemotherapy, prolonged antibiotic therapy, and blood components. Although blood sampling from a CVC site that is being used for PN administration is thought to increase the risk of contamination, risks may be diminished by strict use of aseptic technique.[10]

Central venous access can be temporary or permanent. In neonates, umbilical vessels may be used temporarily as a central route for TPN. Risk of thrombosis increases if umbilical artery catheters are used beyond 5 days or if umbilical venous catheters are used beyond 14 days.[5] To avoid complications associated with their use, many institutions restrict use of umbilical catheters to lab and blood pressure monitoring, and PN is administered through a peripherally inserted central catheter (PICC) if central access is required.[23]

A PICC line provides reliable central venous access and may be inserted at the bedside using strict sterile techniques.[24–26] Insertion-related complications inherent in the surgically placed CVC, such as pneumothorax and hemothorax, are virtually eliminated with the PICC line. Some studies have also found that sepsis rates tend to be lower in neonates and children with PICC lines versus surgically placed central catheters.[27,28] PICC lines are being used in increasing numbers in both neonates and older children because they provide central venous access less invasively, with lower risks, and at lower cost than surgically placed CVCs or multiple insertions of peripheral lines.[10,29–32]

Permanent catheters are indicated when long-term access (over 3 weeks) is needed.[29] The surgically placed right atrial catheter (e.g., Broviac, Hickman) is the most suitable CVC for pediatric patients who require long-term or home TPN. The catheter is placed in the external jugular or the facial vein and threaded through the internal jugular vein and down into the superior vena cava. Tip placement outside the pericardial sac avoids the risk of pericardial tamponade.[10] Location of the catheter tip should be verified every 6 to 12 months for children undergoing significant linear growth.[33] The distal end of the catheter is tunneled subcutaneously and exits mid-chest. The Dacron cuff affixed to the tunneled portion of the catheter helps secure the catheter because subcutaneous fibrous tissue adheres to the cuff. The major complications associated with CVC insertion and use include infection and thrombosis.[29,34]

Although a single-lumen CVC is the venous access device most often used for the pediatric PN patient, two- and three-lumen CVCs also have been used in the pediatric population. Double- and triple-lumen catheters are particularly useful in patients who require frequent infusions of blood products and medications in addition to the nutrition solution. Designating one port exclusively for PN or PN with compatible medications and using the other ports for blood drawing, blood product delivery, and central venous pressure measurements may help decrease the risk for sepsis associated with multiple lumen catheters.[10] Lumens not in use must be heparinized and capped. Multiple-lumen catheters may be more suitable for the larger child rather than the neonate because of total catheter size. Strict aseptic technique is critical when a multiple-lumen CVC is in place.[35,36]

In order to avoid some of the problems associated with the externalized CVC, a totally implantable vascular device consisting of a catheter connected to a chamber or port can be used.[37] The advantages of the implantable port are that it eliminates daily dressing changes when not in use and it is not as disruptive to body image.

For the child on home PN, the implanted CVC requires daily access. Daily percutaneous puncture or leaving a Huber needle in place with a dressing for days at a time may negate the overall benefits of the implanted device. Skin irritation and breakdown have been associated with frequent port access, and other CVC-related complications, such as occlusion and infection, remain risks with the implanted CVC.[26]

PN Administration Factors

Due to the wide range in nutrient needs, fluid requirements, and clinical conditions of infants and children who require PN, individualized solutions are generally preferred over standard solutions.[10] Standard solutions may be used for short periods of time, particularly during the neonatal period, provided that electrolyte adjustment is possible and laboratory monitoring is consistent.[10,38] For individualized solutions, nutrient doses are calculated based on the infant or child's weight (per kg) or daily need and ordered per unit of volume, usually per liter, or per day in a specified volume. Recommendations for writing PN prescriptions are provided in **Exhibit 20-2**. Software programs and online tools also are available to simplify order entry for PN.[39–41]

PN solutions may be prepared as 2-in-1 solutions or as 3-in-1 or total nutrient admixtures (TNAs). In 2-in-1 solutions, dextrose and amino acids are combined with electrolytes, minerals, and trace elements. This solution is infused through one arm of a Y-connector, while lipids are infused in the other arm. Administering lipids separately allows for the visualization of potential calcium phosphate precipitates in the dextrose/amino acid solution, but increases the risk for increased bacterial growth in the lipid emulsion, especially if lipid is transferred from the original bottle into smaller syringes.[42] Vitamin stability may be greater if dosed in the lipid emulsion rather than the dextrose and amino acid solution. Administration tubing and extension sets for dextrose and amino acid solutions should be changed at least every 72 hours, or as recommended by the manufacturer. Infusion sets for TNAs or lipids administered separately should be changed as soon as the infusion is delivered or, if a second infusion is given, at least every 24 hours.[10,43]

A 3-in-1 or TNA combines the lipid emulsion, amino acid, and dextrose solutions in the same container. Although the TNA is more convenient to use, there has been concern about the stability and safety of these solutions. TNAs, unlike 2-in-1 solutions, are emulsions and therefore are more significantly influenced by pH and temperature.[44,45] Another concern is the potential peroxidation of lipid emulsions by phototherapy lights.[46] Using aluminum foil to shield the bag and the tubing from phototherapy lights can prevent this from happening. Opaque tubing is also available.[47] Infusion of a multivitamin (MVI) preparation along with shielding the tubing may fully protect the solution from peroxidation.[48] Tubing for TNA should be changed every 24 hours.[10,43]

EXHIBIT 20-2 Recommendations for Writing Parenteral Nutrition Prescriptions

1. Use standard order forms specifically developed for infants and children.
2. Identify prescription with patient's name and date of birth.
3. Provide patient's current weight; provide dosing weight if different than current weight due to malnutrition, edema, or obesity.
4. Identify whether intravenous access route is peripheral or central because this determines dextrose concentration limitations.
5. Include fluid prescription, accommodating other fluids needed for administration of flushes, medications, other intravenous fluids, and/or enteral feedings.
6. Specify total daily volume, hourly rate of delivery, and number of hours of delivery.
7. Each nutrient should be clearly identified, including chloride and acetate.
8. Include guidelines for nutrient requirements for various ages and/or acceptable ranges of nutrient concentration in admixture, including mineral content compatibility.
9. The list of nutrients in the prescription should be in the same order and units as in the guidelines and on the label. For example, do not use "mEq" for calcium in the prescription list but "mg" of calcium in the guidelines or "mL" of calcium gluconate on the label.
10. Avoid using percent concentration. Use amount per volume, amount per kg, or amount per day.
11. Use one zero before the decimal to hold a place, but do not use trailing zeros. For example, use 0.5, but do not use .5; use 5, but do not use 5.0.
12. Complete the form for all subsequent orders, even if only one nutrient is changed.
13. If standard solutions are used, provide options for adjusting electrolytes; decreasing lipid, copper, and manganese; and other modifications that may be clinically indicated.
14. Establish standard guidelines for laboratory monitoring.

Three main variables affect the overall stability of the final TNA:

1. The final concentration of the macronutrients
2. The amount of added cations (especially polyvalent cations such as iron, magnesium, calcium, and zinc)
3. The compounding order[43,49,50]

If parenteral medications are to be infused simultaneously via a Y-site, compatibility with the TNA solution should be verified.[51] Care must be taken to identify any precipitates or emulsion breakdown in the TNA before infusion occurs. The most commonly found precipitate is calcium phosphate. Emulsion breakdown or "creaming" (liberation of free oil) can result when higher amounts of cations are used in the mixture. The presence of yellow-brown oil droplets at or near the TNA surface is an indicator that the solution is unsafe for administration.[43] Compounding PN solutions, either manually or using an automated compounding device, requires meticulous adherence to standards that ensure safety, sterility, accuracy, quality, and labeling.[52,53]

Of greatest concern with neonatal and pediatric PN solutions is the solubility of calcium and phosphorus.[48] Although the addition of lipids to the PN solution does not directly affect the solubility of calcium and phosphorus, the opacity of the admixture makes visual detection of precipitates difficult. Software programs and online tools are available to help calculate the amount of calcium and phosphorus that can be provided safely in PN solutions.[40,43]

For neonates and children receiving home PN, the stability of the PN needs to be assured for longer periods of time. Using dual-chamber bags to separate the lipid from the rest of the solution and adding vitamins and trace minerals just before infusion helps improve the shelf-life of TNAs used in this setting.[49,54] Use of an MCT/LCT-based TNA also may improve stability.[55,56] Caretakers administering PN in the home need to be trained on how to visually assess the stability of the emulsion.

The use of filters with PN provides additional safety.[10,43,57] Filters can prevent the infusion of particulate matter, air, and microorganisms. Different size filters are available. These filters remove microorganisms and pyrogens (gram-negative endotoxins) and reduce the risk of air embolism. For TNAs, larger 1.2-micron filters are used to allow administration of lipid droplets. These filter out particulate matter and larger organisms, such as *Candida albicans*, but are unable to filter out common smaller bacterial contaminants. Infusion sets for 2-in-1 solutions should be changed at least every 72 hours, or per manufacturer's instruction.

PN solutions should be initiated slowly and advanced gradually as the child's fluid and glucose tolerance permits. Infusion pumps are used to maintain a constant flow rate, thereby maintaining steady glucose delivery. If the PN infusion is interrupted or discontinued abruptly, a 10% dextrose solution may be infused to maintain euglycemia (or to prevent hypoglycemia) until the PN solution can be replaced.

Cycling PN

Administration of PN in cycles provides for planned interruption of the nutrient infusion. Cycling more closely simulates normal patterns of food ingestion and fasting and may help prevent PN-associated hepatic complications.[58] Cyclic PN allows a more normal daytime routine, enhancing mobility and activity patterns and also leaving a window of time for lipid clearance.

The nutrition needs of the child, compared with the ability to tolerate oral/enteral feedings, should be taken into consideration when deciding on cyclic PN. Infants younger than 4 to 6 months of age who are receiving all of their nutrition parenterally may be able to tolerate breaks from PN of up to only 4 hours. Older infants and children may tolerate interruptions of up to 6 to 8 hours. Infants and children who are receiving enteral feedings or who are eating in addition to their PN may receive adequate PN in shorter spans of time. Supplemental PN can usually be provided over 8 to 12 hours. Children who are more tolerant of the necessary fluid load can receive their total required nutrition and fluid loads condensed into 10- to 16-hour cycles.

Glucose infusion rate should not exceed 20 mg/kg/min (1.2 g/kg/hr) to prevent wide variations in serum glucose.[10] Gradually increasing the rate when starting the infusion and slowly weaning the rate at the end of the infusion may lessen the likelihood of hyper/hypoglycemia. The rate is adjusted over a period of 1 to 2 hours (i.e., run at half rate for the first hour and last hour) to maintain euglycemia. Infusion pumps that can be programmed to accomplish the gradual introduction and weaning of PN are available. A rate adjustment for cycling may not be necessary in children older than 2 years of age.[59]

Transitioning Off PN

Minimal enteral feedings should be given whenever possible to prevent bowel atrophy and improve adaptation for tolerance of feeding advancement.[10] When increasing enteral feedings, making one change at a time in substrate, volume, or rate makes it easier to assess tolerance. Newborn infants are best weaned to mother's milk, although fortification may be needed for preterm infants to adequately meet their nutrient needs. Older infants and children who recover gastrointestinal function quickly may be weaned to an age-appropriate diet. When bowel function is expected to return gradually or remain somewhat compromised, mother's milk or hydrolyzed protein– or amino acid–based enteral products may be better tolerated.[10]

As an infant or child is able to make the transition to enteral/oral feedings, the volume of PN is gradually weaned by decreasing the hourly rate and/or decreasing the infusion time.[10] Total energy intake is adjusted as the percentage of enteral nutrition increases. Enteral energy needs are usually higher than PN needs because energy is required for digestion and absorptive losses may be small or significant, depending on gastrointestinal function. When PN is cycled, providing PN at night offers supplemental nutrition with limited suppression of appetite during the day, which may better support a transition to oral feedings.

Fluid and Nutritional Considerations

Guidelines for the administration of parenteral fluids to infants and children are based on normal maintenance estimates with adjustments for increased or decreased losses due to disease or environmental conditions (see **Table 20-1**).

Fluid losses through urine and the gastrointestinal tract may be relatively easy to measure, although insensible water loss (IWL) through the respiratory tract and skin is more elusive and may be affected by environmental conditions. Radiant heat warmers and ultraviolet light therapy may increase IWL 20–25%.[60] Use of double-walled isolettes may prevent this increase in water loss.[61] Use of mist tents and humidified air may decrease IWL. In older infants and children, hyperventilation and visible sweating often associated with fever may increase IWL 20–25%.[62]

Frequent monitoring of fluid and electrolyte intake, serum and urine electrolyte levels, weight changes, and urine output may be needed to appropriately manage fluid and electrolyte balance during the neonatal period. Beyond the first week of life and throughout childhood, maintenance fluid and electrolyte requirements are directly related to metabolic rate.[63] Infants and children generally require at least 115 mL of fluid for every 100 kcal of energy provided[64] (see Table 20-1). The amount of fluid needed to maintain adequate hydration often does not provide adequate nutrition when using peripheral venous access, though administration of fluids 30–50% above maintenance levels are usually well tolerated. Older infants and children may initially require fluids and electrolytes in excess of maintenance requirements to establish normal hydration if they have had prolonged or excessive vomiting or diarrhea.

TABLE 20-1 Daily Maintenance Fluid Requirements

Clinical Condition	Fluids Required per Day
Sick newborn, day 1	40–80 mL/kg
Sick newborn, week 1	80–150 mL/kg
Newborn to 1 year, stable growth	140–160 mL/kg/day
Anuria, extreme oliguria	45 mL/kg
Diabetes insipidus	Up to 400 mL/100 kcal
1–10 kg body weight	100 mL/kg
11–20 kg body weight	1000 mL + 50 mL/kg above 10 kg
Body weight above 20 kg	1500 mL + 20 mL/kg above 20 kg
Body surface area	1500–1800 mL/m^2

Sources: Data from Koletzko B, Goulet O, Hunt J, et al. for the Parenteral Nutrition Guidelines Working Group. Guidelines on paediatric parenteral nutrition of the European Society of Paediatric Gastroenterology, Hepatology and Nutrition (ESPGHAN) and the European Society for Clinical Nutrition and Metabolism (ESPEN), supported by the European Society of Paediatric Research (ESPR). *J Pediatr Gastroenterol Nutr.* 2005;41:S1–S87; Mirtallo J, Canada T, Johnson D, et al. for the Task Force for the Revision of Safe Practices for Parenteral Nutrition. Safe practices for parenteral nutrition formulations. *J Parenter Enteral Nutr.* 2004;28:S39–S70; Kerner JA Jr (ed). *Manual of Pediatric Parenteral Nutrition.* New York: John Wiley and Sons; 1983; Nelson WE, Behrman RE, Vaughan VC (eds). *Nelson's Textbook of Pediatrics,* 12th ed. Philadelphia: WB Saunders; 1983:231; and Baumgart S, Costarino AT. Water and electrolyte metabolism of the micropremie. *Clin Perinatol.* 2000;27:131–146.

Loss of fluids and electrolytes through the GI tract in disease states may be measured directly for replacement or estimated by monitoring changes in body weight every 8 or 24 hours. GI losses may be due to vomiting, nasogastric suctioning, diarrhea, or ostomy drainage.[65] Due to the wide range in electrolyte composition of various GI fluids, direct measurement may be required to provide adequate replacement.

Urinary losses of fluid and electrolytes depend largely on intake and renal maturity. Infants younger than 1 year of age can dilute urine to 50 mOsm/kg of water. Concentrating ability at birth is about 600 mOsm/kg of water and gradually increases to 1000–1200 mOsm/kg of water during the first year. During periods of growth, the renal solute load is lower because nitrogen, phosphorus, sodium, potassium, and chloride are retained as constituents of body tissues. During periods of stress and tissue catabolism, the renal solute load is higher.

Various conditions may alter urinary loss of fluid and electrolytes. Preterm infants have an immature capacity to either excrete or retain electrolytes and maintain acid–base balance.[10,66,67] Excessive sodium losses are common and may require up to 12 mmol/kg/day of sodium.

Fluid and electrolyte restriction may be necessary in disease states such as congestive heart failure, head trauma, and renal insufficiency. Medications may be a significant source of fluid and/or electrolytes. Saline flushes used in routine care of intravenous lines may be a significant source of sodium and chloride.[68] Some medications may cause increased excretion or retention of various electrolytes. Direct measurement of urine volume and electrolytes may be necessary to provide appropriate replacement.

Parenteral energy needs are probably about 10–15% lower than estimated enteral needs for most infants and children due to reduced fecal losses and reduced energy required for digestion and absorption (see **Table 20-2**). Various equations that incorporate length, age, body temperature, and heart rate have been developed to estimate individual energy needs.[10] Whatever method is used to estimate energy needs, frequent monitoring of anthropometric, clinical, and laboratory parameters allows adjustment of energy delivery to meet individual needs.

General guidelines for energy distribution are 8–15% protein, 45–60% carbohydrate, and 25–40% fat.[69] Positive nitrogen balance is best achieved when the nonprotein calorie to nitrogen ratio is 150–300:1.[70,71]

TABLE 20-2 Recommendations for Daily Parenteral Administration of Macronutrients, Electrolytes, and Minerals

	Dose Unit	Premature Infants	Term Infants	1–3 Years	4–6 Years	7–10 Years	11–18 Years	Maximum Dose
Fluid	mL/kg	140–160	120–150	80–120	80–100	60–80	50–70	
Basal energy[1]	kcal/kg	46–55	55	40–55	38–40	25–38	23–25	
Total energy[2]	kcal/kg	90–120	80–105	75–90	65–80	55–70	30–55	
Dextrose[3]	mg/kg/min	5–15	5–15	5–12	5–11	6–10	4–7	See text
Carbohydrate	g/kg	8–21	8–21	8–18	8–16	8–14	6–10	See text
Protein[4]	g/kg	2.5–4	2–3	1–2	1–2	1–2	0.8–1.5	4
Fat[5]	g/kg	0.6–3	0.6–3	0.6–2.5	0.5–2.5	0.5–2.5	0.4–1.8	4
Sodium	mEq/kg	2–5	2–3	1–5	1–5	1–5	60–150 mEq/d	150 mEq/d
Potassium	mEq/kg	2–4	2–3	2–4	2–4	2–4	70–180 mEq/d	180 mEq/d
Chloride	mEq/kg	2–5	2–3	2–4	2–4	2–4	60–150 mEq/d	150 mEq/d
Calcium[6]	mEq/kg	2.5–3	1–2	0.5–1	0.5–1	0.5–1	10–20 mEq/d	See text
Phosphorus[7]	mmol/kg	1–1.5	1–1.5	0.5–1.3	0.5–1.3	0.5–1.3	10–40 mEq/d	See text
Magnesium[8]	mEq/kg	0.5–1	0.25–1	0.25–0.5	0.25–0.5	0.25–0.5	10–30 mEq/d	See text
Zinc[9]	μg/kg	325–400	100–250	100	100	50	2000–5000 μg/d	5000 μg/d
Copper[9]	μg/kg	20	20	20	20	5–20	200–300 μg/d	300 μg/d
Chromium[9]	μg/kg	0.05–0.2	0.14–0.2	0.14–0.2	0.14–0.2	0.14–0.2	5–15 μg/d	15 μg/d
Manganese[9]	μg/kg	1	1	1	1	1	40–50 μg/d	50 μg/d
Selenium[9]	μg/kg	2–3	2	2	2	1–2 μg/d	40–60 μg/d	60 μg/d
Molybdenum[9]	μg/kg	0.25–1	0.25	0.25	0.25	0.25	5 μg/d	5 μg/d
Iron[10]	mg/kg	See text	0.1/See text	See text	See text	See text	See text	See text

[1]Basal energy needs increase: 12% for every degree of fever, 15–25% in cardiac failure, 20–30% in traumatic injury or major surgery, 25–30% in severe respiratory distress or bronchopulmonary dysplasia, 40–50% in severe sepsis, 6 kcal/g weight gain for catch-up growth.

[2]Total parenteral energy needs include basal energy needs, activity, and growth but do not include energy required for digestion or energy losses in stool that occur with enteral feeding. Adjust energy intake if activity or growth needs are higher or lower than normal. Although surgery may increase basal needs temporarily, total energy needs may not increase due to inactivity and temporary interruption of growth.

[3]Peripheral venous access limits dextrose concentration to 12% solutions due to high osmolality and increased risk of tissue damage. Central venous access allows up to 25% dextrose solutions.

[4]Protein needs may vary with diagnoses: 0.8–2 g/kg/day for renal failure; 3 g/kg/day for necrotizing enterocolitis, major surgery, traumatic injury, or sepsis; 4–8 g/kg/day for thermal injury. Most efficient protein utilization occurs when nonprotein/calorie ratio is 150–250:1 (100–150:1 in burns and multiple trauma).

[5]Minimum fat dose to meet essential fatty acid requirements varies depending upon fat source and total energy needs. See text.

[6]Calcium conversions: 1 mEq = 0.5 mmol = 20 mg elemental calcium; 1 mL calcium gluconate 10% contains 100 mg calcium gluconate = 9.3 mg elemental calcium = 0.47 mEq = 0.25 mmol calcium.

[7]Phosphorus conversions: 1 mmol = 31 mg elemental phosphorus; 1 mL sodium phosphate contains 3 mmol or 93 mg elemental phosphorus (and 4 mEq sodium); 1 mL potassium phosphate contains 3 mmol or 93 mg elemental phosphorus (and 4.4 mEq potassium).

[8]Magnesium conversions: 1 mEq = 0.5 mmol = 12.5 mg elemental magnesium; magnesium sulfate 50% contains 500 mg magnesium sulfate heptahydrate or 4.1 mEq (or 51.3 mg) elemental magnesium.

[9]Trace mineral additives are currently available individually and in various combinations/concentrations for various ages. Doses vary. Copper and manganese needs may be lower with cholestasis.

[10]Many institutions do not routinely include iron in parenteral admixtures due to incompatibility with other nutrients, contraindication during sepsis, and risks associated with overdose with multiple blood transfusions.

Sources: Data from Koletzko B, Goulet O, Hunt J, et al. for the Parenteral Nutrition Guidelines Working Group. Guidelines on paediatric parenteral nutrition of the European Society of Paediatric Gastroenterology, Hepatology and Nutrition (ESPGHAN) and the European Society for Clinical Nutrition and Metabolism (ESPEN), supported by the European Society of Paediatric Research (ESPR). *J Pediatr Gastroenterol Nutr.* 2005;41:S1–S87; American Society for Parenteral and Enteral Nutrition. Guidelines for the use of parenteral and enteral nutrition in adult and pediatric patients. *J Parenter Enteral Nutr.* 1993;17(Suppl):27SA–52SA; Mirtallo J, Canada T, Johnson D, et al. for the Task Force for the Revision of Safe Practices for Parenteral Nutrition. Safe practices for parenteral nutrition formulations. *J Parenter Enteral Nutr.* 2004;28:S39–S70; Kerner JA Jr (ed). *Manual of Pediatric Parenteral Nutrition.* New York: John Wiley and Sons; 1983; Heimler R, Doumas BT, Jendrzejcak BM, et al. Relationship between nutrition, weight change, and fluid compartments in preterm infants during the first week of life. *J Pediatr.* 1993;122:110–114; Tilden SJ, Watkins S, Tong TK, Jeevanandam M. Measured energy expenditure in pediatric intensive care patients. *Am J Dis Child.* 1989;143:490–492; Lowery GH. *Growth and Development of Children,* 6th ed. Chicago: Year Book Medical Publishers; 1973:331–332; Heird WC, Kashyap S, Gomez MR. Parenteral alimentation of the neonate. *Semin Perinatol.* 1991;15:493–502; Greene HL, Hambidge KM, Schanler R, et al. Guidelines for the use of vitamins, trace elements, calcium, magnesium, and phosphorus in infants and children receiving total parenteral nutrition: report of the Subcommittee on Pediatric Parenteral Nutrient Requirements from the Committee on Clinical Practice Issues of the American Society for Clinical Nutrition. *Am J Clin Nutr.* 1988;48:1324. (Revised in 1990.); Kleinman RE (ed). *Pediatric Nutrition Handbook.* Elk Grove Village, IL: American Academy of Pediatrics; 1998:285–305; Khaldi N, Coran AG, Wesley JR. Guidelines for parenteral nutrition in children. *Nutr Supp Serv.* 1984;4:27; Sunehag AL, Haymond MW. Glucose extremes in newborn infants. *Clin Perinatol.* 2002;29:245–260; Prelack K, Sheridan RL. Micronutrient supplementation in the critically ill patient: strategies for clinical practice. *J Trauma.* 2001;51:601–620; and Illingworth RS, Lister J. The critical or sensitive period, with special reference to certain feeding problems in infants and children. *J Pediatr.* 1964;65:839–848.

Glucose (dextrose monohydrate, 3.4 kcal/g) is the primary source of parenterally administered carbohydrate and generally provides 60–75% of nonprotein calories. Glycerol, found in parenterally administered fat emulsions, is also a source of carbohydrate. Glucose dose recommendations for infants and children are found in Table 20-2. Glucose infusions of less than 2 mg/kg/min (3 g/kg/day) may be insufficient to prevent ketosis caused by mobilization of fat stores as a source of energy. Glucose utilization by infants (6–8 mg/kg/min or 8.6–11.5 g/kg/day) is significantly different from adults (2 mg/kg/min or 3 g/kg/day), primarily due to brain metabolism. The brain requires glucose as the primary source of energy, and the ratio of brain to body weight in infants is 12%, compared to 2% in adults.[72,73] Brain utilization of glucose may account for as much as 90% of basal glucose needs. In addition, infants and children require glucose to support normal growth. Prematurely born infants may require as much as 16 mg/kg/min (24 g/kg/day) of glucose if fat is poorly tolerated as a source of energy.[71,72]

Maximum glucose tolerance varies with age, total energy expenditure, and clinical condition.[41,72,73] Net fat synthesis is shown to occur in infants when glucose intake exceeds 12.5 mg/kg/min (18 g/kg/day) or 6 mg/kg/min (8.6 g/kg/day) in older children. Premature infants or severely malnourished children often require lipogenesis because they may lack adequate fat stores.[10] Glucose intake for full-term infants and children up to 2 years of age should not exceed 13 mg/kg/min (18 g/kg/day). Glucose given in excess of need may be associated with hyperglycemia, hepatic steatosis, and/or increased carbon dioxide production and minute ventilation.[1,70,74] During periods of critical illness, glucose tolerance may be limited to 5 mg/kg/min (7.2 g/kg/day).[10]

Generally, insulin is not added to parenteral nutrient admixtures because dose response varies widely, particularly in the low-birth-weight infant. Insulin, when needed, may be given in a separate infusion starting at 0.1 U/kg/hour and increased or decreased as needed to maintain euglycemia.[75,76] Small glycogen stores in low-birth-weight infants and undernourished infants and children place them at a greater risk of developing hypoglycemia following abrupt cessation of parenteral glucose. Gradual weaning from parenteral glucose and adequate enteral feeding help prevent the development of hypoglycemia.

The recommended dose of carbohydrate may be delivered while meeting normal fluid requirements by using a 10–12.5% dextrose solution. This concentration is compatible with peripheral intravenous infusion. Greater concentrations of carbohydrate are given by central venous infusion, generally up to a maximum concentration of 25%.[77] These may be needed when caloric needs are greater than normal, when parenterally administered fat is poorly tolerated, or when fluid restriction is necessary.

Parenteral administration of 1.1–2.5 g/kg/day along with 30–60 kcal/kg/day supports neutral or positive nitrogen balance in very-low-birth-weight (VLBW) infants during the first 24 hours of life. Subsequently, 3.0–3.5 g/kg/day (3.5–4.0 g/kg/day in infants less than 1000 g) is needed to support normal tissue accretion.[78–84] Early amino acid delivery may improve glucose tolerance by enhancing endogenous insulin secretion.[74,83] Insulin-like growth factor I (IGF-1) is lower in premature infants and may be further reduced by inadequate protein intake. Low levels of IGF-1 are associated with increased risk of retinopathy of prematurity, bronchopulmonary dysplasia, intraventricular hemorrhage, and necrotizing enterocolitis.[85] General recommendations for protein administration for infants and children are given in Table 20-2. Protein usually comprises 10–15% of total energy intake. Individual protein needs can be determined from nitrogen balance studies.

The administration of amino acids during periods of acute stress does not completely prevent endogenous protein catabolism, but, in conjunction with enough energy to meet basal requirements, helps maintain normal plasma amino acid concentrations, increases nitrogen retention, and may stimulate endogenous insulin secretion to improve glucose tolerance.[10,74,83] A reasonable and safe protein intake during critical illness is 3 g/kg/day for infants and children and up to 2 g/kg/day for adolescents.[10,43] Protein status is generally evaluated by monitoring serum total protein and albumin levels, although changes in serum prealbumin, transferrin, retinol binding protein, or blood urea nitrogen (BUN) levels may identify changes in protein status more quickly. Monitoring acid–base balance and BUN or ammonia levels helps identify excess protein intake. Recommendations concerning monitoring are found in **Table 20-3**. Metabolic complications of hyperammonemia and prerenal azotemia can occur with a need to reduce the protein infusion and/or increase nonprotein calories.

Crystalline amino acid (CAA) products have been developed for infants reflecting the amino acid composition of human milk or plasma aminograms of healthy term infants fed mature human milk. Metabolic immaturity also has been considered because cystine, taurine, tyrosine, and histidine may be essential amino acids for neonates and young children.[86–90] Methionine, phenylalanine, and glycine concentrations have been decreased in these solutions while histidine, tyrosine, taurine, arginine, glutamic acid, and aspartic acid may be added or their concentrations increased.[90] Although cystine may be a conditionally essential amino acid, it is not included in CAA solutions because it is unstable in solution for prolonged periods of time.[91] It is available as L-cystine hydrochloride to be added separately at the time of administration. Cystathionase activity matures to 70% of adult activity by 9 days of age in preterm infants and by 3 days of age in

TABLE 20-3 Suggested Laboratory Monitoring During Pediatric Parenteral Nutrition

Laboratory Index	Initial	Stable	Home Monitoring
Blood glucose	Daily	Daily to 3×/week	Daily to 3×/week
Acid–base status	Daily to weekly	Every other week	Monthly < 6 months Every 3 months < 1 year Every 6 months > 1 year
Electrolytes Na, K, Cl, CO_2	Daily	Weekly or every other week	
Chemistry profile: total protein albumin BUN, creatinine Ca, P, Mg triglyceride	Weekly	Weekly or every other week	Monthly < 6 months Every 3 months < 1 year Every 6 months > 1 year
Liver profile: total bilirubin alkaline phosphatase LDH, ALT, AST PTT	Weekly	Monthly	Monthly < 6 months Every 3 months < 1 year Every 6 months > 1 year
Hematology profile: HBG/HCT platelet count	Baseline	Weekly	Monthly < 6 months Every 3 months < 1 year Every 6 months > 1 year
CBC w/diff	Weekly	Monthly or as indicated*	As above or as indicated*
iron/TIBC/ferritin	As indicated*	As indicated*	As indicated*
Other: trace minerals vitamins carnitine	As indicated*	As indicated*	As indicated*
Urine glucose specific gravity pH	2–4 times a day	Daily to weekly	As indicated*

*As indicated by clinical condition or symptoms indicating deficiency, imbalance, or abnormality
Abbreviations: BUN, blood urea nitrogen; LDH, lactic dehydrogenase; ALT, alanine amino transferase; AST, aspartate amino transferase; PTT, prothrombin time; HGB, hemoglobin; HCT, hematocrit; CBC, complete blood count; TIBC, total iron binding capacity.

term infants. Cystine supplementation does not increase overall nitrogen retention or improve growth in neonates when 120 mg methionine per kilogram per day is provided, suggesting that cystine may not be needed beyond the neonatal period.[92,93] However, children 1 to 7 years of age with short bowel syndrome receiving home PN demonstrate low serum taurine levels that are increased to within normal reference range by the addition of cystine to their pediatric amino acid preparation, even though the preparation itself contains taurine.[94] The most commonly recommended dose for cystine is 30–40 mg/g of protein for pediatric CAA products, although cystine may not be needed for standard solutions due to higher methionine content.[93–96]

Although glutamine is not routinely added to PN solutions due to solubility problems, it may be conditionally essential during periods of sepsis, trauma, surgery, or shock when circulating levels decrease and needs, particularly in maintaining GI mucosal cell integrity, are increased.[97,98] For extremely low-birth-weight infants, glutamine added to PN solutions in amounts of 0.3–0.5 g/kg/day (or 20% of amino acid intake) appears safe and may support lower occurrence rates of GI dysfunction and severe neurological sequelae and promote earlier achievement of full enteral feedings.[99,100]

Pediatric CAA products may be of benefit to the prematurely born infant or the infant who requires long-term PN. Pediatric CAA products may require cystine supplementation of 55–77 mg/kg/day for infants younger than 4 months of age due to inadequate cystathionase activity. All other infants and children may need 3–22 mg cystine per gram of total amino acid content due to reduced methionine content.[75,91,93–96]

Special solutions of L-isomer CAA formulated for adults with severe hepatic or renal failure appear to be efficacious in children with severe hepatic or chronic renal failure, although standard CAA solutions may better meet the amino acid needs of children with acute renal failure.[101–105] Older children with sepsis or traumatic injury may benefit from using formulations with increased amounts of branched-chain amino acids.[106]

Fat is included in PN regimens for infants and children as a source of essential fatty acids (EFA) and to provide 25–40% of nonprotein energy intake. Linoleic acid (LA) deficiency is clinically manifested as the following:

- Dry, flaky skin
- Dry hair
- Poor growth
- Decreased platelets
- Impaired wound healing

Biochemical deficiency of LA precedes these clinical manifestations. Plasma levels of LA and arachidonic acid (AA) decline, and the ratio of plasma eicosatrienoic acid to AA (triene:tetraene) becomes elevated. Numbness, paresthesia, weakness, inability to walk, and blurring of vision may occur if linolenic acid (LNA) deficiency is present, and docosapentaenoic acid (DPA) levels increase while docosahexaenoic acid (DHA) levels decrease.[10,107,108] The long-chain polyunsaturated acids AA and DHA are involved in the structure and function of cell membranes, specifically retinal and central nervous system structures, and dietary intake of these fatty acids may be essential during infancy.[109] Very-low-birth-weight infants or infants and children with depleted body stores of fat or with a chronic history of fat malabsorption are at greatest risk of developing EFA deficiencies.[110]

Providing as little as 2–4% of the total daily caloric intake as LA (0.25 g/kg/day for infants and 0.1 g/kg/day in older children) and 0.25–0.5% of the total daily caloric intake as LNA can prevent deficiency in most infants and children.[10,11,43,69,111] Parenteral lipids currently available in the United States contain soy oil (Intralipid and Liposyn III) or safflower oil and soy oil (Liposyn II). Soy oil preparations provide 0.5 g LA and 0.09 g LNA per gram of fat. Safflower oil and soy oil mixtures contain 0.65 g LA and 0.04 g LNA per gram of fat. Usual recommendations for prevention of EFA deficiency using these emulsions are 0.5–1 g/kg/day or 2.5–5 mL of 20% lipid emulsion/kg/day. Children older than 4 years require 0.5 g/kg/day and adolescents require 0.4 g/kg/day to meet estimated essential fatty acid needs.

Limitations of glucose or fluid tolerance and high energy needs usually dictate a greater intake of lipid than that which prevents deficiency. Parenteral lipid doses of 2.5–3.0 g/kg/day provide infants with only 25–35% of total energy intake as fat, but higher doses may be poorly tolerated, especially in premature or small-for-gestational-age infants.[69,70,112,113] In children older than 2 years of age, it may be advisable to limit fat to 30% of total calories (generally 1.0–2.5 g/kg/day), as recommended by the American Academy of Pediatrics.[114] Fat should not provide more than 60% of total calories in any patient because ketotic acidosis may occur.[115]

The rate of administration may be just as significant a factor in lipid tolerance as daily dose. Adverse effects of intravenous fat when given in boluses or in doses exceeding 0.15 g/kg/hour or 3.6 g/kg/day have been reported, including the following:

- Altered pulmonary function
- Impaired neutrophil function
- An increased risk of kernicterus in infants with elevated serum bilirubin level[116–118]

Preterm or malnourished infants and children may be at greater risk for impaired fat tolerance due to decreased adipose tissue mass, reduced lipoprotein lipase activity, hepatic immaturity, or carnitine deficiency.

Parenteral lipid emulsions contain egg phospholipid as an emulsifying agent. Because phospholipids interfere with enzymes that help metabolize and clear plasma lipids, 20% emulsions are recommended over 10% emulsions due to their lower phospholipid-to-lipid ratio. Parenteral lipid emulsions also contain glycerol and are relatively isotonic and pH neutral, providing a favorable environment for the proliferation of several common pathogens. When infused separately, lipid emulsions are associated with an increased incidence of coagulase-negative staphylococcal bacteremia, particularly when hang times exceed 12 hours. When administered as a component of a TNA, this association is no longer apparent, likely due to the hypertonic and relatively acidic environment provided by the presence of other nutrients.[118] Both of these factors may decrease the stability of the lipid emulsion, causing separation, particularly when higher amounts of amino acids and minerals are used, as for low-birth-weight infants. The opacity of TNAs also may mask the presence of incompatibilities and precipitates, resulting in adverse outcomes, although use of a 1.2-micron filter can remove larger organisms, particles, precipitates, and fat globules.[119]

Intravenous fat may be safely given if:

- The initial dose is 0.5 g/kg/day and is gradually increased by 0.25 or 0.5 g/kg/day.
- The highest dose is less than 0.12–0.15 g/kg/hour (3–3.6 g/kg/day) or less than 0.08 g/kg/hour (2 g/kg/day) during periods of acute sepsis.
- Serum triglycerides are monitored and kept within the normal range, although various recommendations are given in the literature for the acceptable upper limit of normal, ranging from 100–200 mg/dL.[111,116,117]

- Whenever possible, lipids are administered as a component of a TNA over 24 hours using a 1.2-micron filter to best maintain physiochemical stability and minimize infectious risk.[119,120]

When lipids must be infused separately due to higher protein and mineral needs, such as for low-birth-weight infants, recommendations for reducing risk of nosocomial bacteremia include the following:

1. Aseptic transfer of lipid emulsion from the original container directly to infusion devices by pharmacy personnel under a class A laminar air flow hood
2. Hang times limited to 12 hours whenever possible[121]

Limiting hang times to 12 hours ultimately limits total lipid dose to 1.8 g/kg/day or 17–20% of total energy intake. When energy needs exceed 95 kcal/kg/day and fluid tolerance is limited to 120–150 mL/kg/day, dextrose solutions of 15–18% given through centrally placed catheters may be required. Because this may exceed glucose tolerance, particularly in extremely low-birth-weight infants, using administration sets up to 24 hours to accommodate a second lipid infusion has been suggested.[120]

If serum bilirubin levels are greater than 8–10 mg/dL (while the serum albumin level is 2.5–3 g/dL), lipids should be given only in amounts adequate to prevent EFA deficiency.[118] If intravenous fat is given in greater amounts or given in bolus doses, the molar ratio of free fatty acid to serum albumin should be maintained at less than 6 while bilirubin levels remain elevated.[69] (See Chapter 4 for further discussion on this issue.)

Carnitine facilitates transport of long- and medium-chain fatty acids across mitochondrial membranes. Carnitine is normally synthesized by the liver from methionine and lysine. Pediatric amino acid solutions are lower in methionine than in standard solutions, and patients at risk for carnitine deficiency demonstrate lower plasma concentrations of carnitine when receiving carnitine-free parenteral products as their single source of nutrition.[122] Patients at highest risk for carnitine depletion include those who are less than 30 weeks' gestation, have a birth weight less than 1500 g or a history of fetal malnutrition, or have hepatic or renal dysfunction, infection, or medium-chain acetyl-dehydrogenase deficiency.[123]

Carnitine supplementation may be considered in patients identified at high risk if PN is expected to be the single source of nutrition for longer than 2 weeks or if hypertriglyceridemia, hypoglycemia, and low serum carnitine are present.[10,123,124] Dose recommendations for oral or intravenous supplementation of carnitine vary from 50–100 mmol/kg/day (approximately 10–20 mg/kg/day).[124–128] Doses of 300 mmol/kg/day (50 mg/kg/day) or greater are not recommended, because these doses are associated with increased metabolic rate, decreased protein deposition, and impaired growth.[123,128]

Recommendations for term infants and children up to 11 years of age are available[129] and are based on the 1974 recommended dietary allowances (RDAs). Recommendations for adolescents are based on guidelines for adults. Vitamin requirements of prematurely born infants may vary from those of term infants due to the immaturity of vitamin absorption, excretion, enterohepatic recirculation, and renal tubular reabsorption mechanisms. Current estimates of need are based on numerous studies and extrapolations from term infant data.[130] Two different vitamin dose regimens for infants who weigh less than 2500 g have been suggested. Doses based on broad weight categories are more likely to underdose larger infants and/or overdose smaller infants, particularly with vitamins E and K and B-complex vitamins.[131–133] Either dose regimen is likely to underdose vitamin A, particularly for smaller infants, although vitamin A is often dosed separately for these infants and given intramuscularly.[131,134] The vitamin content of MVI Pediatric for Infusion and MVI-12 Multivitamin Infusion (Astra USA, Inc.) are compared to the current vitamin dose recommendations in **Table 20-4**.

Levels of several vitamins may decrease over time in parenteral nutrient admixtures due to light degradation, decomposition in the presence of bisulfite (an antioxidant additive) or varying pH, and adsorbance to plastic or glass. For these reasons, multivitamins should be added to TNA solutions immediately prior to administration, excessive light exposure (direct sunlight or phototherapy light) should be avoided, and administration of these admixtures should be completed within 24 hours. If lipids are given separately, adding both fat- and water-soluble vitamins to the lipid emulsion may increase vitamin stability and delivery.[10]

It is important to monitor key minerals such as magnesium, calcium, and phosphorus as well as trace minerals and adjust their intake as needed while on PN. Magnesium deficiency is identified by decreased serum levels. Hypomagnesemia can occur in many conditions, such as protein-calorie malnutrition, chronic malabsorption, proximal jejunal resection, ileostomy, cystic fibrosis, neonatal hepatitis, congenital biliary atresia, DiGeorge's syndrome, and hypokalemia; in infants born to diabetic mothers; or during chronic diuretic therapy, aminoglycoside therapy, or chemotherapy.[135] If serum levels are below 1.4 mg/dL or if seizures occur, the repletion dose is 0.2 mEq/kg given intramuscularly or intravenously every 6 hours until symptoms subside. Older children may require 0.8–1 mEq/kg/day for repletion or during critical illness.[136] Blood pressure should be monitored when providing intravenous magnesium repletion because hypotension may occur.[69]

Parenteral doses of 0.5–1 mEq of magnesium/kg/day may be needed for adequate retention in prematurely born infants, although general dose recommendations for all other infants and children are 0.25–0.5 mEq/kg/day of magnesium, with a maximum allowable dose of 24 mEq/day.[69,71,113]

TABLE 20-4 Recommendations for Pediatric Parenteral Daily Vitamin Dosage

	A IU	D IU	E mg	K μg	C mg	B_1 mg	B_2 mg	B_3 mg	B_6 mg	B_{12} μg	FA μg	PA mg	Biotin μg
Recommended amount/kg/day													
Preterm infant (≤ 2.5 kg)	500–1700	32–160	2.8–3.5	10–80	15–25	0.35–0.5	0.15–0.2	4–6.8	0.15–0.2	0.3	56	1–2	5–8
MVI Pediatric** doses													
30% dose/day (0.5–1 kg)	700–1400	120–240	2.1–4.2	60–120	24–48	0.4–0.7	0.3–0.6	5–10	0.3–0.6	0.3–0.6	42–84	1.5–3	6–12
65% dose/day (1–2.5 kg)	600–1500	100–260	1.8–4.5	50–130	21–52	0.3–0.8	0.4–0.9	4–11	0.3–0.6	0.3–0.6	36–90	1.5–3	5–13
40% dose/kg/day (≤ 2.5 kg)*	920	160	2.8	80	32	0.48	0.56	6.8	0.4	0.4	56	2	8
Recommended amount/day													
Preterm infant (> 2.5 kg)	700–1500	40–160	2–4	6–10	35–50	0.3–0.8	0.4–0.9	5–12	0.3–0.7	0.3–0.7	40–90	2–5	6–13
Term infant/child (age 1–11 yrs)	2300	400	5–7	200	80	1.2	1.4	17	1	1	140	5	20
MVI Pediatric,** 1 dose/day	2300	400	7	200	80	1.2	1.4	17	1	1	140	5	20
Recommended amount/day													
Adolescents (11–18 yrs)	3300	200	10	150–700	100	3	3.6	40	4	5	400	15	60
MVI–12,** 1 dose/day	3300	200	10	150	100	3	3.6	40	4	5	400	15	60

*Maximum dose not to exceed 1 full dose per day.

**Pediatric MVI (pediatric parenteral multivitamin) and MVI-12 Injection or Unit Vial, Astra USA, Inc., Westboro, MA.

Abbreviations: A, retinol; D, cholecalciferol; E, alpha-tocopherol; K, phytonadione; B1, thiamin; B2, riboflavin; B3, niacin; B6, pyridoxine; B12, cyanocobalamin; FA, folic acid; PA, pantothenic acid.

Sources: Data from Koletzko B, Goulet O, Hunt J, Krohn K, Shamir R for the Parenteral Nutrition Guidelines Working Group. Guidelines on paediatric parenteral nutrition of the European Society of Paediatric Gastroenterology, Hepatology and Nutrition (ESPGHAN) and the European Society for Clinical Nutrition and Metabolism (ESPEN), supported by the European Society of Paediatric Research (ESPR). *J Pediatr Gastroenterol Nutr.* 2005;41:S1–S87; Storm HM, Young SL, Sandler RH. Development of pediatric and neonatal parenteral nutrition order forms. *Nutr Clin Pract.* 1995;10:54–59; John E, Klavdianou M, Vidyasagar D. Electrolyte problems in neonatal surgical patients. *Clin Perinatol.* 1989;16:219–232; Greene HL, Hambidge KM, Schanler R, et al. Guidelines for the use of vitamins, trace elements, calcium, magnesium, and phosphorus in infants and children receiving total parenteral nutrition: report of the Subcommittee on Pediatric Parenteral Nutrient Requirements from the Committee on Clinical Practice Issues of the American Society for Clinical Nutrition. *Am J Clin Nutr.* 1988;48:1324. (Revised in 1990.); Friedman Z, Danon A, Stahlman MT, et al. Rapid onset of essential fatty acid deficiency in the newborn. *Pediatrics.* 1976;58:640–649; Magnusson G, Boberg M, Cederblad G, et al. Plasma and tissue levels of lipids, fatty acids, and plasma carnitine in neonates receiving a new fat emulsion. *Acta Paediatr.* 1997;86:638–644; and McDonald CM, MacKay MW, Curtis J, et al. Carnitine and cholestasis: nutritional dilemmas for the parenterally nourished newborn. *Support Line.* 2003;25:10.

Upper-range doses may be needed during rapid growth phases, diuretic therapy, or chronic malabsorption. Lower-range doses may be indicated if renal function is impaired. Magnesium is added to parenteral admixtures as magnesium sulfate (50% $MgSO_4$), which contains 4.1 mEq (49.3 mg) of magnesium per milliliter. Excessive doses may cause central nervous system depression and hypotonia.[130] Serum magnesium levels may be transiently elevated in preterm infants whose mothers received significant amounts of magnesium sulfate to prevent premature labor or treat preeclampsia. Magnesium may be withheld from PN solutions for these infants until serum levels are within normal limits.

Calcium deficiency is not usually identified by low serum levels because serum calcium is usually maintained at the expense of bone stores.[130] Hypocalcemia is most common during the neonatal period, particularly in infants born prematurely, due to their relatively low calcium stores and inappropriately low parathyroid hormone levels. This initial hypocalcemia usually resolves within the first few days of life when treated with intravenous administration of calcium 1–2 mEq/kg/day.[86]

Nutrition recommendations for parenteral calcium administration to prematurely born infants range from 50–80 mg/kg/day (which is 1.3–2 mmol/kg/day or 2.5–3 mEq/kg/day).[117,130,137,138] Most published sources empirically recommend 10–50 mg/kg/day (which is 0.25 to 1.3 mmol/kg/day or 0.5 to 2 mEq/kg/day) for all other ages[45] (see Table 20-2). Calcium should be administered over 24 hours, because parenteral calcium administered chronically as bolus doses over 20 minutes to 1 hour has been associated with hypercalcemia and hypercalciuria.[139,140] Nephrolithiasis and hypercalciuria have been associated with furosemide therapy and inadequate phosphorus intake.[137,141] Older children receiving cyclic parenteral nutrition may have greater urinary losses of calcium due to higher rates of infusion.[142]

Calcium gluconate is generally the additive of choice, but there is some concern about aluminum contamination, especially at higher doses.[143] Solutions that deliver 15–30 μg aluminum/kg/day may result in tissue loading and are considered unsafe.[130,144] Calcium gluconate 10% contains 100 mg of calcium gluconate per 1 mL, providing 0.5 mEq, 0.25 mmol, or 10 mg of elemental calcium per 1 mL.

Phosphorus depletion has been reported in infants and children; it may be more pronounced when calcium is given without phosphorus, or it may occur during chronic aminoglycoside or vancomycin therapy.[145] Phosphorus depletion is characterized by hypercalciuria (at least 4 mg calcium/kg/day), hypophosphatemia (serum levels less than 4 mg/dL), and undetectable levels of urinary phosphorus excretion.[130,137,146] Parenteral repletion of phosphorus may be accomplished by an initial one to two doses of 5–11 mg/kg (0.15–0.36 mmol/kg), each given over 6 hours. When refeeding malnourished individuals, the initial 7 to 10 days of the anabolic phase is accompanied by increased needs for phosphorus, and, to a lesser extent, potassium and magnesium, because these electrolytes are incorporated into cells of lean tissue. Phosphorus needs may be twice the normal recommended allowance during this time, though consistent monitoring is recommended to prevent excessive phosphorus administration, which can cause hyperphosphatemia, hypocalcemia, and secondary hyperparathyroidism.[130]

Recommendations for parenteral administration of phosphorus to infants and children are given in Table 20-2. Doses for phosphorus are often given in proportion to calcium as 1–1.3:1 molar ratio or 1.3–1.7:1 calcium/phosphorus ratio by weight.[130] Phosphorus is added to parenteral nutrient solutions as potassium phosphate or sodium phosphate salts. Potassium phosphate contains 93 mg (3 mmol) of phosphorus and 4.4 mEq of potassium per mL. Sodium phosphate contains 93 mg (3 mmol) of phosphorus and 4 mEq of sodium per mL.

The greatest difficulty in providing adequate calcium and phosphorus parenterally is their relative insolubility in the same admixture, limited further by increasing pH and temperature. Alternating calcium and phosphorus administration is not recommended due to adverse effects, including alternating elevations of serum mineral levels, increased mineral losses due to urinary excretion, and altered mineral homeostasis.[147–149] Recommendations for compounding to minimize precipitation usually include adding phosphate salts early in the process and calcium salts late (but before the lipid emulsion in 3-in-1 admixtures).[149,150] Adherence to compounding protocol is particularly important when lipid is present because precipitates are more difficult to identify due to the opacity of the admixture. The addition of L-cysteine increases mineral solubility; the use of calcium glycerophosphate or monobasic phosphate formulations may also improve solubility.[48] Filters are recommended to prevent precipitate delivery: a 1.2-micron air-eliminating filter for lipid-containing admixtures and a 0.22-micron air-eliminating filter for non–lipid-containing admixtures.[150] The higher doses of minerals needed for young infants are given through central intravenous access to prevent vascular damage and tissue sloughs. Separate administration of lipid may be needed to allow higher concentrations of calcium and phosphorus for prematurely born infants.

Recommendations for daily parenteral doses of trace minerals are given in Table 20-2.[130,151] Zinc, copper, chromium, manganese, selenium, and iodine are available singly or in combination for use in PN admixtures. Product concentrations and dose recommendations are given in **Table 20-5**. Neither clinical nor biochemical deficiency of molybdenum or iodine with parenteral nutrition has been reported, and they are generally not included in PN admixtures. Transdermal absorption of iodine from cleansing or disinfecting solutions or ointments may be an adequate source of

TABLE 20-5 Dose Concentrations and Recommendations for Combined Trace Mineral Products

Product Category	Dose mL	Zinc µg	Copper µg	Chromium µg	Manganese µg	Selenium[1] µg
Neonatal[2]	1	1500	100	0.85	25	—
	0.2/kg	300/kg[3]	20/kg	0.17/kg	5/kg[4]	—
Pediatric	1	500 or 1000	100	0.85 or 1	25	0 or 15
	0.1/kg	50 or 100/kg	10/kg	~ 0.1/kg	2.5/kg	0 or 1.5/kg
	0.2/kg	100 or 200/kg	20/kg	~ 0.2/kg	5/kg[4]	0 or 2/kg
	2[5]	2000	200	2	50	30
	5[5]	2500 or 5000	500	4.25 or 5	125	0
Adult[6,7] (standard)	1	1000	400	4	100	0 or 20
	0.05/kg	50/kg	20/kg	0.2/kg	5/kg[4]	0 or 1/kg
Adult[6] (concentrate)	1	5000	1000	10	500	0 or 60
	0.01/kg	50/kg	10/kg	0.1/kg	5/kg[4]	0 or 0.6/kg

[1]Neonatal and select pediatric and adult products do not contain selenium or molybdenum. These may be added separately when total parenteral nutrition is required for longer than 4 weeks.

[2]Neonatal products are generally recommended for preterm infants until term age. Maximum dose is 3 mL/day.

[3]Additional zinc is needed to meet recommendations for preterm neonates.

[4]Manganese dose may be excessive in cholestatic jaundice.

[5]Maximum dose of pediatric product with selenium is limited by the amount of selenium. Maximum dose of pediatric product without selenium is limited by cwopper content.

[6]Adult products are generally used for adolescents, or children over 10 years of age.

[7]Iodine is included in one standard and one concentrated adult product in concentrations of 25 and 75 mcg/mL respectively; molybdenum is included in one standard adult product in a concentration of 25 µg/mL.

Source: Intravenous nutritional therapy: trace metals. In: Killion KH, Kastrup EK (eds). *Drug Facts and Comparisons*, 57th ed. St. Louis, MO: Wolters Kluwer Health; 2003;125.

iodine.[141] Fluorine is not added because its role in human nutrition is limited primarily to dental health and may be of greater benefit when administered topically once teeth have erupted around 6 months of age.[152]

Very-low-birth-weight infants and infants and children with protein-calorie malnutrition, thermal injury, neoplasms, chronic diarrhea, enterocutaneous fistulas, or bile salt malabsorption are at greatest risk for developing trace element deficiency.[151,153–155] Zinc supplementation without copper supplementation may interfere with copper metabolism.[153] Copper doses are reduced or eliminated and manganese often is withheld for infants and children who develop cholestatic jaundice because these minerals are excreted primarily through bile and their accumulation is potentially hepatotoxic and, in the case of magnesium, neurotoxic.[69,156–158] However, serum copper and manganese levels may not correlate with serum direct bilirubin levels.[159] Hepatic copper content has been shown to decrease as evidence of cholestasis increases, and copper deficiency has been reported when omitted from PN due to presence of cholestasis.[160–162] Serum manganese levels may become markedly elevated after several months of PN. A contributory role of manganese in the development of PN-related cholestasis has been considered, particularly in individuals receiving PN for longer than 30 days.[163] Both serum copper and manganese should be monitored and supplemented as needed to maintain serum levels within the normal range.[59] Selenium and molybdenum are not generally used when PN is required for only a short period of time. Selenium is present as a contaminant in parenteral dextrose solutions, providing up to 0.9 mg/dL. Parenteral selenium toxicity has not been reported, though lower doses may be indicated when renal function is impaired.[130]

Iron deficiency is probably the most common trace mineral deficiency. It manifests as microcytic hypochromic anemia and is characterized by low serum hemoglobin and ferritin levels, low hematocrit, and low percent transferrin saturation. Infants and children at risk for iron deficiency include those who are prematurely born, chronically ill, protein-calorie malnourished, have significant unreplaced blood loss, or who receive unsupplemented PN for long periods of time.

Controversy exists over whether iron should be routinely included in PN therapy. Intramuscular injections of iron may not be the best choice in the small prematurely born infant or the protein-calorie malnourished patient due to small muscle mass and increased risk of sarcoma at the site of injection.[164] Anaphylaxis can occur with administration of iron dextran.[164] Iron may be safely given daily in PN admixtures or in bolus doses given intravenously over 2 to 3 hours weekly or monthly.[164–167] Often, iron is given parenterally only in treatment of iron deficiency anemia.

Although standard dose recommendations for prematurely born infants are 0.1–0.2 mg/kg/day,[130,168] trials of recombinant erythropoietin have used iron supplements of 1 mg/kg/day without evidence of harmful side effects.[169,170] Iron toxicity may be difficult to ascertain because iron is stored quickly in hepatic tissue, and serum iron levels may not reflect overload. Excess iron may also increase risk of gram-negative septicemia and raise antioxidant requirements. These risks do not preclude use of standard doses of parenteral iron, but higher doses must be used with caution beyond 4 weeks duration.[130] Very-low-birth-weight infants who have received blood transfusion of at least 180 mL of packed cells may not need additional iron supplementation.[171] Doses of 0.1 mg/kg/day up to 1 mg/day are recommended for all other infants and children. Iron dextran is available as the source of iron for parenteral use. Guidelines for dosage and administration of iron dextran in treatment of iron deficiency are given in the manufacturer's package insert.

Monitoring

A comprehensive monitoring program for infants and children receiving PN includes evaluating laboratory measurements of metabolic and electrolyte status (see Table 20-3), assessing growth (see **Table 20-6**), and evaluating other clinical parameters (see **Table 20-7**). Baseline and regularly scheduled laboratory measurements enable timely identification of metabolic complications and assessment of nutritional adequacy. Some of the metabolic complications that may occur during parenteral nutrition support include the following:

- Hypokalemia
- Hyperkalemia
- Hypocalcemia
- Hypomagnesemia
- Hypophosphatemia
- Anemia
- Hyperglycemia
- Metabolic acidosis/alkalosis

Laboratory monitoring should take into consideration smaller blood volumes in pediatric patients, using microtechniques whenever possible and avoiding unnecessary blood work. For patients on long-term PN, the need and frequency for some tests can be reevaluated once a stable regimen has been established. See also Chapter 3 on nutrition assessment and Appendix G for biochemical evaluation of nutritional status.

Temperature instability, apnea, bradycardia, and increased respiration rate and pulse may be early signs of sepsis in the pediatric patient. Records of intake provide documentation that actual administration equals planned intake. Documentation of output establishes a basis for evaluation of fluid balance, as do evaluation of skin turgor and the presence of edema. Insertion sites are monitored for redness, swelling, leaking, or other signs of infection or infiltration. Changes in behavior and/or mental status may precede other signs of sepsis or fluid and electrolyte balance.

Other Concerns

When normal feeding is replaced with PN, parents may feel helpless or useless. An infant or child of any age may feel frustrated at not being able to eat. Older children may have

TABLE 20-6 Growth Parameters Monitored During Pediatric Parenteral Nutrition

Parameter	Frequency
Weight	Daily (neonates up to 1 month corrected age) Weekly (1–6 months corrected age) Monthly (infants, 6 months corrected age; children)
Length or height	Weekly (infants, 6 months corrected age) Monthly (infants, 6 months corrected age) Every 3 months (ages 1–3) Every 6 months (ages 4–18)
Head circumference	Weekly (infants, 6 months corrected age) Monthly (infants, 6 months corrected age) Every 3 months (ages 1–3)
Body composition triceps skinfold arm muscle area	As clinically indicated; comparison against established norms is more useful in children over 3 years than in younger children

TABLE 20-7 Clinical Monitoring During Pediatric Parenteral Nutrition

Clinical Parameter	Initial	Stable
Temperature Pulse/respirations	Hourly, then every 4–8 hr	Daily or as indicated
Intake	Hourly, then every 4–8 hr	Daily
Output	Hourly, then every 4–8 hr	As indicated
Administration system	Hourly, then every 4–8 hr	Daily
Infusion site/dressing	Hourly, then every 4–8 hr	Daily
Mental status, behavioral status, edema, skin turgor	Every 4–8 hr	Daily or as indicated

fears or insecurities about body function or body image. The ability of an infant or child and his or her family to accept and adapt to PN depends on the presenting diagnosis, the acuity or chronic nature of the disease or condition, the duration and complexity of the hospitalization, the duration of nutrition support therapy, and the physical and emotional development of the infant or child.[172–174] When long-term or home PN is needed, the stability of the family unit and its financial, physical, and emotional resources are important factors as well.

Members of the hospital-based multidisciplinary team, including the physician, nurse, dietitian, pharmacist, social worker, and developmental specialist, must plan a program of home PN that is feasible, given family and community resources. Resources that support success of home PN are listed in **Table 20-8**. Education of family members must take into account their readiness and ability to learn. Assessment of learning includes measuring the family's ability to accurately repeat instructions or demonstrate techniques. Communication with home healthcare providers is essential for continuity of care.

The technical nature of PN must not overshadow the infant or child and his or her developmental progress. Occupational and physical therapists, speech pathologists, and other healthcare team members ensure the hospital setting is modified as much as possible to support the normal development of the child on PN.

For neonates whose feedings are limited or who are unable to take oral feedings, pleasant oral stimulation, non-nutritive sucking, and other sensory stimulation are needed to support normal oral development. Prolonged early oral deprivation can lead to increased oral sensitivity and abnormal tongue movements that can adversely influence the development of future speech patterns.[175] Infants use their mouths to explore much of their environment. Sucking on fingers or toys can be encouraged to help infants experience and develop trust in their environment.

Parents, particularly mothers, may feel responsible for their infant's problems and may suffer loss of self-esteem or have feelings of inadequacy at being unable to perform the simple caregiving task of feeding. Healthcare professionals can enhance the parents' involvement in "feeding" the PN-dependent infant by encouraging them to hold, cuddle, and offer other forms of oral stimulation during "normal" feeding times. When possible, the infant on PN should be offered some type of oral feeding, if only in very small amounts. If totally deprived of oral sustenance, the introduction of oral feedings may be met with gagging, vomiting, swallowing difficulties, or other signs of feeding aversion.

Toddlers present many challenges to the safe delivery of PN. These challenges may include temperament, mobility, and the development of other normal milestones, such as toileting. Creative strategies to allow toddlers some control and independence in their environment can promote

TABLE 20-8 Resources that Support Successful Home Parenteral Nutrition

Environment	Grounded electrical outlets. Backup electricity, either battery, generator, or power company priority for loss of power. Lack of physical barriers to maneuvering equipment or storing supplies. Refrigeration to store adequate supplies of solutions. Reliable telephone service. Convenient and safe water supply and hand-washing facilities.
Medical support	Convenient and reliable home healthcare agency for nursing care. Ongoing nutritional assessment, supplies, laboratory assessment. Local physician experienced and amenable to home parenteral nutrition. Responsive local community emergency care, both ambulance and local emergency room.
Family characteristics	At least two responsible adults are competent to provide all care associated with home parenteral nutrition; extended family support. All children (both the patient and siblings, particularly small children) are protected from harm associated with home parenteral nutrition, such as needle sticks; damage to catheter, tubing, or other equipment; removal of catheter; etc.
Financial	Adequate medical insurance coverage with certified medical necessity for home parenteral nutrition.
Attitude	Family and patient must see home parenteral nutrition as having a positive influence on the life of the child. Respect for risks and safety issues associated with parenteral nutrition. Ability and willingness to comply with medical plan and techniques.

autonomy and lessen the negative impact of hospitalization or home PN on normal development. A backpack that contains solution, pump, and tubing in fastened compartments can allow mobility and prevent toddlers from handling equipment but offer parents easy access for managing PN. Nocturnal cyclic PN may reduce interference with developmental needs.

The school-age child who is frequently hospitalized and requires PN needs to stay involved with school and with friends, to have some conformity with peers in appearance, and to have as much control over personal issues as possible. In-hospital teachers or private tutors may be needed to maintain educational progress. An established routine that allows the child to accomplish as many aspects of care as possible is important to avoid feelings of inferiority and prevent excessive dependency. During home PN, children are encouraged to resume as many normal school and play activities as their clinical condition allows.

Although the technical aspects of PN in the adolescent may be easier to manage, other issues may present greater challenges. The adolescent may have concerns, fears, and/or anxiety regarding many issues, including the following:

- Loss of control
- Altered body image or appearance
- Peer acceptance or isolation
- Technical failures or malfunctions
- Health and life expectancy
- Ability to participate in sports and other peer group activities
- Financial issues
- The effects on other family members

Sleep disturbances may occur due to anxiety or frequent urination that occurs with nocturnal fluid administration. Many of these issues may cause anger or depression and lead to poor compliance with the therapeutic regimen.

Backpacks or vests designed to hold PN solutions and equipment may be used to maximize mobility and minimize changes in physical appearance. Nocturnal cyclic PN circumvents changes in appearance during the day and places less limitation on activities with peers.

Home Care Considerations

PN is a complex and expensive therapy. Costs include the following:

- Nutrient solutions
- Technical equipment, such as catheters, tubing, and automated pumps
- Laboratory monitoring
- Healthcare providers, such as physicians, nurses, dietitians, pharmacists, and developmental therapists

Though PN administered at home may generate fewer costs, it is still expensive.

In efforts to contain healthcare costs, many third-party payers have developed regulations that restrict who can be reimbursed and what is reimbursed and place a capitation on reimbursement for PN. Because PN is not a directly reimbursed service, reimbursement often depends on the assigned primary diagnosis or specific diagnosis-related group (DRG) or comorbid condition (CC). DRGs or CCs that include the presence of malnutrition or nonfunctioning gastrointestinal tract with malabsorption are often required, particularly in the home setting. Medical necessity for PN must be justified by the prescribing physician at the initiation of therapy and periodically throughout the course of therapy. Even then, reimbursement is usually less than 100%, which leaves the family (or supplemental insurance) with the remaining costs.

Case Study

Nutrition Assessment of Child on Parenteral Nutrition

Patient history: HC, an 8-year, 4-month-old male, is admitted to the hospital with a medical history of blunt abdominal trauma 4 years ago with ruptured duodenum and gastrojejunostomy with pyloric exclusion. Current radiologic findings indicate possible partial bowel obstruction.

Assessment

Weight: 22.2 kg, 10th percentile, gaining only 0.3 kg over the past year when weight was 21.9 kg, 25th percentile. Normal gain over this time at this age is 2.1–2.4 kg, which would maintain the 25th percentile.

Height: 125 cm, 25th percentile

Body mass index: 14.2 kg/m^2, 7th percentile

Ideal weight: For height and age, given previous growth, ideal weight is likely 24 kg.

Lab work: All within normal limits for age.

Diet order: Clear liquids. Physician has recommended parenteral nutrition and peripheral IV placement. RD consulted for TPN recommendations.

Intake: Oral intake provides less than 200 kcal/day and is not adequate to meet estimated needs at this time. Patient experiences severe abdominal cramps with food and beverage intake at this time. No known food allergies.

Nutrition Diagnosis

The nutrition diagnosis is inadequate oral intake related to pain associated with eating, as evidenced by low weight gain and intake records.

Nutrition Intervention/Recommendations

Nutritional needs at this time can be met by the following PN delivery:

- Start parenteral nutrition at 55 mL/hour to meet minimum fluid requirements and gradually increase over the next 2 to 3 days to 92 mL/hour to meet estimated nutritional needs.
- Goal volume is 2208 mL, providing approximately 100 mL/kg/day at a rate of 92 mL/hour.
- Provide 10% dextrose, 1.5% protein with standard amino acids, 2% liposyn at goal volume supplies: 60 kcal/kg/day, 1.5 g protein/kg/day, 2 g fat/kg/day; energy source: 57% cholesterol, 10% protein, 33% fat.
- 30 mEq/L sodium chloride with sodium phosphate provides 3.8 mEq/kg/day sodium (normal level is 1–5 mEq/kg/day).
- 6 mmol/L sodium phosphate provides 0.6 mmol/kg/day phosphorus (normal level is 0.5–1.3 mmol/kg/day).
- 10 mEq/L potassium chloride with sodium chloride provides a total chloride dose of 4 mEq/kg/day (normal level is 2–4 mEq/kg/day).
- 10 mEq/L potassium acetate with potassium chloride provides a total potassium dose of 2 mEq/kg/day (normal level is 2–4 mEq/kg/day).
- 3 mEq/L magnesium sulfate provides 0.3 mEq/kg/day magnesium (normal level is 0.25–0.5 mEq/kg/day).
- 6 mEq/L calcium gluconate provides 0.6 mEq/kg/day calcium (normal level is 0.5–1 mEq/kg/day).
- Provide a dose of pediatric multivitamins and 0.2 mL pediatric trace mineral package/kg/day.

This provides 100% of needs peripherally. If oral intake provides a significant amount of nutrients, the rate can be reduced, although a clear liquid diet does not meet many nutritional needs and the patient's weight is lower than expected for growth history and current height.

Nutrition Monitoring/Evaluation

Although the patient should not experience refeeding syndrome, because he does not appear to be in a malnourished state, standard laboratory assessment for PN will be monitored as well as changes in weight (normal weight gain is 0.24 kg/month). Follow up in 3 to 5 days.

Questions for the Reader

1. Lab work on day 3 includes a serum phosphorus level of 3.4 g/dL (normal level is 3.6–5.6 mg/dL). What is one possible nutrition diagnosis or problem?
2. What changes would you make in this patient's PN prescription to address his current nutrition diagnosis?
3. On day 5, the patient is taken to surgery, and laparoscopic surgical findings are significant. A large colon mesenteric rent was found with rotation of cecum through the defect. Rotation was corrected, and venous congestion was relieved. Lysis of adhesions and reconstruction of the previous gastrojejunostomy was performed. After surgery, what adjustments might be necessary in this patient's TPN?
4. Lab work on day 7 includes a serum triglyceride level of 250 mg/dL (normal level < 150 mg/dL). What adjustment would you recommend in this patient's PN prescription?

REFERENCES

1. Steinhorn DM. Nutrition in the PICU: who needs it?! Guidelines for nutritional support of critically ill children. In: Green TP, Zucher AR (eds). *Current Concepts in Pediatric Critical Care.* Chicago: Society of Critical Care Medicine; 1996:77–86.
2. Archer S, Burnett R, Fischer J. Current uses and abuses of total parenteral nutrition. In: *Advances in Surgery.* Chicago: Mosby-Year Book; 1996;29:165–189.
3. Chellis MJ, Sanders SV, Webster H, et al. Early enteral feeding in the pediatric intensive care unit. *J Parenter Enteral Nutr.* 1996;20:71–73.
4. Acra S, Rollins C. Principles and guidelines for parenteral nutrition in children. *Pediatr Ann.* 1999;28:113–120.
5. Davis A. Pediatrics. In: Matarese LE, Gottschlich MM (eds). *Contemporary Nutrition Support Practice.* Philadelphia: WB Saunders; 1998:349–351.
6. Fisher G, Opper F. An interdisciplinary nutrition support team improves quality of care in a teaching hospital. *J Am Diet Assoc.* 1996;96:176–178.
7. Fisher A, Poole R, Machie R, et al. Clinical pathway for pediatric parenteral nutrition. *Nutr Clin Pract.* 1997;12:76–80.
8. Phillips S. Pediatric parenteral nutrition clinical pathway. *Building Block Life.* 2003;Winter:1.
9. Trujillo EB, Young LS. Metabolic and monetary costs of avoidable parenteral nutrition use. *J Parenter Enteral Nutr.* 1999;23:109–113.
10. Koletzko B, Goulet O, Hunt J, et al. for the Parenteral Nutrition Guidelines Working Group. Guidelines on paediatric parenteral nutrition of the European Society of Paediatric Gastroenterology, Hepatology and Nutrition (ESPGHAN) and the European Society for Clinical Nutrition and Metabolism (ESPEN), supported by the European Society of Paediatric Research (ESPR). *J Pediatr Gastroenterol Nutr.* 2005;41:S1–S87.
11. American Society for Parenteral and Enteral Nutrition. Guidelines for the use of parenteral and enteral nutrition in adult and pediatric patients. *J Parenter Enteral Nutr.* 1993;17(Suppl):27SA–52SA.
12. Sitrin MD. Nutrition support in inflammatory bowel disease. *Nutr Clin Pract.* 1992;7:53–60.
13. Rickard KA, Grosfield JL, Kirksey A, et al. Reversal of protein-energy malnutrition in children during treatment of advanced neoplastic disease. *Ann Surg.* 1979;190:771–781.

14. Filler RM, Dietz W, Suskind RM, et al. Parenteral feeding in management of children with cancer. *Cancer.* 1979;43(Suppl): 2117–2120.
15. Copeland EM, MacFadgen BV, Dudrick SJ. Effect of intravenous hyperalimentation on established delayed hypersensitivity in the cancer patient. *Ann Surg.* 1976;184:60–64.
16. Copeland EM, Daly JM, Ota DM, et al. Nutrition, cancer, and intravenous hyperalimentation. *Cancer.* 1979;43:2108–2116.
17. Andrassay RJ, Chwals WJ. Nutritional support of the pediatric oncology patient. *Nutrition.* 1998;14:124–129.
18. Christensen ML, Hancock ML, Gattuso J, et al. Parenteral nutrition associated with increased infection rate in children with cancer. *Cancer.* 1993;72:2732–2738.
19. Copeman MC. Use of total parenteral nutrition in children with cancer: a review and some recommendations. *Pediatr Hematol Oncol.* 1994;11:463–470.
20. Perl M. TPN and the anorexia nervosa patient. *Nutr Supp Serv.* 1981;1:13.
21. Pertschuk MJ, Forster J, Buzby G, et al. The treatment of anorexia nervosa with total parenteral nutrition. *Biol Psychiatr.* 1981;16:539–550.
22. Pereira-da-Silva L, Virella D, Henriques G, et al. A simple equation to estimate the osmolarity of neonatal parenteral nutrition solutions. *J Parenter Enteral Nutr.* 2004;28:34–37.
23. Kanarek KS, Kuznicki MB, Blair RC. Infusion of total parenteral nutrition via the umbilical artery. *J Parenter Enteral Nutr.* 1991;15:71–74.
24. Chathas MK. Percutaneous central venous catheters in neonates. *J Obstet Gynecol Neonatal Nurs.* 1986;15:324–332.
25. Goodwin ML. The Seldinger method of PICC insertion. *J Intraven Nurs.* 1989;12:238–243.
26. Brown JM. Peripherally inserted central catheters: use in home care. *J Intraven Nurs.* 1989;12:144–147.
27. Yeung CY, Lee HC, Huang FY, Wang CS. Sepsis during total parenteral nutrition: exploration of risk factors and determination of the effectiveness of peripherally inserted central venous catheters. *Pediatr Infect Dis J.* 1998;17:135–142.
28. Chathas MK, Paton JB. Sepsis outcomes in infants and children with central venous catheters: percutaneous versus surgical insertion. *J Obstet Gynecol Neonatal Nurs.* 1996;25:500–506.
29. Chung D, Ziegler M. Central venous catheter access. *Nutrition.* 1988;14:119–123.
30. Dubois J, Garel L, Tapiero B, et al. Peripherally inserted central catheters in infants and children. *Radiology.* 1997;204:622–626.
31. Pettit J. Assessment of infants with peripherally inserted central catheters: part 1. Detecting the most frequently occurring complications. *Adv Neonatal Care.* 2002;2:304–315.
32. Liossis G, Bardin C, Papageorgiou A, et al. Comparison of risks from percutaneous central venous catheter and peripheral lines in infants of extremely low birth weight: a cohort controlled study of infants, 1000 g. *J Matern Fetal Neonatal Med.* 2003;13:171–174.
33. Reed T, Phillips S. Management of central venous catheter occlusions and repairs. *J Intraven Nurs.* 1996;19:289–294.
34. Kakzanov V, Monagle P, Chan AKC. Thromboembolism in infants and children with gastrointestinal failure receiving long-term parenteral nutrition. *J Parenter Enteral Nutr.* 2008; 32:88–93.
35. Pemberton LB, Lyman B, Lander V, et al. Sepsis from triple versus single lumen catheters during total parenteral nutrition in surgical or chronically ill patients. *Arch Surg.* 1986;121:591.
36. Yeung C, May J, Hughes R. Infection rate for single lumen versus triple lumen subclavian catheters. *Inf Control Hosp Epidemiol.* 1988;9:154.
37. Hughes CB. A totally implantable central venous system for chemotherapy administration. *NITA.* 1985;8:523–527.
38. Valentine CJ, Puthoff TD. Enhancing parenteral nutrition therapy for the neonate. *Nutr Clin Pract.* 2007;22:183–193.
39. Puangco M, Nguyen H, Sheridan M. Computerized PN ordering optimizes timely nutrition therapy in a neonatal intensive care unit. *J Am Diet Assoc.* 1997;97:258–261.
40. Schloerb PR. Electronic parenteral and enteral nutrition. *J Parenter Enteral Nutr.* 2000;24:23–29.
41. Lehmann CU, Conner KG. Preventing provider errors: online total parenteral nutrition calculator. *Pediatrics.* 2004;113:748–753.
42. Hardy G, Puzovic M. Formulation, stability, and administration of parenteral nutrition with new lipid emulsions. *Nutr Clin Pract.* 2009;24:616–625.
43. Mirtallo J, Canada T, Johnson D, et al. for the Task Force for the Revision of Safe Practices for Parenteral Nutrition. Safe practices for parenteral nutrition formulations. *J Parenter Enteral Nutr.* 2004;28:S39–S70.
44. Mirtallo J. Should the use of total nutrient admixtures be limited? *Am J Hosp Pharm.* 1994;51:2831–2836.
45. Lee MD, Yoon JE, Kim, SI, et al. Stability of total nutrient admixtures in reference to ambient temperatures. *Nutrition.* 2003;19:886–890.
46. Neuzil J, Darlow BA, Inder TE, et al. Oxidation of parenteral lipid emulsion by ambient and phototherapy lights: potential toxicity of routine parenteral feeding. *J Pediatr.* 1995;126:785–790.
47. Laborie S, Lavoie JC. Protecting solutions of parenteral nutrition from peroxidation. *J Parenter Enteral Nutr.* 1999;23:104–108.
48. Silvers KM, Sluis KB. Limiting light-induced lipid peroxidation and vitamin loss in infant parenteral nutrition by adding multivitamin preparations to Intralipid. *Acta Paediatr.* 2001;90:242–249.
49. Alwood M, Driscoll D, Sizer T, Ball P. Physicochemical assessment of total nutrient admixture stability and safety: quantifying the risk. *Nutrition.* 1998;14:166–167.
50. Skouroliakou M, Matthaiou C, Chiou A, et al. Physicochemical stability of parenteral nutrition supplied as all-in-one for neonates. *J Parenter Enteral Nutr.* 2008;32:201–209.
51. Trissel LA, Gilbert DL. Compatibility of medications with 3-in-1 parenteral nutrition admixtures. *J Parenter Enteral Nutr.* 1999;23:67–74.
52. Pharmaceutical compounding—sterile preparations. In: *Revision Bulletin, The United States Pharmacopeia.* Rockville, MD: United States Pharmacopeial Convention; 2008:1–61.
53. Curtis C, Sacks GS. Compounding parenteral nutrition: reducing the risks. *Nutr Clin Pract.* 2009;24:441–446.
54. Steger PJ, Muhlebach SF. Lipid peroxidation of intravenous lipid emulsions and all-in-one admixtures in total parenteral nutrition bags: the influence of trace elements. *J Parenter Enteral Nutr.* 2000;24:37–41.
55. Driscoll DF, Bacon MN. Physicochemical stability of two types of intravenous lipid emulsion as total nutrient admixtures. *J Parenter Enteral Nutr.* 2000;24:15–22.

56. Driscoll DF, Nehne J, Peterss H, et al. Physicochemical stability of intravenous lipid emulsions as all-in-one admixtures intended for the very young. *Clin Nutr.* 2003;22:489–495.
57. Driscoll D, Bacon M, Bistrian B. Effects of in-line filtration on lipid particle size distribution in total nutrient admixtures. *J Parenter Enteral Nutr.* 1996;20:296–301.
58. Muller MJ. Hepatic complications in parenteral nutrition. *Z Gastroenterol.* 1996;34:36–40.
59. Slicker J, Vermilyea S. Pediatric parenteral nutrition: putting the microscope on macronutrients and micronutrients. *Nutr Clin Pract.* 2009;24:481–486.
60. Oh W, Karechi H. Phototherapy and insensible water loss in the newborn infant. *Am J Dis Child.* 1972;124:230–232.
61. Yeh TF, Voora S, Lillien J. Oxygen consumption and insensible water loss in premature infants in single versus double walled incubators. *J Pediatr.* 1980;97:967–971.
62. Gruskin AB. Fluid therapy in children. *Urol Clin North Am.* 1976;3:277–291.
63. Rao M, Koenig E, Li S, et al. Estimation of insensible water loss in low birth weight infants by direct calorimetric measurement of metabolic heat release. *Pediatr Res.* 1989;25:295A.
64. Ford EG. Nutrition support of pediatric patients. *Nutr Clin Pract.* 1996;11:183–191.
65. Carlson S. Acid/base balance in special care nurseries. *Support Line.* 2002;24:17.
66. Aperia A, Broberger O, Elinder G, et al. Postnatal development of renal function in pre-term and full-term infants. *Acta Paediatr Scand.* 1981;70:183–187.
67. Peters O, Ryan S, Matthew L, et al. Randomised controlled trial of acetate in preterm neonates receiving parenteral nutrition. *Arch Dis Child.* 1997;77:F12–F15.
68. Groh-Wargo S, Ciaccia A, Moore J. Neonatal metabolic acidosis: effect of chloride from normal saline flushes. *J Parenter Enteral Nutr.* 1988;12:159–161.
69. Kerner JA Jr (ed). *Manual of Pediatric Parenteral Nutrition.* New York: John Wiley and Sons; 1983.
70. Khaldi N, Coran AG, Wesley JR. Guidelines for parenteral nutrition in children. *Nutr Supp Serv.* 1984;4:27.
71. Zlotkin SH, Bryan MH, Anderson GH. Intravenous nitrogen and energy intakes required to duplicate in utero nitrogen accretion in prematurely born human infants. *J Pediatr.* 1981;99:115–120.
72. Sunehag AL, Haymond MW. Glucose extremes in newborn infants. *Clin Perinatol.* 2002;29:245–260.
73. Kalhan SC, Kilic I. Carbohydrate as nutrient in the infant and child: range of acceptable intake. *Eur J Clin Nutr.* 1999;53:S94–S100.
74. Adamkin DH. Total parenteral nutrition. *Neonatal Intensive Care.* 1997;Sept/Oct:24.
75. Cochran EB, Phelps SJ, Helms RA. Parenteral nutrition in pediatric patients. *Clin Pharm.* 1988;7:351–366.
76. Sajbel TA, Dutro MP, Radway PR. Use of separate insulin infusions with total parenteral nutrition. *J Parenter Enteral Nutr.* 1987;11:97–99.
77. Groh-Wargo S. Prematurity/low birth weight. In: Lang C (ed). *Nutritional Support in Critical Care.* Gaithersburg, MD: Aspen Publishers; 1987:287.
78. Rubecz I, Mestyan J, Varga P, Klujber L. Energy metabolism, substrate utilization, and nitrogen balance in parenterally fed postoperative neonates and infants. *J Pediatr.* 1981;98:42–46.
79. Thureen PJ, Anderson AH, Baron KA, et al. Protein balance in the first week of life in ventilated neonates receiving parenteral nutrition. *Am J Clin Nutr.* 1998;68:1128–1135.
80. Poindexter BB, Denne SC. Protein needs of the preterm infant. *NeoReviews.* 2003;4:E52.
81. Thureen PJ, Hay WW Jr. Intravenous nutrition and postnatal growth of the micropremie. *Clin Perinatol.* 2000;27:197–219.
82. Kalhan SC, Iben S. Protein metabolism in the extremely low-birth-weight infant. *Clin Perinatol.* 2000;27:23–56.
83. Micheli J-L, Schultz Y, Junod S, et al. Early postnatal intravenous amino acid administration to extremely-low-birth-weight infants. In: Hay WW Jr (ed). *Seminars in Neonatal Nutrition and Metabolism,* vol 2. Columbus, OH: Ross Products Division; 1994:1–3.
84. Zlotkin SH, Stallings VA, Pencharz PB. Total parenteral nutrition in children. *Pediatr Clin North Am.* 1985;32:381–400.
85. Hellstrom A, Engstrom E, Hard A-L, et al. Postnatal serum insulin-like growth factor I deficiency is associated with retinopathy of prematurity and other complications of premature birth. *Pediatr.* 2003;112:1016–1020.
86. Coran AG, Drongowski RA. Studies on the toxicity and efficacy of new amino acid solution in pediatric parenteral nutrition. *J Parenter Enteral Nutr.* 1987;11:368–377.
87. Helms RA, Christensen ML, Mauer EC, Storm MC. Comparison of a pediatric versus standard amino acid formulation in preterm neonates requiring parenteral nutrition. *J Pediatr.* 1987;110:466–470.
88. Chessex P, Zebiche H, Pineault M, et al. Effect of amino acid composition of parenteral solutions on nitrogen retention and metabolic response in very-low-birth weight infants. *J Pediatr.* 1985;106:111–117.
89. Heird WC, Dell RB, Helms RA, et al. Amino acid mixture designed to maintain normal plasma amino acid patterns in infants and children requiring parenteral nutrition. *Pediatrics.* 1987;80:401–408.
90. Intravenous nutritional therapy: crystalline amino acid infusions. *Drug Facts and Comparisons.* St. Louis, MO: *Drug Facts & Comparisons*; 2010;96–97.
91. Heird WC. Essentiality of cyst(e)ine for neonates. Clinical and biochemical effects of parenteral cysteine supplementation. In: Kinney JM, Borum PR (eds). *Perspectives in Clinical Nutrition.* Munich, Germany: Urban Schwarzenberg; 1989:275–282.
92. Gaull GE, Sturman JA, Raiha NCR, Sturman JA. Development of mammalian sulfur metabolism. Absence of cystathionase in human fetal tissues. *Pediatr Res.* 1972;6:538–547.
93. Zlotkin SH, Bryan H, Anderson H. Cysteine supplementation to cysteine-free intravenous feeding regimens in newborn infants. *Am J Clin Nutr.* 1981;34:914–923.
94. Helms RA, Storm MC, Christensen ML, et al. Cysteine supplementation results in normalization of plasma taurine concentrations in children receiving home parenteral nutrition. *J Pediatr.* 1999;134:358–361.
95. Heird WC, Hay W, Helms RA, et al. Pediatric parenteral amino acid mixture in low birth weight infants. *Pediatrics.* 1988;81:41–50.

96. Heird WC, Dell RB, Helms RA, et al. Amino acid mixture designed to maintain normal plasma amino acid patterns in infants and children requiring parenteral nutrition. *Pediatrics.* 1987;80:401–408.
97. Lowe DK, Benfell K, Smith RJ, et al. Safety of glutamine-enriched parenteral nutrient solutions in humans. *Am J Clin Nutr.* 1990;52: 1101–1106.
98. Wischmeyer PE. Clinical applications of L-glutamine: past, present, and future. *Nutr Clin Pract.* 2003;18:377.
99. Lacey JM, Crouch JB, Benfell K, et al. The effects of glutamine-supplemented nutrition in premature infants. *J Parenter Enteral Nutr.* 1996;20:74–80.
100. Vaughn P, Thomas P, Clark R, et al. Enteral glutamine supplementation and morbidity in low birth weight infants. *J Pediatr.* 2003;142:662–668.
101. Abitbol CL, Holliday MA. Total parenteral nutrition in anuric children. *Clin Nephrol.* 1976;5:153–158.
102. Holliday MA, Wassner S, Ramirez J. Intravenous nutrition in uremic children with protein-energy malnutrition. *Am J Clin Nutr.* 1978;31:1854–1860.
103. Motil KJ, Harmon WE, Grupe WE. Complications of essential amino acid hyperalimentation in children with acute renal failure. *J Parenter Enteral Nutr.* 1980;4:32–35.
104. Takala J. Total parenteral nutrition in experimental uremia: studies of acute and chronic renal failure in the growing rat. *J Parenter Enteral Nutr.* 1984;8:427–432.
105. Helms RA, Phelps SJ, Mauer EC, et al. Parenteral protein use in liver disease. *Pediatr Res.* 1989;25:115A.
106. Maldonato J, Gil A, Faus MJ, et al. Differences in the serum amino acid pattern of injured and infected children promoted by two parenteral nutrition solutions. *J Parenter Enteral Nutr.* 1989;13:41–46.
107. Holman RT, Johnson SB, Hatch TF. A case of human linolenic acid deficiency involving neurologic abnormalities. *Am J Clin Nutr.* 1982;35:617–623.
108. Uauy R, Mena P, Rojas C. Essential fatty acid metabolism in the micropremie. *Clin Perinatol.* 2000;27:71–93.
109. Jensen CL, Heird WC. Lipids with an emphasis on long-chain polyunsaturated fatty acids. *Clin Perinatol.* 2002;29:261–281.
110. Friedman Z, Danon A, Stahlman MT, et al. Rapid onset of essential fatty acid deficiency in the newborn. *Pediatrics.* 1976;58:640–649.
111. Baugh N, Recupero MA, Kerner JA Jr. Nutritional requirements for pediatric patients. In: Merritt RJ (ed). *The ASPEN Nutrition Support Practice Manual.* Silver Spring, MD: American Society for Parenteral and Enteral Nutrition; 1998:1–13.
112. American Academy of Pediatrics, Committee on Nutrition. Commentary on parenteral nutrition. *Pediatrics.* 1983;71:547–552.
113. Levy JS, Winters RW, Heird WC. Total parenteral nutrition in pediatric patients. *Pediatr Rev.* 1980;2:99.
114. American Academy of Pediatrics, Committee on Nutrition. Prudent life-style for children: dietary fat and cholesterol. *Pediatrics.* 1986;78:521–525.
115. Sapsford A. Energy, carbohydrate, protein, and fat. In: Groh-Wargo S, Thompson M, Cox JH (eds). *Nutritional Care for High-Risk Newborns.* Chicago: Precept Press; 1994:83.
116. Mitton SG. Amino acids and lipid in the total parenteral nutrition for the newborn. *J Pediatr Gastroenterol Nutr.* 1994;18:25–31.
117. Pereira GR. Nutritional care of the extremely premature infant. *Clin Perinatol.* 1995;22:61–75.
118. American Academy of Pediatrics, Committee on Nutrition. Use of intravenous fat emulsions in pediatric patients. *Pediatrics.* 1981;68:738–743.
119. Driscoll DF, Bacon MN, Bistrian BR. Effects of in-line filtration on lipid particle size distribution in total nutrient admixtures. *J Parenter Enteral Nutr.* 1996;20:296–301.
120. Sacks GS, Driscoll DF. Does lipid hang time make a difference? Time is of the essence. *Nutr Clin Prac.* 2002;17:284–290.
121. Pearson ML, Hospital Infection Control Practices Advisory Committee. Guideline for prevention of intravascular-device-related infections. *Infect Control Hosp Epidemiol.* 1996;17:438–479.
122. Magnusson G, Boberg M, Cederblad G, et al. Plasma and tissue levels of lipids, fatty acids, and plasma carnitine in neonates receiving a new fat emulsion. *Acta Paediatr.* 1997;86:638–644.
123. McDonald CM, MacKay MW, Curtis J, et al. Carnitine and cholestasis: nutritional dilemmas for the parenterally nourished newborn. *Support Line.* 2003;25:10.
124. Borum P. Carnitine in neonatal nutrition. *J Child Neurol.* 1995; 10(Suppl 2):S25–S31.
125. Helms RA, Mauer EC, Hay WW Jr, et al. Effect of intravenous L-carnitine on growth parameters and fat metabolism during parenteral nutrition in neonates. *J Parenter Enteral Nutr.* 1990; 14:448–453.
126. Winter SC, Szabo-Aczel S, Curry CJR, et al. Plasma carnitine deficiency: clinical observations in 51 pediatric patients. *Am J Dis Child.* 1987;141:660–665.
127. Coran AG, Drongowshi RA, Baker PJ. The metabolic effects of oral L-carnitine administration in infants receiving total parenteral nutrition with fat. *J Pediatr Surg.* 1985;20:758–764.
128. Crill CM, Wang B, Storm MC, et al. Carnitine: a conditionally essential nutrient in the neonatal population? *J Pediatr Pharmacol Ther.* 2001;6:225.
129. American Medical Association, Nutrition Advisory Group. Multivitamin preparations for parenteral use. *J Parenter Enteral Nutr.* 1979;3:258–262.
130. Greene HL, Hambidge KM, Schanler R, et al. Guidelines for the use of vitamins, trace elements, calcium, magnesium, and phosphorus in infants and children receiving total parenteral nutrition: report of the Subcommittee on Pediatric Parenteral Nutrient Requirements from the Committee on Clinical Practice Issues of the American Society for Clinical Nutrition. *Am J Clin Nutr.* 1988;48:1324. (Revised in 1990.)
131. Greer FR. Vitamin metabolism and requirements in the micropremie. *Clin Perinatol.* 2000;27:95–118.
132. Kumar D, Greer FR, Super DM, et al. Vitamin K status of premature infants: implications for current recommendations. *Pediatrics.* 2001;108:1117–1122.
133. Brion LP, Bell EF, Raghuveer TS, et al. What is the appropriate intravenous dose of vitamin E for very-low-birth-weight infants? *J Perinatol.* 2004;24:205–207.
134. Darlow BA, Graham PJ. Vitamin A supplementation for preventing morbidity and mortality in very low birthweight infants. *Cochrane Database Syst Rev.* 2002;4:CD000501.
135. Sondheimer JM, Cadnapaphornchai M, Sontag M, et al. Predicting the duration of dependence on parenteral nutrition after neonatal intestinal resection. *J Pediatr.* 1998;132:80–84.

136. Prelack K, Sheridan RL. Micronutrient supplementation in the critically ill patient: strategies for clinical practice. *J Trauma.* 2001;51:601–620.
137. Greer FR, Tsang RC. Calcium and vitamin D metabolism in term and low-birth-weight infants. *Perinatol Neonatol.* 1986:14.
138. Koo WWK, Tsang RC. Mineral requirements for low-birth-weight infants. *J Amer Coll Nutr.* 1991;10:474–486.
139. Changaris DG, Purohit DM, Balentine JD, et al. Brain calcification in severely stressed neonates receiving parenteral calcium. *J Pediatr.* 1984;104:941–946.
140. Goldsmith MA, Bhatia SS, Kanto AP, et al. Gluconate calcium therapy and neonatal hypercalciuria. *Am J Dis Child.* 1981;135:538–543.
141. Hufnagle KF, Khan SN, Penn D, et al. Renal calcifications: a complication of long-term furosemide therapy in preterm infants. *Pediatrics.* 1982;70:360–363.
142. Wood RJ, Bengoa JM, Sitrin MD, Rosenberg IH. Calciuretic effect of cyclic versus continuous total parenteral nutrition. *Am J Clin Nutr.* 1985;41:614–619.
143. Koo WWK, Kaplan LA, Horn J, et al. Aluminum in parenteral nutrition solution—sources and possible alternatives. *J Parenter Enteral Nutr.* 1986;10:591–595.
144. Moreno A, Dominguez C, Ballabriga A. Aluminum in the neonate related to parenteral nutrition. *Acta Paediatr.* 1994;83:25–29.
145. Giapros VI, Papdimitriou FK, Andronikou SK. Tubular disorders in low birth weight neonates after prolonged antibiotic treatment. *Neonatology.* 2007;91:140–144.
146. Aladjem M, Lotan D, Biochis H, et al. Changes in the electrolyte content of serum and urine during total parenteral nutrition. *J Pediatr.* 1980;97:437–439.
147. Kimura S, Nose O, Seino Y, et al. Effects of alternate and simultaneous administrations of calcium and phosphorus on calcium metabolism in children receiving total parenteral nutrition. *J Parenter Enteral Nutr.* 1986;10:513–516.
148. Pelegano JF, Rowe JC, Carey DE, et al. Effect of calcium/phosphorus ratio on mineral retention in parenterally fed premature infants. *J Pediatr Gastroenterol Nutr.* 1991;12:351–355.
149. Hoehn GJ, Carey DE, Rowe JC, et al. Alternate day infusion of calcium and phosphate in very low birth weight infants: wasting of the infused mineral. *J Pediatr Gastroenterol Nutr.* 1987;5:752–757.
150. U.S. Department of Health and Human Services. *FDA Safety Alert: Hazards of Precipitation Associated with Parenteral Nutrition.* Rockville, MD: Food and Drug Administration; 1994.
151. Shils ME, Burke AW, Greene HL, et al. Guidelines for essential trace element preparations for parenteral use: a statement by an expert panel. *JAMA.* 1979;241:2051–2054.
152. Kleinman RE (ed). *Pediatric Nutrition Handbook.* Elk Grove Village, IL: American Academy of Pediatrics, Committee on Nutrition; 1998:285–305.
153. Pyati SP, Ramamurthy RS, Krauss MT, Pildes RS. Absorption of iodine in the neonate following topical use of povidone iodine. *J Pediatr.* 1977;91:825–828.
154. Shaw JC. Trace elements in the fetus and young infant II. Copper, manganese, selenium and chromium. *Am J Dis Child.* 1980;134:74–81.
155. Triplett WC. Clinical aspects of zinc, copper, manganese, chromium and selenium metabolism. *Nutr Int.* 1985;1:60.
156. American Academy of Pediatrics, Committee on Nutrition. Zinc. *Pediatrics.* 1978;62:408–412.
157. Reynolds AP, Keily E, Meadows N. Manganese in long term paediatric parenteral nutrition. *Arch Dis Child.* 1994;71:527–528.
158. Hardy G. Manganese in parenteral nutrition: who, when and why should we supplement? *Gastroenterology.* 2009;137:S29–S35.
159. McMillan NB, Mulroy C, MacKay MW, et al. Correlation of cholestasis with serum copper and whole-blood manganese levels in pediatric patients. *Nutr Clin Pract.* 2008;23:161–165.
160. Hurwitz M, Garcia MG, Poole RL, et al. Copper deficiency during parenteral nutrition: a report of four pediatric cases. *Nutr Clin Pract.* 2004;19:305–308.
161. Fuhrman MP, Herrmann V, Masidonski P, et al. Pancytopoenia after removal of copper from total parenteral nutrition. *J Parenter Enteral Nutr.* 2000;24:361–366.
162. Zambrano E, El-Hennawy M, Ehrenkranz RA, et al. Total parenteral nutrition induced liver pathology: an autopsy series of 24 newborn cases. *Pediatr Dev Pathol.* 2004;7:425–432.
163. Fok TF, Chui KK, Cheung R, et al. Manganese intake and cholestatic jaundice in neonates receiving parenteral nutrition: a randomized controlled study. *Acta Paediatr.* 2001;90:1009–1115.
164. Seashore JH. Metabolic complications of parenteral nutrition in infants and children. *Surg Clin North Am.* 1980;60:1239.
165. Reed MD, Bertino JS, Halpin TC. Use of intravenous iron dextran injection in children receiving total parenteral nutrition. *Am J Dis Child.* 1981;135:829–831.
166. Wan KK, Tsallas G. Dilute iron dextran formulation for addition to parenteral nutrient solutions. *Am J Hosp Pharm.* 1980;37:206.
167. Halpin T, Reed M, Bertino J. Use of intravenous iron dextran in children receiving TPN for nutritional support of inflammatory bowel disease. *J Parenter Enteral Nutr.* 1980;4:600.
168. Ehrenkranz RA. Iron requirements of preterm infants. *Nutrition.* 1994;10:77.
169. Ohls RK, Harcum J, Schibler KR, et al. The effect of erythropoietin on the transfusion requirements of preterm infants weighing 750 grams or less: a randomized, double-blind, placebo-controlled study. *J Pediatr.* 1995;126:421–426.
170. Meyer MP, Haworth C, Meyer JH, et al. A comparison of oral and intravenous iron supplementation in preterm infants receiving recombinant erythropoietin. *J Pediatr.* 1996;129:258–263.
171. Ng PC, Lam CWK, Lee CH, et al. Hepatic iron storage in very low birthweight infants after multiple blood transfusions. *Arch Dis Child Fetal Neonatal Ed.* 2001;84:F101–F105.
172. Bastian C, Driscoll R. Enteral tube feeding at home. In: Rombeau JL, Caldwell MD (eds). *Enteral and Tube Feeding.* Philadelphia: WB Saunders; 1984:494–512.
173. Beghin L, Michaud L. Total energy expenditure and physical activity in children treated with home parenteral nutrition. *Pediatr Res.* 2003;53:684–690.
174. Johnson T, Sexton E. Managing children and adolescents on parenteral nutrition: challenges for the nutritional support team. *Proc Nutr Soc.* 2006;65:217–221.
175. Illingworth RS, Lister J. The critical or sensitive period, with special reference to certain feeding problems in infants and children. *J Pediatr.* 1964;65:839–848.

CHAPTER 21

Botanicals

John Westerdahl

Since the beginning of time, botanicals have played an important part in the diet and well-being of every major culture. The Greek physician Hippocrates (ca. 468–ca. 377 BC), known as the Father of Medicine, used herbs extensively with his patients and wrote about their healing benefits. In the first century, another Greek physician, Dioscorides, listed 500 plant medicines in his classic herbal guide, *De Materia Medica*. Many of the currently popular medicinal herbs were once listed in official monographs in the United States Pharmacopoeia (USP) and the National Formulary (NF) and were used extensively by physicians. Today, some 25% of prescription drugs marketed in the United States are derived from plants,[1,2] and 80% of the world's population currently relies mainly on traditional medicines, most of which utilize medicinal plants.[3] **Table 21-1** lists the botanicals that are currently approved by the U.S. Food and Drug Administration (FDA) as effective over-the-counter (OTC) drug ingredients. Note, however, that the FDA does not regulate herbal supplements.

During the past three decades, the use of herbs and phytomedicines has increased as consumers have become more aware of their uses. This can be attributed both to increased published scientific research documenting the therapeutic efficacy of many medicinal herbs and to the passing of the Dietary Supplement Health and Education Act of 1994 (DSHEA), which created a regulatory framework for dietary supplement products. It allows herbal manufacturers to make truthful, nonmisleading claims about the herb's effect on the structure and function of the body. These claims are required to be accompanied by a disclaimer that states, "This statement has not been evaluated by the Food and Drug Administration. This product is not intended to diagnose, treat, cure, or prevent any disease."[4]

When using commercial herbal products, look for standardized versions with measured amounts of active ingredients. Consumers interested in using herbs should seek reputable manufacturers' products and contact companies to ascertain the source of their herbs and their manufacturing procedures. Pregnant or nursing women should not use herbal supplements without first consulting a knowledgeable physician.

Consumers have shown a growing interest in trying natural alternatives rather than synthetic drugs to address their health concerns.[5] As a result, the herbal market has experienced steady growth. Some of the best-selling herbal products sold in the United States are cranberry, soy, garlic, saw palmetto, and gingko. Health professionals should be aware of the types of herbs that many patients are using today.

An increasing number of parents are using botanical medicines with their children. Several herbal product companies now market phytomedicines specially formulated for children. Many parents perceive herbal remedies as more effective and as being "gentler" and having fewer side effects than most conventional drugs. In the United States, the majority of doctors and pharmacists recognize that there is a growing consumer interest in herbal medicine. Doctors, pharmacists, registered dietitians, and other healthcare practitioners need to increase their knowledge about herbal products to better assist their patients who use them.

Definitions

In the world of herbs and phytomedicines, the health professional should be familiar with some basic nomenclature when working with patients who use these preparations. This starts with adequately defining the word *herb*. Depending on the context, the term *herb* can be defined in a few different ways.

An herb is defined botanically as a seed-producing, nonwoody plant that dies down to its roots at the end of its growing season. Others have described an herb simply as a useful plant. In the culinary arts field, the term *herb* is described as a vegetable product that is used in cooking to add flavor and/or aroma to foods.[1] However, in the field of herbal medicine, the term *herb* takes on a more medical meaning. Perhaps the most precise and accurate definition of the term *herb* as it pertains to medicinal values is the definition offered by the late Dr. Varro E. Tyler: "a crude drug of vegetable origin utilized for the treatment of disease states, often

TABLE 21-1 Botanicals Approved as OTC Drug Ingredients

Herb	Approved Use
Capsicum (*Capsicum* spp.)	Counterirritant
Ipecac root (*Cephaelis ipecacuanha*)	Emetic
Peppermint oil (*Mentha piperita*)	Antitussive
Psyllium (*Plantago psyllium*)	Bulk laxative
Senna (*Senna alexandrina; Cassia senna*)	Stimulant laxative
Slippery elm (*Ulmus fulva*)	Demulcent
Witch hazel (*Hamamelis virginiana*)	Astringent

Source: Food and Drug Administration. *OTC Drug Review Ingredient Status Report.* Rockville, MD: Food and Drug Administration; July 2003.

of a chronic nature, or to attain or maintain a condition of improved health."[6]

Commercial herbal and phytomedicine preparations are available in several different forms. Some of the key forms are defined as follows:[1]

- *Extract:* An herbal concentrate that contains the phytochemical constituents found in the herb. Extracts are made when the plant constituents are extracted from the plant by physical and/or chemical means.
- *Standardized extract:* An herbal extract that is guaranteed to provide a standardized level of a particular phytochemical constituent. In many cases, this phytochemical constituent is considered to be the key active compound.
- *Infusion:* An herbal tea. An herbal extract is prepared by steeping dried plant parts in hot water.
- *Decoction:* An herbal extract prepared by putting the plant material (usually hard or woody parts) in water and boiling the water, then allowing it to simmer gently for extended periods of time. The liquid is then cooled and strained for use.
- *Tincture:* An herbal extract prepared by mixing the herb with a solvent (usually an alcohol and water mixture) for a specified period of time (hours to days). The solvent extracts phytochemical constituents from the herb. Any remaining solids are removed, and the solution that results is used medicinally.
- *Glycerite:* An herbal extract that is similar to a tincture; however, glycerol is used as the solvent in preparation instead of alcohol. Because they are alcohol-free, glycerites have recently become very popular for use with children.
- *Fluid extract:* Liquid preparations that usually contain a ratio of one part solvent to one part herb. They are much more concentrated than tinctures, and their alcohol content can vary.
- *Solid extract:* Made by evaporating all the residual solvent or liquid used during the extraction process. (Also called *powdered extract.*)
- *Powder:* A preparation in the form of finely divided, sieved herbal particles made from dried and finely milled herbs for use in herbal preparations such as tablets and capsules.
- *Syrup:* A water and sugar solution to which flavoring and an herbal extract may be added. Syrups are often used to relieve coughs or to mask the unpleasant flavor of a tincture. Syrups are a popular form of herbal medicine in pediatrics.

Use in Pediatrics

The scientific data examining the use of herbs with children are limited. As a result, herbal medicine experts do not have a consensus of opinion as to the appropriate use of botanicals for children, particularly very young ones. In general, the safety of most responsibly formulated commercial herb products has been well established. However, there are situations in which specific herbs should not be used. If a child has an allergy to a specific herb, it must be avoided. Certain plants in the Asteraceae, Apiaceae, and other plant families possess a high degree of allergenicity with some children. It is advised to observe caution in the consumption of plants classified as ragweeds, especially flowers found in the Asteraceae family, such as chamomile.

Parents should observe the child who takes an herbal preparation for the first time for several hours for any adverse reactions. Watery, itchy eyes; sneezing; wheezing; coughing; or hives could be signs of allergy. Pediatricians who utilize herbal remedies in their practice recommend to concerned parents of allergy-prone children that they introduce an herb in the same way they would introduce new foods to an infant. The pediatrician's advice is to try only one herb at a time, administered in very small doses.

Herbs should not be given by the parent to a child who is currently taking a medication without first consulting a doctor. The interaction of an herb with medicinal substances should always be considered. Although little data are available on herb–drug interactions, some important information in this area is known by the medical profession, such as the risks of using St. John's Wort with other antidepressants and using garlic while taking other anticoagulants.

There is debate among herbal medicine experts as to which herbal remedies are safe and appropriate for use by children. In Germany, Commission E, an interdisciplinary expert committee on herbal medicines, is responsible for evaluating the scientific data on the safety and efficacy of phytomedicines. Most experts regard these monographs as the most accurate scientific information available in the world on the safety and efficacy of herbs and phytomedicines. Although the monographs describe the medicinal use of herbs primarily for adults, they also identify herbs and herbal products that are contraindicated for children. Some of these include aloe, camphor, fennel oil, peppermint oil, and senna leaf.[7] **Table 21-2** gives an overview of

TABLE 21-2 Common Herbal Remedies Used in Pediatrics

Common and Latin Names	Internal and External Uses	Contraindications/Precautions
Aloe (*Aloe vera*)	External use: wound healing, minor skin irritation, burns	Not recommended internally for pediatrics.
Anise (*Pimpinella anisum*)	Internal use: common colds, coughs, bronchitis, indigestion	Rare allergic reactions to anise and its constituent anethole.
Bilberry (*Vaccinium myrtillus*)	Internal use: diarrhea	None known.
Calendula flowers (*Calendula officinalis*)	Internal use: inflammation of mouth and pharynx External use: wounds and burns	Rare allergic reactions through frequent skin contact.
Catnip (*Nepeta cataria*)	Internal use: nervous disorders, sleep aid, common colds, colic	None known.
Chamomile flowers (*Matricaria chamomilla*)	Internal use: carminative, sleep aid External use: inflammation and irritations of the skin, wounds, burns	Rare allergic reactions.
Cherry bark (*Prunus sp.*)	Internal use: coughs, common colds	None known.
Comfrey leaf (*Symphytum officinale*)	External use: minor wounds, ulcers, inflammations, bruises, and sprains; used as poultice for skin disorder	Not to be taken internally. Internal use promotes hepatotoxic effects.
Echinacea (*Echinacea angustifolia*) (*Echinacea purpurea*)	Internal use: common colds, flu, coughs, bronchitis, fever, immune stimulant External use: wounds, burns	Allergic reactions may occur with some individuals. Not recommended for individuals with autoimmune diseases.
Elder flowers (*Sambucus nigra*)	Internal use: common colds, antiviral, diaphoretic	None known.
Eucalyptus (*Eucalyptus globulus*)	Internal use: expectorant, coughs, congestion of the respiratory tract	Nausea, vomiting, and diarrhea may occur after ingestion in rare cases. Eucalyptus preparations should not be applied to the face or nose of infants and very young children.
Fennel seed (*Foeniculum vulgare*)	Internal use: carminative, indigestion, coughs, bronchitis, gastrointestinal afflictions	Allergic reactions may occur with some individuals.
Garlic (*Allium sativum*)	Internal use: common colds, bronchitis, fever External use: antibacterial, antifungal, ear infections	Intake of large quantities can lead to stomach complaints. Rare allergic reactions.
Ginger (*Zingiber officinale*)	Internal use: carminative, antinausea, indigestion	None known.
Goldenseal (*Hydrastis canadensis*)	Internal use: common colds, flu, inflammation of mucous membranes External use: antiseptic, antimicrobial, cuts, wounds, ear infections	Internal use can cause nausea, vomiting, and diarrhea, and may disrupt intestinal flora. Internal use is not recommended for young children by many experts due to the herb's alkaloid (berberine and hydrastine) content.
Hops (*Humulus lupulus*)	Internal use: nervous disorders, sleep aid	Rare allergic reactions.
Horehound (*Marrubium vulgare*)	Internal use: coughs, bronchitis	None known.
Hyssop (*Hyssopus officinalis*)	Internal use: coughs, common colds	None known.

(continues)

TABLE 21-2 *(Continued)*

Common and Latin Names	Internal and External Uses	Contraindications/Precautions
Lemon balm (*Melissa officinalis*)	Internal use: nervous disorders, sleep aid	None known.
Licorice root (*Glycyrrhiza glabra*)	Internal use: coughs, bronchitis	Prolonged use with high doses may promote hypertension, edema, and hypokalemia.
Marshmallow root (*Althaea officinalis*)	Internal use: coughs, bronchitis, sore throat	None known.
Mullein leaf (*Verbascum thapsus*)	Internal use: coughs, bronchitis, common colds, flu	None known.
Oat straw (*Avena sativa*)	External use: inflammation of the skin, itching	None known.
Passion flower (*Passiflora incarnata*)	Internal use: nervous disorders, sleep aid	None known.
Peppermint leaf (*Mentha piperita*)	Internal use: carminative, indigestion, nausea, gastrointestinal disorders, common colds, cough, bronchitis	Preparations containing peppermint oil should not be applied to the face or nose of infants or very young children.
Pleurisy root (*Asclepias tuberosa*)	Internal use: coughs, pleurisy	Excessive amounts can be toxic due to the herb's cardioactive steroid content that can lead to digitalis-like poisonings. High doses can promote vomiting.
St. John's wort (*Hypericum perforatum*)	Internal use: emotional upsets, including anxiety and depressive moods. External use: cuts and abrasions	Safety of internal use with children has not been established. The safety and ethics of the use of herbal antidepressants with children without the consultation of a doctor is questionable. Should not be taken by children already taking prescription medications for depression without first consulting a doctor. May cause sun sensitivity in some individuals.
Thyme (*Thymus vulgarus*)	Internal use: cough, bronchitis, common colds	None known.
Valerian root (*Valeriana officinalis*)	Internal use: nervous disorders, sleep aid	The safety and ethics of the use of herbal sedatives with children without the consultation of a doctor is questionable.

Note: Clinical efficacy for each of these herbs has not necessarily been established.

several of the internal and external uses of many of the medicinal herbs commonly used in pediatrics.

Most herbal medicine experts caution against the use of herbal stimulant laxatives by children younger than 12 years of age. Herbal stimulant laxatives include aloe (*Aloe ferox*), buckthorn bark (*Rhamnus frangula*), cascara sagrada bark (*Rhamnus purshiana*), and senna leaf or pod (*Cassia senna*). Stimulants such as caffeine-containing herbs are also generally contraindicated for young children.[7,8]

Herbs that are classified as stimulants include not only coffee and black and green tea (*Camellia sinensis*), but also cola nut (also called kola nut; *Cola nitida*), guarana (*Paullinia cupana*), and maté (*Ilex paraguariensis*). Ma huang (also known as ephedra) is also a potent stimulant and is contraindicated for young children. It has been taken off the U.S. market. Asian ginseng (*Panax ginseng*) and American ginseng (*Panax quinquefolium*), traditionally regarded as herbal stimulants, are also not recommended for young children by many herbal medicine authorities.[1,8]

Many plants have traditionally been used for their sedative properties. Most health authorities would agree that any sedative, herbal or otherwise, should be given to a child only under medical direction. Many herbal medicine experts would agree that strong sedative herbs such as valerian (*Valeriana officinalis*) should not be given to young children. There is no consensus of opinion on the use of some of the other popular traditional sedative herbs for children, despite the fact that many of them have been used with children for centuries. These herbs include catnip (*Nepeta cataria*), German chamomile (*Matricaria recutita*), hops (*Humulus lupulus*), lemon balm (*Melissa officinalis*), and passion flower (*Passiflora incarnata*). St. John's wort (*Hypericum perforatum*), an herb that has proven efficacy in treating mild and moderate depression in adults, has not been adequately studied for use by children.

Many herbal experts have concerns about children's use of herbs that contain powerful alkaloids. One of the alkaloids of concern is berberine. Berberine is a key phytochemical constituent found in several of the currently popular herbal products sold in natural food and drug stores. Herbs containing berberine include goldenseal root (*Hydrastis canadensis*), Oregon grape root (*Mahonia aquifolium*), and barberry root (*Berberis vulgaris*). Berberine has antibacterial properties. Overuse of herbs containing this and other alkaloids could disrupt the normal flora in a child's gastrointestinal tract.[8] In addition, alkaloids that affect the central nervous system (caffeine, ephedrine, pseudoephedrine, and others) are generally not recommended for young children except under a doctor's direction.[8]

Few studies have been done with infants using herbal preparations. However, an herbal tea containing chamomile (*Matricaria chamomilla*), vervain (*Verbena officinalis*), licorice root (*Glycyrrhiza glabra*), fennel (*Foeniculum vulgare*), and lemon balm (*Melissa officinalis*) was found to be effective in treating infants with colic. None of the infants in the study experienced any adverse effects from the herbal tea.[9]

Additional studies demonstrating the effectiveness of herbal remedies with children have been published. For example, standardized ginger root has been shown to be effective in treating motion sickness in children ages 4 to 8 years of age.[10] Enteric-coated peppermint oil capsules have been demonstrated to be safe and effective as a treatment for pain associated with the acute phases of irritable bowel syndrome (IBS) in older children and adolescents.[11] Herbal ear drops containing a combination of mullein, marigold (calendula), St. John's wort, lavender, and garlic in an olive oil base reduced ear pain associated with acute otitis media (AOM) in children and was as effective as standard anesthetic eardrops.[12] Ivy leaf extract (*Hedra helix*) preparations may improve the respiratory functions of children with chronic asthma.[13]

The benefits of many phytomedicines outweigh the risks because they have a relatively good benefit/risk ratio. Many combinations of naturally occurring compounds in herbs have been experimentally established and/or clinically confirmed, with minimal or negligible side effects. Other advantages of herbal remedies are that herbs have gentle medicinal actions and that their common methods of administration (inhalation, baths, ointments, syrups) are particularly appropriate for children. As a result, this can provide for good compliance. Herbal medicines in pediatrics may be used at a preventive level, not just for treating symptoms. As a general rule, phytomedicines are less expensive than conventional medicines.[14]

EXHIBIT 21-1 How to Calculate a Child's Dosage for Herbal Medicines

The following are two classic rules used to calculate the approximate dosage for a child.

Clark's Rule: Divide the child's weight by 150. The example given is for a 50-pound child:

$$\frac{50}{150} = \frac{1}{3} \text{ adult dosage}$$

Young's Rule: Divide the child's age by the child's age + 12. The example given is for a 4-year-old child:

$$\frac{4}{4+12} = \frac{4}{16} = \frac{1}{4} \text{ adult dosage}$$

Dosage for Medicinal Herbs

Little scientific, or even traditional, information is available on the proper dosage of herbs and phytomedicines in pediatrics. Because most clinical trials using herbs have been with adults, official dosages have been established for only the adult population. A general pediatric guide used for determining the dosage of phytotherapeutic drugs is one-third of the adult dose (as established in the Commission E monographs) for very young and young children and one-half the adult dose for school-age children.[14] Two classic pharmacy rules used to calculate the dosage for a child are known as *Clark's Rule* and *Young's Rule*. **Exhibit 21-1** illustrates how they are calculated. Because children have lower body weight than adults and do not have the sufficient development of liver enzymes necessary to metabolize many medications, their dosages of conventional as well as herbal medicines must be reduced. The proper pediatric dosage is best determined by an experienced and trained health professional. In recent years, some herbal product manufacturers have formulated their preparations for dosage levels appropriate for children.

Case Study

Nutritional Assessment of Child with Dyspepsia

Patient history: A 7-year-old female visited her pediatrician for digestive problems, including feelings of nausea. The pediatrician diagnosed the patient with having a mild case of dyspepsia (i.e., indigestion, upset stomach). The patient has a history of remarkable good health throughout her childhood. On one previous occasion, about 7 months ago, the patient had a similar episode of mild dyspepsia associated with eating a rich meal. The patient's parents are interested in complementary and alternative medicine approaches to treating their child's dyspepsia.

Family history: No family history of any serious digestive problems.

Medical/lab tests: No medical or lab tests were performed.

Food allergies: No known food allergies.

Anthropometrics

Height: 122.0 cm
Weight: 23.0 kg
BMI: 15.5 kg/m^2

Nutrition History

Patient and her family typically follow a very healthy, low-fat vegetarian diet that includes three vegetarian meals with healthy vegetarian snacks throughout the day. This typical diet is routinely followed with the exception of occasional holidays, parties, and special social events when the vegetarian diet is not always followed.

The child's diet on the day with dyspepsia was as follows:

- *Breakfast:* Granola cereal with blueberries and soy milk, whole-wheat toast with whole-fruit strawberry jam, and a small glass of fresh-squeezed orange juice. Children's multivitamin taken with breakfast.
- *Lunch:* Birthday party lunch included a vanilla milkshake, cheeseburger, French fries, nachos, candy, birthday cake, and chocolate ice cream cone.
- *Dinner:* Could not eat dinner that evening due to indigestion and stomach ache.

Nutrition Diagnosis

Based on the above information, a nutrition diagnosis or problem is determined.

Nutrition and Botanical Medicine Intervention

Goal: To alleviate patient's dyspepsia and offer plan to avoid future episodes.

Food/nutrient delivery: Patient will temporarily avoid solid foods. Tolerable clear liquids will be advised and recommended, starting with an appropriate warm herbal tea/beverage.

Nutrition education: Educate parents and patient about a recommended clear liquid diet and how to begin using an appropriate warm herbal tea/beverage to help alleviate symptoms of dyspepsia.

Nutrition counseling: Patient to remain on appropriate clear liquid diet and warm herbal tea/beverage until symptoms of dyspepsia have resolved. Then reinstitute the healthy diet plan the family regularly follows. Counsel parents and patient to be moderate in consumption of rich foods at parties and celebrations to avoid future episodes of dyspepsia.

Nutrition Monitoring and Evaluation

Should symptoms persist or later reoccur, follow up with the patient with an appropriate diet plan and nutrition counseling in conjunction with recommendations from the patient's pediatrician.

Questions for the Reader

1. What percentiles on the CDC growth chart are the patient's height and weight?
2. Based on the list of herbs in Table 21-2, what appropriate herbs (herbal remedies) can be used in the preparation of a warm herbal tea or beverage for the treatment of symptoms of dyspepsia (indigestion, upset stomach)?

REFERENCES

1. Westerdahl J. *Medicinal Herbs: A Vital Reference Guide.* Dallas, TX: Bruce Miller Enterprises; 1998.
2. Principe PP. The economic significance of plants and their constituents as drugs. *Econ Med Plant Res.* 1989;3:1–17.
3. Farnsworth NR, Akerele O, Bingel AS, et al. Medicinal plants in therapy. *Bull World Health Org.* 1985;63:965–981.
4. Dietary Supplement Health and Education Act of 1994 (DHEA), Pub.LNo. 103-417, 108 Stat, 1994. U.S. Food and Drug Adminis-

tration, Center for Food Safety and Applied Nutrition. Available at: http://www.vm.cfsan.fda.gov/ndMS/dietsupp.html. Accessed August 23, 2010.

5. Eisenberg DM, Kessler RC, Foster C, et al. Unconventional medicine in the United States. *N Engl J Med.* 1993;328:246–252.
6. Awang DVE. *Tyler's Herbs of Choice: The Therapeutic Use of Phytomedicinals,* 3rd ed. Boca Raton, FL: CRC Press; 2009:1.
7. Blumenthal M, Busse WR, Goldberg A, et al. (eds). Klein S, Rister RS (trans). *The Complete German Commission E Monographs: Therapeutic Guide to Herbal Medicines.* Austin, TX: American Botanical Council; 1998.
8. Gruenwalk J, Brendler T, Jaenicke C (eds). *PDR for Herbal Medicines,* 4th ed. Montvale, NJ: Thomson Healthcare; 2007.
9. Weizman Z, Alkrinawi S, Goldfarb D, Bitran C. Efficacy of herbal tea preparation in infantile cholic. *J Pediatr.* 1993;122:650–652.
10. Careddu P. Motion sickness in children: results of a double-blind study with ginger (*Zintona*) and dimenhydrinate. *European Phytotherapy.* 1999;2:102–107.
11. Kline RM, Kline JJ, Di Palma J, Barbero GJ. Enteric-coated, pH-dependent peppermint oil capsules for the treatment of irritable bowel syndrome in children. *J Pediatr.* 2001;138: 125–128.
12. Sarrel FM, Cohen HA, Kahan E. Naturopathic treatment for ear pain in children. *Pediatrics.* 2003;111:574–579.
13. Hofmann D, Hecker M, Volp A. Efficacy of dry extract of ivy leaves in children with bronchial asthma—a review of randomized controlled trials. *Phytomedicine.* 2003;10:213–220.
14. Schilcher H. *Phytotherapy in Pediatrics: Handbook for Physicians and Pharmacists.* Stuttgart, Germany: MedPharm Scientific Publishers; 1997.

Index

Note: Page numbers followed by *f* indicate figures; page numbers followed by *t* indicate tables; and page numbers followed by *e* indicate exhibits.

D

E

Printed in the USA
CPSIA information can be obtained
at www.ICGtesting.com
CBHW062302131223
2510CB00005B/22

9 781284 289992